Headache: Evaluation and Management

Headache: Evaluation and Management

Editor: Sienna West

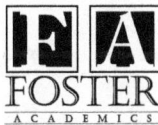

FA
FOSTER
ACADEMICS

www.fosteracademics.com

www.fosteracademics.com

FA
FOSTER
ACADEMICS

Cataloging-in-Publication Data

Headache : evaluation and management / edited by Sienna West.
    p. cm.
Includes bibliographical references and index.
ISBN 978-1-63242-733-5
1. Headache. 2. Headache--Treatment. 3. Nervous system--Diseases. I. West, Sienna.
RC392 .H43 2019
616.849 1--dc23

Foster Academics,
118-35 Queens Blvd., Suite 400,
Forest Hills, NY 11375, USA

ISBN 978-1-63242-733-5 (Hardback)

Contents

Preface

Pain in the region of the head and the neck is termed as a headache. It can occur as migraines, cluster headaches and tension-type headaches. Headaches may be caused due to a variety of reasons. Dehydration, fatigue, sleep deprivation, effects of drugs, infections and head injuries are some of these reasons. Most headaches are diagnosed on the basis of the clinical history itself. It is determined if a headache pertains to low-risk, benign or high-risk headaches. Although the management of headaches is based on its diagnosis, its treatment generally involves pain medication. This book is compiled in such a manner, that it will provide in-depth knowledge about the incidence of headaches and their underlying causes. It presents researches and studies performed by experts across the globe. For someone with an interest and eye for detail, this book covers the most significant topics in the evaluation and management of headache.

This book is a result of research of several months to collate the most relevant data in the field.

When I was approached with the idea of this book and the proposal to edit it, I was overwhelmed. It gave me an opportunity to reach out to all those who share a common interest with me in this field. I had 3 main parameters for editing this text:

1. Accuracy – The data and information provided in this book should be up-to-date and valuable to the readers.

2. Structure – The data must be presented in a structured format for easy understanding and better grasping of the readers

3. Universal Approach – This book not only targets students but also experts and innovators in the field, thus my aim was to present topics which are of use to all

Thus, it took me a couple of months to finish the editing of this book.

I would like to make a special mention of my publisher who considered me worthy of this opportunity and also supported me throughout the editing process. I would also like to thank the editing team at the back-end who extended their help whenever required.

Editor

Undifferentiated headache: broadening the approach to headache in children and adolescents, with supporting evidence from a nationwide school-based cross-sectional survey in Turkey

Christian Wöber[1], Çiçek Wöber-Bingöl[2], Derya Uluduz[3], Tuna Stefan Aslan[3], Uğur Uygunoglu[3], Ahmet Tüfekçi[4], Selen Ilhan Alp[5], Taşkın Duman[6], Fidan Sürgün[6], Gülser Karadaban Emir[7], Caner Feyzi Demir[8], Ferhat Balgetir[8], Yeliz Bahar Özdemir[9], Tanja Auer[10], Aksel Siva[3] and Timothy J. Steiner[11,12]*

Abstract

Background: Headache is a leading disabler in adults worldwide. In children and adolescents, the same may be true but the evidence is much poorer. It is notable that published epidemiological studies of these age groups have largely ignored headaches not fulfilling any specific set of ICHD criteria, although such headaches appear to be common. A new approach to these is needed: here we introduce, and investigate, a diagnostic category termed "undifferentiated headache" (UdH), defined in young people as recurrent mild-intensity headache of < 1 h's duration.

Methods: We conducted a nationwide cross-sectional survey in 31 schools in six regions of Turkey selected by mixed convenience-based and purposive modified cluster-sampling. A validated, standardised self-completed structured questionnaire was administered by a physician-investigator to entire classes of pupils aged 6–17 years.

Results: Of the identified sample of 7889 pupils, 7088 (89.8%) participated. The 1-year prevalence of UdH was 29.2%, of migraine (definite and probable) 26.7%, and of tension-type headache (TTH) (definite and probable) 12.9%. UdH differed with respect to almost all headache features and associated symptoms from both migraine and TTH. Burden of headache and use of acute medication were lower in UdH than in migraine and TTH. Headache yesterday was less common in UdH than migraine (OR 0.32; 95% CI 0.28–0.37) and TTH (OR 0.64; 95% CI 0.56–0.77). Quality of life (QoL) was better in UdH (33.6 ± 5.2) than in migraine (30.3 ± 5.6; $p < 0.001$) and TTH (32.4 ± 5.3; $p < 0.001$), but worse than in pupils without headache (35.7 ± 4.7; $p < 0.001$).

(Continued on next page)

* Correspondence: t.steiner@imperial.ac.uk
[11]Department of Neuromedicine and Movement Science, NTNU Norwegian University of Science and Technology, Edvard Griegs Gate, Trondheim, Norway
[12]Division of Brain Sciences, Imperial College London, London, UK
Full list of author information is available at the end of the article

(Continued from previous page)

Conclusions: This large nationwide study in Turkey of pupils aged 6–17 years has shown that many children and adolescents have a headache type that does not conform to existing accepted diagnostic criteria. This new diagnostic category of presumably still-evolving headache (*undifferentiated headache*) is common. UdH differs in almost all measurable respects from both migraine and TTH. Although characterised by mild headaches lasting < 1 h, UdH is associated with significant adverse impact on QoL. Longitudinal cohort studies are needed to evaluate the prognosis of UdH but, meanwhile, recognition of UdH and its distinction from migraine and TTH has implications for epidemiological studies, public-health policy and routine clinical practice.

Keywords: Headache, Undifferentiated headache, Migraine, Tension-type headache, Headache yesterday, Burden of headache, Quality of life, Children, Adolescents, Population-based study, Nationwide, Turkey, Global Campaign against Headache

Background

In the Global Burden of Disease Study 2010 (GBD2010) [1], tension-type headache (TTH) and migraine were revealed as second and third most prevalent disorders in the world. In GBD2013, headache disorders collectively were third among the leading causes of disability [2]. In GBD2016, migraine came top – the single most disabling disorder – in the age group 15–49 years [3].

The data underpinning these statistics were derived in the main from studies in adults aged 18–65 years. In children (6–11 years) and adolescents (12–17 years), the prevalence of headache disorders is not well established and the burdens attributable to them are poorly characterised. Multiple factors explain this. First, there are relatively few published epidemiological studies [4] and, second, most of these have been conducted in middle- or high-income Western countries, leaving very large geographical gaps [4]. Third, substantial methodological differences between them limit their comparability. Nonetheless, extrapolations to these age groups in these global surveys put migraine among the top 10 global causes of years lived with disability (YLDs) in the 50 most populous countries [5].

An additional factor arises from the operational diagnostic criteria set out in the universally accepted International Classification of Headache Disorders (ICHD), now in its third edition (ICHD-3) [6]. While ICHD recognises > 200 headache disorders, only migraine and TTH among the primary headache disorders have public-health importance [1–4]. Medication-overuse headache (MOH), with an adult mean global prevalence of 1.5–2% [7], also contributes substantially to global disability [2, 3]. The ICHD diagnostic criteria for migraine in adults specify recurrent moderate-to-severe headache of 4–72 h' duration, with a range of specific characteristics (unilaterality, pulsating quality, aggravation by physical activity) and accompanying symptoms (photophobia *and* phonophobia; nausea and/or vomiting) [6]. In children it is noted that the headache may be of shorter duration (2–72 h). The criteria for TTH specify mild-to-moderate headache lasting from 30 min to 7 days, with neither the specific characteristics nor the accompanying symptoms of migraine [6]. In our pilot school-based prevalence survey conducted in Turkey and Austria, mild headache of < 1 h's duration was reported by a large proportion (37.2%) of participants aged 6–17 years, often with migraine-like features [8].

Such headache could not be given a definite diagnosis of migraine or, when there were migraine-like features, of TTH. Furthermore, although ICHD criteria for TTH have, from the first edition onwards [9], specified a lower duration limit of 30 min, we questioned whether this disorder existed in a form in which headache was *typically* of < 1 h's duration. Therefore, in the context of epidemiological studies, we found ourselves in doubt as to how this common presentation of headache should be labelled.

The literature offered no guidance. In the most recent survey [10] and a Medline search (using the terms "migraine", "tension-type headache", "children", "adolescents", "prevalence" and "epidemiology" without language restrictions), we found 59 relevant studies. The majority (54: 91.5%) reported only selected diagnoses (most often definite migraine), and, crucially, did not specify the proportion of unclassifiable headaches. However, among the five studies that did report them [11–15], unclassifiable headaches were common, with an average prevalence of almost 20%. In other words, the problem we encountered had been recognised previously – but ignored.

In the present study, we investigate whether a new approach is required in children and adolescents, recognising that the characteristics of adult migraine (and perhaps TTH) may be undeveloped in 6–17 year-olds. We introduce an additional diagnostic category defined by headache duration of < 1 h and mild intensity, which we have termed "undifferentiated headache" (UdH). In a nationwide school-based epidemiological survey in Turkey, we compare the clinical features of UdH with those of migraine and TTH. We also compare the burdens attributable to each, including impact on quality of life (QoL). Our purpose is to establish whether or not UdH should be regarded for epidemiological and perhaps clinical purposes as distinct from migraine and TTH.

The survey was conducted under the auspices of the Global Campaign against Headache [16], which is directed by the UK-registered non-governmental organisation *Lifting The Burden* (LTB) in official relations with the World Health Organization [17], and of Dr. Gönül Bingöl-Dr Muammer Bingöl Çocuk ve Ergen Başağrısı Derneği.

Methods

Ethics and approvals

The protocol was approved by the ethics committee of the co-ordinating centre (Istanbul University no. 83045809/604/02–12,472). Since the study involved multiple schools nationwide, approval was also obtained from the Ministry of National Education. Copies of these approvals were sent to the school managers to obtain permissions to visit.

Informed consent, in terms agreed within these approvals, was given by or on behalf of each child or adolescent before his or her participation.

Data were collected anonymously and managed in accordance with data-protection legislation.

Study design

The cross-sectional survey applied the methods developed and tested in pilot studies performed in Istanbul and Vienna [8]. Conducted nationwide in selected schools, it employed a self-completed structured questionnaire administered to entire classes. It was performed within one academic term, avoiding examination periods, between April 4th and June 13th 2014.

Sampling and subjects

We used mixed convenience-based and purposive modified cluster-sampling. The procedure was multistage: (1) selection of sites in each of six regions of Turkey, reflecting the country's geographical and socioeconomic diversity; (2) identification by the local investigators of three or more schools within each site to reflect, as far as possible, its socioeconomic and urban/rural diversity; (3) selection of classes in each school across the age ranges 6–11 and/or 12–17 years (randomly, when there were more than one for any particular year); and (4) inclusion of all eligible children in the classes.

The survey sites were six cities and their environs: Elâzığ (eastern Anatolia, in uppermost Euphrates valley); Hatay (southern Turkey, close to the Syrian border) Istanbul (north-western Turkey, astride the Bosphorus); Muğla (south-western Turkey, close to the Aegean coast); Rize (north-eastern Turkey, on the Black Sea coast), and Tekirdağ (European side, on the northern coast of the Sea of Marmara).

Selected schools were invited to participate. Within each class, all eligible pupils were included except for those who refused, were unable to take part for any reason, or were absent from school on the interview day.

Questionnaires

The questionnaire was an adaptation of the HARDSHIP questionnaire [18] in separate versions for children and adolescents. These were translated into Turkish language in accordance with LTB's translation protocol for hybrid documents to capture exact meaning rather than simple linguistic equivalence [19]. Each version had been evaluated with satisfactory results in the pilot studies [8], requiring < 30 min to complete. The questionnaires were administered to the pupils in class by trained medical residents, introduced by their teacher (the mediator). The mediator took steps to prevent any participant copying the responses of another.

Questions were included on demographics, headache occurrence, ICHD-3 beta diagnostic criteria (no different, with respect to migraine and TTH, from those of ICHD-3 [6]), burden attributable to headache, and QoL. A short questionnaire completed by the mediator recorded details about the school and its local environment. A further very brief questionnaire also completed by the mediator documented non-participation. Both these questionnaires have been published previously [8].

Headache diagnosis

Diagnoses were made using the HARDSHIP algorithm [18], but we modified the process to include UdH. First, we applied the criteria for UdH (duration < 1 h, intensity mild). Among remaining participants, we separated those reporting headache on ≥15 days/month, diagnosing probable MOH (pMOH) when acute medication was reportedly used on ≥15 days/month or, otherwise, "other headache on ≥15 days/month" (these cases were not included in this analysis). To those still remaining (with episodic headache of duration ≥1 h and/or intensity moderate or severe), we applied the criteria, in order, for definite migraine, definite TTH, probable migraine and finally probable TTH [20]; criterion B for TTH [6] was modified by raising the lower limit of duration to 1 h.

Statistics and analyses

Recommendations on sample-size calculation for headache *prevalence* suggest limited gain from samples of > 2000 participants [20]. For *burden*, larger numbers may be more informative, but there is no good basis for power calculation. We aimed for 4000 evaluable participants per age range, spread as evenly overall as possible by recruiting across the age groups in each school.

Completed questionnaires were conveyed to and held securely at Istanbul University, where data were transferred into a secure electronic database.

Many questions required "yes/no" responses. Headache duration was reported in hours and intensity as "not bad", "quite bad" or "very bad", which we equated to mild, moderate and severe. Frequencies were reported in days per week or 4 weeks. Emotional impact and QoL questions required selection from the response options "never", "sometimes", "often" and "always" in the preceding 4 weeks; these were scored 1–4, and summed to generate impact (potential range 6–24; high being adverse) and QoL scores (12–48; low being adverse).

For descriptive analyses we generated proportions (%) and, where appropriate, means and standard deviations (SDs). In comparative analyses, we applied Student's t-test to parametric variables, Kruskal Wallis test to nonparametric continuous variables and chi-squared test to categorical variables. We used bivariate analysis to estimate odds ratios (ORs) with 95% confidence intervals (CIs).

We used IBM SPSS Statistics, Version 23, for all calculations. To adjust for multiple comparisons, Bonferroni correction was performed online [21] following the suggestions of Sankoh et al. [22]. In the case of correlated outcome variables, Bonferroni correction is too conservative; the variables in our study were highly correlated with each other: calculating Pearson correlation coefficients we found a statistically significant correlation in 227 of 253 correlations (90%). Therefore, the p-value for significance required adjustment only to $p < 0.03$.

Results

Study population

We invited 31 schools (2–10 [mean 5.2 ± 2.6] per site), 288 classes (2–32 [mean 9.4 ± 6.6] per school) and 7889 pupils (3–167 [27.4 ± 16.1] per class). None of the invited schools or classes declined to participate. Of the 7889 invited pupils, 7088 (89.8%) participated and 7068 (99.7%; 89.6% overall) completed questionnaires were evaluable (2551 children, 4517 adolescents). We did not achieve the intended $N = 4000$ children because of skewed age-distributions within the schools. Mean participation proportion of pupils per class was $90.8 \pm 12.1\%$ with no gender difference (girls $91.1 \pm 14.4\%$; boys $90.5 \pm 13.6\%$) and similar across age-groups (lowest [$86.9 \pm 17.7\%$] in pupils aged 15–16 and highest [$95.1 \pm 5.6\%$] in those aged 11–12 years). Pupil numbers per site ranged from 578 to 1855, and per age group from 290 (6–7 years) to 1146 (13–14 years).

Reasons for non-participation in the 10.2% were inadequately established despite the mediator's questionnaire for this purpose, and cannot be reported.

Schools

The proportions of schools in urban, semiurban and rural regions were 42.4%, 43.1% and 14.6% (compared with national urban and rural proportions extrapolated from 2011 data of about 77% and 23% [23]). The proportions in high-income, upper middle-, lower middle- and low-income districts were 2.8%, 27.1%, 68.4% and 1.7%.

Headache prevalence

Headache during the previous year was reported by 73.7% of participants. We found the following 1-year prevalences: UdH 29.2%; migraine 26.7% (7.3% definite, 19.4% probable); TTH 12.9% (definite 6.7%, probable 6.2%); pMOH 0.9%; other headache on ≥15 days/month 3.4%; unclassifiable headache 0.5%. With concern for possible interest bias among responders, we also calculated prevalences with reference to the target sample of 7889 pupils: UdH 26.2%; migraine 23.9% (definite 6.5%, probable 17.4%); TTH 11.6% (definite 6.2%, probable 5.4%); pMOH 0.8%; other headache on ≥15 days/month 3.0%; unclassifiable headache 0.5%.

Further analyses focus on UdH, migraine and TTH, combining definite and probable cases of the latter two as recommended in guidelines [20].

Headache characteristics and associated symptoms

Classifying UdH according to frequency analogously to TTH, we recorded infrequent episodic UdH in 26.7%, frequent episodic UdH in 72.0% and chronic UdH in 1.3% of cases.

UdH differed with respect to almost all headache features and associated symptoms from both migraine and TTH (Table 1). Headache days both in the previous week and in the previous 4 weeks were fewer in UdH than in migraine and TTH; in keeping with this, headache yesterday was less common in UdH than in migraine and TTH (Table 2). Intensity of headache yesterday was lower in UdH than in migraine and TTH. In contrast to the general rating of headache intensity as mild in UdH, 16.3% of pupils with the diagnosis of UdH rated headache yesterday as moderate or severe (Table 2).

ICHD criteria

Criterion B (duration < 1 h) was predefined for UdH. Criterion C for migraine without aura was fulfilled by 57.4% of UdH cases and criterion C for episodic TTH by 86.1%. Criterion D for each was fulfilled by 55.1% and 44.9% of UdH cases. The proportions of pupils with UdH fulfilling none, one or two of criteria C and D for migraine without aura were 20.7%, 45.7% and 33.5%. The proportions who fulfilled none, one or two of criteria C and D for episodic TTH were 8.7%, 52.0% and 39.3%.

Burden of headache

The proportions of pupils who missed school lessons because of headache yesterday did not differ between the three groups (Table 2), but impact on school attendance and leisure-time activities in the preceding 4 weeks was lower in UdH than in migraine and TTH. UdH was less likely than migraine, but not TTH, to cause a parent to leave work (Table 3).

Table 1 Headache features in undifferentiated headache, migraine and tension-type headache

	Undifferentiated headache		Migraine[a]		Tension-type headache[a]		Undifferentiated headache vs migraine[a]		Undifferentiated headache vs tension-type headache[a]	
	N = 2066		N = 1888		N = 911		OR [95% CI]	p[b]	OR [95% CI]	p[b]
	n	%	n	%	n	%				
Headache in previous week	2036		1864		899					
No	949	46.6	417	22.4	322	35.8	reference		reference	
≥ 1 day	1087	53.4	1447	77.6	577	64.2	0.33 [0.29–0.38]	< 0.001	0.64 [0.54–0.75]	< 0.001
Headache in previous 4 weeks	2050		1880		898					
No	548	26.7	207	11.0	161	17.9	reference		reference	
≥ 1 day	1502	73.3	1673	89.0	737	82.1	0.34 [0.29–0.40]	< 0.001	0.60 [0.49–0.73]	< 0.001
Duration (hr)	2066		1877		910					
< 1	2066	100	317	16.9	145	15.9	NA	NA	NA	NA
1–2	0	0	989	52.7	657	7.2				
> 2 and < 4	0	0	370	19.7	77	8.5				
≥ 4	0	0	201	10.7	31	3.4				
Intensity	2066		1877		907					
Mild	2066	100	537	28.5	516	56.9	NA	NA	NA	NA
Moderate	0	0	1046	55.4	319	35.2				
Severe	0	0	304	16.1	72	7.9				
Quality	2044		1885		908					
Pulsating	1437	70.3	1478	78.4	555	61.1	reference		reference	
Pressing	607	29.7	407	21.6	353	38.9	1.5 [1.3–1.8]	< 0.001	0.66 [0.56–0.78]	< 0.001
Localisation	2048		1887		906					
Unilateral	645	31.5	463	24.5	158	17.4	0.90 [0.76–1.07]	NS	1.7 [1.4–2.1]	< 0.001
Middle	652	31.8	421	22.3	269	29.7	reference		reference	
Bilateral	751	36.7	1003	53.2	479	52.9	0.48 [0.41–0.56]	< 0.001	0.65 [0.54–0.78]	< 0.001
Aggravation by physical activity	2059		1886		910					
No	1356	65.9	596	31.6	509	55.9	reference		reference	
Yes	703	34.1	1290	68.4	401	44.1	0.24 [0.21–0.27]	< 0.001	0.66 [0.56–0.77]	< 0.001
Avoidance of physical activity	2060		1888		911					
No	1009	49.0	319	16.9	408	44.8	reference		reference	
Yes	1051	51.0	1569	83.1	503	55.2	0.21 [0.18–0.25]	< 0.001	0.85 [0.72–0.99]	0.04
Nausea	2053		1887		909					
No	1381	67.3	578	30.6	751	82.6	reference		reference	
Yes	672	32.7	1309	69.4	158	17.4	0.22 [0.19–0.25]	< 0.001	2.3 [1.9–2.8]	< 0.001
Vomiting	2054		1887		902					
No	1842	89.7	1364	72.3	845	93.7	reference		reference	
Yes	212	10.3	523	27.7	57	6.3	0.30 [0.25–0.36]	< 0.001	1.7 [1.3–2.3]	< 0.001
Photophobia	2058		1883		908					
No	1385	67.3	622	33.0	752	82.8	reference		reference	
Yes	673	32.7	1261	67.0	156	17.2	0.24 [0.21–0.24]	< 0.001	2.3 [1.9–2.9]	< 0.001
Phonophobia	2062		1887		909					
No	257	12.5	72	3.8	125	13.8	reference		reference	
Yes	1805	87.5	1815	96.2	784	86.2	0.28 [0.21–0.37]	< 0.001	1.1 [0.89–1.4]	0.3

[a]Including definite and probable; [b]chi-squared test

Table 2 Headache yesterday in undifferentiated headache, migraine and tension-type headache

Headache yesterday	Undifferentiated headache		Migraine[a]		Tension-type headache[a]		Undifferentiated headache vs migraine[a]		Undifferentiated headache vs tension-type headache[a]	
	N = 2066		N = 1888		N = 911		OR [95% CI]	p[b]	OR [95% CI]	p[b]
	n	%	n	%	n	%				
Present	2027		1872		895					
No	1624	80.1	1053	56.3	645	72.1	reference			
Yes	403	19.9	819	43.7	250	29.9	0.32 [0.28–0.37]	< 0.001	0.64 [0.56–0.77]	< 0.001
Intensity	403		819		250					
Mild	328	83.7	408	50.6	151	62.7	3.9 [2.8–5.4]	< 0.001	2.8 [1.9–4.2]	< 0.001
Moderate	55	14.0	265	32.9	72	29.9	reference		reference	
Severe	9	2.3	133	1.5	18	7.4	0.33 [0.16–0.68]	0.002	0.66 [0.27–1.6]	0.3
Loss of lessons at school	403		819		250					
No	360	90.2	693	87.3	217	89.7	reference		reference	
Yes	39	9.8	101	12.7	25	10.3	0.74 [0.50–1.1]	0.1	0.94 [0.55–1.6]	0.8

[a]Including definite and probable; [b]chi-squared test

UdH imposed less emotional impact (summed impact score 11.3 ± 2.7) than migraine (13.6 ± 3.0; $p < 0.001$) and TTH (11.9 ± 2.7; $p < 0.001$).

Quality of life
UdH adversely affected QoL (summed QoL score 33.6 ± 5.2 versus 35.7 ± 4.7 [$p < 0.001$] in pupils without headache), but to a lesser extent than migraine (30.3 ± 5.6; $p < 0.001$) and TTH (32.4 ± 5.3; $p < 0.001$).

Use of acute medication
Pupils with UdH took acute medication on fewer days than those with migraine or TTH. Nevertheless, large proportions of those with UdH reported use of acute

medication in the previous week (38.9%) and 4 weeks (43.2%) (Table 4).

Discussion
In this large nationwide sample of pupils aged 6–17 years in Turkey, we identified a headache type which we termed "undifferentiated headache" (UdH). UdH differed measurably with respect to almost all headache features and associated symptoms from both migraine and TTH. Although characterised by mild headaches lasting < 1 h, UdH was associated with significant burden, including adverse impact on QoL. Crucially, UdH was common, affecting almost 30% of the pupils.

Table 3 Burden of undifferentiated headache, migraine and tension-type headache (preceding 4 weeks)

Burden measure	Undifferentiated headache		Migraine[a]		Tension-type headache[a]		Undifferentiated headache vs migraine[a]		Undifferentiated headache vs tension-type headache[a]	
	N = 2066		N = 1888		N = 911		OR [95% CI]	p[b]	OR [95% CI]	p[b]
	n	%	n	%	n	%				
School absence	2046		1866		900					
No	1792	87.6	1439	76.2	753	83.7	reference		reference	
≥ 1 day	254	12.4	427	23.8	147	16.3	0.48 [0.40–0.57]	< 0.001	0.73 [0.59–0.91]	0.004
School left early	1997		1818		884					
No	1819	91.1	1479	81.4	766	86.7	reference		reference	
≥ 1 day	17	8.9	339	18.6	118	13.3	0.43 [0.35–0.52]	< 0.001	0.64 [0.50–0.81]	< 0.001
Impact on activity	2015		1800		887					
No	1261	62.6	582	32.3	459	51.7	reference		reference	
≥ 1 day	754	37.4	1218	67.7	428	48.3	0.29 [0.25–0.33]	< 0.001	0.64 [0.55–0.75]	< 0.001
Parent took work leave	2044		1880		902					
No	1906	93.2	1607	85.5	832	92.2	reference		reference	
≥ 1 Day	138	6.8	273	14.5	70	7.8	0.43 [0.34–0.53]	< 0.001	0.86 [0.64–1.2]	0.3

[a]Including definite and probable; [b]chi-squared test

Table 4 Use of acute medication in undifferentiated headache, migraine and tension-type headache

Use of acute medication	Undifferentiated headache N = 2066		Migraine[a] N = 1888		Tension-type headache[a] N = 911		Undifferentiated headache vs migraine[a]		Undifferentiated headache vs tension-type headache[a]	
	n	%	n	%	n	%	OR [95% CI]	p^b	OR [95% CI]	p^b
Previous week	1074		1390		566					
None	656	61.1	555	39.9	279	49.3	reference		reference	
≥ 1 day	418	38.9	835	60.1	287	50.7	0.42 [0.36–0.50]	< 0.001	0.62 [0.50–0.76]	< 0.001
Previous 4 weeks	1490		1620		725					
None	846	56.8	513	31.7	324	44.7	reference		reference	
≥ 1 day	644	43.2	1107	68.3	401	55.3	0.35 [0.31–0.41]	< 0.001	0.62 [0.51–0.76]	< 0.001

[a] Including definite and probable; [b] chi-squared test

It is arguable that UdH meeting two criteria of migraine without aura (as did one third of the cases diagnosed as UdH) might better be classified as probable migraine, and UdH meeting two criteria of TTH (almost 40% of cases) might better be classified as probable TTH. Longitudinal studies suggest, however, that a considerable proportion (8.3–71%) of children and adolescents with migraine evolve to TTH or vice versa [24]. In a 7-month follow-up study, diagnostic stability was higher in definite migraine (76.7%) and definite TTH (57.1%) than in probable migraine (44.7%) or probable TTH (43.3%) [25]. The findings of our study reflect this, and support the concept of UdH as a more appropriate diagnosis among these age groups than probable migraine or probable TTH.

With respect to headache duration, in order to accommodate the diagnosis of UdH, we necessarily modified the ICHD criteria for TTH, raising the minimum duration from 30 min to 1 h. As we noted earlier, we question whether TTH – in children or adults – really exists in a form in which headache of < 1 h's duration is *typical*. Although epidemiological studies indicate that it does, we suggest that such reported occurrences are the consequence of treatment: many participants may not have experienced untreated attacks for many years [20].

In previous epidemiological studies of headache in children and adolescents, we were interested in whether authors classified headache in every participant who screened positively for headache or, instead, selectively reported cases fulfilling any specific set of ICHD diagnostic criteria. To clarify this, we re-reviewed all 50 studies included in the most recent review [10] and nine later studies focusing on TTH identified in a literature search up to April 2016 [11, 26–33]. Only five of the 59 studies reliably reported headache that was not classifiable by ICHD criteria [11–15], with prevalences of 2.9–35.5% (mean 18.3 ± 14.1) but with participation proportions ranging between 54.0% and 98.3% (mean 76.2 ± 19.8). In summary, past studies have generally ignored headaches not fulfilling ICHD criteria for migraine or TTH, which nonetheless appear to be common. There is no evidence

from the publications that they met our criteria for UdH, but we offer this as a likely possibility.

There are implications in our proposal both for ICHD and for future epidemiological studies in these age groups, which may need to recognise UdH. There are also clinical implications if UdH, while clearly distinct from migraine, is in fact a precursor or immature form of it. We should emphasise that we propose UdH at this stage as a new diagnostic category, *not* as a new entity. Future research is needed, both to characterise UdH more comprehensively and, especially, to evaluate its prognosis. Only longitudinal cohort studies, ideally into adulthood and perhaps subdividing UdH according to the associated symptoms, can achieve the latter.

Strengths and limitations

The strengths of this study lay in the large numbers of schools, classes and participants, the wide age range, the even distribution of girls and boys, the participants' geographical and socio-economic diversity, the use of a validated questionnaire presented to the pupils in class by a physician and a high participation proportion.

The study was limited by its convenience-based rather than random sampling. Schools from urban regions (41%) were underrepresented (the national urban proportion is 77% [23]) and those from lower-middle income regions (68%) were overrepresented (Turkey is an upper-middle income country [34]). With respect to the features of UdH, we believe these deviations were not important. We relied on questionnaires, and, as in all such studies, were dependent on participants' recall and accurate reporting. This is imperfect methodology [20], but it is not easily improved. While young children in particular may report imprecisely, enquiry of parents not only requires greatly increased resources but also, since it involves second-hand reporting, may not be more reliable. Lastly, our study refers to pupils from Turkey, and UdH needs to be assessed in other countries.

Conclusion

Undifferentiated headache characterised by mild headaches lasting < 1 h is common in children and adolescents. It differs measurably with respect to almost all headache features and associated symptoms from both migraine and TTH and has significant adverse impact on QoL. This new diagnostic category in these age groups offers an alternative to jamming an evolving headache disorder that is neither clearly migraine nor clearly TTH into either of these diagnoses. Future longitudinal studies will show whether UdH represents those headaches that are in a shifting state between migraine and TTH before maturing by adulthood into one or the other. Differentiating UdH from migraine and TTH therefore has implications not only for epidemiology but also in routine clinical practice, since patients diagnosed with UdH call for closer follow-up with regard to their headache characteristics and associated symptoms, and a different therapeutic approach.

Funding

No external funding was received in support of this study.

Authors, contributions

CW contributed to conception and design of the study, analysed the data, contributed to data interpretation and drafted the manuscript. ÇWB conceived and initiated the study and contributed to data interpretation and drafting of the manuscript. DU contributed to design of the study, acted as project coordinator in Turkey and contributed to data interpretation. TSA contributed to data collection, undertook data management and cleansing, and contributed to data analysis and interpretation. UU contributed to data collection, management and cleansing, and to data analysis and interpretation. AT, SIA, TD, FS, GKE, CFD and FB contributed to project management at the survey sites, and to data collection. YBÖ and TA contributed to data management and cleansing, and to data analysis and interpretation. AS contributed to design of the study and drafting of the manuscript. TJS conceived the study, contributed to data interpretation and revised the manuscript critically. All authors commented on and revised the manuscript, and approved the final version.

Competing interests

CW is paid consultant to Curelator, Inc. and has received personal fees from St Jude, Allergan, Pfizer and Apomedica.
AS has received honoraria for presentations at national or international congresses and/or consultation fees from Bayer, Biogen Idec, Genzyme, Merck Serono, Novartis and Teva, and reimbursement of travel expenses and/or registration fees for attendances at national or international congresses from Biogen Idec and GenPharma of Turkey, Genzyme, Merck Serono, Novartis and Teva.
TJS is a director of *Lifting The Burden*, but otherwise declares no competing interests.
All other authors declare no competing interests.

Author details

[1]Department of Neurology, Medical University of Vienna, Vienna, Austria. [2]Dr Gönül Bingöl-Dr Muammer Bingöl Çocuk ve Ergen Başağrısı Derneği, Istanbul, Turkey. [3]Neurology Department, Cerrahpaşa School of Medicine, Istanbul University, Istanbul, Turkey. [4]Neurology Department, Recep Tayyip Erdoğan University School of Medicine, Rize, Turkey. [5]Neurology Department, Namık Kemal University School of Medicine, Tekirdağ, Turkey. [6]Neurology Department, Mustafa Kemal University School of Medicine, Hatay, Turkey. [7]Neurology Department, Sıtkı Kocaman University School of Medicine, Mugla, Turkey. [8]Neurology Department, Fırat University School of Medicine, Elazığ, Turkey. [9]Department of Physical Medicine and Rehabilitation, Marmara University Medical School, Istanbuk, Turkey. [10]Department of Child and Adolescent Psychiatry, Medical University of Vienna, Vienna, Austria. [11]Department of Neuromedicine and Movement Science, NTNU Norwegian University of Science and Technology, Edvard Griegs Gate, Trondheim, Norway. [12]Division of Brain Sciences, Imperial College London, London, UK.

References

1. Vos T, Flaxman AD, Naghavi M, Lozano R, Michaud C et al (2012) Years lived with disability (YLD) for 1160 sequelae of 289 diseases and injuries 1990-2010: a systematic analysis for the global burden of disease study 2010. Lancet 380: 2163–2196

2. Global Burden of Disease Study 2013 Collaborators (2015) Global, regional, and national incidence, prevalence, and years lived with disability for 301 acute and chronic diseases and injuries in 188 countries, 1990-2013: a systematic analysis for the global burden of disease study 2013. Lancet 386: 743–800

3. Vos T, Abajobir AA, Abbafati C, Abbas KM, Abate KH, Abd-Allah F et al (2017) Global, regional, and national incidence, prevalence, and years lived with disability for 328 diseases and injuries for 195 countries, 1990-2016: a systematic analysis for the global burden of disease study 2016. Lancet 390: 1211–1259

4. Stovner LJ, Hagen K, Jensen R, Katsarava Z, Lipton R, Scher A, Steiner TJ, Zwart JA (2007) The global burden of headache: a documentation of headache prevalence and disability worldwide. Cephalalgia 27:193–210

5. Global Burden of Disease Pediatrics Collaboration, Kyu HH, Pinho C, Wagner JA, Brown JC, Bertozzi-Villa A et al (2016) Global and National Burden of diseases and injuries among children and adolescents between 1990 and 2013: findings from the global burden of disease 2013 study. JAMA Pediatr 170:267–287

6. Headache Classification Committee of the International Headache Society (2018) The international classification of headache disorders, 3rd edition. Cephalalgia 38:1–211

7. Westergaard ML, Hansen EH, Glumer C, Olesen J, Jensen RH (2014) Definitions of medication-overuse headache in population-based studies and their implications on prevalence estimates: a systematic review. Cephalalgia 34:409–425

8. Wöber-Bingöl Ç, Wöber C, Uluduz D, Uygunoğlu U, Aslan TS, Kernmayer M et al (2014) The global burden of headache in children and adolescents - developing a questionnaire and methodology for a global study. J Headache Pain 15:86

9. Headache Classification Subcommittee of the International Headache Society (1988) Classification and diagnostic criteria for headache disorders, cranial neuralgias and facial pain. Cephalalgia 8(Suppl 7):1–96

10. Wöber-Bingöl Ç (2013) Epidemiology of migraine and headache in children and adolescents. Curr Pain Headache Rep 17:341

11. Krogh AB, Larsson B, Linde M (2015) Prevalence and disability of headache among Norwegian adolescents: a cross-sectional school-based study. Cephalalgia 35:1181–1191

12. Chong SC, Chan YH, Ong HT, Low PS, Tay SK (2010) Headache diagnosis, disability and co-morbidities in a multi-ethnic, heterogeneous paediatric Asian population. Cephalalgia 30:953–961

13. Heinrich M, Morris L, Kröner-Herwig B (2009) Self-report of headache in children and adolescents in Germany: possibilities and confines of questionnaire data for headache classification. Cephalalgia 29:864–872

14. Kong CK, Cheng WW, Wong LY (2001) Epidemiology of headache in Hong Kong primary-level schoolchildren: questionnaire study. Hong Kong Med J 7:29–33

15. Rho YI, Chung HJ, Lee KH, Eun BL, Eun SH, Nam SO et al (2012) Prevalence and clinical characteristics of primary headaches among school children in South Korea: a nationwide survey. Headache 52:592–599

16. Steiner TJ (2004) Lifting the burden: the global campaign against headache. Lancet Neurol 3:204–205

17. Steiner TJ, Birbeck GL, Jensen R, Katsarava Z, Martelletti P, Stovner LJ (2011) The global campaign, World Health Organization and Lifting The Burden: collaboration in action. J Headache Pain 12:273–274

18. Steiner TJ, Gururaj G, Andree C, Katsarava Z, Ayzenberg I et al (2014) Diagnosis, prevalence estimation and burden measurement in population surveys of headache: presenting the HARDSHIP questionnaire. J Headache Pain 15:3

19. Peters M (2007) Translation protocols. In: Steiner TJ, Martelletti P (eds) aids for management of common headache disorders in primary care. J Headache Pain 8(Suppl 1):S45–S47

20. Stovner LJ, Al Jumah M, Birbeck GL, Gururaj G, Jensen R, Katsarava Z, Queiroz L-P, Scher AI, Tekle-Haimanot R, Wang S-J, Steiner TJ (2014) The methodology of population surveys of headache prevalence, burden and cost: principles and recommendations. A product of the global campaign against headache. J Headache Pain 15:5

21. SISA – Simple Interactive Statistical Analysis http://www.quantitativeskills.com/sisa/calculations/bonfer.htm (Accessed 8 Dec 2017)

22. Sankoh AJ, Huque MF, Dubey SD (1997) Some comments on frequently used multiple endpoint adjustment methods in clinical trials. Stat Med 16: 2529–2542

23. Index Mundi. Turkey demographics profile 2014. At: http://www.indexmundi.com/turkey/demographics_profile.html (Accessed 9 Sept 2016)

24. Antonaci F, Voiticovschi-Iosob C, Di Stefano AL, Galli F, Özge A, Balottin U (2014) The evolution of headache from childhood to adulthood: a review of the literature. J Headache Pain 15:15

25. Albers L, Straube A, Landgraf MN, Heinen F, von Kries R (2014) High diagnostic stability of confirmed migraine and confirmed tension-type headache according to the ICHD-3 beta in adolescents. J Headache Pain 15:36

26. Anttila P, Metsähonkala L, Aromaa M, Sourander A, Salminen J, Helenius H et al (2002) Determinants of tension-type headache in children. Cephalalgia 22:401–408

27. Kaynak Key FN, Donmez S, Tuzun U (2004) Epidemiological and clinical characteristics with psychosocial aspects of tension-type headache in Turkish college students. Cephalalgia 24:669–674

28. Russell MB, Levi N, Saltyte-Benth J, Fenger K (2006) Tension-type headache in adolescents and adults: a population based study of 33,764 twins. Eur J Epidemiol 21:153–160

29. Winkler A, Stelzhammer B, Kerschbaumsteiner K, Meindl M, Dent W, Kaaya J et al (2009) The prevalence of headache with emphasis on tension-type headache in rural Tanzania: a community-based study. Cephalalgia 29:1317–1325

30. Kóbor J, Nyári T, Benedek G, Túri S (2013) Age-related prevalence and features of migraine headache in Hungarian schoolchildren and adolescents. Eur J Paediatr Neurol 17:600–607

31. Waldie KE, Thompson JM, Mia Y, Murphy R, Wall C, Mitchell EA (2014) Risk factors for migraine and tension-type headache in 11 year old children. J Headache Pain 15:60

32. Abdollahpour I, Salimi Y, Shushtari ZJ (2015) Migraine and quality of life in high school students: a population-based study in Boukan, Iran. J Child Neurol 30:187–192

33. Poyrazoğlu HG, Kumandas S, Canpolat M, Gümüs H, Elmali F, Kara A, Per H (2015) The prevalence of migraine and tension-type headache among schoolchildren in Kayseri, Turkey: an evaluation of sensitivity and specificity using multivariate analysis. J Child Neurol 30:889–895

34. World Bank. http://data.worldbank.org/country/turkey (Accessed 8 Dec 2017)

2

Anodal frontal tDCS for chronic cluster headache treatment: a proof-of-concept trial targeting the anterior cingulate cortex and searching for nociceptive correlates

Delphine Magis[1]* (iD), Kevin D'Ostilio[1], Marco Lisicki[1], Chany Lee[2] and Jean Schoenen[1]

Abstract

Background: Percutaneous occipital nerve stimulation (ONS) is effective in refractory chronic cluster headache (rCCH) patients. Responders to ONS differ from non-responders by greater glucose metabolism in subgenual anterior cingulate cortex (sgACC). We reasoned that transcranial direct current stimulation (tDCS), a non-invasive approach, might be able to activate this area and thus improve rCCH patients. Our objective was to explore in a pilot trial the therapeutic potential of tDCS (anode at Fz, cathode over C7) and its possible effects on pain perception, frontal executive functions and mood in rCCH patients.

Methods: Thirty-one patients were asked to apply daily 20-min sessions of 2 mA tDCS for 4 or 8 weeks after a 1-month baseline. CH attacks were monitored with paper diaries. The primary outcome measure was change in weekly attacks between baseline and the last week of tDCS. Twenty-three patients were available for a modified ITT analysis, 21 for per-protocol analysis. We also explored treatment-related changes in thermal pain thresholds and nociceptive blink reflexes (nBR), frontal lobe function and mood scales.

Results: In the per-protocol analysis there was a mean 35% decrease of attack frequency ($p = 0.0001$) with 41% of patients having a $\geq$ 50% decrease. Attack duration and intensity were also significantly reduced. After 8 weeks ($n = 10$), the 50% responder rate was 45%, but at follow-up 2 weeks after tDCS ($n = 16$) mean attack frequency had returned to baseline levels. The treatment effect was significant in patients with high baseline thermal pain thresholds in the forehead ($n = 12$), but not in those with low thresholds ($n = 9$). The Frontal Assessment Battery score increased after tDCS ($p = 0.01$), while there was no change in depression scores or nBR.

Conclusion: tDCS with a Fz-C7 montage may have a preventive effect in rCCH patients, especially those with low pain sensitivity, suggesting that a sham-controlled trial in cluster headache is worthwhile. Whether the therapeutic effect is due to activation of the sgACC that can in theory be reached by the electrical field, or of other prefrontal cortical areas remains to be determined.

Keywords: Chronic cluster headache, Transcranial direct current stimulation, Subgenual anterior cingulate cortex

* Correspondence: dmagis@chuliege.be
[1]Headache Research Unit, University Department of Neurology CHR, CHU de Liège, Boulevard du 12ème de Ligne 1, 4000 Liège, Belgium
Full list of author information is available at the end of the article

Background

Cluster headache affects 0.2–0.3% of the general population [1] and is characterized by attacks of excruciating unilateral periorbital/temporal pain associated with ipsilateral autonomic symptoms, lasting 15 to 180 min. 70–80% of patients have the episodic form of the disorder where attacks occur in bouts (clusters) lasting some weeks or months separated by periods of remission of ≥1 month with a circannual periodicity (ICHD-3 beta 3.1.1) [2]. The remaining patients suffer from chronic cluster headache (CCH) where remissions are inexistent or last < 1 month (ICHD-3 beta 3.1.2 [2]). CCH is a dreadful and highly disabling condition, for which available pharmacological treatments [3] often become ineffective and/or induce intolerable side effects. Such refractory patients (rCCH) represent up to 10% of the CCH population [4] and have a high incidence of depression [5], severe sleep disruption, and suicide [6].

Various surgical therapies, including destructive lesions of the trigeminal nerve or the sphenopalatine ganglion, have therefore been applied with disappointing results in terms of efficacy and/or adverse effects [7]. More recently, non-destructive neurostimulation techniques like deep hypothalamic brain stimulation [8], occipital nerve stimulation (ONS) [9] or sphenopalatine ganglion stimulation [10] were found effective in a proportion of rCCH patients. These methods, however, are invasive, may cause serious adverse events [11, 12] and are not universally accessible, partly because of their high cost and need for surgical expertise [11].

Neuroimaging studies clearly suggest that the ipsilateral postero-ventral hypothalamus plays a seminal role during cluster headache attacks [13, 14]. Between attacks, however, there is evidence that frontal brain areas, including the medial frontal [15] and cingulate gyri [16], are dysfunctioning, suggesting a deficient top-down pain control. The precise mode of action of the various neurostimulation techniques in rCCH is not fully understood, but neuroimaging studies provide some insight into possible mechanisms. Using FDG-PET we found that the only difference in brain metabolism between responders and non-responders after 3 and 6 months of ONS treatment was increased glucose uptake in the subgenual portion of the anterior cingulate cortex (sgACC) in responders [16]. Besides other cortical and subcortical structures, the ACC and adjacent inferior medial frontal cortex also showed respectively increased blood flow during hypothalamic deep brain stimulation on $H_2^{15}O$-PET [17] and connectivity with the effective hypothalamic surgical target on fMRI [18].

Transcranial direct current stimulation (tDCS) is able to directly activate (under the anode) or inhibit (under the cathode) the underlying cerebral cortex. Since its first description by Nitsche & Paulus in 2000 [19], tDCS has been widely studied in a number of neurological and psychiatric disorders [20, 21], including migraine [22, 23], with varying results and an excellent safety profile [24]. The effects of tDCS on the brain might be more complex than initially thought. Most importantly, tDCS can induce changes in brain areas remote from the electrode location. Besides preferential spread of the electric field to the depth of sulci rather than to the surface of cortical gyri [25], tDCS can influence deep structures trans-synaptically including the cingulate cortex [26, 27] and modify cortico-subcortical functional connectivity [27, 28]. Moreover, when applied daily for several days, tDCS is able to modify perceptual functions for several weeks [29, 30]. In an electrophysiological study, tDCS over the primary motor and dorsolateral prefrontal cortex decreased the amplitude of nociceptive laser-evoked potentials [31] and in an FDG-PET study, daily tDCS (20 min, 2 mA) over the motor cortex for 10 days to treat neuropathic pain significantly increased metabolism in the subgenual anterior cingulate cortex [32].

Given the imaging results in ONS responders and the known anatomical spread of tDCS-induced effects, we found it worthwhile to explore in a pilot-trial the therapeutic potential of anodal tDCS over the frontal cortex in rCCH, hypothesizing that it would be able to activate the sgACC, i.e. the area of the brain metabolically activated in clinical responders to ONS therapy [16]. We combined the clinical evaluation with quantitative sensory testing and nociceptive blink reflex recordings searching for possible tDCS-induced changes in pain processing, as well as with an assessment of frontal functions and mood.

Methods

Patients

Thirty-one patients (9 females) suffering from rCCH were recruited in our headache clinic (University Department of Neurology, CHR Citadelle, Liège, Belgium). Six patients dropped out during the first week of tDCS treatment because of local skin abrasion and/or inefficacy (n = 4), or unrelated health problems (n = 2). Two patients did not perform the treatment. These 8 patients were not included in the efficacy analysis.

All patients suffered from the chronic form of cluster headache (CCH, ICHD 3 beta 3.1.2 [2]) (mean chronic phase duration: 11 ± 9 yrs) and had been refractory to at least 3 adequate preventive treatments [4], including methylprednisolone, verapamil, lithium carbonate, topiramate and suboccipital betametasone-lidocaine infiltrations. At the beginning of the study, 19 out of the 23 patients were under preventive treatment (stable for at least 2 months) and were allowed to continue it throughout the trial. One patient had percutaneous occipital nerve stimulation for 8 years (Tables 1 and 2).

Table 1 Clinical characteristics of patients included in the analysis

Patients	Age (years)	Gender	CH Side	Baseline weekly attack frequency	CH duration (years)	Chronic phase duration (years)	Ongoing prophylaxis at time of tDCS
1	56	F	R	5	6	2	verapamil - lithium
2	35	M	R/L	30	17	8	verapamil - lithium
3	48	M	R	12	13	13	verapamil - lithium
4	60	M	L	39	9	9	verapamil- clomipramine
5	51	M	L	4	10	10	none
6	46	M	R	7	13	3	carbamazepine - amitriptyline
7	55	M	R	9	20	16	verapamil
8	57	M	L	13	?	?	none
9	56	M	R	13	9	9	duloxetine
10	50	M	R/L	11	18	18	clomipramine
11	41	M	R	12	1.5	1.5	none
12	29	M	R	5	4	4	lithium
13	57	M	L	16	21	18	topiramate
14	50	F	L	4	2.5	2.5	lithium carbonate
15	48	M	L	8	5	3	verapamil - lithium - melatonin
16	59	F	R	60	22	14	ONS
17	63	M	R	17	15	1	verapamil
18	42	M	R	8	16	16	verapamil
19	30	M	R	5	11	5	verapamil - lithium - topiramate
20	53	M	R	18	40	40	verapamil
21	59	M	L	25	14	14	none
22	34	M	L	14	15	15	none
23	40	M	R	22	7	4	verapamil
Mean	48,65				14,25	11,10	
SD	9,97				8,03	8,85	

CH cluster headache, *R* right, *L* left, *M* male, *F* female, *ONS* percutaneous occipital nerve stimulation, *tDCS* transcranial direct current stimulation

To be included in the trial, patients had to provide a 4-week headache baseline paper diary and to suffer at least 4 CH attacks per week. Other inclusion criteria were absence of other significant medical or psychiatric conditions and personal or family history of seizures. The 23 patients who treated themselves for more than a week (mean age: 49 ± 10 yrs.; 3 females; mean disease duration: 14 ± 8 yrs) were included in the intention-to-treat (ITT) analysis. Twenty-one out of them achieved 4 weeks of treatment while two patients dropped out before this

time period because of treatment inefficacy. The 10 patients first enrolled among the 21 stopped tDCS treatment after 4 weeks and were followed for 2 weeks afterwards. The 11 following patients continued tDCS for another 4 weeks to complete a total treatment of 8 weeks, except for 1 patient who dropped out due to lack of efficacy. In this sub-group, subsequent follow-up information was available in 6 patients. Thus, 21 patients (mean age 49 ± 10 years) were available for a per-protocol (PP) analysis of a 4-week treatment effect, and 10

Table 2 Clinical outcome measures: per protocol analysis

	4 weeks tDCS ($n = 21$)		8 weeks of tDCS ($n = 10$)	
	Pre-treatment	Post-treatment	Pre-treatment	Post-treatment
CH attack frequency/week	$15,33 \pm 13,12$	$9,91 \pm 11,72$***	$18,90 \pm 16,01$	$12,30 \pm 16,57$*
CH attack duration (min)	$47.7 \pm 50,6$	32.6 ± 28.4*	$32,8 \pm 22,0$	$28,9 \pm 28,0$
CH attack intensity (0–4)	3.2 ± 0.8	2.5 ± 1.3*	$2,6 \pm 0,7$	$2,3 \pm 1,2$
N° of acute treatments/week	$13,8 \pm 13,8$	$8,0 \pm 8,8$**	$11,9 \pm 6,7$	$5,9 \pm 6,2$

*$p < 0.05$; **$p < 0.01$; ***$p < 0.001$

patients for a PP analysis of 8 weeks of treatment. The patients' allocation and disposition are depicted in Fig. 1.

Transcranial direct current stimulation (tDCS)

Bipolar transcutaneous tDCS was applied with a novel portable user-friendly battery-driven device developed by Cefaly Technology® (Seraing, Belgium). The first 4 patients were provided with sticking electrodes containing a special conductive gel (Spes Medica®, Genova, Italy – anode: 35×45 mm, cathode: 40×90 mm), but developed a transient electro-chemical skin irritation under the cathode after a few days, therefore the treatment was immediately discontinued in these patients. In subsequent patients we employed sponge-electrodes (80×60 mm, Spes Medica®, France), moistened with saline, we had used previously in a migraine study with a non-portable tDCS device [23]. The anode was fixed with elastic straps (width 100 mm, Spes Medica®, France) over Fz (10–20 system), the cathode over the spinous process of C7 (Fig. 2). No local skin irritation was seen with sponge electrodes.

All patients were trained to adequately position the electrodes and use the device before starting the trial. Stimulation intensity was set at 2 mA, and patients were asked to apply tDCS outside an attack as a preventive treatment, once daily during 20 min where after the device switched off automatically. The stimulation parameters were set in accordance with safety recommendations [24, 33]. Adherence to the tDCS treatment was monitored with an in-built software designed by Cefaly Technology®. During the trial patients could treat their CH attacks as usual, the majority of them using injectable sumatriptan and oxygen inhalation.

Simulations of absolute value of electric field intensity and electric potential distributions were performed using COMETS [34], a MATLAB (The MathWorks Inc.) toolbox for simulation of local electric fields generated by tDCS, based on the electrostatic finite element method (FEM). Parameters of tDCS (electrode size and placement as well as current intensity) introduced in the model were those applied to patients (described in detail above). Simulation results were imported in Tecplot® (Tecplot Inc., WA, US) for 3D visualization (Fig. 2).

Clinical assessment

The patients filled in cluster headache paper diaries at least one month before beginning the trial (baseline), during the whole tDCS 4- or 8-week therapy and at least 2 weeks after the end of the treatment. Attack occurrence, intensity (rated 1-mild to 4-worst), duration (minutes) and use of acute treatment (injectable sumatriptan, oxygen inhalation, analgesics) were recorded.

There are unfortunately no clinical biomarkers of ACC activation. Searching for changes in frontal functions associated with tDCS, we determined in all patients a Frontal Assessment Battery (FAB) score before and after treatment [35]. The FAB consists of six subtests exploring conceptualization, mental flexibility, motor programming, sensitivity to interference, inhibitory control and environmental autonomy [35].

Depression scores were also determined before and after tDCS with Beck's Depression Inventory (BDI) [36].

Patients were interrogated about possible side effects of tDCS at each visit and asked to immediately inform the Headache Research Unit team in case of any adverse event.

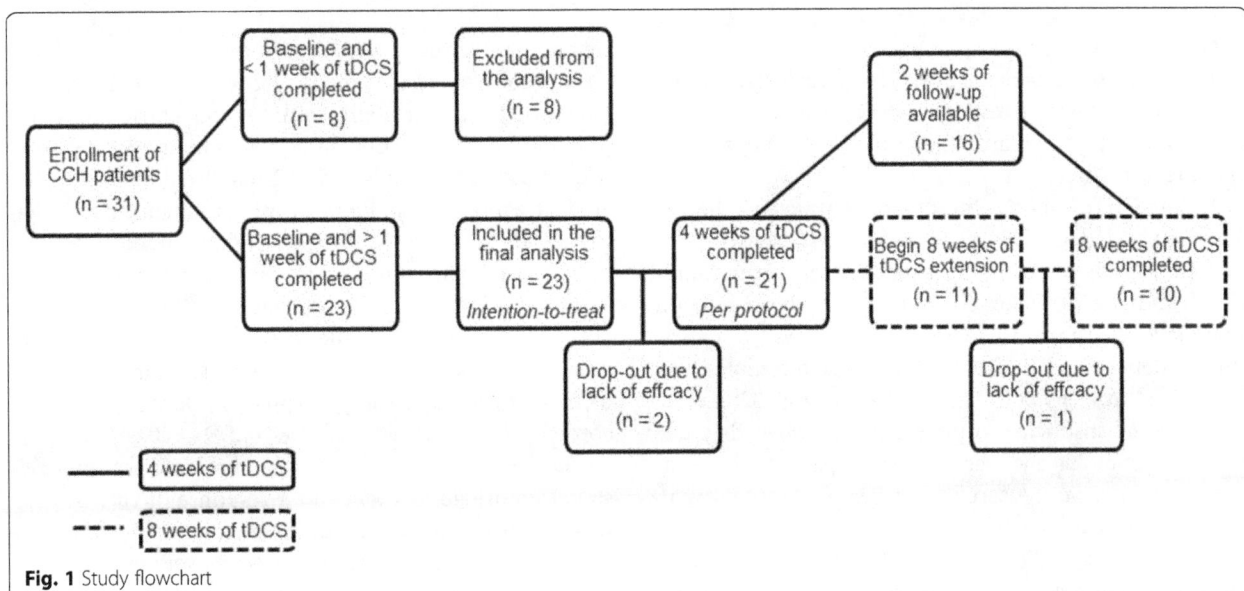

Fig. 1 Study flowchart

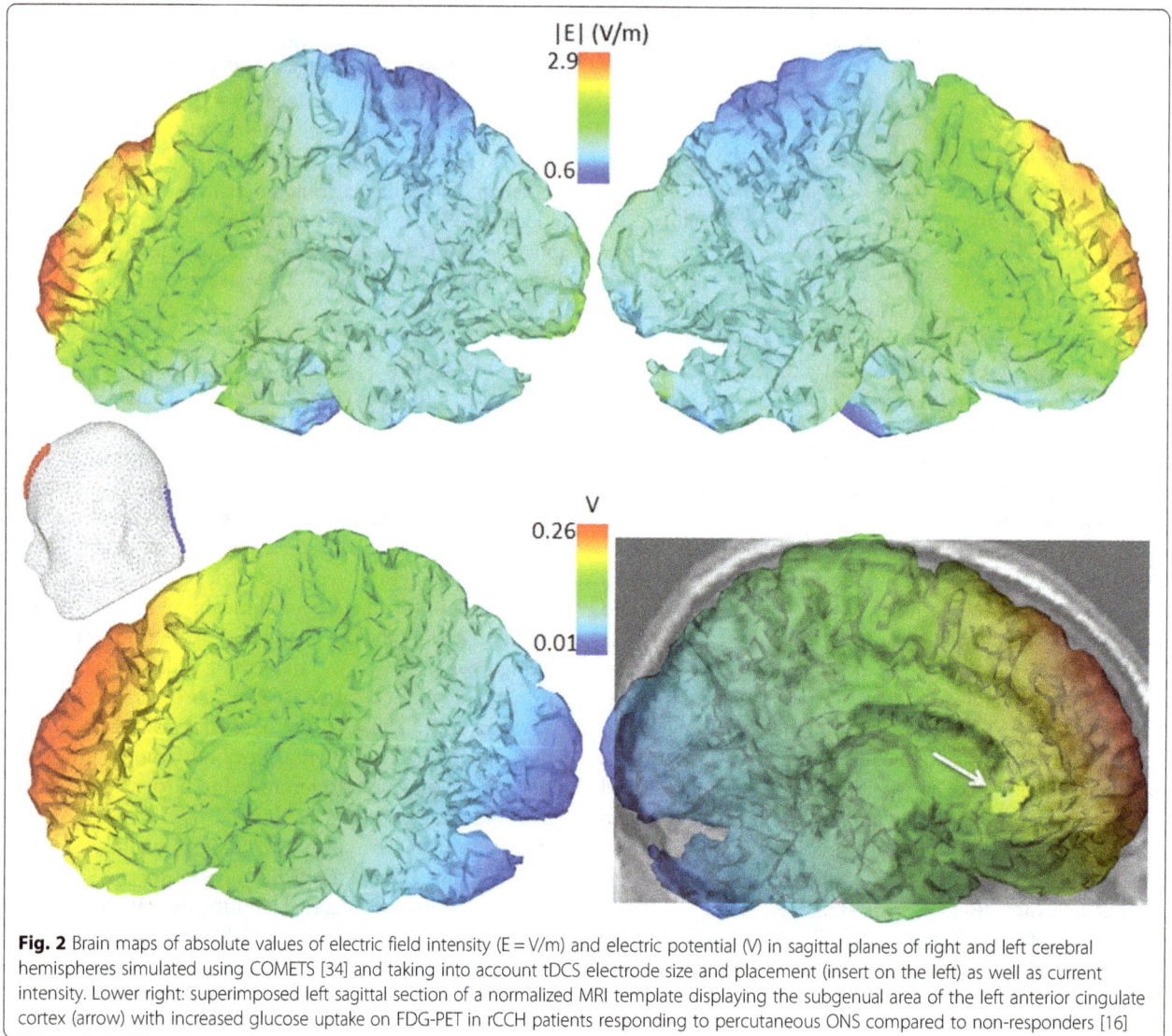

Fig. 2 Brain maps of absolute values of electric field intensity (E = V/m) and electric potential (V) in sagittal planes of right and left cerebral hemispheres simulated using COMETS [34] and taking into account tDCS electrode size and placement (insert on the left) as well as current intensity. Lower right: superimposed left sagittal section of a normalized MRI template displaying the subgenual area of the left anterior cingulate cortex (arrow) with increased glucose uptake on FDG-PET in rCCH patients responding to percutaneous ONS compared to non-responders [16]

Nociceptive tests

Eighteen out of 21 patients accepted to undergo thermal quantitative sensory testing (QST) and 11 to have nociception-specific blink reflex (nBR) recordings before and after treatment.

During QST, using a thermode (Advanced Thermal Stimulator-Medoc™ USA), we determined sensory and pain thresholds to cold (CST and CPT) or warm stimuli (WST and WPT) bilaterally over the forehead and the volar side of the wrist. The device allows to deliver stimuli between – 10 °C and + 54 °C. The thresholds were determined in steps of 1 °C/second starting at 32 °C. The subjects were instructed to press a button when they perceived the stimulus and when it became painful. The mean of three successive measures was taken as threshold value for each variable.

Nociception-specific blink reflexes (nsBR) were recorded as previously described [37]. Briefly, surface recording electrodes were placed bilaterally over orbicularis oculi muscles, and electrical stimulation was performed supraorbitally with a concentric electrode (central cathode: 1 mm; insert: 8 mm; anode: 23 mm). Monopolar square pulses of 0.2 ms duration were delivered at a pseudo randomized interstimulus interval between 15 and 17 s. We first determined electrical sensory and pain thresholds using ascending and descending steps of 0.2 mA intensity (Digitimer stimulator DS7A). To elicit the nsBR, the final stimulus intensity was set at 1.5 times the individual pain threshold. Sixteen rectified electromyographic responses were recorded and averaged off-line (CED 1401 and 1902 devices, Signal 4.11 Software, Cambridge Electronic Design, Cambridge, UK). The first response of each session was discarded to avoid contamination with startle responses. The remaining 15 sweeps were averaged in three sequential blocks of five responses. The amplitude of the R2 response was calculated for each block and expressed as area under the curve (AUC). Results were normalized using R2 AUC divided by the square of stimulus intensity (AUC/i^2). Habituation of the nsBR was calculated as the percentage change of the R2 AUC between the 3rd and the 1st block of averages and also expressed as the regression slope of the R2 AUC over the three successive blocks of five responses.

Data analysis

The primary outcome measure was the change of weekly CH attack frequency during and following tDCS treatment, compared to the mean weekly frequency during the 4-week baseline. Secondary outcome measures were change in attack intensity and duration, and acute medication use.

As mentioned above, 8 patients were not included in the analysis because they applied tDCS for less than 1 week. Two patients stopped treatment before the 4-week term and were considered protocol violators; their data were handled on a "last value carried forward" basis for the ITT analysis. Twenty-three patients were thus available for intention-to-treat (ITT), 21 for per-protocol (PP) analysis of the effects of daily tDCS treatment during 4 weeks. A subgroup of 10 patients was available for assessing the effect of an 8-week treatment.

PP and ITT outcomes were analysed with the Wilcoxon signed-rank test and Friedman's Anova (Statistica 8.0, StatSoft, France). The Wilcoxon signed-rank test was also used to compare electrophysiological values and psycho-behavioural scores before and after tDCS. A p value ≤0.05 was considered significant.

Like in a study on neuropathic pain [38], QST data were first standardized and then entered in a non-hierarchical K-means cluster analysis. This analysis was employed in order to identify subgroups of patients with distinct sensory profiles and their possible correlation with treatment outcome. We searched if the tDCS treatment effect was correlated with pre-treatment pain thresholds using Pearson's correlation analysis and if tDCS had an effect on pain thresholds with mixed-design ANOVA.

Results

Clinical outcome

The changes in outcome measures in the *per-protocol* (PP) analysis ($N = 21$) over 4 weeks of treatment are graphically depicted in Fig. 3. Mean weekly attack frequency decreased significantly from 15.33 ± 13.12 at baseline to 9.91 ± 11.72 after 4 weeks of tDCS (− 5.43/35%, $p < 0.001$). The 50% responder rate was 38%. Mean attack duration decreased from 47.70 ± 50.55 min at baseline to 32.62 ± 28.38 min ($p = 0.020$) and mean attack intensity from 3.2 to 2.5 ($p = 0.016$). Weekly use of abortive treatments decreased from 13.82 ± 13.83 at baseline to 8.00 ± 8.81 at 4 weeks ($p = 0.006$) (Fig. 3).

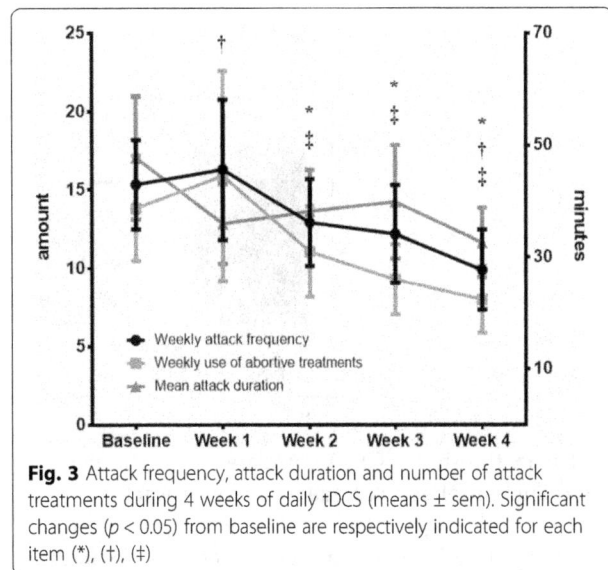

Fig. 3 Attack frequency, attack duration and number of attack treatments during 4 weeks of daily tDCS (means ± sem). Significant changes ($p < 0.05$) from baseline are respectively indicated for each item (*), (†), (‡)

Favourable outcomes were sustained over time (Friedman test $p = 0.049$) (Fig. 3). In the subgroup of patients who treated themselves with tDCS for 8 weeks ($N = 10$), weekly CH attack frequency decreased from 18.90 ± 16.01 at baseline to 12.30 ± 16.57 ($p = 0.041$, Fig. 4). The 50% responder rate was 50%. Reductions in mean attack duration, severity and acute treatment use did not reach the statistical level of significance in this smaller subset of patients.

In the *intention-to-treat* analysis of all patients who performed at least 1 week of tDCS ($N = 23$) the results were similar showing a significant decrease of attack frequency after 4 weeks of treatment ($p < 0.001$).

Follow-up headache diaries were available for 16 patients, as five subjects stopped filling them in after the end of tDCS therapy. In this subgroup of 16 patients, weekly CH attack frequency returned to pre-treatment levels 2 weeks after tDCS (13.38 ± 15.88) despite a significant decrease with respect to baseline during the treatment period (from 15.06 ± 14.59 to 10.81 ± 14.27; $p = 0.007$).

A pooled analysis of compliance revealed that patients who completed the protocol (4 or 8 weeks) had used the tDCS device 87% of the recommended time.

Nociceptive tests

Overall, thermal QST results were not modified by tDCS whatever modality (cold/warmth), threshold (sensory/painful), side (right/left) or stimulus location (forehead/wrist) was considered (all $p > 0.1$). Along the same line, electrical thresholds and nsBR results were not modified by tDCS (all $p > 0.1$).

Searching for correlations between treatment response and baseline thermal pain thresholds, we found that patients who perceived pain at more extreme temperatures exhibited a better response to tDCS. Individual baseline

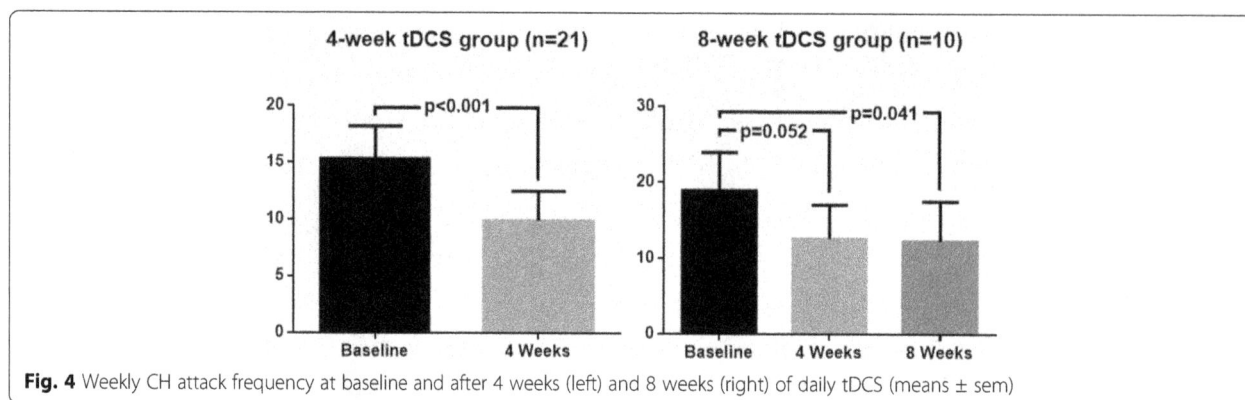

Fig. 4 Weekly CH attack frequency at baseline and after 4 weeks (left) and 8 weeks (right) of daily tDCS (means ± sem)

cold pain threshold (CPT) correlated with the percentage reduction of attack frequency after 4 weeks of tDCS ($N = 21$, $r = 0.45$, $p = 0.042$) and concordantly, heat pain threshold (HPT) anti-correlated with tDCS-induced attack frequency reduction ($r = -0.45$, $p = 0.041$, Fig 5). A data-driven K-means cluster analysis revealed 2 distinct QST profiles: patients with low ('hypersensitive', $N = 9$) and patients with high pain thresholds ('hyposensitive', $N = 12$). The tDCS-induced reduction in CH attack frequency was greater in 'hyposensitive' (-6.67 attacks/week, $p = 0.014$) than in 'hypersensitive' patients (-3.78 attacks/week, $p = 0.049$).

The mean frontal assessment battery (FAB) score significantly increased after tDCS, (from 16.58 ± 1.46 to 17.16 ± 1.17, $N = 19$, $p = 0.01$). There were no significant changes in BDI scores (13.18 ± 18.88 before vs 12.41 ± 9.22 after tDCS, $p > 0.1$).

Adverse events

The sponge electrodes were well tolerated and did not produce any skin abrasion, like in our previous tDCS study in migraine [23]. Besides a slight and transient tingling sensation at the electrode site, frequently reported with tDCS [24], there were no treatment-related adverse effects. Among the 8 patients who stopped tDCS during the 1st week, 2 had actually not switched on the device at all while the 4 others applied tDCS only for a few days because of electrochemical skin irritation related to the use of sticking electrodes. These electrodes had been tested with the tDCS device by the manufacturer before the study. We hypothesize that the repetition of tDCS could be responsible for this skin irritation. Conversely, sponge electrodes were very well tolerated at long–term. Two patients dropped out for unrelated health problems: ENT cancer and peritonitis.

Discussion

Our study suggests for the first time that excitatory tDCS over the frontal cortex targeting the anterior cingulate cortex could be a useful non-invasive, well tolerated add-on therapy for attack prevention in patients suffering from chronic cluster headache refractory to preventive treatments (rCCH). After 4 weeks of one daily 20-min session of tDCS there was on average a

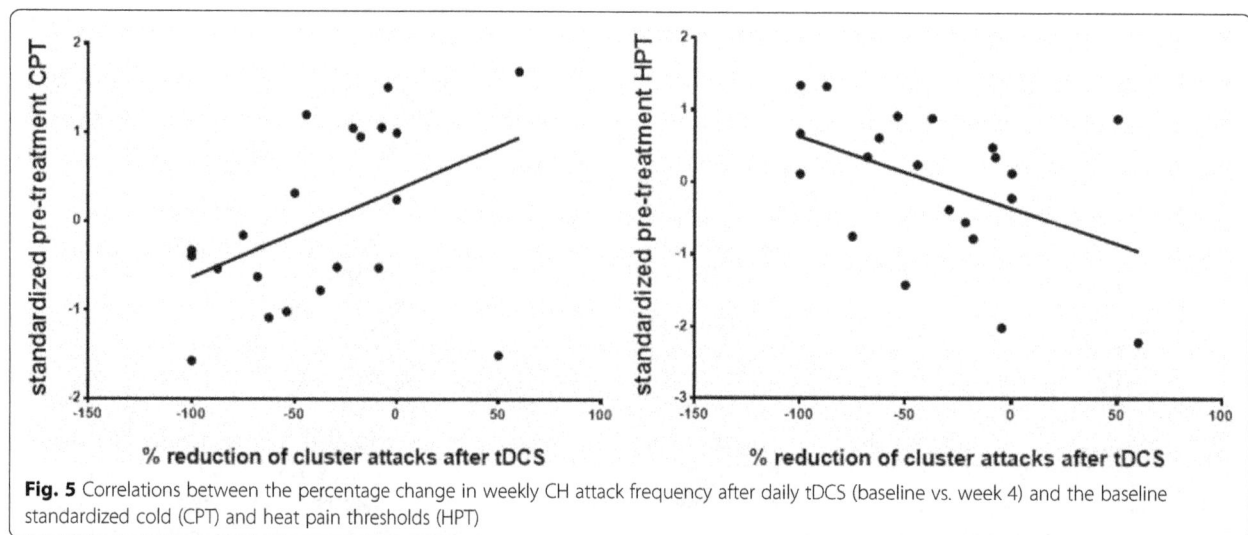

Fig. 5 Correlations between the percentage change in weekly CH attack frequency after daily tDCS (baseline vs. week 4) and the baseline standardized cold (CPT) and heat pain thresholds (HPT)

37% reduction in weekly attack frequency (– 5.39) and a 50% frequency responder rate of 43%, when patients who completed at least 1 week of treatment were included in the analysis. As this was an open label proof-of-concept trial, we excluded from the outcome analysis subjects who dropped during the first week. Despite the relatively small size of the subgroup of patients who completed 8 weeks of treatment, our study was able to detect a sustained beneficial effect of tDCS on the number of weekly attacks (– 6,60 attacks or 35.6% reduction). As illustrated in Fig. 3, there was overall no significant clinical change during the 1st week of treatment, or even a slight numerical increase in attack frequency. This may suggest that it takes some time for tDCS to induce plastic changes [39] in frontal networks [14, 15]. The lack of improvement during 1st week may also explain some of the early drop-outs and should be explained to patients in future tDCS trials. Future study protocols should also consider extending the treatment period beyond eight weeks, since in the present study clinical improvement did not last for more than 2 weeks after interrupting tDCS.

These outcomes may appear modest at first sight. One has to take into account, however, that rCCH patients are most difficult patients to treat and that tDCS is an accessible and safe therapy devoid of serious adverse effects [40]. There was great variation of attack frequency between patients reflecting clinical practice and of treatment effects, which could in part be related to the known inter-individual variability of physiological tDCS changes [41]. Needless to say that a randomized, sham-controlled trial is warranted to confirm the results of this open label study. Given the excellent safety and tolerability of tDCS, however, such a trial could target a less- or non-refractory population of chronic and episodic cluster headache patients, which might increase the effect size.

Up to now transcutaneous cervical vagus nerve stimulation (nVNS) is the only other non-invasive neurostimulation method that was studied in cluster headache, though not in patients refractory to preventive drugs. Similar benefits were reported with nVNS in CCH attack prevention after 4 weeks of daily stimulations (– 5.9 attacks/week [42]) and for the acute treatment of episodic, but not chronic CH [43].

Baseline scores on the Frontal Assessment Battery (FAB) were non significantly lower (16.58 ± 1.46) in our patients than available normative values matched for age (17.1 ± 1) [44]. After tDCS therapy FAB scores increased significantly. Although we cannot rule out a learning effect, this may be due to an excitatory effect of anodal tDCS on frontal and prefrontal areas that are known to be dysfunctioning in CH according to behavioural [45] and fMRI studies [46].

The fact that tDCS had no effect on thermal pain thresholds or on amplitude of the nociceptive blink reflex suggests that it has no direct anti-nociceptive effect. The therapeutic effect of tDCS, however, was greater in patients with high baseline pain thresholds than in those belonging to the low threshold subgroup. Whether this is related to allodynia that is prevalent during CH attacks and may outlast the attack [47] and/or to different underlying brain activation states known to influence tDCS effects [48] remains to be determined. It suggests nevertheless that baseline pain thresholds could have predictive value for tDCS treatment success in future clinical trials.

The rationale of this proof-of-concept study was that Fz anode-C7 cathode tDCS would be able to activate the anterior cingulate cortex (ACC) of which we found the subgenual portion (sgACC) to be hypermetabolic in rCCH patients responding to percutaneous ONS [16]. Simulations using the COMETS [34] toolbox indicate indeed that our tDCS protocol generates an electric field able to reach this area of the deep frontal cortex. As illustrated in Fig. 2, however, the electrical field generated by tDCS spreads largely over several prefrontal areas that are implicated in cluster headache pathophysiology [14, 15, 18, 45, 46], and may even exert a lesser effect in other subcortical structures like the hypothalamus, known to be pivotal in this disorder [49]. Current density maps suggest that tDCS-related brainstem activation is probably negligible. Moreover, we didn't observe any signs specific to brainstem modulation (like visual disturbances or vertigo, or nsBR modifications). Although the prefrontal cortex is involved in pain control, a comprehensive review shows that tDCS trials targeting areas such as the dorsolateral prefrontal cortex are overall ineffective in chronic pain disorders [21]. Thus, although increased cortical excitability has been demonstrated in episodic (not chronic) cluster headache patients [50], it is likely that the activation of prefrontal cortices in our tDCS protocol was not involved directly in the beneficial therapeutic effect, but rather via its connexions with subcortical structures including the ACC [25–27]. Unfortunately, we had no access to functional neuroimaging nor laser evoked potentials, which would have allowed a more straightforward anatomo-clinical interpretation.

Conclusions

To conclude, this proof-of-concept study suggests that daily tDCS (2 mA, 20 min) with the anode at Fz and the cathode at C7 could be a useful and well-tolerated therapy in difficult-to-treat chronic cluster headache patients, refractory to medical treatment. The beneficial effect takes 1 week to appear and is short-lasting after the treatment period. The mechanism of action could be an activation of the subgenual anterior cingulate cortex either directly via the generated electrical field or via activation of prefrontal areas. It remains to be determined if the effect size could be greater in less disabled cluster headache patients. We are aware that these results need to be confirmed in a randomized sham-controlled trial, for which our study has provided several methodological hints.

Abbreviations
CH: Cluster Headache; CPT: Cold pain threshold; CST: Cold sensory threshold; FAB: Frontal Assessment Battery; ITT: Intention-to-treat; nBR: nociceptive blink reflexes; ONS: Occipital nerve stimulation; PET: Positron emission tomography; QST: Thermal quantitative sensory testing; rCCH: refractory chronic cluster headache; sgACC: subgenual anterior cingulate cortex; tDCS: transcranial direct current stimulation; WST: Warm sensory threshold

Acknowledgements
The authors wish to wholeheartedly acknowledge Dr. Anna Cosseddu for her help in data collection.

Funding
This study was supported by a research grant of the Fondation Roi Baudouin, Fonds Malou Malou. The portable tDCS devices were generously provided by Cefaly Technology™.

Availability of data and materials
Further data from the underlying research material can be obtained upon request to the corresponding author.

Authors' contributions
DM conceived and designed the study, recruited and followed-up patients, participated in data analysis and statistics, and wrote the manuscript. KD followed-up patients, performed electrophysiological recordings, participated in data analysis and performed the statistics. ML performed electrophysiological recordings and participated in data analysis.
CL performed the simulations of electric field intensity and electric potential distribution. JS conceived the study, recruited and followed-up patients, participated in data analysis, and contributed to writing and correcting the manuscript. All authors reviewed and approved the manuscript.

Competing interests
Delphine Magis has received travel and research grants from electroCore LLC.
Kevin D'Ostilio has nothing to disclose.
Marco Lisicki has nothing to disclose.
Chany Lee has nothing to disclose.
Jean Schoenen is a consultant for Cefaly Technology, Chordate and Neuramodix.

Author details
[1]Headache Research Unit, University Department of Neurology CHR, CHU de Liège, Boulevard du 12ème de Ligne 1, 4000 Liège, Belgium. [2]Department of Biomedical Engineering, Hanyang University, 222 Wangsimni-ro, Seongdong-gu, Seoul 04763, South Korea.

References
1. Fischera M, Marziniak M, Gralow I, Evers S (2008) The incidence and prevalence of cluster headache: a meta-analysis of population-based studies. Cephalalgia 28:614–618
2. Headache Classification Committee of the International Headache Society (IHS) (2013) The international classification of headache disorders, 3rd edition (beta version). Cephalalgia 53:137–146. https://doi.org/10.1177/0333102413485658
3. Obermann M, Holle D, Naegel S et al (2015) Pharmacotherapy options for cluster headache. Expert Opin Pharmacother 16:1177–1184. https://doi.org/10.1517/14656566.2015.1040392
4. Mitsikostas DD, Edvinsson L, Jensen RH et al (2014) Refractory chronic cluster headache: a consensus statement on clinical definition from the European headache federation. J Headache Pain 15:79. https://doi.org/10.1186/1129-2377-15-79
5. Louter MA, Wilbrink LA, Haan J et al (2016) Cluster headache and depression. Neurology 87:1899–1906. https://doi.org/10.1212/WNL.0000000000003282
6. Trejo-Gabriel-Galan JM, Aicua-Rapún I, Cubo-Delgado E, Velasco-Bernal C (2017) Suicide in primary headaches in 48 countries: a physician-survey based study. Cephalalgia 333102417714477. doi: https://doi.org/10.1177/0333102417714477
7. Rozen TD (2002) Interventional treatment for cluster headache: a review of the options. Curr Pain Headache Rep 6:57–64. https://doi.org/10.1007/s11916-002-0025-6
8. Leone M, Franzini A, Cecchini AP, Bussone G (2012) Efficacy of hypothalamic stimulation for chronic drug-resistant cluster headache. Cephalalgia 32:267–268
9. Magis D, Allena M, Bolla M et al (2007) Occipital nerve stimulation for drug-resistant chronic cluster headache: a prospective pilot study. Lancet Neurol 6:314–321. https://doi.org/10.1016/S1474-4422(07)70058-3
10. Schoenen J, Jensen RH, Lantéri-Minet M et al (2013) Stimulation of the sphenopalatine ganglion (SPG) for cluster headache treatment. Pathway CH-1: a randomized, sham-controlled study. Cephalalgia 33:816–830. https://doi.org/10.1177/0333102412473667
11. D'Ostilio K, Magis D (2016) Invasive and non-invasive electrical Pericranial nerve stimulation for the treatment of chronic primary headaches. Curr Pain Headache Rep 20:61
12. Schoenen J, Di Clemente L, Vandenheede M et al (2005) Hypothalamic stimulation in chronic cluster headache: a pilot study of efficacy and mode of action. Brain 128:940–947. https://doi.org/10.1093/brain/awh411
13. May A, Bahra A, Büchel C et al (1998) Hypothalamic activation in cluster headache attacks. Lancet 352:275–278. https://doi.org/10.1016/S0140-6736(98)02470-2
14. Yang FC, Chou KH, Fuh JL et al (2015) Altered hypothalamic functional connectivity in cluster headache: a longitudinal resting-state functional MRI study. J Neurol Neurosurg Psychiatry 86:437–445. https://doi.org/10.1136/jnnp-2014-308122
15. Sprenger T, Ruether KV, Boecker H et al (2007) Altered metabolism in frontal brain circuits in cluster headache. Cephalalgia 27:1033–1042. https://doi.org/10.1111/j.1468-2982.2007.01386.x
16. Magis D, Bruno M-A, Fumal A et al (2011) Central modulation in cluster headache patients treated with occipital nerve stimulation: an FDG-PET study. BMC Neurol 11:25. https://doi.org/10.1186/1471-2377-11-25
17. May A, Leone M, Boecker H et al (2006) Hypothalamic deep brain stimulation in positron emission tomography. J Neurosci 26:3589–3593. https://doi.org/10.1523/JNEUROSCI.4609-05.2006
18. Owen SLF, Green AL, Davies P et al (2007) Connectivity of an effective hypothalamic surgical target for cluster headache. J Clin Neurosci 14:955–960. https://doi.org/10.1016/j.jocn.2006.07.012
19. Nitsche MA, Paulus W (2000) Excitability changes induced in the human motor cortex by weak transcranial direct current stimulation. J Physiol 527:633–639. https://doi.org/10.1111/j.1469-7793.2000.t01-1-00633.x
20. Lefaucheur J-P (2016) A comprehensive database of published tDCS clinical trials (2005—2016) MOTS CLÉS. Neurophysiol Clin 46:319–398. https://doi.org/10.1016/j.neucli.2016.10.002
21. Lefaucheur J-P, Antal A, Ayache SS et al (2017) Evidence-based guidelines on the therapeutic use of transcranial direct current stimulation (tDCS). Clin Neurophysiol 128:56–92. https://doi.org/10.1016/j.clinph.2016.10.087

22. Antal A, Kriener N, Lang N et al (2011) Cathodal transcranial direct current stimulation of the visual cortex in the prophylactic treatment of migraine. Cephalalgia 31:820–828. https://doi.org/10.1177/0333102411399349

23. Viganò A, D'Elia TS, Sava SL et al (2013) Transcranial direct current stimulation (tDCS) of the visual cortex: a proof-of-concept study based on interictal electrophysiological abnormalities in migraine. J Headache Pain 14:23. https://doi.org/10.1186/1129-2377-14-23

24. Antal A, Alekseichuk I, Bikson M et al (2017) Low intensity transcranial electric stimulation: safety, ethical, legal regulatory and application guidelines. Clin Neurophysiol 128:1774–1809

25. Miranda PC, Mekonnen A, Salvador R, Ruffini G (2013) The electric field in the cortex during transcranial current stimulation. Neuroimage 70:48–58. https://doi.org/10.1016/j.neuroimage.2012.12.034

26. DaSilva AF, Truong DQ, DosSantos MF et al (2015) State-of-art neuroanatomical target analysis of high-definition and conventional tDCS montages used for migraine and pain control. Front Neuroanat 9:89. https://doi.org/10.3389/fnana.2015.00089

27. Weber MJ, Messing SB, Rao H et al (2014) Prefrontal transcranial direct current stimulation alters activation and connectivity in cortical and subcortical reward systems: a tDCS-fMRI study. Hum Brain Mapp 35:3673–3686. https://doi.org/10.1002/hbm.22429

28. Polanía R, Paulus W, Nitsche MA (2012) Modulating cortico-striatal and thalamo-cortical functional connectivity with transcranial direct current stimulation. Hum Brain Mapp 33:2499–2508. https://doi.org/10.1002/hbm.21380

29. Behrens JR, Kraft A, Irlbacher K et al (2017) Long-lasting enhancement of visual perception with repetitive noninvasive transcranial direct current stimulation. Front Cell Neurosci 11. https://doi.org/10.3389/fncel.2017.00238

30. Olma MC, Dargie RA, Behrens JR et al (2013) Long-Term Effects of Serial Anodal tDCS on Motion Perception in Subjects with Occipital Stroke Measured in the Unaffected Visual Hemifield. Front Hum Neurosci 7. https://doi.org/10.3389/fnhum.2013.00314

31. Vecchio E, Ricci K, Montemurno A et al (2016) Effects of left primary motor and dorsolateral prefrontal cortex transcranial direct current stimulation on laser-evoked potentials in migraine patients and normal subjects. Neurosci Lett 626:149–157. https://doi.org/10.1016/j.neulet.2016.05.034

32. Yoon EJ, Kim YK, Kim H-R et al (2014) Transcranial direct current stimulation to lessen neuropathic pain after spinal cord injury: a mechanistic PET study. Neurorehabil Neural Repair 28:250–259. https://doi.org/10.1177/1545968313507632

33. Poreisz C, Boros K, Antal A, Paulus W (2007) Safety aspects of transcranial direct current stimulation concerning healthy subjects and patients. Brain Res Bull 72:208–214

34. Jung Y-J, Kim J-H, Im C-H (2013) COMETS: a MATLAB toolbox for simulating local electric fields generated by transcranial direct current stimulation (tDCS). Biomed Eng Lett 3:39–46. https://doi.org/10.1007/s13534-013-0087-x

35. Dubois B, Slachevsky A, Litvan I, Pillon B (2000) The FAB: a frontal assessment battery at bedside. Neurology 55:1621–1626. https://doi.org/10.1212/WNL.55.11.1621

36. Robinson BE, Kelley L (1996) Concurrent validity of the Beck depression inventory as a measure of depression. Psychol Rep 79:929–930

37. Di Clemente L, Coppola G, Magis D et al (2005) Nociceptive blink reflex and visual evoked potential habituations are correlated in migraine. Headache 45:1388–1393. https://doi.org/10.1111/j.1526-4610.2005.00271.x

38. Freeman R, Baron R, Bouhassira D et al (2014) Sensory profiles of patients with neuropathic pain based on the neuropathic pain symptoms and signs. Pain 155:367–376. https://doi.org/10.1016/j.pain.2013.10.023

39. Huang YZ, Lu MK, Antal A et al (2017) Plasticity induced by non-invasive transcranial brain stimulation: a position paper. Clin Neurophysiol 128:2318–2329

40. Nikolin S, Huggins C, Martin D et al. (2018) Safety of repeated sessions of transcranial direct current stimulation: a systematic review. Brain Stimul 11(2):278–288.

41. Woods AJ, Antal A, Bikson M et al (2016) A technical guide to tDCS, and related non-invasive brain stimulation tools. Clin Neurophysiol 127:1031–1048

42. Gaul C, Diener H-C, Silver N et al (2016) Non-invasive vagus nerve stimulation for PREVention and acute treatment of chronic cluster headache (PREVA): a randomised controlled study. Cephalalgia 36:534–546. https://doi.org/10.1177/0333102415607070

43. Goadsby PJ, de Coo IF, Silver N et al (2017) Non-invasive vagus nerve stimulation for the acute treatment of episodic and chronic cluster headache: a randomized, double-blind, sham-controlled ACT2 study. Cephalalgia 0:333102417744362. https://doi.org/10.1177/0333102417744362

44. Appollonio I, Leone M, Isella V et al (2005) The frontal assessment battery (FAB): normative values in an Italian population sample. Neurol Sci 26:108–116. https://doi.org/10.1007/s10072-005-0443-4

45. Dresler T, Lürding R, Paelecke-Habermann Y et al (2012) Cluster headache and neuropsychological functioning. Cephalalgia 32:813–821. https://doi.org/10.1177/0333102412449931

46. Chou K-H, Yang F-C, Fuh J-L et al (2017) Bout-associated intrinsic functional network changes in cluster headache: a longitudinal resting-state functional MRI study. Cephalalgia 37:1152–1163. https://doi.org/10.1177/0333102416668657

47. Wilbrink LA, Louter MA, Teernstra OPM et al (2017) Allodynia in cluster headache. Pain 158:1113–1117. https://doi.org/10.1097/j.pain.0000000000000891

48. Thibaut A, Zafonte R, Morse LR, Fregni F (2017) Understanding negative results in tDCS research: the importance of neural targeting and cortical engagement. Front Neurosci 11:707

49. May A, Schwedt TJ, Magis D et al (2018) Cluster headache. Nat Rev Dis Prim 4. https://doi.org/10.1038/nrdp.2018.6

50. Cosentino G, Brighina F, Brancato S et al (2015) Transcranial magnetic stimulation reveals cortical hyperexcitability in episodic cluster headache. J Pain 16:53–59. https://doi.org/10.1016/j.jpain.2014.10.006

3

NR2B-Tyr phosphorylation regulates synaptic plasticity in central sensitization in a chronic migraine rat model

Xue-Ying Wang[1], Hui-Ru Zhou[1], Sha Wang[1], Chao-Yang Liu[1], Guang-Cheng Qin[1], Qing-Qing Fu[1], Ji-Ying Zhou[2] and Li-Xue Chen[1]* ⓘ

Abstract

Background: Although the mechanism of chronic migraine (CM) is unclear, it might be related to central sensitization and neuronal persistent hyperexcitability. The tyrosine phosphorylation of NR2B (NR2B-pTyr) reportedly contributes to the development of central sensitization and persistent pain in the spinal cord. Central sensitization is thought to be associated with an increase in synaptic efficiency, but the mechanism through which NR2B-pTyr regulates synaptic participation in CM-related central sensitization is unknown. In this study, we aim to investigate the role of NR2B-pTyr in regulating synaptic plasticity in CM-related central sensitization.

Methods: Male Sprague-Dawley rats were subjected to seven inflammatory soup (IS) injections to model recurrent trigeminovascular or dural nociceptor activation, which is assumed to occur in patients with CM. We used the von Frey test to detect changes in mechanical withdrawal thresholds, and western blotting and immunofluorescence staining assays were performed to detect the expression of NR2B-pTyr in the trigeminal nucleus caudalis (TNC). NR2B-pTyr was blocked with the Src family kinase inhibitor 4-amino-5-(4-chlorophenyl)-7-(t-butyl)-pyrazolo [3,4-d] pyrimidine (PP2) and the protein tyrosine kinase inhibitor genistein to detected the changes in calcitonin gene-related peptide (CGRP), substance P (SP), and the synaptic proteins postsynaptic density 95 (PSD95), synaptophysin (Syp), synaptotagmin1 (Syt-1). The synaptic ultrastructures were observed by transmission electron microscopy (TEM), and the dendritic architecture of TNC neurons was observed by Golgi-Cox staining.

Results: Statistical analyses revealed that repeated infusions of IS induced mechanical allodynia and significantly increased the expression of NR2B Tyr-1472 phosphorylation (pNR2B-Y1472) and NR2B Tyr-1252 phosphorylation (pNR2B-Y1252) in the TNC. Furthermore, the inhibition of NR2B-pTyr by PP2 and genistein relieved allodynia and reduced the expression of CGRP, SP, PSD95, Syp and Syt-1 and synaptic transmission.

Conclusions: These data indicate that NR2B-pTyr might regulate synaptic plasticity in central sensitization in a CM rat model. The inhibition of NR2B tyrosine phosphorylation has a protective effect on threshold dysfunction and migraine attacks through the regulation of synaptic plasticity in central sensitization.

Keywords: Chronic migraine, Central sensitization, NR2B-Tyr phosphorylation, Synaptic plasticity, TEM, Golgi-cox staining

* Correspondence: chenlixue@hospital.cqmu.edu.cn
[1]Laboratory Research Center, The First Affiliated Hospital of Chongqing Medical University, Chongqing, China 1st You Yi Road, Yu Zhong District, Chongqing 400016, China
Full list of author information is available at the end of the article

Background

Migraine is an incapacitating neurovascular disorder that substantially affects the quality of both life and work of patients. According to the number of headache days suffered per month, migraine can be classified as episodic migraine (EM) or chronic migraine (CM). The prevalence of CM is 1–3% in the general population and 2.5% of migraine patients develop CM each year, which seriously affects their life and work of patients [1, 2]. In addition, the high medical expenses and the decreased ability of CM patients to work place an enormous financial burden on society. The severe headache and high morbidity in CM seriously harm patients' physical and mental health. Therefore, the World Health Organization (WHO) has listed CM as one of the four most serious chronic dysfunction diseases [3].

The physiopathology of CM is poorly understood. Most research conducted to date has suggest that activation of the trigeminovascular system (TGVS) contributes to the migraine development [4, 5]. Hyperexcitability of neurons lead to neuropathic pain and trigger central sensitization. Central sensitization refers to increased synaptic efficacy in somatosensory neurons in the dorsal horn of the spinal cord following intense peripheral noxious stimuli, tissue injury or nerve damage. This heightened synaptic transmission can lead to a reduction in the pain threshold, the spread of pain sensitivity to non-injured areas and amplification of the pain responses [6]. In chronic migraine, the release of calcitonin gene-related peptide (CGRP) and other excitatory neurotransmitters from the central terminals of trigeminal ganglion (TG) neurons could repetitively excite second-order neurons in the trigeminal nucleus caudalis (TNC), leading to central sensitization and the manifestation of hyperalgesia and allodynia [7, 8]. Therefore, the neuron activation caused by enhanced synaptic transmission in central sensitization may plays a very important role in the maintenance of CM.

Additionally, most studies have suggested that the development and maintenance of central sensitization are largely dependent on the activation of the glutamate N-methyl-D-aspartate (NMDA) receptors [9]. The combination of NMDA receptors and transmitters leads to an intracellular cascade that triggers a series of biochemical reactions resulting in alterations in the structure and function of the synapse, and these synaptic changes greatly enhance excitatory synaptic transmission and thus contribute to chronic pain [10]. Some research on the brain has shown that the N-methyl D-aspartate receptor subtype 2B (NR2B) subunit is the most important tyrosine-phosphorylated protein, and the phosphorylation of NR2B receptor subunits has been proposed to lead to increased Ca2+ entry through the receptor in both central sensitization and NMDA-dependent

synaptic plasticity [11, 12]. However, the mechanism through which NR2B participates in CM-related central sensitization by altering synaptic plasticity has not been reported. We conducted a preliminary study and found that NR2B-pTyr might contribute to CM in rats, which manifested as decreased pain thresholds and exaggerated pain responses [13]. Based on our previous studies, NR2B-pTyr was blocked by the administration of PP2 and genistein to investigate synaptic plasticity-related protein expression, the synapse ultrastructure, and the dendritic spine numbers and thus illustrate the resulting changes in the structural plasticity of the synapse. According to our data, NR2B-pTyr participates in the central sensitization-related mechanism of CM by regulating synaptic plasticity.

In this study, we aimed to explore the possible activity-dependent synaptic plasticity of NMDA receptors in CM, and our findings indicated that inhibition of NR2B-pTyr regulation of synaptic plasticity in central sensitization might be a novel and promising candidate for future treatment or prevention of CM.

Methods

Animals

Total up to 149 male adult Sprague-Dawley rats (250–300 g) were provided by the Experimental Animal Center of Chongqing Medical University (Chongqing, China). The experimental groups are shown in Table 1. Rats were allowed free access to water and food and were housed at 23 ± 1 °C under a 12/12 h light-dark cycle. Before any experimental procedures, all animals were acclimated for at least 7 days. All the experiments were conducted in accordance with the National Institutes of Health Guide for the Care and Use of Laboratory Animals (NIH Publications No. 80–23, revised 1996). Because this model induces pain in animals, the number of rats used was the minimum necessary to achieve a sufficient level of power for the statistical power.

Craniotomy and cannula fixation

Rats were fitted with a cranial chamber, deeply anaesthetized with 10% chloral hydrate (i.p., 0.4 g/kg body weight), and placed in a stereotaxic apparatus (ST-51603; Stoelting Co, Chicago, IL, USA). Following disinfection with iodophor and alcohol, an incision was made along the midline of each rat's head to fully expose the skull. A skull drill was used to perform a 1-mm-diameter craniotomy in the right frontal bone (+ 1.5 mm from the bregma and + 1.5 mm lateral to the bregma), and a sterile stainless-steel cannula with a plastic cup (RWD, Shenzhen, China) was affixed to the bone using dental cement. The end of the cannula opened onto the dura, allowing inflammatory

Table 1 Animal numbers in each group

Experimental group	Animals used					Mortality	Total
	VFT	WB	IF	TEM	Golgi-Cox		
sham	10[a]	6	6	6	6		24
CM	10[a]	6	6	6	6	2	26
CM + DMSO	10[a]	6	6	6	6	2	26
CM + PP2 (7.3 nmol)	10					1	11
CM + PP2 (73 nmol)	10[a]	6	6	6	6	1	25
CM + genistein (100 ng/g)	10					1	11
CM + genistein (300 ng/g)	10[a]	6	6	6	6	2	26
Total	20	30	30	30	30	8	149

[a]Indicates shared with other experiments, do not count

soup (IS) or phosphate-buffered saline (PBS) to contact the dura. A matched obturator cap was used to seal the cannula. After surgery, antibiotics were topically applied to prevent any infections in the operation region. The rats were then maintained at approximately 37 °C on an electric heating blanket and housed separately until complete recovery from anaesthesia. The rats were allowed recover for at least 7 days prior to dural infusions. All the rat experiments were approved by the Ethics Committee of the Department of First Affiliated Hospital of Chongqing Medical University Medical Research.

Repeated dura infusions

A CM rat model was established by repeated infusions of IS to the dura in conscious rats. We modeled recurrent trigeminovascular or dural nociceptor activation that is assumed to occur in patients with CM, as described previously [14]. Rats were placed in a box that allowed free movement for the infusion of IS or PBS to the dura. The IS contained 1 mM histamine, 1 mM serotonin, 1 mM bradykinin, and 0.1 mM prostaglandin E2 in PBS (pH 7.4). What is said above chemicals were obtained from Sigma-Aldrich (St. Louis, MO, USA). We provided a steady infusion of 2 µl of IS or PBS was provided through the cannula for 10 min while each rat was freely moving. The tube was left in place for at least 5 min after the infusion to allow the IS or PBS to diffuse into the tissue surrounding the dura, and the cap was returned to the cannula after the infusion. In addition, we inspected the skin and dental cement seal around the cap to ensure no leakage of IS or PBS outside the dura onto the skin. The rats were randomly divided into two groups and infused with IS or PBS for 7 days.

Animal groups and treatment

Animals were randomly divided into the following groups: the (1) sham group, (2) CM group, (3) CM + dimethyl sulphoxide (DMSO) group, (4) CM + PP2 group,

and (5) CM + genistein group. The animals in the sham group were slowly infused with 2 µL of PBS (pH 7.4) into the dura, as described above, whereas those in the CM group were infused with 2 µL of IS. To investigate the role of NR2B-pTyr in the intracellular events after CM, we dissolved the NR2B-pTyr inhibitor PP2 (Abcam, USA) or genistein (Beyotime, China) in DMSO and injected it into the lateral ventricle (− 1.0 mm rear from the rear of the bregma, + 1.5 mm lateral to the bregma, 4.0 mm from the skull plane) with the designated treatment solution (5 µL). An equivalent volume of DMSO was injected into the lateral ventricle as a control. The doses of PP2 (7.3 and 73 nmol) and genistein (100 and 300 ng) used in this study were based on previous studies [13, 15].

Tactile sensory testing

As previously described, we used the von Frey test to detect the mechanical threshold in the periorbital and hind paw regions. Mechanical thresholds were tested before the first IS or PBS infusion to serve as the baseline. In addition, the test was performed 24 h after each dural infusion and before the next IS or PBS stimulation ($n = 10$, each group). Tactile sensory testing was performed 24 h after the administration of PP2, genistein or DMSO (n = 10, each group) to determine these infusions on mechanical thresholds. Briefly, the rats were placed in the testing apparatus and were acclimated to the testing apparatus during training periods before and after the cannula implantation surgery. Pressure thresholds were determined by applying an electronic von Frey device (Electrovonfrey, model no: 2391, IITC Inc., Woodland Hills, CA, USA), and the assigned force values ranged from 0 to 800 g. According to the manufacturer's instructions, the pressure probe tip was applied to the periorbital region and hindpaw region of the rats, and the threshold was automatically recorded when the rat quickly retracted its head or hind paw away from the rigid tip. The results for the PBS group were considered to indicate the control mechanical threshold. Threshold values were measured at least three times at each site, with an interval of at least 1 min between tests. The results are presented as the thresholds in g ± standard deviations (SDs). The data were recorded separately for each time point.

Western blot analysis

We examined the expression of total NR2B (tNR2B), pNR2B-Y1472, pNR2B-Y1252, PSD95, Syp, Syt-1, and CGRP through a western blot assay ($n = 6$ in each group). Twenty-four hours after the administration of PP2 and genistein, the rats were euthanized, and the brains were removed. The TNC tissue was then separated. Cut TNC tissues into pieces and homogenized in radioimmunoprecipitation assay (RIPA) lysis buffer (sc-24,948, Beyotime, China) with protease inhibitor (Beyotime, China) and phosphatase inhibitor (Beyotime, China) at 4 °C for 2 h. The homogenate was centrifuged at 14,000 rpm at 4 °C for 20 min, and the protein concentrations were then determined using a Bicinchoninic Acid (BCA) Protein Assay Kit (Beyotime, China). The supernatant was used as a whole-cell protein extract. Equal amounts of protein were loaded onto a sodium dodecyl sulphate-polyacrylamide gel electrophoresis (SDS-PAGE) gel (Beyotime, China), electrophoresed, and transferred to a polyvinylidene difluoride (PVDF) membrane (Millipore, USA). The membrane was then blocked with 5% nonfat milk at 37 °C for 2 h and incubated with primary antibodies, including anti-NR2B (1:1000, Proteintech), anti-NR2B phospho Y1252 (1:500, Abcam), anti-NR2B phospho Y1472 (1:500, Abcam), anti-PSD95 (1:1000, Abcam), anti-synaptophysin (1:5000, Abcam), anti-synaptotagmin1 (1:500, Bioss), anti-CGRP (1:2000, Abcam), and anti-β-actin (1:5000, Proteintech, USA) at 4 °C overnight. The membranes were washed with Tris-buffered saline Tween 20 (TBST) buffer three times and incubated with a secondary antibody (1:5000, Zhongshan Golden Bridge Bio, China) at 37 °C for 2 h. The immunoblots were probed with a western blot detection kit (Advansta, USA) and visualized with an imaging system (Fusion, Germany). β-actin was used as a loading control to normalise the protein levels.

Immunofluorescence staining

Rats were anaesthetized and transcardially perfused with 0.9% saline, followed by 4% paraformaldehyde in 0.1 M PBS 1 day after the administration of PP2 or genistein. Regions from the medulla oblongata to the first cervical cord were separated immediately, post-fixed in 4% paraformaldehyde for 24 h, and then sequentially immersed in solutions of sucrose with increasing concentrations (20% to 30%) until the tissue sank to the bottom. Segments of the TNC were cut into 10-μm-thick sections with a cryostat (Leica, Japan). All the sections were stored at – 80 °C for later use. For immunofluorescence staining, the sections were washed three times with PBS and permeabilised with 0.3% Triton X-100 (Beyotime, China) in 0.1 M PBS at 37 °C for 10 min and then incubated with 10% normal goat serum (Boster, China) at 37 °C for 30 min, using a neuronal marker (anti-neuronal nuclei (NeuN), mouse, 1:200, Novus), anti-PSD95 (1:500, rabbit, Abcam), anti-synaptophysin (1:500, rabbit, Abcam), anti-synaptotagmin1 (1:200, rabbit, Bioss), anti-CGRP (1:50, mouse, Santa Cruz Biotechnology, Santa Cruz, CA, USA), and anti-SP (1:50, mouse, Abcam) at 4 °C overnight. Then, after three washes with PBS, the sections were incubated with secondary antibodies Alexa Fluor 488-conjugated goat anti-rabbit immunoglobulin G (IgG, 1:200, Beyotime, China), Alexa Fluor 488-conjugated goat anti-mouse IgG (1:200, Beyotime, China), and Cy3-conjugated goat anti-mouse IgG (1:200, Beyotime, China) at 37 °C for 90 min. Microphotographs were obtained analysed with a fluorescent confocal microscope (ZEISS, Germany). PBS rather than primary antibody was applied to the negative control sections, and no positive signals were detected. The expression levels of CGRP, SP, PSD95, Syp and Syt-1 in the TNC were detected by immunofluorescence staining ($n = 6$ in each group, five images per animal), and five sections from each rat were randomly selected. A 20x objective was used to capture PSD95- and Syt-1-immunoreactive cells and the intensity of Syp immunoreactivity. A 10x objective was used to capture bilateral CGRP and SP immunoreactivity in the TNC, and CGRP and SP expression did not differ between the two sides. The number of positive cells was calculated as the mean of the numbers obtained from five images.

Transmission electron microscopy

Six rats per group were anaesthetized and perfused with 2.5% glutaraldehyde, and their brains were dissected and removed. The TNC was separated and incubated overnight in 4% glutaraldehyde at 4 °C for 24 h. Then, the TNC was cut into 1-mm^3 pieces with a blade. Post fixing, embedding, sectioning and staining were performed at Chongqing Medical University. Briefly, the 1-mm^3 tissue blocks from the TNC were washed three times with PBS and fixed in 1% osmium tetroxide for two hrs. In addition, the tissue blocks were dehydrated in a series of graded aqueous ethanol for 10 min each (50%/70%/90%/2 × 100%). In addition, the tissue blocks were transferred to 100% propylene oxide for 15 min, followed by graded resin infiltration and embedding. Ultrathin sections were prepared on a Leica Ultracut T using a 45-degree diamond histoknife. The tissue was washed two times with distilled water and stained en bloc with 2% uranyl acetate and lead citrate for 45 min. Images were taken using a JEM-1400 PLUS transmission electron microscope (TEM) and analysed using Image Pro Plus. Synaptic morphology parameters were measured at 50000x. The width of the synaptic cleft and the thickness of the postsynaptic density (PSD) were measured using a multi-point averaging method and Guldner's [16] method. The synaptic interface curvature was obtained using Jones' [17] method ($n = 6$ in each group, five images per animal).

Golgi-cox staining

One day after the administration of PP2 or genistein, the rats were injected intraperitoneally with a lethal dose of chloral hydrate to induce anaesthestia ($n = 6$ in each group, five images per animal). The brains were removed as soon as possible without perfusion, and the tissue was rinsed in double-distilled water for 2–3 s to remove blood from the surface. An FD Rapid Golgi Stain Kit™ (FD NeuroTechnologies—Columbia, MD, USA) was used for the tissue preparation and staining procedure. The entire Golgi-Cox staining procedure was conducted in strict accordance with the manufacturer's user manual and material safety datasheet. The extracted brains were immersed in Rapid Golgi-Cox solution ("Solutions A/B") for 14 days (the solution was changed once after 24 h) at room temperature (RT) with low ambient light, transferred into cutting solution ("Solution C"), sectioned on a vibratome (Leica VT 1200S, Japan) at 200 μm to ensure that whole (untransected) neuronal arbours could be accommodated and then mounted on gelatine-coated slides. The slides were further developed and processed according to the manufacturer's instructions and then coverslipped with Permount™ Mounting Medium (Fisher Scientific Co, Waltham, MA, USA). Briefly, the dendrites within the region were imaged with a Zeiss microscope (Axio Imager A2) using 40x and 64x objectives, and the dendritic

spines were quantified by an experimenter who was blinded to the group of each sample [18].

Statistical analysis

The data are expressed as the means ± SDs. Statistical analyses were performed with SPSS 22.0 (SPSS Inc., Chicago, IL, USA), and graphs were generated by GraphPad Prism 7 (GraphPad Software, San Diego, CA, USA). The mechanical thresholds of the sham and CM groups were assessed using two-way analysis of variance (ANOVA) followed by a Bonferroni post hoc test. One-way ANOVA followed by a Bonferroni post hoc test was used to compare the differences among multiple groups. Statistical differences between two groups were analysed using independent-sample t-tests. $P < 0.05$ was considered to indicate statistical significance.

Results

The mechanical threshold is reduced after the induction of CM in rats

We used von Frey monofilaments to test the mechanical threshold of the periorbital and hindpaw regions of rats, and the results are shown in Fig. 1. The PBS group was used as a control. Prior to injection, there was no difference in the withdrawal responses to mechanical stimuli in the periorbital (Fig. 1a) or hindpaw (Fig. 1b) region between the IS and PBS groups. The basal pain threshold of the PBS group did not change over time. Compared with the PBS group, the mechanical thresholds of the periorbital and hindpaw regions were significantly reduced in the IS group starting on the third day.

Changes in total NR2B and phosphorylated NR2B at tyrosine 1472 and 1252 in the TNC after CM in rats

To investigate the changes in NR2B and its phosphorylated forms in CM, we observed the expression of

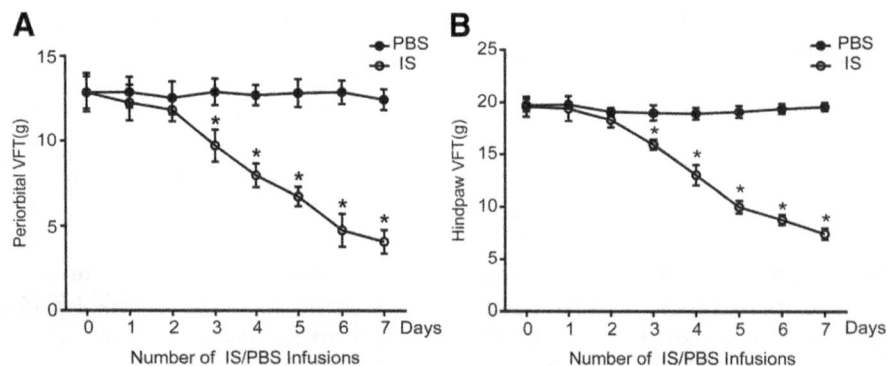

Fig. 1 Development of mechanical allodynia in rats. **a** The pain thresholds of the periorbital region were significantly decreased after three days of IS infusions compared with those detected after three days of PBS infusions. **b** A significant decrease in the hindpaw thresholds was observed after three days of IS infusions compared with those detected after three days of PBS infusions ($n = 10$ each group, *$P < 0.01$)

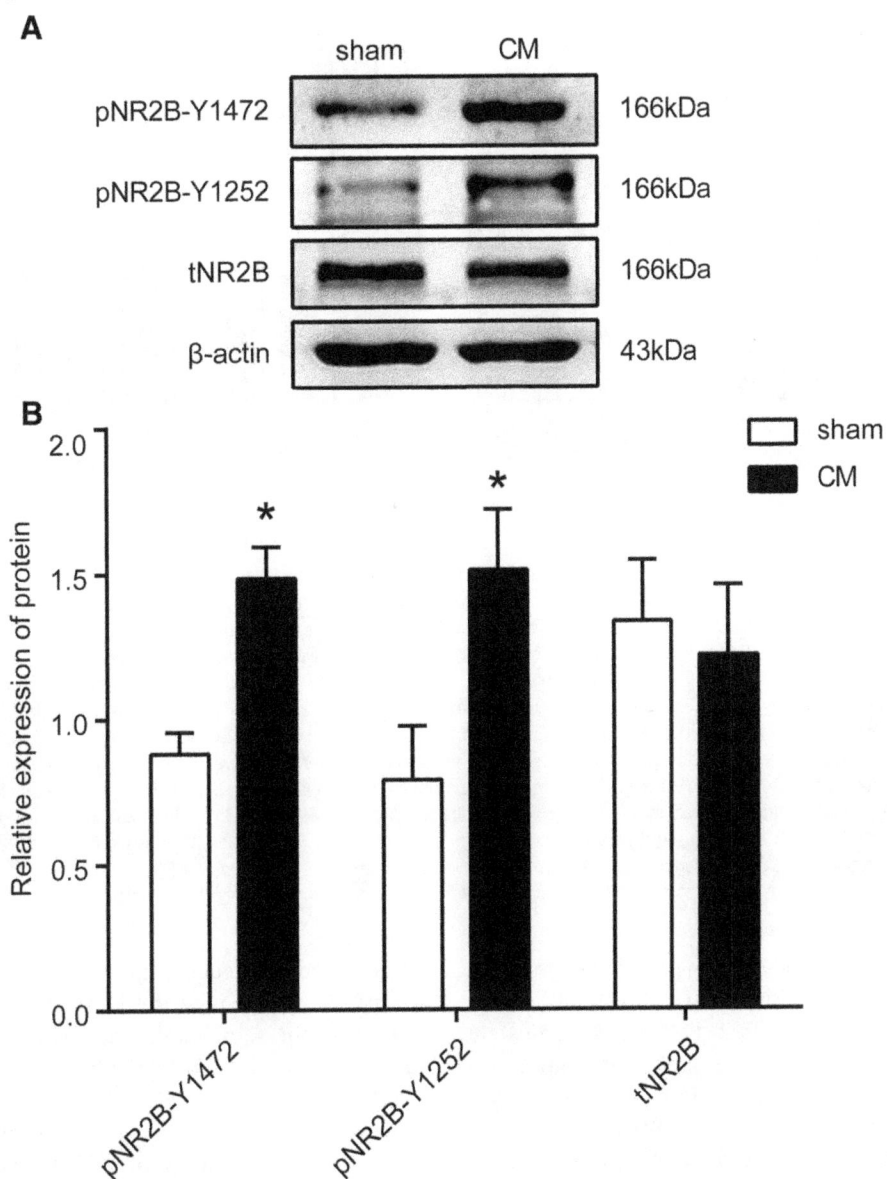

Fig. 2 Expression of NR2B and tyrosine-phosphorylated NR2B in the TNC of CM rats. **a** Representative western blots of NR2B-Y1472, NR2B-Y1252 and tNR2B. **b** The phosphorylation of the NR2B receptor subunit at tyrosine 1472 and 1252 was significantly increased in the CM group compared with the sham group. However, the expression of tNR2B in the CM group was indistinguishable from that in the sham group ($n = 6$ in each group, *$P < 0.05$)

tNR2B and the levels of NR2B-pTyr in CM rats. For these experiments, the rats were killed, their TNC tissues were dissected, and the expression levels of NR2B and NR2B-pTyr were analysed by a western blot analysis. The results revealed that the phosphorylation levels of the NR2B receptor subunit phosphorylated at tyrosine 1472 and 1252 were significantly increased in the CM group compared with those in the sham group ($P < 0.05$). However, the expression of NR2B in the CM group was indistinguishable from that in the sham group ($P > 0.05$) (Fig. 2).

NR2B-Tyr phosphorylation was associated with allodynia

The von Frey monofilament-based approach was used to determine whether NR2B-pTyr is related to allodynia in CM rats. As shown in Fig. 3a and b, the periorbital pressure thresholds and paw withdrawal thresholds to mechanical stimulation decreased after CM. However, there was no significant difference in the hind paw pain thresholds and between the CM and CM + DMSO groups. The administration of PP2 and genistein significantly improved periorbital pressure thresholds and paw withdrawal thresholds.

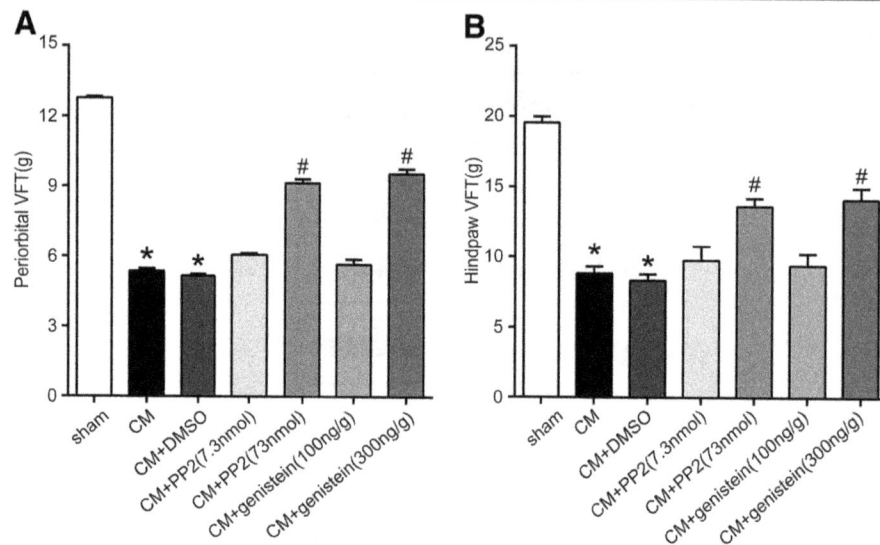

Fig. 3 Periorbital pressure and paw withdrawal thresholds after the administration of PP2 and genistein. **a** Periorbital pressure thresholds of the different groups. Compared with the sham group, the CM group showed a significant decrease in the periorbital pressure thresholds, but no significant difference in the von Frey test was found between the CM and CM + DMSO groups. Compared with that found for the CM + DMSO group, the administration of PP2 and genistein significantly increased the periorbital pressure thresholds. There was no significant difference in the von Frey test results among the CM + PP2 (7.3 nmol), genistein (100 ng/g) and CM + DMSO groups. The pain thresholds of the periorbital region obtained in the CM + PP2 (73 nmol) and genistein (300 ng/g) groups were significantly increased compared with those in the CM + DMSO group. **b** Paw withdrawal thresholds of the different groups. Compared with the sham group, the CM group showed a significant decrease in the paw withdrawal thresholds, but there was no significant difference in the von Frey test results between the CM and CM + DMSO groups. Compared with that found for the CM + DMSO group, the administration of PP2 and genistein significantly increased the periorbital pressure thresholds. There was no significant difference in the von Frey test results among the CM + PP2 (7.3 nmol), genistein (100 ng/g) and CM + DMSO groups, but there were significant differences in the von Frey test results mong the CM + PP2 (73 nmol), genistein (300 ng/g) and CM + DMSO groups ($n = 10$, each group, *$P < 0.01$ compared with the sham group, #$P < 0.01$ compared with the CM + DMSO group)

No significant differences in the periorbital pressure thresholds or paw withdrawal thresholds were detected among the CM + PP2 (7.3 nmol), genistein (100 ng/g) and CM + DMSO groups, but high doses of PP2 (73 nmol) and genistein (300 ng/g) exerted a significant protective effect against allodynia. We then performed western blot and immunofluorescence staining analyses of the high-dose (PP2/genistein) group.

Changes in NR2B and phosphorylated NR2B at tyrosine 1472 and 1252 in the TNC after PP2 and genistein administration

To investigate the changes in NR2B and its phosphorylated forms after the administration of PP2 and genistein, we measured the tNR2B and tyrosine-phosphorylated NR2B (pNR2B-Y1472 and pNR2B-Y1252) expression levels in CM rats 1 day after the administration of PP2 and genistein by western blotting (Fig. 4a). The level of pNR2B-Y1472 was significantly higher in the CM group than in the sham group. However, our data did not show a significant difference in the phosphorylation level of this subunit between the CM and CM + DMSO groups, which suggests that

intracerebroventricular injections of DMSO (control group) did not change the level of pNR2B-Y1472. PP2 and genistein significantly decreased the phosphorylation level of pNR2B-Y1472 (Fig. 4b), and the same result was also observed with pNR2B-Y1252 (Fig. 4c). However, we did not observe any significant differences in the expression of tNR2B among the groups (Fig. 4d).

NR2B-pTyr was associated with CGRP and SP expression

CGRP and SP are important in migraine pathophysiology, and the synthesis and release of CGRP and SP by primary afferent neurons are very important for the induction of central sensitization following peripheral injury, as well as the maintenance of central sensitization in inflammatory pain [19, 20]. A western blot analysis showed that the CGRP levels were significantly increased in the CM group compared with those in the sham group. However, our data did not show a significant difference in CGRP expression between the CM and CM + DMSO groups, suggesting that intracerebroventricular injections of DMSO (control group) did not change CGRP expression in the TNC. The inhibition of NR2B-Tyr

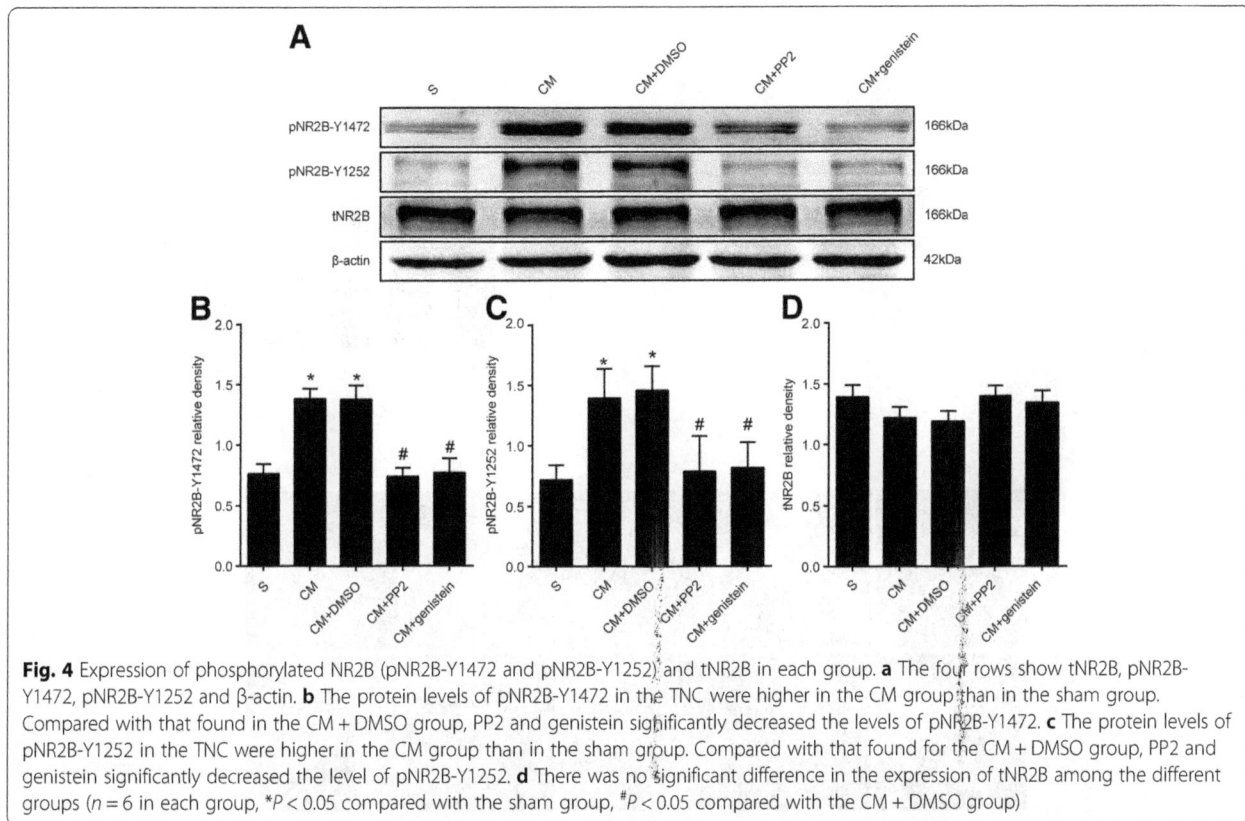

Fig. 4 Expression of phosphorylated NR2B (pNR2B-Y1472 and pNR2B-Y1252) and tNR2B in each group. **a** The four rows show tNR2B, pNR2B-Y1472, pNR2B-Y1252 and β-actin. **b** The protein levels of pNR2B-Y1472 in the TNC were higher in the CM group than in the sham group. Compared with that found in the CM + DMSO group, PP2 and genistein significantly decreased the levels of pNR2B-Y1472. **c** The protein levels of pNR2B-Y1252 in the TNC were higher in the CM group than in the sham group. Compared with that found for the CM + DMSO group, PP2 and genistein significantly decreased the level of pNR2B-Y1252. **d** There was no significant difference in the expression of tNR2B among the different groups ($n = 6$ in each group, *$P < 0.05$ compared with the sham group, #$P < 0.05$ compared with the CM + DMSO group)

phosphorylation by PP2 and genistein reduced the levels of CGRP (Fig. 5a). CGRP and SP immunoreactivity in the TNC was then evaluated by immunofluorescence staining (Fig. 5b). The fluorescence intensity of CGRP was higher in the CM group than in the sham group, and PP2 and genistein treatment weakened the elevation of CGRP immunoreactivity induced by IS infusions, which was consistent with the western blotting results (Fig. 5c). The same result was also obtained for SP (Fig. 5d).

Tyrosine phosphorylation of NR2B was involved in the mechanism of chronic migraine through synaptic plasticity
The level of NR2B-pTyr regulated the expression of the synapse-associated proteins PSD95, Syp and Syt-1
To test whether NR2B-pTyr affects synaptic plasticity in CM rats, we first measured the expression of the synapse-associated proteins PSD95, Syp, and Syt-1 (Fig. 6a). A western blot analysis showed that the expression levels of PSD95 (Fig. 6b), Syp (Fig. 6c) and Syt-1 (Fig. 6d) were significantly increased in the CM group compared with those in the sham group, and no significant difference was found between the CM and CM + DMSO groups. In addition, PP2 and genistein significantly decreased the expression levels of PSD95, Syp, and Syt-1. The immunoreactivity of PSD95, Syp and Syt-1 in the TNC was then evaluated

by immunofluorescence staining (Fig. 6e). The fluorescence intensity of Syp (Fig. 6g) and the numbers of PSD95 (Fig. 6f) and Syt-1 (Fig. 6h)-positive cells were elevated in the CM group compared with those in the sham group, but there were no obvious differences between the CM + DMSO and CM groups. PP2 and genistein treatment weakened the elevation of Syp immunoreactivity induced by IS infusions and reduced the numbers of PSD95- and Syt-1-immunoreactive cells. These findings were consistent with the results of the western blot analysis.

The level of NR2B-pTyr regulated the synaptic ultrastructure observed by TEM
The synaptic structure of TNC neurons in each group was observed under a TEM, and representative images are shown in Fig. 7.

In the sham control group, the presynaptic and postsynaptic membranes were clear and had complete outlines, the synaptic cleft was clear, and abundant PSD was detected. Compared with the sham control group, the CM group exhibited vague presynaptic membranes, augmented synaptic clefts, thicker postsynaptic densities, longer active zones, and an increased synaptic interface curvature. The administration of PP2 and genistein restored the related synapse morphological indicators (Table 2).

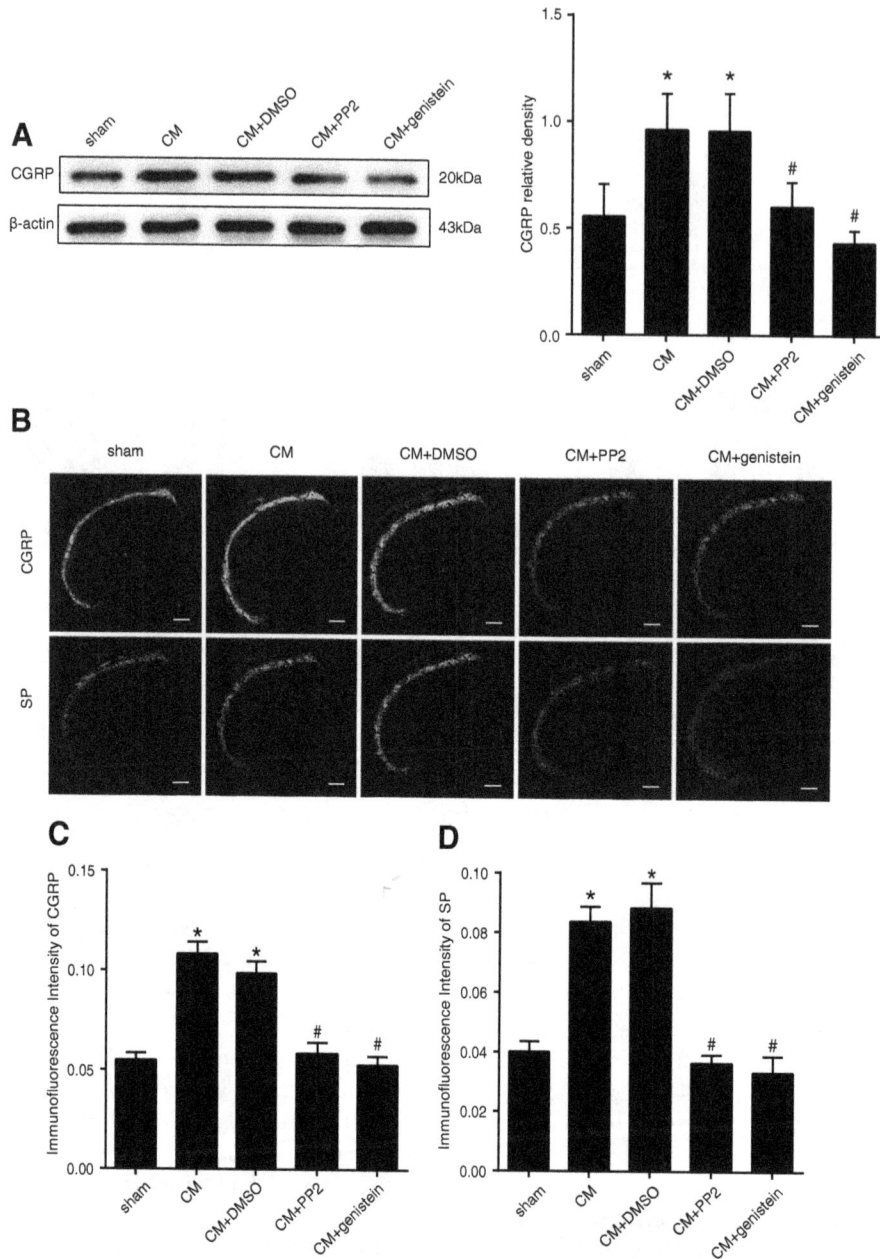

Fig. 5 Expression levels of CGRP in the TNC and immunofluorescence staining for CGRP and SP in the TNC. **a** The expression of CGRP was significantly increased in the CM group compared with that in the sham group, and no significant difference in the expression of CGRP was found between the CM and CM + DMSO groups. The expression of CGRP in CM rats was significantly decreased after the administration of PP2 and genistein ($n = 6$ in each group, five images per animal, *$P < 0.05$ compared with the sham group, #$P < 0.05$ compared with the CM + DMSO group). **b** The bilateral immunoreactivity of CGRP and SP in the TNC was investigated by immunofluorescence staining (the image shows only one side because no difference was found between the two sides). **c** The fluorescence intensities of CGRP in the TNC were elevated in the rats belonging to the CM groups compared with those in the sham group, and no significant difference in the expression of CGRP was found between the CM and CM + DMSO groups. PP2 and genistein treatment decreased the CGRP fluorescence intensities. **d** The fluorescence intensities of SP in the TNC were elevated in the rats of the CM groups with those in the sham group, and there was no significant difference in the expression of SP between the CM and CM + DMSO groups. PP2 and genistein treatment decreased the SP fluorescence intensities ($n = 6$ in each group, *$P < 0.05$ compared with the sham group, #$P < 0.05$ compared with the CM + DMSO group, scale bar = 200 μm)

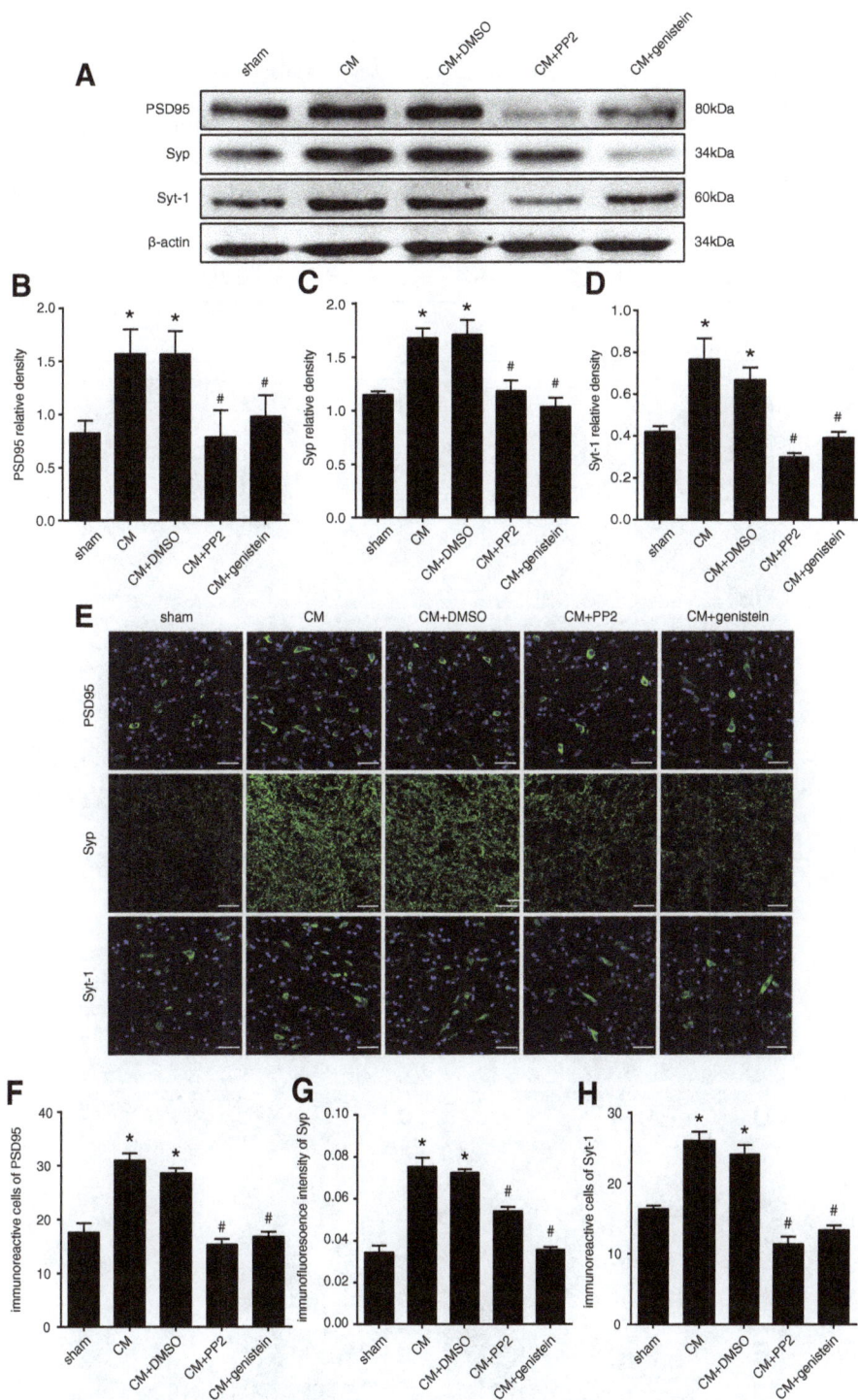

Fig. 6 (See legend on next page.)

(See figure on previous page.)

Fig. 6 Expression and immunofluorescence staining of PSD95, Syp, and Syt-1 in the TNC in each of the five groups. **a** The expression levels of PSD95 (**b**), Syp (**c**), and Syt-1 (**d**) were significantly increased in the CM group compared with those in the sham group, and no significant difference in the expression of PSD95 was found between the CM and CM + DMSO groups. The expression of PSD95 in CM rats significantly decreased following the administration of PP2 and genistein ($n = 6$ in each group, five images per animal, *$P < 0.05$ compared with the sham group, #$P < 0.05$ compared with the CM + DMSO group). **e** Immunofluorescence staining for PSD95, Syp, and Syt-1 in the TNC. Semiquantitative analyses showed that the numbers of PSD95 (**f**) and Syt-1 (**h**)-positive cells were significantly increased in the CM group compared with those in the sham group; moreover, PP2 and genistein significantly reduced the numbers of PSD95- and Syt-1-positive cells. Semiquantitative analyses showed that the fluorescence intensity of Syp (**g**) in the TNC was higher in the rats belonging to the CM group than in those of the sham group, and there was no significant difference in the expression of Syp between the CM and CM + DMSO groups. PP2 and genistein treatment decreased the Syp fluorescence intensity ($n = 6$ in each group, *$P < 0.05$ compared with the sham group, #$P < 0.05$ compared with the CM + DMSO group, scale bar = 50 μm)

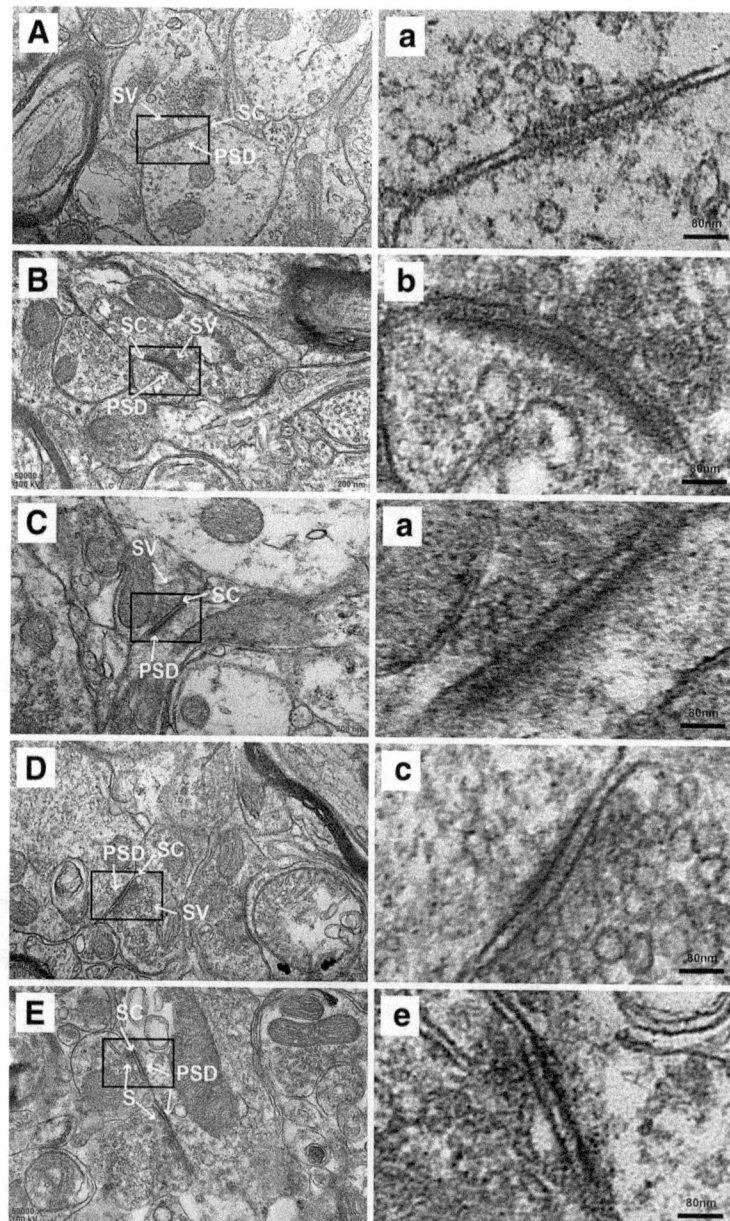

Fig. 7 Synaptic structure of the TNC neurons in each group. **a**, *a*: sham group; **b**, *b*: CM group; **c**, *c*: CM + DMSO group; **d**, *d*: CM + PP2 group; **e**, *e*: CM + genistein group. PSD, postsynaptic density; SC, synaptic cleft; SV, synaptic vesicle. *a-d* show enlarged versions of the images in **a-d**. Scale bars = 200 nm (**a-d**). Scale bars = 40 nm (*a-d*)

Table 2 Parameters of the synaptic interface in each of the five groups in the TNC of CM rats

$n = 6$	Sham	CM	CM + DMSO	CM + PP2	CM + genistein
Thickness of the PSD/nm	22.24 ± 1.2321	40.51 ± 1.9948*	39.64 ± 1.5399*	25.34 ± 0.9563[#]	30.16 ± 0.6379[#]
Width of the synaptic cleft/nm	19.21 ± 0.8048	32.39 ± 0.4477*	32.37 ± 0.4968*	21.56 ± 0.9589[#]	22.63 ± 1.1490[#]
Active zones/nm	289.42 ± 8.31	529.8396 ± 18.6*	538.99 ± 23.15*	382.52 ± 23.51[#]	360.37 ± 22.64[#]
Synaptic interface curvature	1.080 ± 0.0202	1.331 ± 0.0284*	1.3115 ± 0.0184*	1.1643 ± 0.0156[#]	1.1357 ± 0.0125[#]

n, the number of rats. Data are presented as the means ± SDs. *$P < 0.05$ compared with the sham control group. [#]$P < 0.05$ compared with the CM + DMSO control group

The level of NR2B-pTyr regulated the number of dendritic spines in TNC neurons

We performed Golgi-Cox staining to quantify the number of dendritic spines in the five groups (Fig. 8). All neurons selected from each group for the analysis fulfilled the following criteria: (1) the dendrites showed dark and consistent Golgi-Cox staining across their entire length, (2) the dendrites were visibly intact, and (3) the neurons had sufficient space between them to prevent interference during the analysis [21]. A significant increase in the dendritic spine density in the TNC was observed in the rats of the CM group compared with that of the rats belonging to the sham group, and no significant differences were found between the CM and CM + DMSO groups. The administration of PP2 and genistein significantly decreased the dendritic spine

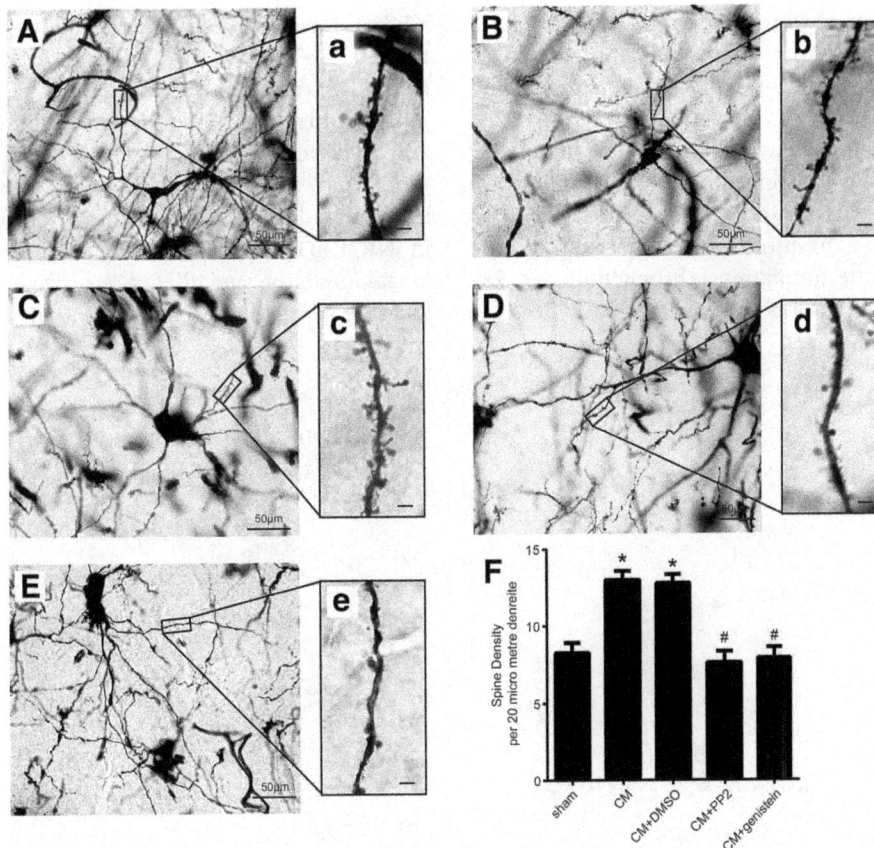

Fig. 8 Dendritic spine density of the TNC neurons in each group. **a-e** Low magnification of Golgi-Cox staining in the five groups (**a**: sham group; **b**: CM group; **c**: CM + DMSO group; **d**: CM + PP2 group; **e**: CM + genistein group, scale bar = 50 μm). a-e Enlarged images of neurons with dendrites that were used for the quantification of the spine density in the five groups; these images correspond to those shown in **a-e** (a: sham group; b: CM group; c: CM + DMSO group; d: CM + PP2 group; e: CM + genistein group, scale bar = 4 μm). **f** Golgi-Cox staining showed that the dendritic spine density was significantly higher in the CM group compared with that in the sham group, and there was no significant difference between the CM and CM + DMSO groups. PP2 and genistein significantly reduced the dendritic spine density, indicating that tyrosine-phosphorylated NR2B reduces the dendritic spine density in CM rats (n = 6 each group, *$P < 0.05$ compared with the sham group, [#]$P < 0.05$ compared with the CM + DMSO group)

density. These data imply that the dendritic spine density was increased in CM rats and was associated with NR2B-pTyr.

Discussion

In the present study, we used the von Frey test to detect hyperalgesia and allodynia and thus investigate the role of NR2B and NR2B-pTyr in rats with CM induced by repeated infusions of IS. In addition, the use of PP2/genistein to suppress the tyrosine phosphorylation of NR2B ameliorated the hyperalgesia induced by repeated IS stimulation and downregulated the expression of CGRP and SP. Moreover, the inhibition of NR2B-pTyr by PP2/genistein downregulated the expression of the synapse-associated proteins PSD95, Syp, and Syt-1 and even altered the synaptic ultrastructure and the number of dendritic spines to reduce synaptic plasticity. Based on these results, we provide the first evidence showing that NR2B-pTyr in the TNC is involved in the mechanism of CM. The effect of NR2B-pTry was found to be largely associated with its regulation of synaptic plasticity. Therefore, the tyrosine phosphorylation of NR2B and synaptic plasticity might represent potential therapeutic targets in CM.

Central sensitization is a crucial process underlying increased neuronal excitability, and some published evidence indicates that central sensitization plays a role in the maintenance of prolonged migraine pain and might also contribute to migraine chronicity [6, 22, 23]. Repeated dural nociceptor activation specifically leads to

gradual worsening of cutaneous hypersensitivity, general neuronal hyperexcitability, persistent cephalic cutaneous hypersensitivity and trigeminal central sensitization [24]. In the present study, we used a CM rat model established by repeated IS stimulation of the dura to repeatedly activate the assumed nociceptors, We discovered that the periorbital and hind paw pain thresholds gradually declined with repeated infusions of IS. This finding suggests that IS induces cephalic and extracephalic allodynia.

NMDA receptors constitute one of the principal types of ionotropic glutamate receptors that mediate fast excitatory synaptic transmission in the central nervous system (CNS). Abundant evidence indicates that NMDA receptors play critical roles in a range of physiological and pathological processes in the CNS. One of the key mechanisms for regulating NMDA receptor function involves the tyrosine phosphorylation of NR2B subunits by the tyrosine kinase Fyn [25, 26]. NR2B contains three tyrosine phosphorylation sites (Y1252, Y1336 and Y1472), and several studies have suggested that pNR2B-Y1472 plays a significant role in the trafficking of NMDA receptors [25, 27, 28]. In an animal model of inflammatory pain, the development of inflammation and hyperalgesia was found to be associated with a rapid and prolonged increase in the pNR2B-Y1472 level. In addition, the inflammation-induced increase in NR2B-pTyr was abolished by genistein, a tyrosine kinase inhibitor, and PP2, a Src family protein tyrosine kinase inhibitor [29]. In agreement with previous studies,

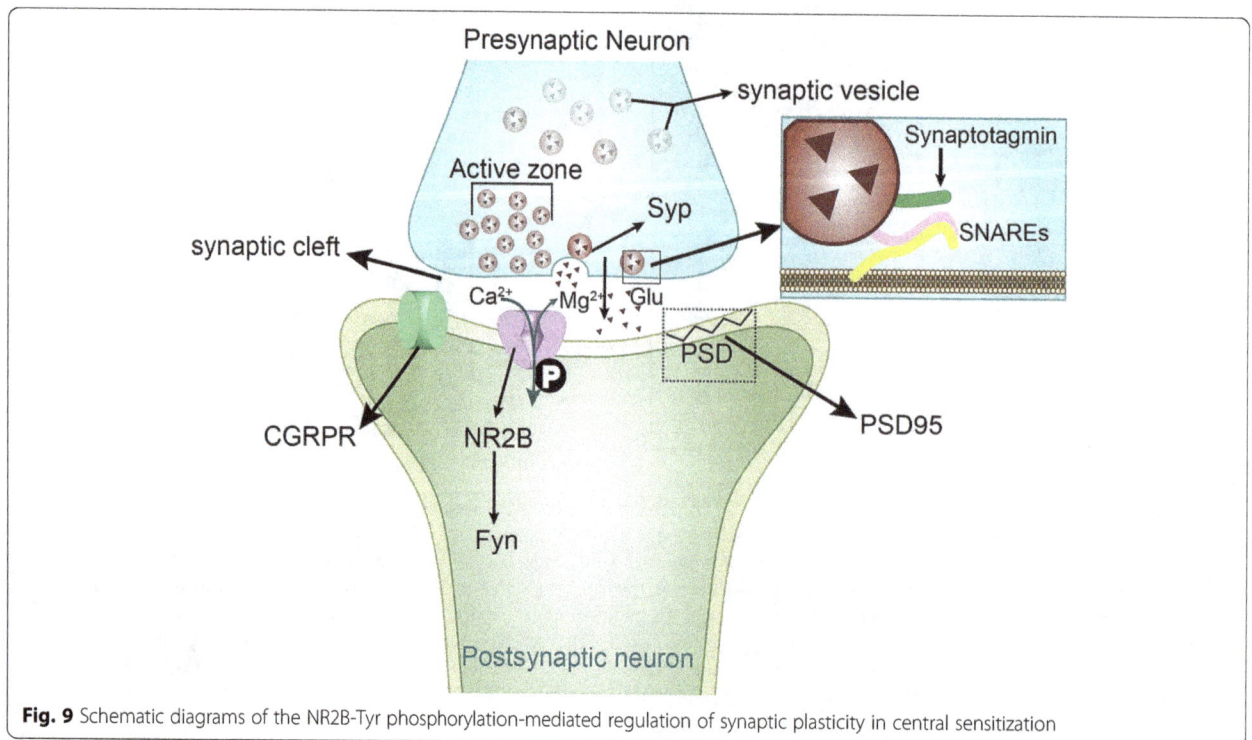

Fig. 9 Schematic diagrams of the NR2B-Tyr phosphorylation-mediated regulation of synaptic plasticity in central sensitization

we found that pNR2B-Y1472 was involved in IS-induced hyperalgesia. The protein levels of pNR2B-Y1472 were overexpressed in the TNC of CM rats, and only high doses of PP2 (73 nmol) and genistein (300 ng) relieved mechanical hyperalgesia. In addition, we found the same changes in the phosphorylation of Y1252 sites. However, other remaining phosphorylation sites should be further investigated. These results suggest that the phosphorylation of NR2B at Y1472 and Y1252 regulated CM activation in TNC neurons.

CGRP and SP are important in migraine pathophysiology, expressed in trigeminal ganglia neurons and involved in trigeminovascular innervation, and modulation of nociceptive transmission. Additionally, these proteins are used as biological markers of neuronal activation and central sensitization [20, 30]. As shown in previous studies, the plasma CGRP and SP levels are increased during a migraine attack [31, 32]. In our study, upregulated expression levels of CGRP and SP were observed in the TNC of CM rats, and CGRP and SP immunoreactivity was mainly detected in the outer laminae of the TNC, which is likely associated with the processing of nociceptive information. This finding is in line with the results of a previous study [30]. In addition, PP2 and genistein downregulated the levels of CGRP and SP in the TNC, which indicates that NR2B phosphorylation might play a prominent role in neuronal activation and central sensitization in the CM model.

In addition, NR2B-pTyr was reported contributes to the development of persistent pain in the spinal cord by regulate synaptic transmission. Therefore, It's very interesting to explore the mechanism of NR2B-pTyr contributes to central sensitization in CM. As is well known, excitatory neurotransmission in somatosensory nociceptive pathways is predominantly mediated by glutamatergic synapses [33]. Recent studies have consistently demonstrated that glutamatergic synapses play an important role in sensory transmission, including pain and itch transmission, and contribute to nociceptive sensitization [34, 35]. Many studies have reported that regulation of synaptic plasticity by NR2B-pTyr may play a role in nociceptive transmission in the chronic visceral pain model and neuropathic pain model [36, 37]. Similar to a previous report, we detected many synaptic-related indicators in the CM model to emphasize that its association with the synaptic plasticity of NMDA receptors. PSD95 is preferentially localized to dendritic spines and plays a critical role in the regulation of the size and shape of dendritic spines [38, 39]. Syp, a major integral membrane protein of presynaptic vesicles, is required for vesicle formation and exocytosis and is widely used as a marker for synaptic activity [40]. Syt-1, which acts as the major Ca^{2+}-sensor for fast presynaptic vesicle exocytosis, is a marker of synaptic transmission. Similar to previous studies, our study revealed that the

expression levels of synaptic function/structure-related proteins PSD95, Syp and Syt-1 were increased in CM rats and that PP2 and genistein downregulated these changes. This finding suggests that the expression of synaptic function/structure-related proteins in the TNC is directly related to CM rats and positively correlated with the level of NR2B-pTyr. However, electrophysiological experiments are necessary to more fully describe these changes in synaptic plasticity changes.

Conclusion

In conclusion, our results demonstrate that NR2B-pTyr contributes to the central sensitization of CM in rats. The inhibition of NR2B tyrosine phosphorylation exerts a protective effect on threshold dysfunction and migraine attacks through the regulation of synaptic plasticity in central sensitization (Fig. 9). This study provides a new perspective on the function of NR2B-pTyr in CM and identifies NR2B as a novel candidate for the treatment of CM in patients.

Abbreviations
CGRP: Calcitonin gene-related peptide; CM: Chronic migraine; CNS: Central nervous system; DMSO: Dimethyl sulfoxide; IS: Inflammatory soup; NMDA: N-methyl-D-aspartate; NR2B-pTyr: Tyrosine-phosphorylated NR2B; PP2: Phosphorylation 4-amino-5-(4-chlorophenyl)-7-(t-butyl)-pyrazolo[3,4-d] pyrimidine; PSD: Postsynaptic density; PSD95: Postsynaptic density 95; SP: Substance P; Syp: Synaptophysin; Syt-1: Synaptotagmin1; TEM: Transmission electron microscope; TG: Trigeminal ganglion; TGVS: Trigeminovascular system; TNC: Trigeminal nucleus caudalis

Acknowledgements
We thank all participants in the study.

Funding
This work was supported by the National Natural Science Foundation of China (No: 81671093 and No: 81671092), and the District Science and Technology Projects of Yuzhong Chongqing (No: 20160107).

Authors' contributions
X-YW conceived and designed the study, collected and analysed the data, and drafted the manuscript. L-XC wrote the proposal, conceived of the study, supervised the experiment and critically revised the manuscript. J-YZ designed the study and critically revised the manuscript. H-RZ, SW and C-YL collected the data and critically revised the manuscript. G-CQ and Q-QF performed the data analysis and reviewed the manuscript. All the authors read and approved the final manuscript.

Competing interests
The authors declare that they have no competing interests.

Author details

[1]Laboratory Research Center, The First Affiliated Hospital of Chongqing Medical University, Chongqing, China 1st You Yi Road, Yu Zhong District, Chongqing 400016, China. [2]Department of Neurology, The First Affiliated Hospital of Chongqing Medical University, Chongqing, China.

References

1. Schwedt TJ (2014) Chronic migraine. BMJ 348:g1416
2. Yamane K (2014) Progression from episodic migraine to chronic migraine. Rinsho Shinkeigaku 54(12):997–999
3. Headache Classification Committee of the International Headache, S (2013) The International Classification of Headache Disorders, 3rd edition (beta version). Cephalalgia 33(9):629–808
4. Oshinsky ML (2014) Sensitization and ongoing activation in the trigeminal nucleus caudalis. Pain 155(7):1181–1182
5. Su M, Yu S (2018) Chronic migraine: a process of dysmodulation and sensitization. Mol Pain 14:1744806918767697
6. Ji RR et al (2003) Central sensitization and LTP: do pain and memory share similar mechanisms? Trends Neurosci 26(12):696–705
7. Youn DH (2018) Trigeminal long-term potentiation as a cellular substrate for migraine. Med Hypotheses 110:27–30
8. Kunkler PE et al (2015) Sensitization of the trigeminovascular system following environmental irritant exposure. Cephalalgia 35(13):1192–1201
9. Latremoliere A, Woolf CJ (2009) Central sensitization: a generator of pain hypersensitivity by central neural plasticity. J Pain 10(9):895–926
10. MacDonald JF, Jackson MF, Beazely MA (2006) Hippocampal long-term synaptic plasticity and signal amplification of NMDA receptors. Crit Rev Neurobiol 18(1–2):71–84
11. Li S et al (2011) NR2B phosphorylation at tyrosine 1472 in spinal dorsal horn contributed to N-methyl-D-aspartate-induced pain hypersensitivity in mice. J Neurosci Res 89(11):1869–1876
12. Qu XX et al (2009) Role of the spinal cord NR2B-containing NMDA receptors in the development of neuropathic pain. Exp Neurol 215(2):298–307
13. Liang X et al (2017) Tyrosine phosphorylation of NR2B contributes to chronic migraines via increased expression of CGRP in rats. Biomed Res Int 2017:7203458
14. Melo-Carrillo A, Lopez-Avila A (2013) A chronic animal model of migraine, induced by repeated meningeal nociception, characterized by a behavioral and pharmacological approach. Cephalalgia 33(13):1096–1105
15. Slack S et al (2008) EphrinB2 induces tyrosine phosphorylation of NR2B via Src-family kinases during inflammatory hyperalgesia. Neuroscience 156(1):175–183
16. Guldner FH, Ingham CA (1980) Increase in postsynaptic density material in optic target neurons of the rat suprachiasmatic nucleus after bilateral enucleation. Neurosci Lett 17(1–2):27–31
17. Jones DG, Devon RM (1978) An ultrastructural study into the effects of pentobarbitone on synaptic organization. Brain Res 147(1):47–63
18. Gibb R, Kolb B (1998) A method for vibratome sectioning of Golgi-cox stained whole rat brain. J Neurosci Methods 79(1):1–4
19. Eftekhari S, Edvinsson L (2011) Calcitonin gene-related peptide (CGRP) and its receptor components in human and rat spinal trigeminal nucleus and spinal cord at C1-level. BMC Neurosci 12:112
20. Tajti J et al (2015) Migraine and neuropeptides. Neuropeptides 52:19–30
21. Groves TR et al (2017) Assessment of Hippocampal Dendritic Complexity in Aged Mice Using the Golgi-Cox Method. J Vis Exp 124:55696
22. Burstein R (2001) Deconstructing migraine headache into peripheral and central sensitization. Pain 89(2–3):107–110
23. Burstein R, Jakubowski M, Rauch SD (2011) The science of migraine. J Vestib Res 21(6):305–314
24. Boyer N et al (2014) General trigeminospinal central sensitization and impaired descending pain inhibitory controls contribute to migraine progression. Pain 155(7):1196–1205
25. Nakazawa T et al (2001) Characterization of Fyn-mediated tyrosine phosphorylation sites on GluR epsilon 2 (NR2B) subunit of the N-methyl-D-aspartate receptor. J Biol Chem 276(1):693–699
26. Chen BS, Roche KW (2007) Regulation of NMDA receptors by phosphorylation. Neuropharmacology 53(3):362–368
27. Liu, Y.N., et al., Fyn kinase-regulated NMDA receptor- and AMPA receptor-dependent pain sensitization in spinal dorsal horn of mice. Eur J Pain, 2014. 18(8): p. 1120–8
28. Takasu MA et al (2002) Modulation of NMDA receptor-dependent calcium influx and gene expression through EphB receptors. Science 295(5554):491–495
29. Ali DW, Salter MW (2001) NMDA receptor regulation by Src kinase signalling in excitatory synaptic transmission and plasticity. Curr Opin Neurobiol 11(3):336–342
30. Iyengar S, Ossipov MH, Johnson KW (2017) The role of calcitonin gene-related peptide in peripheral and central pain mechanisms including migraine. Pain 158(4):543–559
31. Fusayasu E et al (2007) Increased plasma substance P and CGRP levels, and high ACE activity in migraineurs during headache-free periods. Pain 128(3):209–214
32. Messlinger K et al (2012) CGRP and NO in the trigeminal system: mechanisms and role in headache generation. Headache 52(9):1411–1427
33. Luo C, Kuner T, Kuner R (2014) Synaptic plasticity in pathological pain. Trends Neurosci 37(6):343–355
34. Zhuo M (2017) Ionotropic glutamate receptors contribute to pain transmission and chronic pain. Neuropharmacology 112(Pt A):228–234
35. Chen Y, Derkach VA, Smith PA (2016) Loss of ca(2+)-permeable AMPA receptors in synapses of tonic firing substantia gelatinosa neurons in the chronic constriction injury model of neuropathic pain. Exp Neurol 279:168–177
36. Bu F et al (2015) Phosphorylation of NR2B NMDA subunits by protein kinase C in arcuate nucleus contributes to inflammatory pain in rats. Sci Rep 5:15945
37. Ji Y et al (2015) Estradiol modulates visceral hyperalgesia by increasing thoracolumbar spinal GluN2B subunit activity in female rats. Neurogastroenterol Motil 27(6):775–786
38. Ehrlich I et al (2007) PSD-95 is required for activity-driven synapse stabilization. Proc Natl Acad Sci U S A 104(10):4176–4181
39. Moller TC et al (2013) PDZ domain-mediated interactions of G protein-coupled receptors with postsynaptic density protein 95: quantitative characterization of interactions. PLoS One 8(5):e63352
40. Valtorta F et al (2004) Synaptophysin: leading actor or walk-on role in synaptic vesicle exocytosis? Bioessays 26(4):445–453

4

Efficacy and safety of DFN-11 (sumatriptan injection, 3 mg) in adults with episodic migraine: a multicenter, randomized, double-blind, placebo-controlled study

Stephen Landy[1], Sagar Munjal[2*], Elimor Brand-Schieber[2] and Alan M. Rapoport[3]

Abstract

Background: In a previous randomized, double-blind, proof-of-concept study in rapidly escalating migraine, a 3 mg dose of subcutaneous sumatriptan (DFN-11) was associated with fewer and shorter triptan sensations than a 6 mg dose. The primary objective of the study was to assess the efficacy and safety of acute treatment with DFN-11 compared with placebo in episodic migraine.

Methods: This was a multicenter, randomized, double-blind, placebo-controlled efficacy and safety study of DFN-11 in the acute treatment of adults with episodic migraine (study RESTOR). The primary endpoint was the proportion of subjects taking DFN-11 who were pain free at 2 h postdose in the double-blind period compared with placebo. Secondary endpoints included earlier postdose timepoints, assessments of pain relief and subjects' freedom from their most bothersome symptom (MBS) (among nausea, photophobia, and phonophobia). Safety and tolerability were assessed.

Results: A total of 392 subjects was screened, 268 (68.4%) were randomized, and 234 (87.3% of those randomized) completed the double-blind treatment period. The proportion of subjects who were pain free at 2 h postdose was significantly greater in the DFN-11 group than in the placebo group (51.0% vs 30.8%, $P = 0.0023$). Compared with placebo, significantly higher proportions of subjects treated with DFN-11 were also pain free at 30, 60, and 90 min postdose ($P \leq 0.0195$). DFN-11 was significantly superior to placebo for pain relief at 60 min, 90 min, and 2 h postdose ($P \leq 0.0179$). At 2 h postdose, DFN-11 was also significantly superior to placebo for freedom from photophobia ($P = 0.0056$) and phonophobia ($P = 0.0167$). Overall, 33.3% (37/111) who received DFN-11 and 13.4% (16/119) who received placebo experienced at least 1 treatment-emergent adverse event (TEAE), the most common of which were injection site swelling (7.2% vs 0.8%) and pain (7.2% vs 5.9%). Chest discomfort was about half as common in the DFN-11 treatment group as it was in the placebo group (0.9% vs 1.7%).

Conclusions: This study met its primary endpoint, pain freedom at 2 h postdose, with DFN-11 significantly better than placebo, and the incidence of TEAEs and triptan sensations with DFN-11 was low. The 3 mg dose of sumatriptan in DFN-11 appears to be an effective alternative to a 6 mg SC dose of sumatriptan, with good safety and tolerability. (clinicaltrials.gov: NCT02569853; registered 07 October 2015).

Keywords: Episodic migraine, Migraine treatment, Subcutaneous sumatriptan, Sumatriptan autoinjector

* Correspondence: smunjal@drreddys.com
[2]Promius Pharma, a subsidiary of Dr Reddy's Laboratories, 107 College Road East, Princeton, NJ 08540, USA
Full list of author information is available at the end of the article

Background

Migraine is a chronic neurologic disorder characterized by episodic attacks of head pain and associated symptoms, such as photophobia, phonophobia, and gastrointestinal disturbances; attacks are often accompanied by cutaneous allodynia and may be preceded by an aura and/or premonitory symptoms [1]. The International Headache Society recognizes 2 main subtypes: episodic migraine, with fewer than 15 headache days per month, and chronic migraine, in which headache is present on 15 or more days per month [1]. In the United States, nearly 38 million adults have migraine [2, 3], with women about 3 times more likely to be affected than men (18% vs 6%) [4]. For many patients, the burden of migraine includes negative effects on performance and attendance at work, school, family, and leisure activities. Migraineurs have an increased likelihood of unemployment, lack of advancement at work, and occupational disability, as well as elevated risk of developing comorbid conditions (eg, depression, anxiety and other pain disorders) [5–7].

The acute treatment of migraine may involve simple analgesics, combination over-the-counter medications, nonsteroidal anti-inflammatory drugs (NSAIDs), and migraine-specific medications (eg, triptans and ergot alkaloids) [8–13]. Triptans are often considered the best choice for first-line therapy [8, 9, 14]. The most rapidly effective treatment in the class is 6 mg subcutaneous (SC) sumatriptan [15, 16], which reaches peak plasma concentration (t_{max}) in 12 min, has an onset of action of 10 min, and relieves migraine pain in 82% of patients at 2 h postdose [17]. Despite its excellent efficacy profile, fewer than 10% of migraineurs who might benefit from SC sumatriptan use it to treat their condition [18]. This may be because most (59%) SC sumatriptan-treated patients have injection site reactions, and many (42%) experience triptan sensations (eg, tingling, warm/hot, tightness/pressure) that appear to be dose-related [19]. Concerns about drug-related adverse events (AEs) have caused two thirds of migraine patients to delay or avoid treating an attack [18].

DFN-11 (Zembrace® SymTouch®, Promius Pharma, Princeton, NJ) is a low-dose (3 mg) sumatriptan SC injection supplied as a single-dose, ready-to-use, disposable autoinjector [20], which distinguishes it from the 6 mg SC dose of sumatriptan (Imitrex®, GlaxoSmithKline, Research Triangle Park, NC). DFN-11 has less sumatriptan per dose (3 mg vs 6 mg) and is therefore a more dilute formulation (3 mg/0.5 mL vs 6 mg/0.5 mL) [17, 21]. It is stable at controlled room temperature storage and has a 2-year shelf life. In an earlier pilot study in adults with rapidly escalating migraine attacks, DFN-11 was shown to be as effective as a 6 mg SC dose of sumatriptan, and was associated with improved tolerability [22]. Specifically, subjects who received DFN-11 had

effective relief of migraine pain and associated symptoms, a lower incidence of triptan sensations, and no chest pain [22]. The objective of the present study was to assess the efficacy, tolerability, and safety of DFN-11 in the acute treatment of episodic migraine attacks.

Methods

Ethics

This randomized, double-blind, placebo-controlled study, with an open-label extension, evaluated the efficacy, tolerability, and safety of DFN-11 in adults with episodic migraine (study RESTOR). It was conducted at 17 study centers in the United States. The protocol was approved by the institutional review boards at each study site, and the study was conducted in compliance with good clinical practice and in accordance with the ethical principles set forth in the Declaration of Helsinki. Before any study-specific procedures were initiated, investigators explained the nature of the study to the subjects, and subjects provided informed consent. Details about the trial are available online at ClinicalTrials.gov (Identifier: NCT02569853).

Subjects

Subjects included males and females aged 18 to 65 years with a history of episodic migraine with or without aura who experienced 2 to 6 migraine attacks per month for at least the previous 12 months, with no more than 14 headache days per month and a minimum of 48 h of headache-free time between attacks. Individuals with aura lasting longer than 60 min were excluded. Female subjects had to have a negative serum pregnancy test at screening and all subsequent study visits and no plans to become pregnant during the study, and they could not be lactating. Female subjects with male partners and male subjects with female partners had to agree to practice a reliable form of contraception or abstinence during the study.

Subjects were excluded if they had medication overuse headache or any abnormal physiology and/or pathology that would compromise data collection, confound the objectives of the study, be a contraindication for study participation, or not allow the objectives of the study to be met. Complete exclusion criteria are provided in the Additional file 1 (available online).

Study procedures

This study involved 5 site visits: screening, baseline/randomization, end double-blind/begin open-label, week 4, and end of study visit.

Screened subjects who met all the inclusion and none of the exclusion criteria were instructed by the site staff on the proper administration of study medication and randomized (1:1) to receive DFN-11 or placebo via SC autoinjector in a double-blinded fashion.

In the double-blind period, which lasted 4 weeks, subjects self-administered DFN-11 or placebo via SC autoinjector to treat 1 migraine attack within 1 h of experiencing pain of moderate to severe intensity. Subjects who experienced insufficient relief from the first dose of study medication were permitted to take a second dose of study medication or rescue medication if at least 2 h had elapsed since the first dose, and they had completed electronic diary (eDiary) ratings up to and including the 2-h postdose rating. No more than 2 doses of study medication were allowed in any 24-h period. Rescue medications could include prescription and nonprescription drugs (eg, NSAIDs, other acute migraine medications, vitamins, herbal/dietary supplements). At the conclusion of the double-blind treatment period, subjects were re-assessed for eligibility before for continuing into an 8-week open-label period [23].

During the study, eDiaries were used to record data in real-time and transmit it to a web-based data storage system. Diary assessments included onset and duration of headache, predose severity of pain, associated symptoms (including the most bothersome), functional disability, rescue medication use, and injection site reactions.

Assessments

Efficacy

The primary efficacy endpoint was the proportion of subjects with moderate to severe predose pain who were pain free 2 h after the taking first dose of medication, comparing DFN-11 and placebo. Secondary efficacy variables in the double-blind treatment period included freedom from nausea, photophobia, and phonophobia at 10, 15, 20, 30, 60, 90 min, and 2 h postdose; pain relief at 10, 15, 20, 30, 60, 90 min, and 2 h postdose; pain freedom at 10, 15, 20, 30, 60, and 90 min postdose); MBS absent at 10, 15, 20, 30, 60, 90 min, and 2 h postdose; sustained pain freedom at 24 h (2–24 h) postdose; and use of rescue medication or a second dose of the study medication after 2 h (2–24 h) postdose.

Pain intensity was graded on a 4-point Likert-type [24] scale where 0 = no pain, 1 = mild pain, 2 = moderate pain, and 3 = severe pain. Pain free was defined in the double-blind period as a reduction in pain intensity from moderate or severe at baseline to none at 2 h postdose. Pain relief was defined as a reduction from moderate or severe baseline pain to mild or none at 2 h postdose. The MBS was defined as the symptom associated with migraine that was the most bothersome from among nausea, photophobia, and phonophobia identified prior to dosing. Freedom from the MBS was defined as the absence of the baseline MBS at 2 h postdose. Sustained pain freedom was defined as pain-free at 2 h postdose with no use of rescue medication or additional study medication and no recurrence of headache pain within 2 to 24 h postdose.

Safety

The safety endpoints in this study were the proportion of subjects with treatment-emergent AEs (TEAEs) and serious AEs (SAEs), as well as those with changes in clinical laboratory tests, vital signs, and ECG. Triptan related AE terms included, but were not limited to, tingling/prickling, dizziness/vertigo, warm/hot/burning sensation, cold sensation, feeling of heaviness/pressure/tightness, paresthesia, flushing, and numbness. For injection site reactions, terms included injection site swelling, irritation, erythema, hemorrhage, pain, and bruising.

Statistics

The randomization list was generated by study personnel who were not involved with study conduct, and the allocation of randomization numbers to study drug kits was performed by a third-party vendor. In the double-blind portion of the study, all subjects and study personnel involved with study conduct were blinded to the drug assignment. For quantitative variables, descriptive statistics include the number of subjects (n), mean, standard deviation (SD), median, minimum, and maximum. Categorical variables are summarized using the number (n) and percentage (%) of subjects for each category. All data processing, summarization, and analyses were performed using SAS® software, Version 9.2. Adverse events were classified using the Medical Dictionary for Regulatory Activities (MedDRA) dictionary, Version 18.0. All concomitant medications were coded using the World Health Organization Drug Dictionary Enhanced (WHODDE), version Mar2015 further coded against Anatomic Therapeutic Chemical (ATC) classification.

Multiple study populations were analyzed. Subjects who were randomized in the double-blind period were the basis of the subject disposition and baseline summaries. Those who were randomized, received at least 1 dose of double-blind study medication, and recorded at least 1 postdose double-blind efficacy data point were used for the double-blind efficacy analyses.

The analyses comparing proportions were done with 1-sided Fisher's exact test with an alpha level equal to 0.025 to determine statistical significance. Unless noted otherwise, a last observation carried forward (LOCF) imputation method was applied. Baseline data were not carried forward, and only valid data from postbaseline assessments collected before the 2-h postdose time point were carried forward to impute the next missing assessment up to the 2-h postdose time point. Time points beyond 2 h postdose were not carried forward.

The analysis of safety in the double-blind treatment period was based on data from all randomized subjects who received at least 1 dose of study medication in the double-blind period. The efficacy analyses were based on postdose timepoints data captured in real-time in an eDiary for migraine attacks treated. Safety assessment at baseline was defined as the last assessment before receiving the first dose of study medication in the double-blind period. Change from baseline was defined as the postbaseline value minus the baseline value, and the calculations were based on nonmissing data.

One or more interim analyses were planned for the purpose of evaluating potential early stopping for an efficacy conclusion after a minimum of 166 subjects had completed the double-blind period and primary endpoint data were available for approximately 145 subjects. A conservative alpha spending function was used to preserve most of the type I error for the final analysis in case the trial did not stop for an efficacy conclusion at the interim analysis.

Results

Subjects

Sixteen sites in the United States participated and randomized subjects in the study. The first subject was enrolled on 21 September 2015, and the last subject completed the study on 30 May 2017.

A total of 392 subjects was screened, 268 (68.4%) were randomized, and 234 (87.3% of those randomized) completed the double-blind treatment period (Fig. 1). In all, 34 (12.7%) subjects discontinued from the study. Two (0.7%) subjects discontinued from the study due to AEs with DFN-11.

As Table 1 shows, subjects in the DFN-11 and placebo treatment groups were demographically similar. The mean (SD) age of the study population was 41.0 (12.4) years, with subjects in the DFN-11 group slight older than those assigned to receive placebo (41.9 [12.5] vs 40.2 [12.3]). Mean (SD) weight was nearly identical between those receiving DFN-11 and placebo (84.4 [23.9]

kg vs 84.3 [23.6] kg), as was body mass index (30.4 [8.4] kg/m^2 vs 30.7 [8.8] kg/m^2). Overall, most subjects were female (85.4%) and white (75.7%), and the DFN-11 and placebo treatment groups had roughly equal proportions of female (84.7% vs 86.1%, respectively) and white subjects (74.8% vs 76.6%, respectively).

Efficacy

The proportion of subjects who were pain free at 2 h postdose — the prespecified primary endpoint (Fig. 2) — was significantly greater with DFN-11 than placebo (51.0% vs 30.8%, $P = 0.0023$); the odds ratio (95% CI) was 2.57 (1.4–4.9). DFN-11 was also significantly superior to placebo for pain freedom at 30 min (22.3% vs 9.9%, $P = 0.0126$), 60 min (34.6% vs 19.8%, $P = 0.0128$), and 90 min postdose (41.3% vs 26.7%, $P = 0.0195$), as shown in Fig. 2. Compared with placebo, a numerically greater proportion of subjects treated with DFN-11 reported absence of the MBS at 2 h postdose (64.1% vs 48.1%). A post hoc analysis using observed cases instead of LOCF imputation yielded the result that the difference between the proportion of those treated with DFN-11 and placebo for absence of the MBS was statistically significant (65.3% vs 47.4%, $P = 0.0210$).

For pain relief (Fig. 3), DFN-11 was numerically superior to placebo beginning at 15 min postdose, and the differences between treatments were significant at 60 min (67.3% vs 47.5%, $P = 0.0032$); 90 min (73.1% vs 56.4%, $P = 0.0093$); and 2 h postdose (76.0% vs 61.5%, $P = 0.0179$).

As shown in Fig. 4, DFN-11 outperformed placebo for freedom from nausea from 20 min postdose through 2 h postdose, and the separation was significant at 60 min postdose (71.1% vs 48.1%, $P = 0.0178$). Compared with placebo, more subjects who were treated with DFN-11 were photophobia-free from 15 min through 2 h postdose, and

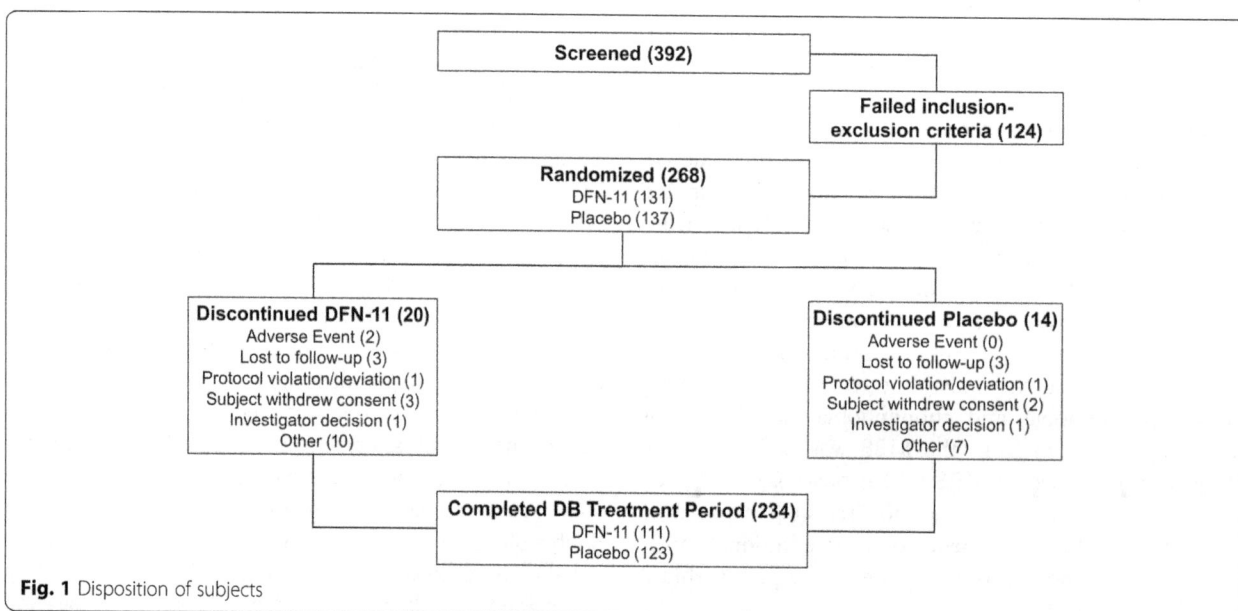

Fig. 1 Disposition of subjects

Efficacy and safety of DFN-11 (sumatriptan injection, 3 mg) in adults with episodic migraine: a multicenter...

39

Table 1 Demographics

	DFN-11 (n = 131) n (%)	Placebo (n = 137) n (%)	Overall (N = 268) n (%)
Age, years[a]	41.9 (12.5)	40.2 (12.3)	41.0 (12.4)
Sex			
Men	20 (15.3)	19 (13.9)	39 (14.6)
Women	111 (84.7)	118 (86.1)	229 (85.4)
Race			
Asian	1 (0.8)	3 (2.2)	4 (1.5)
Black/African-American	29 (22.1)	23 (16.8)	52 (19.4)
Native Hawaiian or Other Pacific Islander	0 (0.0)	2 (1.5)	2 (0.7)
White	98 (74.8)	105 (76.6)	203 (75.7)
Other	3 (2.3)	4 (2.9)	7 (2.6)
Ethnicity			
Not Reported	0 (0.0)	1 (0.7)	1 (0.4)
Hispanic or Latino	10 (7.6)	9 (6.6)	19 (7.1)
Not Hispanic or Latino	121 (92.4)	127 (92.7)	248 (92.5)
Weight, kg[a]	84.4 (23.9)	84.3 (23.6)	84.4 (23.7)
Height, cm[a]	166.7 (8.4)	166.0 (8.7)	166.4 (8.5)
Body Mass Index, kg/m[2a]	30.4 (8.4)	30.7 (8.8)	30.6 (8.6)

[a]Mean (SD)

the differences between DFN-11 and placebo were significant at 30 min (40.0% vs 16.4%, $P = 0.0012$); 60 min (48.7% vs 27.4%, $P = 0.0060$); 90 min (59.2% vs 34.2%, $P = 0.0019$); and 2 h postdose (64.5% vs 42.5%, $P = 0.0056$). Subjects in the DFN-11 group were more likely than those in the placebo group to be phonophobia-free from 10 min through 2 h postdose, and the separations from placebo were significant at 30 min (47.5% vs 27.9%, $P = 0.0183$); 60 min (61.7% vs 38.2%, $P = 0.0066$); and 2 h postdose (70.0% vs 50.0%, $P = 0.0167$).

For sustained pain freedom from 2 through 24 h postdose, DFN-11 was numerically superior to placebo (74.4% vs 66.7%), and a smaller proportion of subjects

took a second dose of study medication or rescue medication (25.2% vs 32.8%). On these endpoints, the differences between DFN-11 and placebo did not reach statistical significance.

Findings from the open-label portion of the study are beyond the scope of this manuscript and are reported elsewhere [23].

Safety

During the double-blind treatment period, 23.0% of subjects (53/230) experienced at least 1 TEAE: 33.3% (37/111) of subjects who received DFN-11 and 13.4% (16/119) of those treated with placebo (Table 2). Most of these subjects

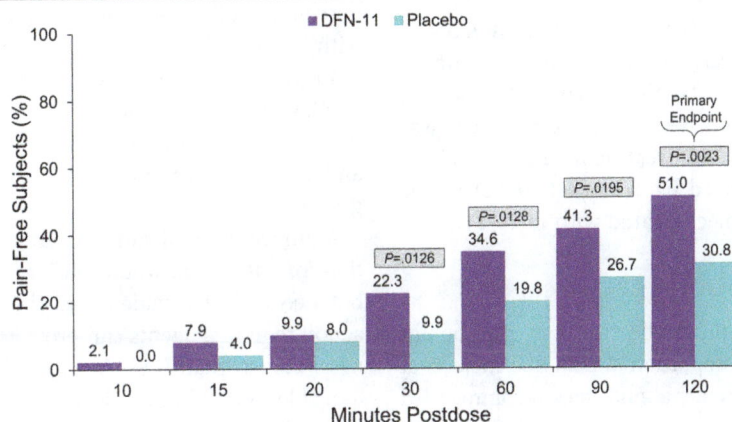

Fig. 2 Proportion of subjects with pain freedom through 2 h postdose

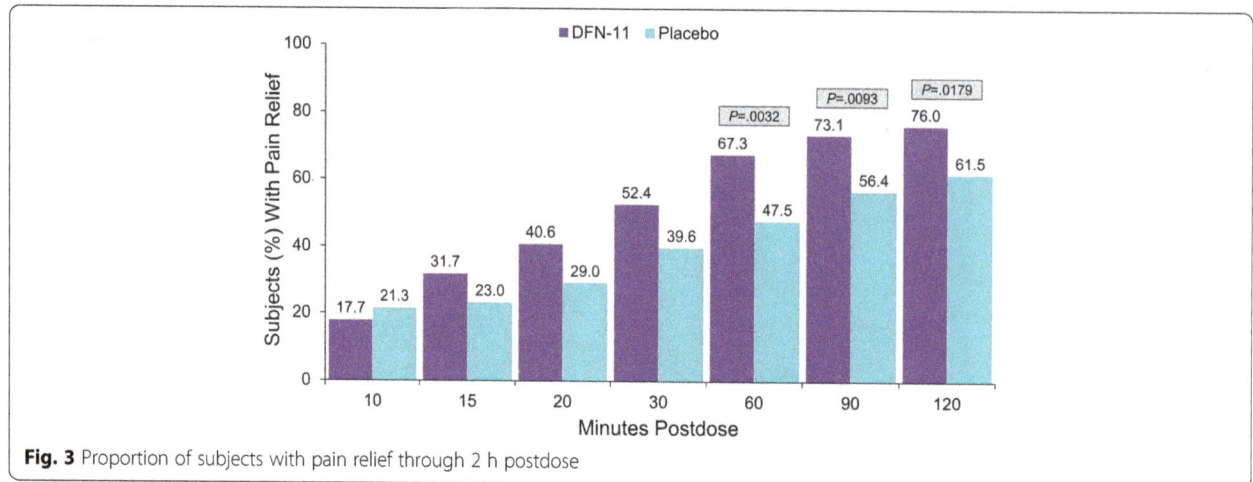

Fig. 3 Proportion of subjects with pain relief through 2 h postdose

(88.7%, 47/53) had events that were mild or moderate in intensity. Two subjects (1.8%) in the DFN-11 group had severe AEs (1 had injection site pain, and 1 had nausea). No subjects in the placebo group experienced severe AEs. Four subjects, 2 in each treatment group, had AEs of unknown severity. There were no serious AEs, but 2 subjects (0.9%) in the DFN-11 group had AEs that led to study discontinuation — worsening of migraine (not treatment-emergent) and a subject with 2 mild TEAEs of abnormal ECG (ventricular extrasystoles and sinus tachycardia), both of which were considered to be unrelated to the study drug.

Injection site reactions

Table 2 shows that the most common TEAEs were associated with the injection site. In total, 17.4% (40/230) of subjects reported at least 1 injection site reaction, with 23.4% (26/111) in the DFN-11 group and 11.8% (14/119) in the placebo group. Compared with placebo, the rate among subjects who received DFN-11 was notably higher for injection site swelling (7.2% vs 0.8%).

Triptan-related adverse events

Triptan-related AEs (Table 3) were reported by 4.3% of subjects overall. They were generally more common among those treated with DFN-11 than with placebo (7.2% vs 1.7%), except for chest discomfort, which was less common in the DFN-11 treatment group (0.9% vs 1.7%), and dyspnea, reported by 1 subject (0.8%) in the placebo group and no subject treated with DFN-11.

Discussion

DFN-11 was significantly more effective than placebo for the primary endpoint, the proportion of pain free subjects at 2 h postdose, which is currently a guidelines-recommended primary measure of efficacy in migraine trials [25]. Significant separation from placebo was seen starting at 30 min

postdose, meeting both patient need for rapid migraine relief [26, 27] and guideline recommendations for measurements of pain freedom before 2 h postdose [25]. DFN-11 was also significantly better than placebo for migraine pain relief from 60 min through 2 h postdose. In addition to significant superiority over placebo on pain free and pain relief outcomes, DFN-11 provided significantly better relief of the symptoms associated with migraine, including the subject-identified MBS (in post hoc analysis). These positive responses on multiple efficacy endpoints suggest that DFN-11 has attributes that are clinically important to migraine sufferers, specifically, fast and effective relief of migraine pain and associated symptoms [26, 27].

As expected, the most common TEAEs were related to the injection site, with a higher overall incidence for DFN-11 than placebo. It is noteworthy, however, that injection site reactions following DFN-11 in the current study were 61% lower than those previously reported for SC sumatriptan (23% vs 59%) [17]. Similarly, the incidence of triptan sensations with the 3 mg dose of sumatriptan in DFN-11 was low. Although not directly comparable, the percentage of subjects with triptan sensations associated with DFN-11 in this study was approximately 80% lower than published estimates for the 6 mg SC dose (7.2% vs 42%), and DFN-11 demonstrated lower rates than placebo on chest discomfort. Treatment-emergent AEs of dyspnea and palpitations were only experienced in the placebo group.

Administration of sumatriptan via SC injection is one option for patients in whom oral medications are suboptimal, but needle-averse patients seeking a more rapid onset of action than oral agents can provide may benefit from intranasal sumatriptan [28]. A novel intranasal powder form is available (ONZETRA® Xsail®, AVANIR Pharmaceuticals, Aliso Viejo, CA, USA), and an intranasal spray (sumatriptan 10 mg with a permeation-enhancing excipient) remains

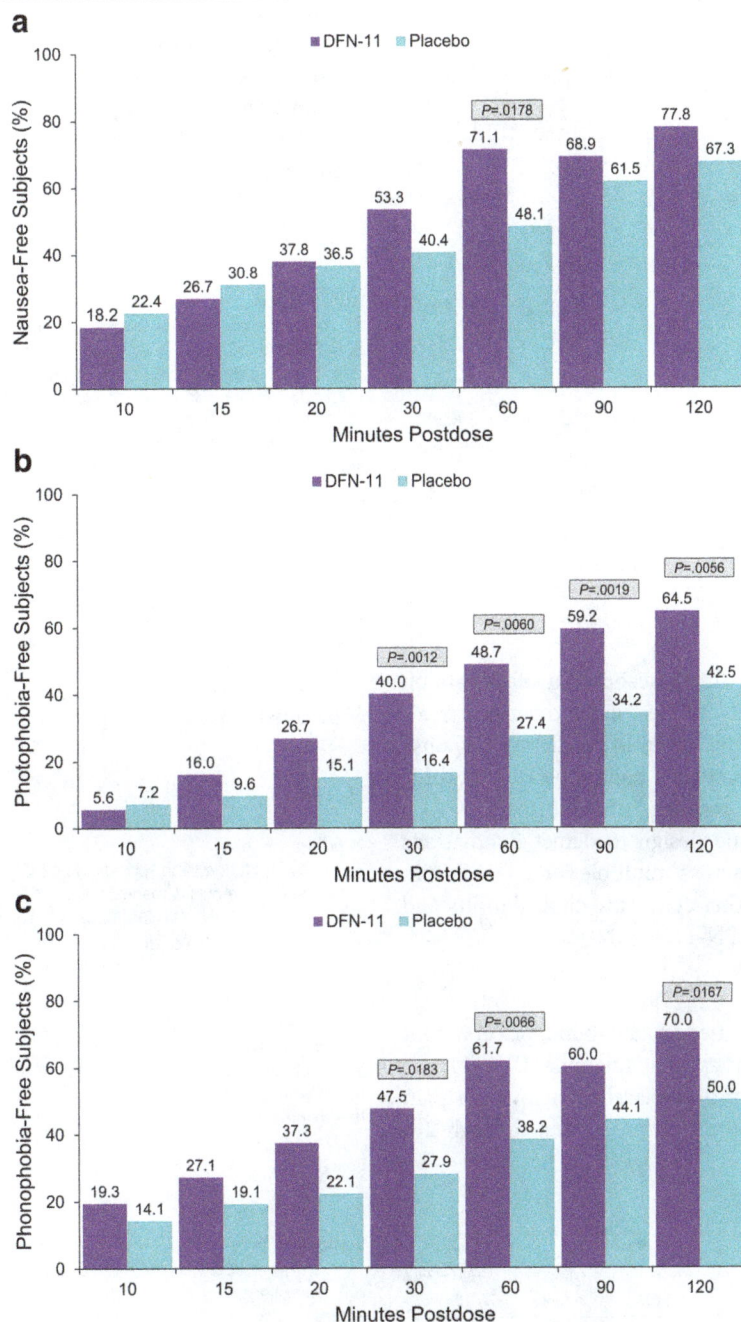

Fig. 4 Proportions of subjects with freedom from nausea (**a**), photophobia (**b**), and phonophobia (**c**)

in development, and both of these agents have a fast onset of action and are effective in the acute treatment of migraine [29–31]. For patients in whom speed of onset is the most important attribute of an acute migraine medication, however, the SC injection of sumatriptan remains the fastest and most effective therapy.

The results of this study support the efficacy and safety of the 3 mg autoinjector dose of sumatriptan, and they complement the results of a previous randomized, double-blind, crossover trial with DFN-11 [22], which

compared the 3 mg dose with a 6 mg dose of DFN-11 [22]. In this pilot trial, a single 3 mg dose of DFN-11 provided relief of migraine pain and associated symptoms comparable to 6 mg and was associated with fewer triptan sensations. Achieving similar efficacy and safety results compared with placebo in the current well-powered, double-blind study supports that patient response to DFN-11 is likely to be reliable and predictable.

This study met its primary efficacy endpoint and demonstrated the efficacy and tolerability of DFN-11. These

Table 2 Treatment-emergent adverse events overall and occurring in at least 2 subjects

	DFN-11 (n = 111) n (%)	Placebo (n = 119) n (%)	Total (N = 230) n (%)
Subjects with ≥1 TEAE	37 (33.3)	16 (13.4)	53 (23.0)
Subjects with ≥1 injection site reaction	26 (23.4)	14 (11.8)	40 (17.4)
Injection site pain	8 (7.2)	7 (5.9)	15 (6.5)
Injection site swelling	8 (7.2)	1 (0.8)	9 (3.9)
Injection site bruising	5 (4.5)	3 (2.5)	8 (3.5)
Injection site irritation	4 (3.6)	3 (2.5)	7 (3.0)
Injection site erythema	2 (1.8)	1 (0.8)	3 (1.3)
Injection site induration	2 (1.8)	0 (0.0)	2 (0.9)
Paresthesia	3 (2.7)	0 (0.0)	3 (1.3)
Nausea	2 (1.8)	0 (0.0)	2 (0.9)
Throat tightness	2 (1.8)	0 (0.0)	2 (0.9)
Chest discomfort	1 (0.9)	2 (1.7)	3 (1.3)

TEAE, treatment-emergent adverse event

results, which provide the first placebo-controlled data on the 3 mg sumatriptan SC autoinjector for the acute treatment of migraine, should be useful in predicting response to DFN-11 in clinical practice. Limitations of the study include the high placebo response and the inability of a single-attack, parallel-group design to detect fluctuations in treatment response across multiple attacks. Future studies, are needed to further clarify the clinical utility and therapeutic potential of DFN-11.

Conclusions

In this multicenter, randomized, double-blind, placebo-controlled study in adults with episodic migraine, DFN-11 was significantly more effective than placebo on multiple pain free and pain relief assessments from 30 min through 2 h

Table 3 Triptan-related adverse events

	DFN-11 (n = 111) n (%)	Placebo (n = 119) n (%)	Total (N = 230) n (%)
Subjects with ≥1 triptan-related AE	8 (7.2)	3 (2.5)	11 (4.8)
Palpitations	0 (0.0)	1 (0.8)	1 (0.4)
Nausea	2 (1.8)	0 (0.0)	2 (0.9)
Chest discomfort	1 (0.9)	2 (1.7)	3 (1.3)
Dizziness	1 (0.9)	0 (0.0)	1 (0.4)
Lethargy	1 (0.9)	0 (0.0)	1 (0.4)
Paresthesia	3 (2.7)	0 (0.0)	3 (1.3)
Dyspnea	0 (0.0)	1 (0.8)	1 (0.4)
Throat irritation	1 (0.9)	0 (0.0)	1 (0.4)
Throat tightness	2 (1.8)	0 (0.0)	2 (0.9)

AE, adverse event

postdose and the relief of migraine associated symptoms, including the subjects' MBS. Taken together with the low incidence of TEAEs and triptan sensations, these findings demonstrate that the 3 mg dose of sumatriptan in DFN-11 may be a useful alternative to the 6 mg SC dose of sumatriptan.

Abbreviations

AE: Adverse event; ATC: Anatomic Therapeutic Chemical; ECG: Electrocardiogram; eDiary: Electronic diary; ICHD: International Classification of Headache Disorders; IRB: Institutional Review Board; LOCF: Last observation carried forward; MBS: Most bothersome symptom; MedDRA: Medical Dictionary for Regulatory Activities; NSAID: Nonsteroidal anti-inflammatory drug; SAE: Serious adverse event; SC: Subcutaneous; SD: Standard deviation; TEAE: Treatment-emergent adverse event; WHODDE: World Health Organization Drug Dictionary Enhanced

Acknowledgements

Medical writing services were provided by Christopher Caiazza. The authors thank the participating patients, the investigators and their staffs, and Katherine D'Angelo (Dr. Reddy's Laboratories, Princeton, NJ) for assisting with the conduct of this study. DRL Publication #834.

Funding

This study was funded and sponsored by the Dr. Reddy's Laboratories group of companies, Princeton, NJ, manufacturer of DFN-11. Its US subsidiary, Promius Pharma, markets DFN-11 as Zembrace®SymTouch®.

Authors' contributions

SM and EBS designed and conducted the study, and all authors contributed to the writing and revision of the manuscript. All authors read and approved the final manuscript.

Competing interests

This study was supported and funded by the Dr. Reddy's Laboratories group of companies, Princeton, NJ, manufacturer of DFN-11. SM and EBS are employed by and own stock in Dr. Reddy's Laboratories Ltd. SL and AMR are paid consultants of Dr. Reddy's Laboratories Ltd., but they were not paid to draft or edit this paper. SL also serves on the speaker's bureau of Allergan, Amgen, Depomed, ElectroCore, Promius Pharma, and Supernus; he is a consultant for Allergan, Amgen, Promius Pharma, and Supernus. AMR is also on the speaker's bureau of Amgen, Avanir, Depomed, Promius Pharma and Teva; he is a consultant for Amgen, Autonomic Technologies, Depomed, ElectroCore, Impax, Pernix, Teva, and Zosano.

Author details

¹Baptist Medical Group Headache Clinic, University of Tennessee Medical School, 6029 Walnut Grove, Suite 210, Memphis, TN 38120, USA. ²Promius Pharma, a subsidiary of Dr Reddy's Laboratories, 107 College Road East, Princeton, NJ 08540, USA. ³The David Geffen School of Medicine at UCLA, 4255 Jefferson Avenue, Suite 27, Woodside, CA 94062, USA.

References

1. Headache Classification Committee of the International Headache Society (IHS). The International Classification of Headache Disorders, 3rd edition (beta version) (2013). Cephalalgia 33:629–808

2. US Census Bureau: QuickFacts United States. Available at: https://www.census.gov/quickfacts/. Accessed 15 June 2018

3. Lipton RB, Stewart WF, Diamond S et al (2001) Prevalence and burden of migraine in the United States: data from the American migraine study II. Headache 41:646–657

4. Lipton RB, Bigal ME, Diamond M et al (2007) Migraine prevalence, disease burden, and the need for preventive therapy. Neurology 68:343–349

5. Blumenfeld AM, Varon SF, Wilcox TK et al (2011) Disability, HRQoL and resource use among chronic and episodic migraineurs: results from the international burden of migraine study (IBMS). Cephalalgia 31:301–315

6. Buse DC, Manack A, Serrano D et al (2010) Sociodemographic and comorbidity profiles of chronic migraine and episodic migraine sufferers. J Neurol Neurosurg Psychiatry 81:428–432

7. Buse DC, Manack AN, Serrano D et al (2008) Summary of disability, treatment and healthcare utilization differences between chronic migraine and episodic migraine populations. Headache 48:S18

8. Silberstein SD (2000) Practice parameter: evidence-based guidelines for migraine headache (an evidence-based review): report of the quality standards Subcommittee of the American Academy of neurology. Neurology 55:754–762

9. Marmura MJ, Silberstein SD, Schwedt TJ (2015) The acute treatment of migraine in adults: the American headache society evidence assessment of migraine pharmacotherapies. Headache 55:3–20

10. Worthington I, Pringsheim T, Gawel MJ et al (2013) Canadian headache society guideline: acute drug therapy for migraine headache. Can J Neurol Sci 40:S1–s80

11. Sarchielli P, Granella F, Prudenzano MP et al (2012) Italian guidelines for primary headaches: 2012 revised version. J Headache Pain 13(Suppl 2):S31–S70

12. Evers S, Afra J, Frese A et al (2009) EFNS guideline on the drug treatment of migraine–revised report of an EFNS task force. Eur J Neurol 16:968–981

13. Haag G, Diener HC, May A et al (2011) Self-medication of migraine and tension-type headache: summary of the evidence-based recommendations of the deutsche Migrane und Kopfschmerzgesellschaft (DMKG), the deutsche Gesellschaft fur Neurologie (DGN), the Osterreichische Kopfschmerzgesellschaft (OKSG) and the Schweizerische Kopfwehgesellschaft (SKG). J Headache Pain 12:201–217

14. Tfelt-Hansen P, Saxena PR, Dahlof C et al (2000) Ergotamine in the acute treatment of migraine: a review and European consensus. Brain 123(Pt 1):9–18

15. Ferrari MD, Roon KI, Lipton RB et al (2001) Oral triptans (serotonin 5-HT(1B/1D) agonists) in acute migraine treatment: a meta-analysis of 53 trials. Lancet 358:1668–1675

16. Lionetto L, Negro A, Casolla B et al (2012) Sumatriptan succinate: pharmacokinetics of different formulations in clinical practice. Expert Opin Pharmacother 13:2369–2380

17. IMITREX (sumatriptan succinate) Injection prescribing information. Available at: https://www.gsksource.com/pharma/content/dam/GlaxoSmithKline/US/en/Prescribing_Information/Imitrex_Injection/pdf/IMITREX-INJECTION-PI-PPI-PIL-COMBINED.PDF. Accessed 12 June 2018

18. Gallagher RM, Kunkel R (2003) Migraine medication attributes important for patient compliance: concerns about side effects may delay treatment. Headache 43:36–43

19. Mathew NT, Dexter J, Couch J et al (1992) Dose ranging efficacy and safety of subcutaneous sumatriptan in the acute treatment of migraine. US Sumatriptan Research Group Arch Neurol 49:1271–1276

20. Andre AD, Brand-Schieber E, Ramirez M, Munjal S, Kumar R (2017) Subcutaneous sumatriptan delivery devices: comparative ease of use and preference among migraineurs. Patient Prefer Adherence 11:121-129

21. ZEMBRACE® SymTouch® (sumatriptan succinate) Injection prescribing information. Available at: http://www.zembrace.com/Content/docs/zembrace-prescribing-information.pdf. Accessed 15 June 2018

22. Cady RK, Munjal S, Cady RJ et al (2017) Randomized, double-blind, crossover study comparing DFN-11 injection (3 mg subcutaneous sumatriptan) with 6 mg subcutaneous sumatriptan for the treatment of rapidly-escalating attacks of episodic migraine. J Headache Pain 18:17

23. Landy S, Munjal S, Brand-Schieber E, Rapoport AM (2018) Efficacy and safety of DFN-11 (sumatriptan injection, 3 mg) in adults with episodic migraine: an 8-week open-label extension study. J Headache Pain. https://doi.org/10.1186/s10194-018-0882-y

24. Likert R (1932) A technique for the measurement of attitudes. Arch Psychol 140:1–55

25. Tfelt-Hansen P, Pascual J, Ramadan N et al (2012) Guidelines for controlled trials of drugs in migraine: third edition. A guide for investigators. Cephalalgia 32:6–38

26. Lipton RB, Hamelsky SW, Dayno JM (2002) What do patients with migraine want from acute migraine treatment? Headache 42(Suppl 1):3–9

27. Gendolla A (2005) Part I: what do patients really need and want from migraine treatment? Curr Med Res Opin 21(Suppl 3):S3–S7

28. Menshawy A, Ahmed H, Ismail A et al (2018) Intranasal sumatriptan for acute migraine attacks: a systematic review and meta-analysis. Neurol Sci 39:31–44

29. Silberstein S, Winner PK, Mcallister PJ et al (2017) Early onset of efficacy and consistency of response across multiple migraine attacks from the randomized COMPASS study: AVP-825 breath powered((R)) exhalation delivery system (sumatriptan nasal powder) vs oral sumatriptan. Headache 57:862–876

30. Munjal S, Gautam A, Offman E et al (2016) A randomized trial comparing the pharmacokinetics, safety, and tolerability of DFN-02, an intranasal sumatriptan spray containing a permeation enhancer, with intranasal and subcutaneous sumatriptan in healthy adults. Headache 56:1455–1465

31. Lipton RB, Munjal S, Brand-Schieber E, Rapoport AM (2018) DFN-02 (sumatriptan 10 mg with a permeation enhancer) nasal spray vs placebo in the acute treatment of migraine: a double-blind, placebo-controlled study. Headache. 58(5):676–687

5

Evidence of an increased neuronal activation-to-resting glucose uptake ratio in the visual cortex of migraine patients: a study comparing [18]FDG-PET and visual evoked potentials

Marco Lisicki[1†], Kevin D'Ostilio[1†], Gianluca Coppola[2], Felix Scholtes[3], Alain Maertens de Noordhout[1], Vincenzo Parisi[2], Jean Schoenen[1] and Delphine Magis[1*] (ID)

Abstract

Background: Migraine attacks might be triggered by a disruption of cerebral homeostasis. During the interictal period migraine patients are characterized by abnormal sensory information processing, but this functional abnormality may not be sufficient to disrupt the physiological equilibrium of the cortex unless it is accompanied by additional pathological mechanisms, like a reduction in energetic reserves. The aim of this study was to compare resting cerebral glucose uptake (using positron emission tomography ([18]fluorodeoxyglucose-PET)), and visual cortex activation (using visual evoked potentials (VEP)), between episodic migraine without aura patients in the interictal period and healthy volunteers.

Methods: Twenty episodic migraine without aura patients and twenty healthy volunteers were studied. [18]FDG-PET and VEP recordings were performed on separate days. The overall glucose uptake in the visual cortex-to-VEP response ratio was calculated and compared between the groups. Additionally, PET scan comparisons adding area under the VEP curve as a covariate were performed. For case-wise analysis, eigenvalues from a specific region exhibiting significantly different FDG-PET signal in the visual cortex were extracted. Standardized glucose uptake values from this region and VEP values from each subject were then coupled and compared between the groups.

Results: The mean area under the curve of VEP was greater in migraine patients compared to healthy controls. In the same line, patients had an increased neuronal activation-to-resting glucose uptake ratio in the visual cortex. Statistical parametric mapping analysis revealed that cortical FDG-PET signal in relation to VEP area under the curve was significantly reduced in migraineurs in a cluster extending throughout the left visual cortex, from Brodmann's areas 19 and 18 to area 7. Within this region, case-wise analyses showed that a visual neuronal activation exceeding glucose uptake was present in 90% of migraine patients, but in only 15% of healthy volunteers.

(Continued on next page)

* Correspondence: dmagis@chuliege.be
[†]Marco Lisicki and Kevin D'Ostilio contributed equally to this work.
[1]Headache Research Unit, University Department of Neurology CHR, CHU de Liège, Boulevard du 12eme de Ligne 1, 4000 Liege, Belgium
Full list of author information is available at the end of the article

(Continued from previous page)

Conclusion: This study identifies an area of increased neuronal activation-to-resting glucose uptake ratio in the visual cortex of migraine patients between attacks. Such observation supports the concept that an activity-induced rupture of cerebral metabolic homeostasis may be a cornerstone of migraine pathophysiology.

This article has been selected as the winner of the 2018 Enrico Greppi Award. The Enrico Greppi Award is made to an unpublished paper dealing with clinical, epidemiological, genetic, pathophysiological or therapeutic aspects of headache. Italian Society for the Study of Headaches (SISC) sponsors this award, and the award is supported through an educational grant from Teva Neuroscience. This article did not undergo the standard peer review process for The Journal of Headache and Pain. The members of the 2018 Enrico Greppi Award Selection Committee were: Francesco Pierelli, Paolo Martelletti, Lyn Griffiths, Simona Sacco, Andreas Straube and Cenk Ayata.

Keywords: Headache, Cerebral energy metabolism, Astrocytes, Neurophysiology

Background

Between attacks, migraine patients often exhibit abnormal sensory information processing [1]. Cortical hyper-responsivity during any kind of sensory stimulus repetition, including visual, is the most common electrophysiological feature found in episodic migraine patients during the interictal state [2]. Such alteration however, although highly prevalent among migraineurs, is by itself insufficient to entirely explain migraine's pathophysiology [3]. The fact that similar cortical reactivity profiles can be found in both migraine patients and their asymptomatic first degree relatives suggests the existence of additional pathologic mechanisms in migraine sufferers that, when associated to visual hyper-responsivity, lead to the development of the disease [3].

In parallel with cortical hyper-responsivity, cerebral metabolism has been suggested to play a major role in migraine [4–6]. Hypotheses argue that reduced mitochondrial energy and ATP levels observed in the cortex of patients between attacks [7–9] might make them unable to deal with an energetically more demanding neuronal activity [5, 10]. This imbalance would later translate into a disruption in cortical homeostasis, with subsequent activation of the trigeminovascular system. Such view is supported by the favourable clinical response to metabolic enhancers [11] and ketogenic diet [12, 13] observed in migraine patients, as well as the capability of metabolic challenges to trigger migraine attacks [6].

[18]Fluorodeoxyglucose-positron emission tomography-(FDG-)PET is an imaging tool used to measure glucose uptake in brain tissue. FDG-studies in migraine patients between attacks have identified regions of reduced metabolism in limbic areas belonging to the pain/salience matrix [14, 15]. Yet, no interictal FDG-PET abnormalities affecting the visual cortex have been reported, with the possible exception of increased glucose uptake in posterior white matter [16] . Nonetheless, in available FDG-PET studies, no attempt was made to correlate cerebral metabolism with sensory processing.

In the present study we sought to determine if interictal glucose metabolism in the visual cortex is proportional to visually-induced neuronal activation. For this purpose, we assessed cerebral glucose uptake, and recorded visual evoked potentials (VEP) in healthy volunteers and migraine patients. Our main hypothesis was that the interictal responsivity of the visual cortex in migraine patients would exceed the resting glucose uptake, rendering migraineurs vulnerable to a disruption of metabolic homeostasis in times of increased neuroenergetic demands.

Methods
Study participants

The study involved twenty episodic migraine without aura patients (MO; mean age (SD): 31.1 (±12.6), 85% fem) diagnosed in accordance with The International Classification of Headache Disorders 3rd edition (Beta version) [17] and twenty healthy volunteers (HV; mean age (SD): 36.1 (±11.4), 75% fem) who did not report having first degree relatives suffering from recurrent headaches of any type. There were no significant differences in age or gender proportions between groups. Participants were recruited among University students or their families or via our headache clinic. None of them took any medication on a daily basis (other than the contraceptive pill), and they were all were free of any systemic or neurological disease other than migraine. Patients were not under any prophylactic treatment at the time of recordings, nor had they been for at least 30 preceding days. The mean number of monthly migraine days determined by headache diary inspection (during the month of the recordings) was 4.3 ± 2.5. All patients were recorded at an interval of at least 72 h before and after an attack. The study was approved by the Institution's ethics committee (Centre Hospitalier Régional de la Citadelle, Liège, Belgium – protocol n°1422) and conducted following the principles of the Declaration of Helsinki. All participants gave their written informed consent.

Visual evoked potentials recordings and analysis

Visual evoked potentials (VEP) were used as a marker of visual cortex responsiveness. Recordings were performed in the electrophysiology laboratory of the Headache Research Unit (Neurology Department, Centre Hospitalier Régional de la Citadelle, Liège, Belgium). Subjects sat on a comfortable armchair, in a quiet room with dimmed light. Needle electrodes were placed at Oz (active) and Fz (reference) of the 10–20 EEG system. With the left eye patched, participants were instructed to fixate on a red dot in the centre of a screen displaying a black and white reversing checkerboard pattern (contrast of 80%, mean luminance 50 cd/m2) at temporal and spatial stimulating frequencies of 1.55 Hz (3.1 reversals/second) and 68° respectively. Six hundred epochs, each lasting 250 ms, were uninterruptedly recorded at a sampling rate of 5.000 Hz using a CED™ power 1401 device (Cambridge Electronic Design Ltd., Cambridge, UK). After DC subtraction, recordings were exported to EEGLAB [18] (an open-source MATLAB (The MathWorks Inc.) toolbox for electrophysiological signal processing), where they were band-pass filtered (low pass 100 Hz, high pass 1 Hz). Artifacted epochs exceeding two standard deviations of the channel mean limit were rejected (< 7% of epochs). We extracted the area under the curve (AUC) of each single trial, and thereafter averaged these individual values. This method is deemed to be less affected by phase synchronization and thus to provide a more straightforward measure of neuronal activation [19].

FDG-PET acquisition and analysis

PET acquisitions were made in the Radiodiagnostics Department of the Centre Hospitalier Universitaire (CHU) Sart Tilman, Liège, Belgium (Prof. R. Hustinx) using a Gemini TF PET/computed tomography (CT) scanner (Philips, Eindhoven, The Netherlands). Resting cerebral metabolism was studied 30 min after intravenous injection of 150 MBq FDG. Mean blood glucose level was 89.5 (range:110–77). Subjects were injected and scanned in a dark room with minimal environmental noise. They were instructed to maintain their eyes closed during the scan. Images were reconstructed using an iterative list mode time-of-flight algorithm. Corrections for attenuation, dead-time, random and scatter events were applied. PET acquisitions were analysed using Statistical Parametric Mapping version 12 (SPM12, Wellcome Trust Centre for Neuroimaging, http://www.fil.ion.ucl.ac.uk/spm) implemented in MATLAB 7.4.0 (MathWorks Inc., Sherborn, MA, USA). Images were first manually reoriented and hen spatially normalised into a standard stereotactic space using an MNI PET template (Montreal Neurological Institute) and smoothed using an 8 mm full-width-half-maximum (FWHM) isotropic kernel. We performed global normalisation by applying proportional scaling. Cerebral regions identification and masks were established using the WFU PickAtlas toolbox (Wake Forest University School of Medicine, Advanced NeuroScience Imaging Research lab (ANSIR), Winston-Salem, NC, U.S.A). PET scans were compared between groups (1) without adding any covariates, and (2) using the interaction with the averaged area under the VEP as regressor. An exploratory ($p < 0.001$ uncorrected) analysis followed by a more stringent comparison (p family-wise error[FWE] < 0.05 correction at a whole brain level) were performed. Only statistically significant clusters within regions of the visual cortex are reported in the results. To estimate the neuronal activation-to-overall resting glucose uptake ratio in the visual cortex, eigenvalues corresponding to Brodmann's areas 17, 18, and 19 were extracted using a volumetric mask. The ratio between these values, and the mean area under the VEP curve was then calculated. In addition, based on the statistical parametric mapping results, for case-wise analysis a specific volumetric mask was generated upon the cluster in the visual cortex exhibiting a statistically significant difference in FDG-uptake between groups when including VEP-AUC as a covariate. By using this volumetric mask, eigenvalues corresponding to this specific region were extracted for each subject.

Statistical analysis

Statistical analyses were performed in Prism version 6.00 for Windows (GraphPad Software, La Jolla, California, USA). Continuous variables were compared using the t-test. The assumption of normality was evaluated using a Shapiro-Wilk normality test. For case-wise analyses, mean area under the VEP curve (accounting for visual activity) and eigenvalues corresponding to the specific cluster of the visual cortex exhibiting significant FDG-uptake differences (accounting for metabolic activity) were Z-transformed and paired for each subject. Proportions of participants with a visual > metabolic Z-score in each group were compared using Fisher's exact test. The significance level was set at $p < 0.05$ for all statistical analyses.

Results

The mean area under the curve of VEP was significantly greater in migraine patients compared to healthy controls (1091 $\mu V^2 \pm 164.8$ vs. 362.8 $\mu V^2 \pm 167.7$; $p < 0.01$) (Fig. 1).

Four clusters of reduced metabolism where initially observed (uncorrected $p < 0.001$ level) in the visual cortex of migraine patients, but they did not withstand the correction for multiple comparisons. No clusters of increased PET signal were found in the visual cortex of migraineurs.

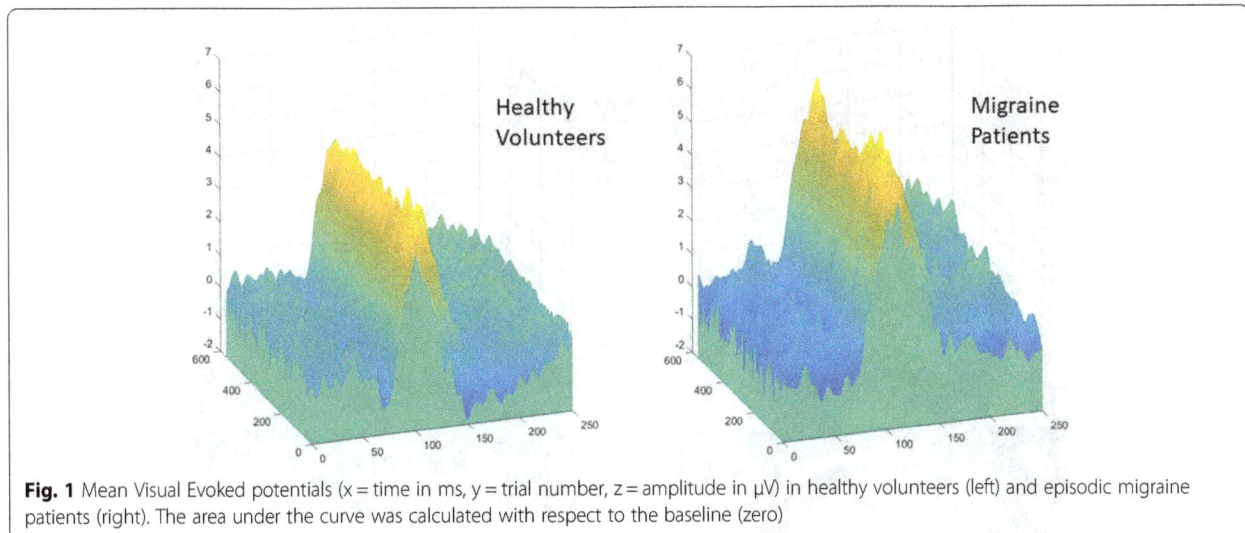

Fig. 1 Mean Visual Evoked potentials (x = time in ms, y = trial number, z = amplitude in µV) in healthy volunteers (left) and episodic migraine patients (right). The area under the curve was calculated with respect to the baseline (zero)

The mean ratio between the VEP-AUC and overall glucose uptake in the visual cortex (BA 17, 18 and 19) was three times higher in migraine patients ($12,73 \pm 1947$ vs. 4.183 ± 1955; $p < 0.01$).

When adding VEP-AUC as a covariate, statistical parametric mapping comparisons revealed a cluster of significantly reduced uptake in patients, with three peaks extending over Brodmann's areas 19, 18 and 7 on the left ($- 20$, $- 78$, 30 $T = 5.66$ peak-level p [FWE-corr] = 0.039; $- 8$, $- 78$, 20 $T = 4.84$; $- 20$, $- 74$, 42 $T = 4.36$, all cluster-level pFWE-corr = 0.021) (Fig. 2). Eigenvalues from this specific cluster were extracted and standardized for case-wise analysis, where a visual activation Z-score exceeding the glucose uptake Z-score was found in 90% of migraine patients, but in only 15% of healthy volunteers ($p < 0.001$, Fisher's exact test) (Fig. 3).

Discussion

In this study, using ^{18}fluorodeoxyglucose-positron emission tomography acquired at rest and pattern reversal-visual evoked potentials, we compared interictal glucose uptake and neuronal activation in the visual cortex of migraine patients and healthy volunteers. Our FDG-PET data confirm the finding of an interictally decreased metabolism in the occipital areas previously shown using phosphorus magnetic resonance spectroscopy [7–9]. An additional, novel finding, is that the ratio between stimulation-induced neuronal activation and resting glucose uptake differs between migraine patients and healthy controls. Using statistical parametric mapping, we identified the specific region of the visual cortex where this difference reaches its maximum. The potential pathophysiological implications of these findings are discussed below.

According to most neurophysiological studies, migraine patients exhibit cortical hyper-responsivity to

repeated sensory stimuli between attacks [20]. Although this may constitute a favourable evolutionary trait [21], enhanced responsivity has a price to be paid in terms of cerebral metabolism. In the brain, the visual system ranks amongst the most energy-consuming systems [22]. This renders it more susceptible to metabolic imbalance when energetic demands increase, energetic supplies decrease, or in a combination of both.

The occurrence of a metabolic strain in the cortex is a plausible hypothesis for igniting a migraine attack [23]. The cornerstone of the metabolic strain model is the unbalanced relationship between enhanced sensory processing and reduced metabolic offers [5]. According to this model, unmet neuronal metabolic demands in the cortex would result in a focal disruption of homeostasis and release of molecules capable of activating the trigemino-vascular system [24–26]. This mechanism, although orchestrated by neurons [26], relies on astrocytes as concertmasters [27]. By determining an area of sensory-metabolic mismatch (suggestive of the presence of a higher cortical responsivity and relatively lower resting energy reserves) in the visual cortex of migraine patients, our results provide supportive experimental evidence to the initiatory phase of the metabolic strain model. Intuitively, energy reserves may be further decreased by daily life stressful and energy consuming events [28], or by the sensory hypersensitivity that patients present even between crises, which extends up to the premonitory phase [29] when, along with the energetic deficit, may worsen up to the tipping point of the attack. This view is supported by a previous study in which the authors simultaneously recorded VEP and cerebral blood flow velocity responses (VEFR) in a group of migraineurs. They observed an interictal increase of neurovascular coupling in patients interictally that, empirically, corresponds to higher neural activity, which

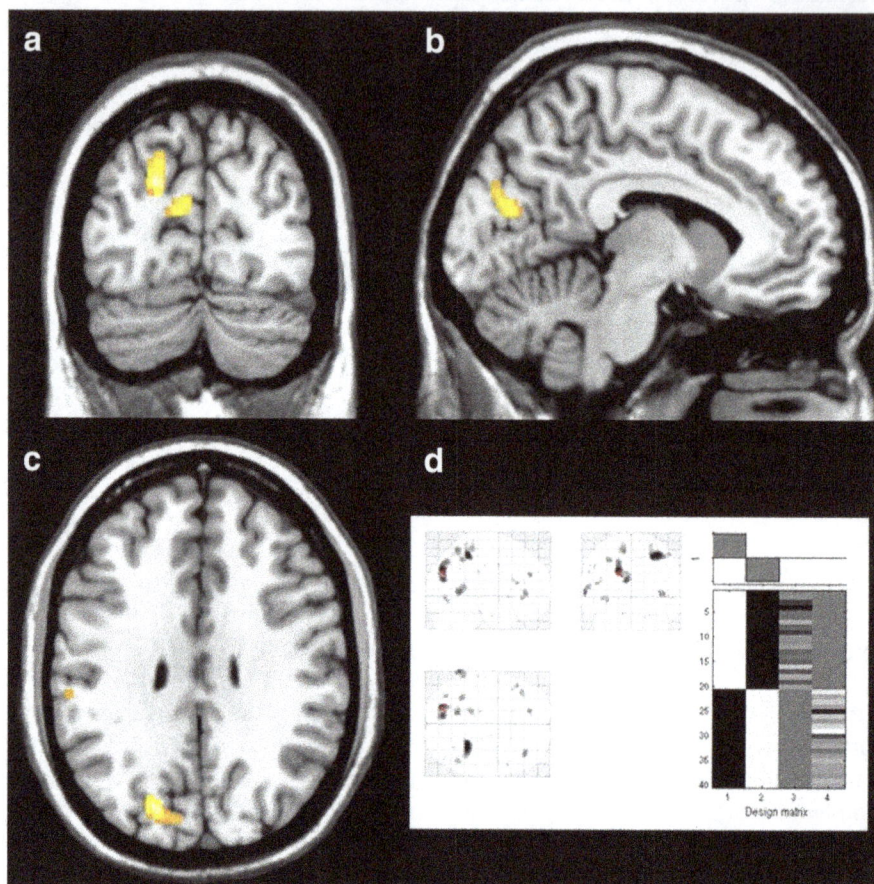

Fig. 2 Areas of increased metabolism in healthy controls compared with migraine patients using the interaction with area under the VEP as regressor. Clockwise from top left: (**a**) coronal view, (**b**) sagittal view, (**c**) axial view, and (**d**) "glass brain" representation and design matrix

might further reduce energy reserves [30]. Hence, the presence of an increase of energetic requirements in the absence of adequate energetic supplies would be a plausible reason for the brain to activate its major alarm system, the trigeminovascular system, that might ignite a migraine attack in order to prevent the system from overloading, and thus re-establish cortical homeostasis [4]. This is supported by three out of four studies where authors positively triggered migraine using sensory overload [31–34]. On the other hand, metabolic challenges have also been shown to provoke migraine attacks. From an observational perspective, skipping meals is the third most common migraine trigger reported by patients [35]. In the laboratory, Schoonman et al. reported provoking headache in six out of fourteen migraine patients exposed to normobaric hypoxia [36], and more recently, in an elegantly designed study also adressing the effects of hypoxia, Arngrim et al. reported migraine-like attacks in eight out of fifteen migraine patients, accompanied by definite aura in three, and possible aura in another four [37].

Our results do not necessarily pull in one direction, favouring sensory over metabolic factors or vice versa, but they rather imply that the physiological sensory-metabolic equilibrium is abnormal in migraine between attacks. However, it is of interest that resting brain energy metabolism remains low even during migraine attacks [38–40] when sensory hyper-responsivity tends to normalize [29]. This suggests that the former might be a trait factor permanently predisposing to the next crisis, while the latter would be more of a state-dependent phenomenon.

As mentioned before, the sensory profile of migraine patients makes them susceptible of sensory overload [1], and therefore in the need of protective mechanisms. Compensatory metaplastic changes have been hypothesized to explain the between-subject variability of electrophysiological responses in migraine groups in previous studies [41]. Thus, it could be debated whether the reduced resting glucose uptake in migraine patients we observed constitutes compensatory mechanism aiming to decrease cortical activation. However, given the heightened visual responsiveness

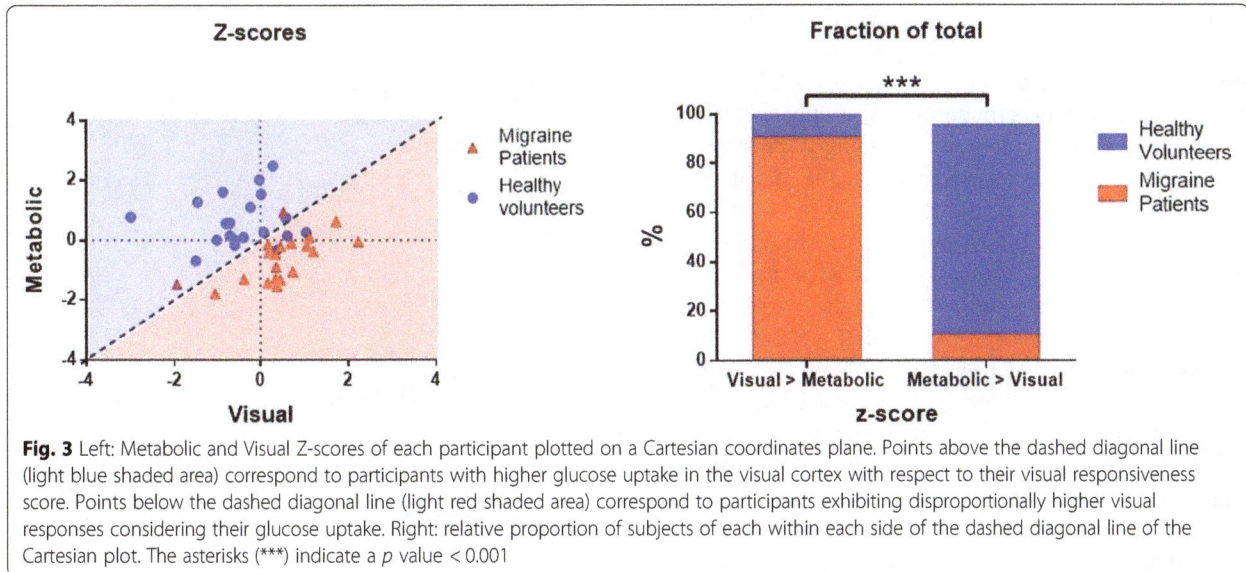

Fig. 3 Left: Metabolic and Visual Z-scores of each participant plotted on a Cartesian coordinates plane. Points above the dashed diagonal line (light blue shaded area) correspond to participants with higher glucose uptake in the visual cortex with respect to their visual responsiveness score. Points below the dashed diagonal line (light red shaded area) correspond to participants exhibiting disproportionally higher visual responses considering their glucose uptake. Right: relative proportion of subjects of each within each side of the dashed diagonal line of the Cartesian plot. The asterisks (***) indicate a p value < 0.001

we recorded in patients, this alternative hypothesis seems unlikely.

One cannot discuss cortical metabolism and homeostasis without considering the role of astrocytes (a deficient uptake of glucose by astrocytes could explain our FDG-PET findings in migraine patients based on current evidence [42–44]). Neurons have a very scarce, if any, energetic reserve. Because of that, their increased metabolic demands upon stimulation basically rely on the energetic supplies provided by astrocytes. Unlike neurons, during rest astrocytes store glucose in the form of glycogen. When the cortex is stimulated, glycogen reserves in astrocytes are rapidly transformed into less complex energetic substrates, which are then provided to neurons in order to fulfil their enhanced metabolic needs (Fig. 4) [42]. In exchange, astrocytes

buffer excessive glutamate molecules released in the synaptic cleft [45]. Other functions of astrocytes, besides regulating neuro-metabolic coupling and glutamate concentrations, include controlling the amount of extracellular potassium [46], and acting as regulators of cerebral blood flow [47]. Indeed, the influence of astrocytes on synaptic transmission is such, that the concept of a tripartite synapse (presynaptic neuron, astrocyte, and postsynaptic neuron) is steadily solidifying [48]. In fact, when altered, deficient clearance of potassium and glutamate by astrocytes seems to explain the pathogenesis of specific forms of migraine with monogenetic inheritance [49]. For the case of more common types of migraine, the pathophysiological implication of astrocytes is less well elucidated, although genetic studies seem to also point in their direction [50, 51].

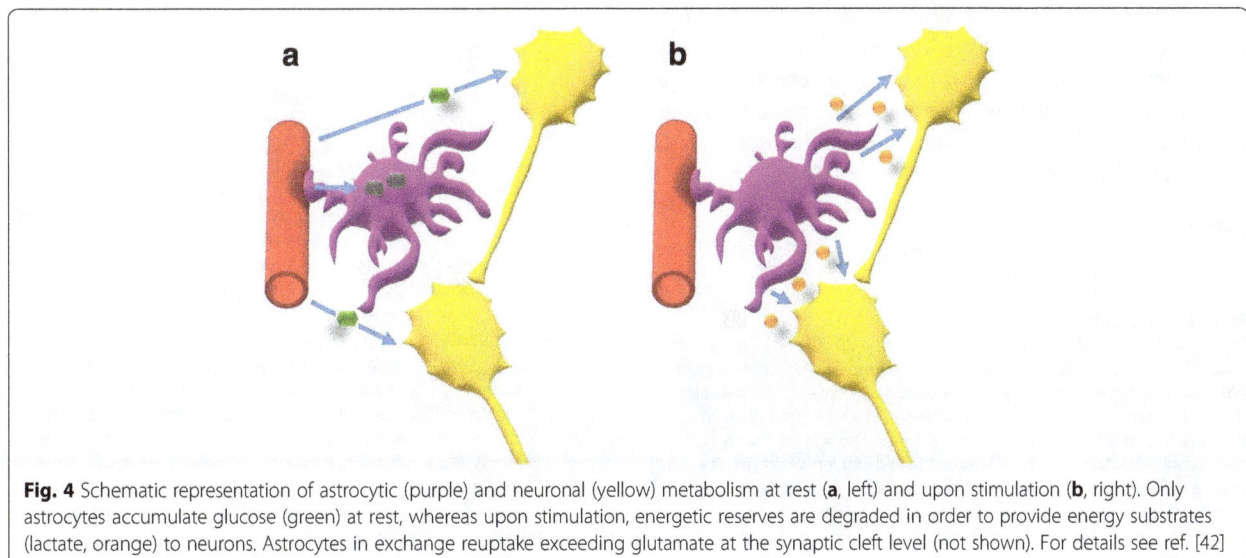

Fig. 4 Schematic representation of astrocytic (purple) and neuronal (yellow) metabolism at rest (**a**, left) and upon stimulation (**b**, right). Only astrocytes accumulate glucose (green) at rest, whereas upon stimulation, energetic reserves are degraded in order to provide energy substrates (lactate, orange) to neurons. Astrocytes in exchange reuptake exceeding glutamate at the synaptic cleft level (not shown). For details see ref. [42]

Interestingly, the visual cortex has the lowest astro-cyte/neuron density in the brain, which renders it more susceptible to homeostatic disturbances [52, 53]. Prior clinical [54] and experimental [55] evidence has suggested that waves of cortical spreading depression, the culprit of migraine aura, originate in the visual cortex. Visual area V3A was specifically pointed to as the initiating region in one report [53]. Another study described increased cortical thickness of this area in migraine without aura patients [56]. It might be worthwhile to mention that the cluster of mismatch we found in the present study extends over visual areas V3A and V7. Whether this observation is coincidental or entails clinical significance remains to be determined.

Our study has several limitations. First, PET scans and VEP where not recorded concomitantly and thus, the possibility of an important compensatory metabolic increase in migraine patients during stimulation remains open. Also, it is worth mentioning that a cycling pattern of increased susceptibility probably determined by the hypothalamus, or its limbic controls, is probably involved in migraine pathogenesis [57], and thus sensory-metabolic coupling might be preserved at one time point and impaired at another. Finally, even if there exists a metabolic imbalance during stimulation in the visual cortex of migraine patients, secondary activation of the trigeminovascular system would need to be further ascertained. In the future, studies addressing these issues would be necessary to clarify the possible role of a disruption in cortical homeostasis due to a sensory-metabolic disequilibrium in migraine pathophysiology.

Conclusion

Our findings indicate the presence of an area of increased neuronal activation-to-resting glucose uptake ratio in the visual cortex of migraine patients between attacks. Despite some methodological reservation, this observation supports the concept that an activity-induced rupture of cerebral metabolic homeostasis may be a cornerstone in migraine pathophysiology. The potential physiopathological implications of such finding should be explored in depth in future studies.

Abbreviations
^{18}FDG-PET: ^{18}fluorodeoxyglucose-positron emission tomography; AUC: Area under the curve; VEP: Visual evoked potentials

Acknowledgements
This article has been selected as the winner of the 2018 Enrico Greppi Award. The Enrico Greppi Award is made to an unpublished paper dealing with clinical, epidemiological, genetic, pathophysiological or therapeutic aspects of headache. The Italian Society for the Study of Headaches (SISC) sponsors this award, and the award is supported through an educational grant from Teva Neuroscience. This article did not undergo the standard peer review process for The Journal of Headache and Pain. The members of the 2018 Enrico Greppi Award Selection Committee were: Francesco Pierelli, Paolo Martelletti, Lyn Griffiths, Simona Sacco, Andreas Straube and Cenk Ayata.

The authors thankfully acknowledge Prof. Roland Hustinx, Chief of the Nuclear Medicine Service at the Centre Hospitalier Universitaire de Liège, for his collaboration on this study (access to FDG-PET).
The contribution of the G.B. Bietti Foundation in this paper was supported by the Italian Ministry of Health and Fondazione Roma.

Funding
This project forms part of the EUROHEADPAIN project - FP7 n° 602633, and received support from the Fonds d'Investissements de Recherche Scientifique (FIRS) of the CHU de Liège.

Authors' contributions
ML contributed in the study design, data acquisition, data processing (focus on electrophysiology), statistical analyses, and wrote the first draft; KDO contributed in the study design, data acquisition, data processing (focus on neuroimaging) and statistical analyses; KD recruited subjects with DM; DM wrote the initial Euroheadpain protocol with JS; GC, AM de N, JS, and DM contributed in the study design and revised the drafts of the manuscript; FS and VP revised the drafts of the manuscript. All authors read and approved the final version.

Competing interests
The authors declare that they have no competing interests.

Author details
^{1}Headache Research Unit, University Department of Neurology CHR, CHU de Liège, Boulevard du 12eme de Ligne 1, 4000 Liege, Belgium. ^{2}G. B. Bietti Foundation IRCCS, Research Unit of Neurophysiology of Vision and Neuro-Ophthalmology, Rome, Italy. ^{3}Departments of Neurosurgery & Neuroanatomy, University of Liège, Liege, Belgium.

References
1. Goadsby PJ, Holland PR, Martins-Oliveira M et al (2017) Pathophysiology of migraine: a disorder of sensory processing. Physiol Rev 97:553–622. https://doi.org/10.1152/physrev.00034.2015
2. Magis D, Vigano A, Sava S et al (2013) Pearls and pitfalls: electrophysiology for primary headaches. Cephalalgia 33:526–539. https://doi.org/10.1177/0333102413477739
3. Lisicki M, Ruiz-Romagnoli E, D'Ostilio K, et al (2017) Familial history of migraine influences habituation of visual evoked potentials. Cephalalgia 37. https://doi.org/10.1177/0333102416673207
4. Schoenen J (1996) Deficient habituation of evoked cortical potentials in migraine: a link between brain biology, behavior and trigeminovascular activation? Biomed Pharmacother 50:71–78. https://doi.org/10.1016/0753-3322(96)84716-0
5. Schoenen J (1994) Pathogenesis of migraine: the biobehavioural and hypoxia theories reconciled. Acta Neurol Belg 94:79–86
6. Schoenen J (2016) Hypoxia, a turning point in migraine pathogenesis? Brain 139:644–647. https://doi.org/10.1093/brain/awv402
7. Reyngoudt H, Paemeleire K, Descamps B et al (2011) 31P-MRS demonstrates a reduction in high-energy phosphates in the occipital lobe of migraine without aura patients. Cephalalgia 31:1243–1253. https://doi.org/10.1177/0333102410394675
8. Montagna P, Cortelli P, Monari L et al (1994) 31P-magnetic resonance spectroscopy in migraine without aura. Neurology 44:666–669
9. Lodi R, Montagna P, Soriani S et al (1997) Deficit of brain and skeletal muscle bioenergetics and low brain magnesium in juvenile migraine: an in vivo 31P magnetic resonance spectroscopy interictal study. Pediatr Res 42: 866–871. https://doi.org/10.1203/00006450-199712000-00024
10. Gantenbein AR, Sandor PS, Fritschy J et al (2013) Sensory information processing may be neuroenergetically more demanding in migraine patients. Neuroreport 24:202–205. https://doi.org/10.1097/WNR.0b013e32835eba81

11. Schoenen J, Jacquy J, Lenaerts M (1998) Effectiveness of high-dose riboflavin in migraine prophylaxis. A randomized controlled trial. Neurology 50:466–470

12. Di Lorenzo C, Coppola G, Sirianni G et al (2015) Migraine improvement during short lasting ketogenesis: a proof-of-concept study. Eur J Neurol 22: 170–177. https://doi.org/10.1111/ene.12550

13. Strahlman RS (2006) Can ketosis help migraine sufferers? A case report. Headache 46:182. https://doi.org/10.1111/j.1526-4610.2006.00321_5.x

14. Kim JH, Kim S, Suh SI et al (2010) Interictal metabolic changes in episodic migraine: a voxel-based FDG-PET study. Cephalalgia 30:53–61. https://doi.org/10.1111/j.1468-2982.2009.01890.x

15. Magis D, D'Ostilio K, Thibaut A et al (2017) Cerebral metabolism before and after external trigeminal nerve stimulation in episodic migraine. Cephalalgia 37:881–891. https://doi.org/10.1177/0333102416656118

16. Kassab M, Bakhtar O, Wack D, Bednarczyk E (2009) Resting brain glucose uptake in headache-free migraineurs. Headache 49:90–97. https://doi.org/10.1111/j.1526-4610.2008.01206.x

17. Headache Classification Committee of the International Headache Society (IHS) (2013) The international classification of headache disorders, 3rd edition (beta version). Cephalalgia 53:137–146. https://doi.org/10.1177/0333102413485658

18. Delorme A, Makeig S (2004) EEGLAB: an open source toolbox for analysis of single-trial EEG dynamics including independent component analysis. J Neurosci Methods 134:9–21. https://doi.org/10.1016/j.jneumeth.2003.10.009

19. Makeig S, Debener S, Onton J, Delorme A (2004) Mining event-related brain dynamics. Trends Cogn Sci 8:204–210. https://doi.org/10.1016/j.tics.2004.03.008

20. de Tommaso M, Ambrosini A, Brighina F et al (2014) Altered processing of sensory stimuli in patients with migraine. Nat Rev Neurol 10:144–155. https://doi.org/10.1038/nrneurol.2014.14

21. Loder E (2002) What is the evolutionary advantage of migraine? Cephalalgia 22:624–632

22. Wong-Riley M (2010) Energy metabolism of the visual system. Eye Brain:99. https://doi.org/10.2147/EB.S9078

23. Paemeleire K, Schoenen J (2013) (31) P-MRS in migraine: fallen through the cracks. Headache 53:676–678. https://doi.org/10.1111/head.12049

24. Zhang X, Levy D, Kainz V et al (2011) Activation of central trigeminovascular neurons by cortical spreading depression. Ann Neurol 69:855–865. https://doi.org/10.1002/ana.22329

25. Kilic K, Karatas H, Dönmez-Demir B et al (2018) Inadequate brain glycogen or sleep increases spreading depression susceptibility. Ann Neurol 83:61–73. https://doi.org/10.1002/ana.25122

26. Karatas H, Erdener SE, Gursoy-Ozdemir Y et al (2013) Spreading depression triggers headache by activating neuronal Panx1 channels. Science 339: 1092–1095. https://doi.org/10.1126/science.1231897

27. Pietrobon D, Moskowitz MA (2014) Chaos and commotion in the wake of cortical spreading depression and spreading depolarizations. Nat Rev Neurosci 15:379–393. https://doi.org/10.1038/nrn3770

28. Lisicki M, Ruiz-Romagnoli E, Piedrabuena R, et al (2017) Migraine triggers and habituation of visual evoked potentials. Cephalalgia 333102417720217. https://doi.org/10.1177/0333102417720217

29. Judit A, Sándor PS, Schoenen J (2000) Habituation of visual and intensity dependence of auditory evoked cortical potentials tends to normalize just before and during the migraine attack. Cephalalgia 20:714–719

30. Zaletel M, Strucl M, Bajrovic FF, Pogacnik T (2005) Coupling between visual evoked cerebral blood flow velocity responses and visual evoked potentials in migraneurs. Cephalalgia 25:567–574. https://doi.org/10.1111/j.1468-2982.2005.00918.x

31. Hougaard A, Amin F, Hauge AW et al (2013) Provocation of migraine with aura using natural trigger factors. Neurology 80:428–431. https://doi.org/10.1212/WNL.0b013e31827f0f10

32. Martin PR, Seneviratne HM (1997) Effects of food deprivation and a stressor on head pain. Health Psychol 16:310–318. https://doi.org/10.1037/0278-6133.16.4.310

33. Cao Y, Aurora SK, Nagesh V et al (2002) Functional MRI-BOLD of brainstem structures during visually triggered migraine. Neurology 59:72–78

34. Cao Y, Welch KM, Aurora S, Vikingstad EM (1999) Functional MRI-BOLD of visually triggered headache in patients with migraine. Arch Neurol 56:548–554

35. Kelman L (2007) The triggers or precipitants of the acute migraine attack. Cephalalgia 27:394–402. https://doi.org/10.1111/j.1468-2982.2007.01303.x

36. Schoonman G, Sándor P, Agosti R et al (2006) Normobaric hypoxia and nitroglycerin as trigger factors for migraine. Cephalalgia 26:816–819. https://doi.org/10.1111/j.1468-2982.2006.01112.x

37. Arngrim N, Schytz HW, Britze J et al (2016) Migraine induced by hypoxia: an MRI spectroscopy and angiography study. Brain 139:723–737. https://doi.org/10.1093/brain/awv359

38. Welch KM, Levine SR, D'Andrea G et al (1989) Preliminary observations on brain energy metabolism in migraine studied by in vivo phosphorus 31 NMR spectroscopy. Neurology 39:538–541

39. Welch KM, Levine SR, D'Andrea G, Helpern JA (1988) Brain pH in migraine: an in vivo phosphorus-31 magnetic resonance spectroscopy study. Cephalalgia 8:273–277. https://doi.org/10.1046/j.1468-2982.1988.0804273.x

40. Ramadan NM, Halvorson H, Vande-Linde A et al (1989) Low brain magnesium in migraine. Headache 29:590–593

41. Cosentino G, Fierro B, Vigneri S et al (2014) Cyclical changes of cortical excitability and metaplasticity in migraine: evidence from a repetitive transcranial magnetic stimulation study. Pain 155:1070–1078. https://doi.org/10.1016/j.pain.2014.02.024

42. Bélanger M, Allaman I, Magistretti PJ (2011) Brain energy metabolism: focus on astrocyte-neuron metabolic cooperation. Cell Metab 14:724–738

43. Zimmer ER, Parent MJ, Souza DG et al (2017) [18F]FDG PET signal is driven by astroglial glutamate transport. Nat Neurosci 20:393–395. https://doi.org/10.1038/nn.4492

44. Figley CR, Stroman PW (2011) The role(s) of astrocytes and astrocyte activity in neurometabolism, neurovascular coupling, and the production of functional neuroimaging signals. Eur J Neurosci 33:577–588. https://doi.org/10.1111/j.1460-9568.2010.07584.x

45. Anderson CM, Swanson RA (2000) Astrocyte glutamate transport: review of properties, regulation, and physiological functions. Glia 32:1–14

46. Kimelberg HK, Nedergaard M (2010) Functions of astrocytes and their potential as therapeutic targets. Neurotherapeutics 7:338–353. https://doi.org/10.1016/j.nurt.2010.07.006

47. Gordon GRJ, Choi HB, Rungta RL et al (2008) Brain metabolism dictates the polarity of astrocyte control over arterioles. Nature 456:745–749. https://doi.org/10.1038/nature07525

48. Araque A, Parpura V, Sanzgiri RP, Haydon PG (1999) Tripartite synapses: glia, the unacknowledged partner. Trends Neurosci 22:208–215. https://doi.org/10.1016/S0166-2236(98)01349-6

49. Capuani C, Melone M, Tottene A, et al (2016) Defective glutamate and K+ clearance by cortical astrocytes in familial hemiplegic migraine type 2. EMBO Mol Med. https://doi.org/10.15252/emmm.201505944

50. Eising E, De Leeuw C, Min JL, et al Involvement of astrocyte and oligodendrocyte gene sets in migraine. https://doi.org/10.1177/0333102415618614

51. Renthal W Localization of migraine susceptibility genes in human brain by single-cell RNA sequencing. https://doi.org/10.1177/0333102418762476

52. Lauritzen M, Dreier JP, Fabricius M et al (2011) Clinical relevance of cortical spreading depression in neurological disorders: migraine, malignant stroke, subarachnoid and intracranial hemorrhage, and traumatic brain injury. J Cereb Blood Flow Metab 31:17–35. https://doi.org/10.1038/jcbfm.2010.191

53. Hadjikhani N, Sanchez Del Rio M, Wu O et al (2001) Mechanisms of migraine aura revealed by functional MRI in human visual cortex. Proc Natl Acad Sci U S A 98:4687–4692. https://doi.org/10.1073/pnas.071582498

54. Lashley KS (1941) Patterns of cerebral integration indicated by the scotomas of migraine. Arch Neurol Psychiatr 46:331–339. https://doi.org/10.1001/archneurpsyc.1941.02280200137007

55. Lauritzen M, Olesen J (1984) Regional cerebral blood flow during migraine attacks by Xenon-133 inhalation and emission tomography. Brain 107(Pt 2): 447–461

56. Granziera C, DaSilva AFM, Snyder J et al (2006) Anatomical alterations of the visual motion processing network in migraine with and without Aura. PLoS Med 3:e402. https://doi.org/10.1371/journal.pmed.0030402

57. Schulte LH, May A (2016) The migraine generator revisited: continuous scanning of the migraine cycle over 30 days and three spontaneous attacks. Brain 139:1987–1993. https://doi.org/10.1093/brain/aww097

6

Efficacy and safety of DFN-11 (sumatriptan injection, 3 mg) in adults with episodic migraine: an 8-week open-label extension study

Stephen Landy[1], Sagar Munjal[2*], Elimor Brand-Schieber[2] and Alan M. Rapoport[3]

Abstract

Background: DFN-11, a 3 mg sumatriptan subcutaneous (SC) autoinjector for acute treatment of migraine, has not been assessed previously in multiple attacks. The objective of this study was to evaluate the efficacy, tolerability, and safety of DFN-11 in the acute treatment of multiple migraine attacks.

Methods: This was an 8-week open-label extension of multicenter, randomized, double-blind, placebo-controlled US study. Subjects averaging 2 to 6 episodic migraine attacks per month were randomized to DFN-11 or placebo to treat a single attack of moderate-to-severe intensity and then entered the extension study to assess the efficacy, tolerability, and safety of DFN-11 in multiple attacks of any pain intensity.

Results: Overall, 234 subjects enrolled in the open-label period, and 29 (12.4%) discontinued early. A total of 848 migraine episodes were treated with 1042 doses of open-label DFN-11 and subjects treated a mean (SD) of 3.9 (2.3) attacks. At 2 h postdose in attacks 1 ($N = 216$), 2 ($N = 186$), 3 ($N = 142$) and 4 ($N = 110$), respectively, pain freedom rates were 57.6%, 64.6%, 61.6%, and 66.3%; pain relief rates were 83.4%, 88.4%, 84.1%, and 81.7%; most bothersome symptom (MBS)-free rates were 69.0%, 76.5%, 77.7%, and 74.7%; nausea-free rates were 78.1%, 84.6%, 86.5%, and 85.7%; photophobia-free rates were 75.3%, 76.4%, 72.3%, and 77.5%; and phonophobia-free rates were 75.2%, 77.5%, 73.6%, and 76.0%. Overall, 40.6% (89/219) of subjects reported treatment-emergent adverse events (TEAE), the most common of which were associated with the injection site: swelling (12.8%), pain (11.4%), irritation (6.4%), and bruising (6.4%). Most subjects (65.2%, 58/89) had mild TEAEs; severe TEAEs were reported by 1 subject (treatment-related jaw tightness). Five subjects (2.1%) discontinued due to adverse events, which included mild throat tightness ($n = 2$), moderate hernia pain ($n = 1$), moderate hypersensitivity ($n = 1$), and 1 subject with mild nausea and moderate injection site swelling. There were no serious TEAEs and no new or unexpected safety findings.

Conclusion: DFN-11 was effective, tolerable, and safe in the acute treatment of 4 migraine attacks over 8 weeks, with consistent responses on pain and associated symptoms. Most TEAEs were mild, with a very low incidence of triptan-related TEAEs. DFN-11 is potentially an effective and safe alternative for the acute treatment of migraine.

Keywords: Low-dose sumatriptan, Multi-attack acute subcutaneous sumatriptan, Consistency of effect

* Correspondence: smunjal@drreddys.com
[2]Promius Pharma, LLC, a subsidiary of Dr. Reddy's Laboratories, 107 College Road East, Princeton, NJ 08540, USA
Full list of author information is available at the end of the article

Background

Migraine is a painful, disabling, and, for most patients, life-long disease [1, 2]. Although migraineurs rate consistent relief with few side effects among the most desirable attributes of an acute migraine medication [3–6], and clinical trial guidelines recommend assessment of the consistency of response to acute medications in multiple-attack studies [7], the effectiveness of acute medications across multiple attacks is not frequently evaluated in clinical trials. Yet the utility of acute treatments depends, in part on their ability to be effective, tolerable, and safe over the long-term [8]; inconsistent relief is an important reason for dissatisfaction with acute therapy [3]. Moreover, confidence that an intervention will reliably relieve migraine pain and associated symptoms is a predictor of adherence to acute therapy [9]. Single-attack studies are not designed to evaluate inter-attack variability of treatment outcomes [10].

DFN-11 (Zembrace® SymTouch®, Promius Pharma, Princeton, NJ) is a low-dose (3 mg) SC sumatriptan injection, supplied as a single-dose, ready-to-use, disposable autoinjector. Compared with the 6-mg SC dose of sumatriptan (Imitrex®, GlaxoSmithKline, Research Triangle Park, NC), DFN-11 has less sumatriptan per 0.5-mL dose (3 mg vs 6 mg) [11, 12]. Other research has shown that DFN-11 provides relief of migraine pain and associated symptoms similar to a 6-mg SC dose of sumatriptan, with fewer triptan sensations and no reports of chest pain, in adults with rapidly-escalating migraine attacks [13]. Subsequent work in episodic migraine found that DFN-11 was significantly more effective than placebo on pain-free and pain relief outcomes from 30 min through 2 h postdose and confirmed the low incidence of TEAEs and triptan sensations [14]. The objective of this study was to evaluate the efficacy, tolerability, and safety of DFN-11 in the acute treatment of multiple migraine attacks in adults with episodic migraine.

Methods

Ethics

This was a randomized, double-blind, placebo-controlled study with an open-label extension to evaluate the efficacy, tolerability, and safety of DFN-11 in adults with episodic migraine at 16 US study centers. The data from the double-blind portion of the study have been presented elsewhere [14]. The protocol was approved by the institutional review boards at each study site, and the study conduct complied with good clinical practice and the ethical principles in the Declaration of Helsinki. Prior to screening, investigators explained the nature of the study and obtained informed consent from subjects. The study is registered at ClinicalTrials.gov (https://clinicaltrials.gov/; Identifier NCT02569853).

Subjects

Subjects included adult males and females (18–65 years of age) with a history of episodic migraine with or without aura (defined by the Second Edition of International Classification of Headache Disorders (ICHD-2) [15]). They had to have 2 to 6 migraine attacks per month for at least the previous 12 months, with no more than 14 headache days per month and a minimum of 48 h of headache-free time between attacks. Subjects had to meet all inclusion and exclusion criteria to be included in the study.

Treatments

DFN-11 (equivalent to 3 mg sumatriptan base in 0.5 mL sterile solution) was provided as an SC injection in a 29-gauge needle-based autoinjector.

Study procedures

This study included site visits for screening, baseline/randomization, end double-blind/begin open-label, week 4 ± 3 days, and week 8 ± 3 days/early termination.

During screening, subjects provided informed consent and staff verified inclusion and exclusion criteria. Subjects were given an electronic diary (eDiary) and instructions on how to complete it, medical and migraine histories were taken, and a physical examination was performed.

At baseline, inclusion and exclusion criteria were re-verified, and medical and treatment histories and physical examinations (including laboratory and vital sign measurements) were repeated. Subjects were randomized (1:1) to receive DFN-11 or placebo via SC autoinjector in a double-blinded fashion to treat 1 migraine attack. Study centers used an Interactive Web Response System to assign drug kits (ie, labeled cartons containing 2 individually labeled autoinjectors) at scheduled and unscheduled visits as needed.

At the conclusion of the double-blind treatment period, subjects were re-examined, and vital signs measurements were repeated. Study staff assessed eligibility for continuing into an open-label period, and eligible subjects entered an 8-week open-label period. During this period, subjects received DFN-11 for 8 weeks and were instructed to treat multiple attacks within 1 h of migraine pain onset at any level of pain intensity. If subjects did not experience sufficient relief 2 h after taking the first dose of study medication, they were allowed a second dose of study medication or rescue medication for the same attack. No more than 2 doses of study medication could be taken in any 24-h period. Rescue medications could include prescription and nonprescription drugs (eg, NSAIDs, other acute migraine medications, vitamins, herbal/dietary supplements).

Adverse events (AEs) were monitored from the time subjects gave informed consent; physical examinations, vital sign measurements, ECGs, and laboratory assessments were performed at designated site visits.

Assessments

In the open-label period, efficacy was assessed for each of the first 4 reported migraine attacks. Efficacy endpoints included the percentage of subjects who had pain-freedom, pain relief, and absence of their most bothersome symptom (MBS) at 10, 15, 20, 30, 60, 90, and 120 min, and the percentage of subjects who were free from nausea, photophobia, and phonophobia at 2 h postdose. The percentage of subjects with sustained pain freedom from 2 to 24 h postdose was also assessed.

Pain freedom was defined as a reduction in migraine pain from a predose rating of moderate (Grade 2) or severe (Grade 3) pain to none (Grade 0). Pain relief was defined as a reduction in migraine pain from predose rating of severe (Grade 3) or moderate (Grade 2) to mild pain (Grade 1) or none (Grade 0), or from mild pain (Grade 1) to none (Grade 0). Absence of MBS was defined as absence of the symptom chosen as most bothersome from among nausea, photophobia, or phonophobia at predose. Sustained pain freedom was defined as pain-free at 2 h postdose with no use of rescue medication or additional study medication and no recurrence of headache pain within 2 to 24 h postdose.

Safety and tolerability were assessed throughout the open-label period. Tolerability included the percentage of subjects with treatment-emergent AEs (TEAEs). Safety endpoints included the percentage of subjects with serious AEs (SAEs), as well as those with changes in vital signs or ECGs. Safety parameters included concomitant medication review; physical examinations; pregnancy tests in females; measurement of vital signs (sitting systolic and diastolic blood pressure, pulse rate, and body temperature); clinical laboratory examination (hematology, chemistry, and urinalysis); urine drug screen; and 12-lead ECG.

Statistics

All data processing, summarization, and analyses were performed using SAS® software, Version 9.2. Adverse events were classified using the Medical Dictionary for Regulatory Activities (MedDRA) dictionary, Version 18.0. Concomitant medications were coded using the World Health Organization Drug Dictionary Enhanced (WHODDE), version Mar2015 further coded against Anatomic Therapeutic Chemical (ATC) classification.

Subjects randomized in the double-blind period comprised the population for subject disposition and baseline summaries. The open-label efficacy analyses included all open-label subjects who received at least 1 dose of active study medication and recorded at least 1 postdose efficacy data point in the open-label period. The open-label safety analysis included all open-label subjects who received at least 1 dose of study medication.

Unless noted otherwise, a last observation carried forward (LOCF) imputation method was applied to pain intensity and the presence of nausea, photophobia, and phonophobia. Baseline data were not carried forward, and only valid data from postbaseline assessments collected before the 2-h postdose time point were carried forward to impute the next missing assessment up to the 2-h postdose time point. Time points beyond 2 h postdose were not carried forward.

The analysis of safety was based on data from all randomized subjects who received at least 1 dose of study medication. The efficacy analyses were based on data captured in the eDiary for migraine attacks treated. Postdosing assessments were collected in real-time. Change from baseline was defined as the postbaseline value minus the predose value, and calculations were based on nonmissing data. Baseline for safety assessments was defined as the last assessment before receiving the first dose of study medication in the double-blind period.

Results

Disposition

A total of 16 US study sites participated and randomized subjects into the study. The duration of the study, from the first subject's enrollment until the last subject's completion, was 618 days (21 September 2015 through 30 May 2017).

As shown in Fig. 1, 392 subjects were screened, 268 (68.4%) were randomized, 234 (87.3% of those randomized) completed the double-blind treatment period and enrolled in the open-label extension. A total of 205 (87.6% of those who enrolled) completed the open-label extension (Table 1).

Of the 234 subjects who entered the open-label extension, 216 (92.3%) treated at least 1 attack, 186 (79.5%) treated at least 2 attacks, 142 (60.7%) treated at least 3 attacks, and 110 (47.0%) treated 4 attacks or more. A total of 29 subjects (12.4%) discontinued: 9 (3.8%) were lost to follow-up, 7 (3.0%) withdrew consent, and 5 (2.1%) discontinued due to AEs.

Demographics

Most subjects were female (85.4%) and white (75.7%), with a mean (SD) age of 41.0 (12.4) years. Mean (SD) weight was 84.4 (23.7) kg and mean (SD) BMI was 30.6 (8.6) kg/m^2.

Exposure

Over the course of the 8-week open-label extension, subjects used 1042 doses of DFN-11 to treat 848 migraine attacks, and they treated a mean (SD) of 3.9 (2.3) attacks per subject. In attacks 1, 2, 3, and 4, respectively, a second dose of DFN-11 (allowed after the completion of the 2-h efficacy assessments) was used by 19.9% (43/

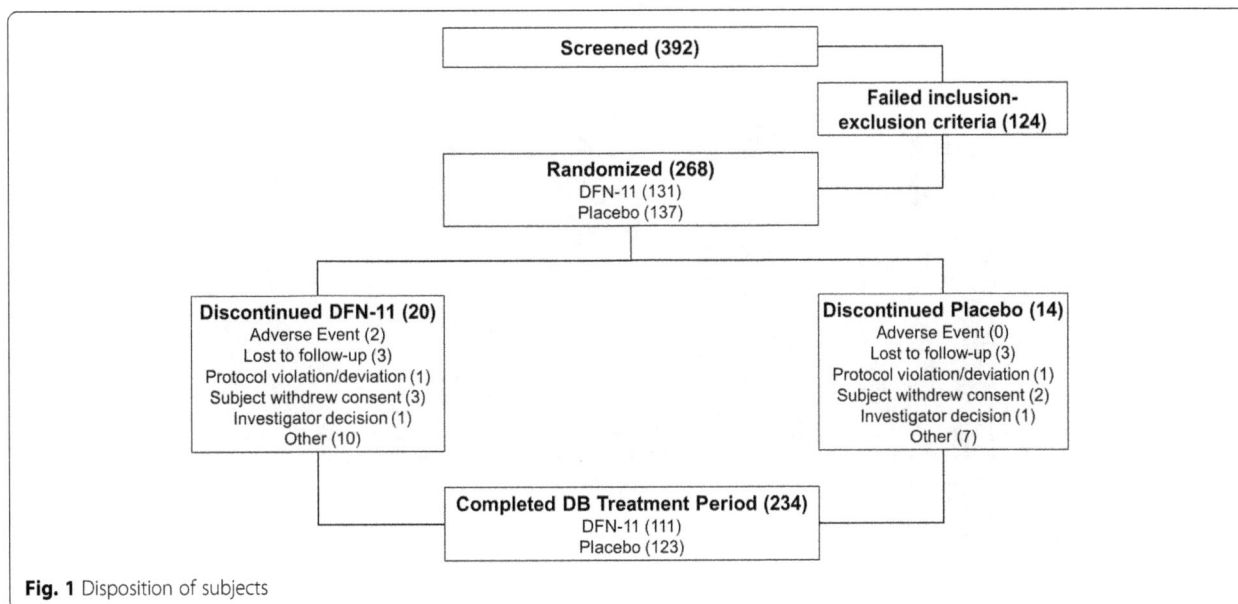

Fig. 1 Disposition of subjects

216), 21.0% (39/186), 15.5% (22/142), and 26.4% (29/110) of subjects.

Efficacy

At 2 h after DFN-11 treatment, the percentages of subjects who were pain-free in attacks 1, 2, 3, and 4, respectively, were 57.6%, 64.6%, 61.6%, and 66.3%. The 2-h pain relief response rates were 83.4% for attack 1, 88.4% for attack 2, 84.1% for attack 3, and 81.7% for attack 4. The percentage

of subjects with 2-h postdose absence of MBS in attacks 1 to 4, respectively, was 69.0%, 76.5%, 77.7%, and 74.7%. Pain-free, pain relief, and MBS responses to DFN-11 for the 4 individual attacks, as well as for the attack treated with DFN-11 in the double-blind period, are presented in Fig. 2.

For freedom from the associated symptoms of migraine, Fig. 3 shows that in attacks 1, 2, 3, and 4, respectively, 78.1%, 84.6%, 86.5%, and 85.7% subjects were free of nausea; 75.3%, 76.4%, 72.3%, and 77.5% were free of

Table 1 Subject disposition

Screened					392	
Double-blind Treatment Period	DFN-11		Placebo		Total	
Randomized	131		137		268	
Completed	111		123		234	
Discontinued	20		14		34	
Open-label Treatment Period (All active DFN-11)	Treatment Received During DB, Prior to OL Period				Overall	
	DFN-11		Placebo			
Enrolled	111[a]		123[a]		234	
Completed	96[a]		109[a]		205	
Discontinued	15[a]		14[a]		29	
Reasons for discontinuation	Discont. During DB	Discont. During OLE[a]	Discont. During DB	Discont. During OLE[a]	OLE Total	DB + OLE
Adverse event	2	3	0	2	5	7
Lost to follow-up	3	8	3	1	9	15
Protocol violation	1	1	1	3	4	6
Withdrew consent	3	2	2	5	7	12
Investigator decision	1	0	1	2	2	4
Other	10	1	7	1	2	19
Total discontinued	20	15	14	14	29	63

DB double-blind treatment period, *OLE* open-label extension period

[a]Treatment group reflects OLE subjects' assignment during the DB period

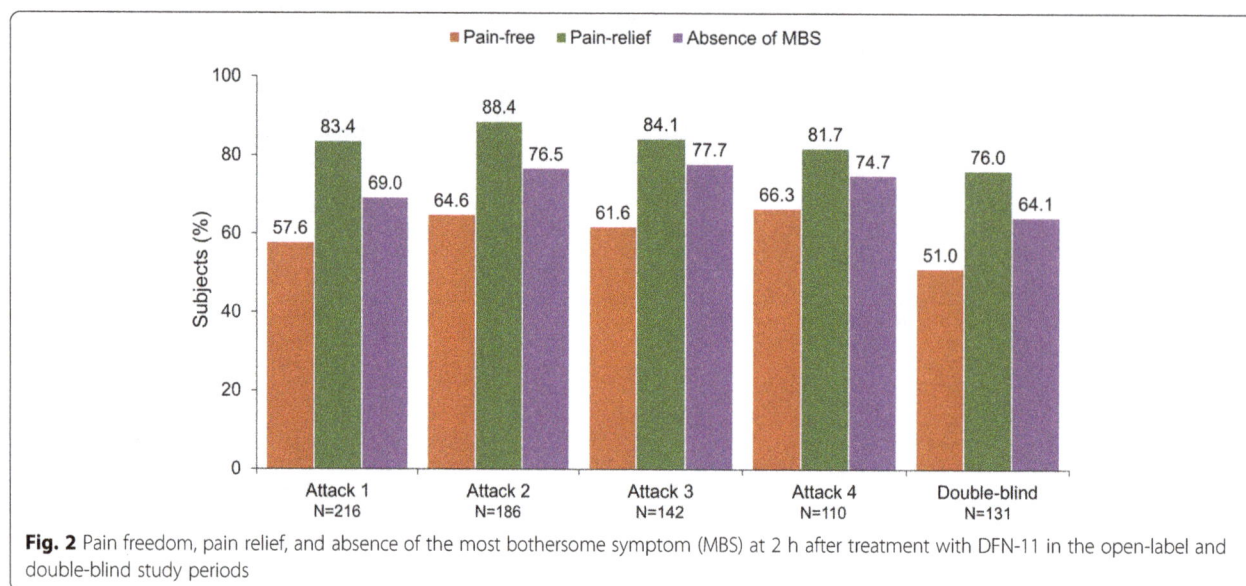

Fig. 2 Pain freedom, pain relief, and absence of the most bothersome symptom (MBS) at 2 h after treatment with DFN-11 in the open-label and double-blind study periods

photophobia; and 75.2%, 77.5%, 73.6%, and 76.0% were free of phonophobia.

Rates of sustained pain freedom from 2 to 24 h postdose in attacks 1, 2, 3, and 4, respectively, were 83.9% (78/93), 76.5% (65/85), 81.3% (52/64), and 77.8% (42/54).

Use of a second dose or rescue medication

The percentage of subjects who took a second dose of study medication, rescue medication, or both, in the 2 to 24 h postdose in attacks 1, 2, 3, and 4, respectively, was 19.4% (42/216), 21.0% (39/186), 16.9% (24/142), and 25.5% (28/110).

Tolerability and safety

During the open-label period, 40.6% (89/219) of subjects reported TEAEs. The most common TEAEs were

injection site swelling (12.8%), injection site pain (11.4%), injection site irritation (6.4%), and injection site bruising (6.4%), as shown in Table 2. Most subjects (65.2%, 58/89) reported a maximum TEAE severity of mild; 24.7% (22/89) reported moderate TEAEs. Eight subjects did not have severity assigned. A single subject reported 10 occurrences of severe joint stiffness (described as injection-related jaw tightness) that was considered definitely related to the study medication. The relationship to DFN-11 was considered by the investigator as definite in 26.9% (59/219) of subjects and probable in 6.4% (14/219) of subjects. Five subjects (2.1%) discontinued due to AEs that included mild throat tightness ($n = 2$); moderate hernia pain ($n = 1$); moderate hypersensitivity ($n = 1$); and mild nausea and moderate injection site swelling ($n = 1$).

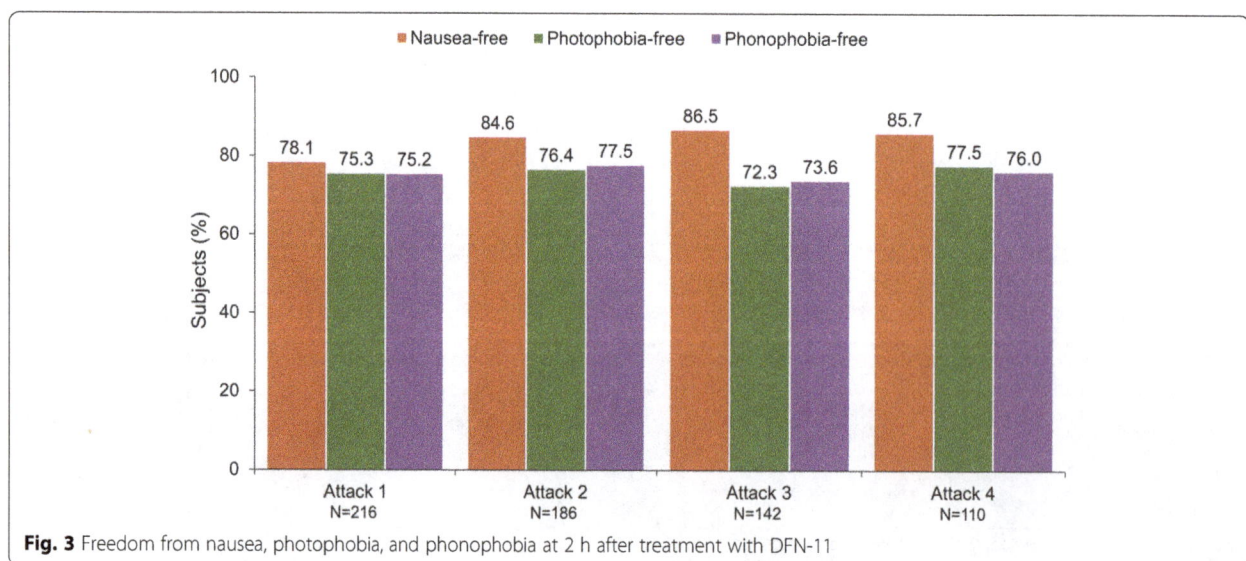

Fig. 3 Freedom from nausea, photophobia, and phonophobia at 2 h after treatment with DFN-11

Table 2 Treatment-emergent adverse events occurring in ≥1% of subjects treated with DFN-11

	(N = 219)
	n (%)
Subjects with ≥1 TEAE	89 (40.6)
Injection site	
Bruising	14 (6.4)
Erythema	8 (3.7)
Induration	6 (2.7)
Irritation	14 (6.4)
Pain	25 (11.4)
Swelling	28 (12.8)
Nausea	6 (2.7)
Chest discomfort	6 (2.7)
Sinusitis	3 (1.4)
Upper respiratory tract infection	7 (3.2)
Burning sensation	3 (1.4)
Dizziness	4 (1.8)
Paresthesia	3 (1.4)
Somnolence	3 (1.4)

TEAE treatment-emergent adverse event

There were no deaths or treatment-emergent SAEs, and no notable shifts in chemistry or hematology parameters, vital signs, or physical examinations; no clinically significant values on these parameters were reported during the study.

Injection site reactions

The most common TEAEs overall were associated with the injection site: swelling (12.8%, 28/219); pain (11.4%, 25/219); and irritation and bruising (both 6.4%, 14/219 each). At least 1 injection site reaction was reported by 27.4% (60/219) of subjects overall, and rates were 19.9% (43/216) in attack 1, 13.4% (25/186) in attack 2, 10.6% (15/142) in attack 3, and 14.5% (16/110) in attack 4.

Triptan-related adverse events

A total of 12.3% (27/219) of subjects had at least 1 triptan-related AE, with 10.6% (23/216), 9.1% (17/186), 7.7% (11/142), and 7.3% (8/110) of subjects experiencing them in attacks 1, 2, 3, and 4, respectively. Chest discomfort was reported 32 times by a total of 6 subjects (2.7%); 5 subjects had 30 mild events, and the sixth had 1 mild and 1 moderate event. These events were described variously by the study investigators as chest tightness, noncardiac; chest tightness after injection, noncardiac; sensation of chest heaviness after injection, noncardiac; and pressure sensation, chest, noncardiac.

Discussion

This open-label extension study was conducted to evaluate the efficacy, tolerability, and safety of DFN-11 in the acute treatment of multiple migraine attacks in adults with episodic migraine. At 2 h postdose, pain-free rates ranged from 57.6% to 66.3%, pain relief response was 81.7% to 88.4%, and absence of the MBS ranged from 69.0% to 77.7% in the first 4 attacks treated with DFN-11. Freedom from migraine associated symptoms at 2 h ranged 78.1% to 86.5% for nausea, 72.3% to 77.5% for photophobia, and 73.6% to 77.5% for phonophobia. DFN-11 had a good tolerability profile, with a predictable but low incidence of TEAEs (ie, injection site reactions) that were mostly mild, and a very low incidence of triptan sensations (all considered noncardiac). These findings show that DFN-11 was consistently effective, tolerable, and safe in the acute treatment of multiple migraine attacks over an 8-week period.

With the caveat that comparing efficacy results from studies with different study populations and methodologies can be misleading, the magnitude of multiple-attack response to DFN-11 appears to be roughly comparable to the 6 mg SC dose of sumatriptan in published reports. For example, an 18-month open-label study of the 6 mg SC dose reported 2-h response rates of 67.0% for pain-free and approximately 72% for pain relief [16]. A trial evaluating sumatriptan SC 6 mg across 455 attacks in 100 consecutive patients found that 84% of subjects had pain relief at 2 h postdose [17]. In the current study of the effects of DFN-11 across 4 attacks, the range of 2-h pain-free rates was narrow and slightly lower (approximately 58–66%), but the range of pain relief responses was considerably higher (approximately 82–88%).

The results of this study confirm and extend the known safety profile of DFN-11. As expected, the overall rate of AEs was low, and only 1 subject experienced severe TEAEs. The most frequently reported TEAEs overall (injection site swelling and pain), as well as those associated with triptans (chest discomfort), decreased in incidence across the 4 treated attacks. Slightly more than one quarter (27.4%) of subjects treated with DFN-11 had at least 1 injection site reaction, which is less than half the rate reported with a 6-mg dose autoinjector (59%) [12] and about one third the incidence in a placebo-controlled study (79%) pooling data from 4 attacks [18]. The rate of injection site TEAEs may be related to the DFN-11 lower dose of active drug, dilute solution, and thin needle — the last of which has been shown to reduce pain and increase patient adherence [19]. Chest discomfort affected only 2.7% of subjects treated with DFN-11, and 5 of the 6 affected subjects reported only mild symptoms. Accounting for differences that might be expected due to the lower dose of sumatriptan in DFN-11 compared with traditional SC sumatriptan (3 mg vs 6 mg), this still represents a reduction from rates observed in earlier multiple-attacks studies of the 6 mg SC dose of sumatriptan. For example, in a previous study over a median of 25 months, 41% of subjects treated with a 6 mg dose of SC sumatriptan experienced chest symptoms in all attacks, and 39% had them in some attacks, leading 10% of subjects to discontinue sumatriptan [20]. In the placebo-controlled study of 4 attacks [18], 15.6% of subjects treated with the 6 mg dose of SC sumatriptan reported chest symptoms, an 83% increase versus DFN-11.

Limitations of this study include the open-label design and a possible selection bias for responders during the open-label period. Also, the study did not assess consistency of response within each individual. Despite these, the size of the study and consistency of response across 4 attacks suggest that DFN-11 will provide predictable migraine relief in clinical practice. In addition, the low incidence of TEAEs that generally decreased across the 4 attacks may increase patient confidence in positive results, encourage patient adherence to professional recommendations (eg, treating at the first sign of migraine pain) and, ultimately, contribute to better efficacy outcomes in clinical practice.

Conclusions

DFN-11 was consistently effective, tolerable, and safe in the acute treatment of multiple migraine attacks over an 8-week period. The responses to DFN-11 at 2 h postdose on migraine pain freedom, pain relief, and associated symptoms (including the most bothersome) endpoints were substantial, and their range across attacks was narrow. TEAEs were predictable and mostly mild, with a very low incidence of triptan sensations. These findings underscore the potential of DFN-11 as an effective and safe SC sumatriptan option for the acute treatment of migraine.

Abbreviations

AE: Adverse event; ECG: Electrocardiogram;; eDiary: Electronic diary; ICHD: International Classification of Headache Disorders; LOCF: Last observation carried forward; MBS: Most bothersome symptom; MedDRA: Medical Dictionary for Regulatory Activities; SAE: Serious adverse event; SC: Subcutaneous; SD: Standard deviation; TEAE: Treatment-emergent adverse event; WHODDE: World Health Organization Drug Dictionary Enhanced

Acknowledgements

Medical writing services were provided by Christopher Caiazza. The authors thank the participating patients, the investigators and their staff and Katherine D'Angelo (Dr. Reddy's Laboratories, Princeton, NJ) for assisting with the conduct of this study. DRL Publication #835.

Funding

This study was supported and funded by Dr. Reddy's Laboratories Ltd., manufacturer of DFN-11. Its US subsidiary, Promius Pharma, markets DFN-11 as Zembrace® SymTouch®.

Authors'contributions

SM and EBS designed and conducted the study, and all authors contributed to the writing and revision of the manuscript. All authors read and approved the final manuscript.

Competing interests

This study was supported and funded by the Dr. Reddy's Laboratories group of companies, Princeton, NJ, manufacturer of DFN-11. SM and EBS are employed by and own stock in Dr. Reddy's Laboratories Ltd. SL and AMR are paid consultants of Dr. Reddy's Laboratories Ltd., but they were not paid to draft or edit this paper. SL also serves on the speaker's bureau of Allergan, Amgen, Depomed, ElectroCore, Promius Pharma, and Supernus; he is a consultant for Allergan, Amgen, Promius and Supernus. AMR is also on the speaker's bureau of Amgen, Avanir, Depomed, Electrocore, Promius Pharma and Teva; he is a consultant for Amgen, Autonomic Technologies, ElectroCore, Impax, Teva, and Zosano.

Author details

[1]Baptist Medical Group Headache Clinic, University of Tennessee Medical School, 6029 Walnut Grove, Suite 210, Memphis, TN 38120, USA. [2]Promius Pharma, LLC, a subsidiary of Dr. Reddy's Laboratories, 107 College Road East, Princeton, NJ 08540, USA. [3]The David Geffen School of Medicine at UCLA, 4255 Jefferson Avenue, Suite 27, Woodside, CA 94062, USA.

References

1. Lipton RB, Stewart WF, Diamond S et al (2001) Prevalence and burden of migraine in the United States: data from the American migraine study II. Headache 41:646–657
2. Lipton RB, Bigal ME, Diamond M et al (2007) Migraine prevalence, disease burden, and the need for preventive therapy. Neurology 68:343–349
3. Lipton RB, Hamelsky SW, Dayno JM (2002) What do patients with migraine want from acute migraine treatment? Headache 42(Suppl 1):3–9
4. Malik SN, Hopkins M, Young WB et al (2006) Acute migraine treatment: patterns of use and satisfaction in a clinical population. Headache 46: 773–780
5. Davies GM, Santanello N, Lipton R (2000) Determinants of patient satisfaction with migraine therapy. Cephalalgia 20:554–560
6. Amoozegar F, Pringsheim T (2009) Rizatriptan for the acute treatment of migraine: consistency, preference, satisfaction, and quality of life. Patient preference and adherence 3:251–258
7. Tfelt-Hansen P, Pascual J, Ramadan N et al (2012) Guidelines for controlled trials of drugs in migraine: third edition. A guide for investigators. Cephalalgia 32:6–38
8. Tansey MJ, Pilgrim AJ, Martin PM (1993) Long-term experience with sumatriptan in the treatment of migraine. Eur Neurol 33:310–315
9. Cady RK, Maizels M, Reeves DL et al (2009) Predictors of adherence to triptans: factors of sustained vs lapsed users. Headache 49:386–394
10. Lipton RB, Bigal ME, Stewart WF (2005) Clinical trials of acute treatments for migraine including multiple attack studies of pain, disability, and health-related quality of life. Neurology 65:S50–S58
11. ZEMBRACE® SymTouch® (sumatriptan succiate) Injection prescribing information. Available at: http://www.zembrace.com/Content/docs/zembrace-prescribing-information.pdf. Accessed June 18, 2018
12. IMITREX (sumatriptan succinate) Injection prescribing information. Available at: https://www.gsksource.com/pharma/content/dam/GlaxoSmithKline/US/en/Prescribing_Information/Imitrex_Injection/pdf/IMITREX-INJECTION-PI-PPI-PIL-COMBINED.PDF. Accessed June 18, 2018
13. Cady RK, Munjal S, Cady RJ et al (2017) Randomized, double-blind, crossover study comparing DFN-11 injection (3 mg subcutaneous sumatriptan) with 6 mg subcutaneous sumatriptan for the treatment of rapidly-escalating attacks of episodic migraine. J Headache Pain 18:17
14. Landy S, Munjal S, Brand-Schieber E et al (2018) Efficacy and safety of DFN-11 injection (sumatriptan 3 mg) in adults with episodic migraine: a multicenter, randomized, double-blind, placebo-controlled study. J headache pain. https://doi.org/10.1186/s10194-018-0881-z
15. (2004) The International Classification of Headache Disorders: 2nd edition. Cephalalgia 24(Suppl 1):9–160

16. Gobel H, Heinze A, Stolze H et al (1999) Open-labeled long-term study of the efficacy, safety, and tolerability of subcutaneous sumatriptan in acute migraine treatment. Cephalalgia 19:676–683 discussion 626

17. Sheftell FD, Weeks RE, Rapoport AM et al (1994) Subcutaneous sumatriptan in a clinical setting: the first 100 consecutive patients with acute migraine in a tertiary care center. Headache 34:67–72

18. Cady RK. Repeat-dose efficacy and laboratory safety trial of subcutaneous GR43175C in migraine patients (Study No. S2B-307). Available at: https://www.gsk-clinicalstudyregister.com/search/?search_terms=S2B-307. Accessed June 18, 2018

19. Gill HS, Prausnitz MR (2007) Does needle size matter? J Diabetes Sci Technol 1:725–729

20. Visser WH, Jaspers NM, De Vriend RH et al (1996) Chest symptoms after sumatriptan: a two-year clinical practice review in 735 consecutive migraine patients. Cephalalgia 16:554–559

7

Effects of topical vs injection treatment of cervical myofascial trigger points on headache symptoms in migraine patients: a retrospective analysis

Giannapia Affaitati[1*], Raffaele Costantini[2], Claudio Tana[3], Domenico Lapenna[4], Cosima Schiavone[4], Francesco Cipollone[5†] and Maria Adele Giamberardino[1†]

Abstract

Background: In migraine patients with cervical myofascial trigger points whose target areas coincide with migraine sites (M + cTrPs), TrP anesthetic injection reduces migraine symptoms, but the procedure often causes discomfort. This study evaluated if a topical TrP treatment with 3% nimesulide gel has similar efficacy as the injection but produces lesser discomfort with higher acceptability by the patients.

Methods: Retrospective analysis of medical charts of M + cTrPs patients in the period January 2012–December 2016 at a single Headache Center. Three groups of 25 patients each were included, all receiving migraine prophylaxis (flunarizine 5 mg/day) for 3 months and symptomatic treatment on demand. Group 1 received no TrP treatment, group 2 received TrP injections (bupivacaine 5 mg/ml at basis, 3rd, 10th, 30th and 60th day), group 3 received daily TrP topical treatment with 1.5 g of 3% nimesulide gel for 15 consecutive days, 15 days interruption and again 15 consecutive days. The following were evaluated: monthly number of migraine attacks and rescue medications, migraine intensity; pain thresholds to skin electrical stimulation (EPTs) and muscle pressure stimulation (PPTs) in TrP and target (basis, 30th, 60th and 180th days); discomfort from, acceptability of and willingness to repeat treatment (end of study). ANOVA for repeated measures and 1-way ANOVA were used to assess temporal trends in each group and comparisons among groups, respectively. Significance level was set at $p < 0.05$.

Results: Migraine improved over time in all groups, but significantly more and earlier in those receiving TrP treatment vs no TrP treatment ($0.02 < p < 0.0001$, 30–180 days for intensity and rescue medication, 60–180 days for number). All thresholds in the non-TrP-treated group did not change over time, while significantly improving in both the injection and nimesulide gel groups ($0.01 < p < 0.0001$, 30–180 days). Improvement of migraine and thresholds did not differ in the two TrP-treated groups. Discomfort was significantly lower, acceptability and willingness to repeat treatment significantly higher ($0.05 < p < 0.0001$) with gel than injection.

Conclusion: In migraine patients, topical treatment of cervical TrPs with 5% nimesulide gel proves equally effective as TrP injection with local anesthetics but more acceptable by the patients. This treatment could be effectively associated to standard migraine prophylaxis to improve therapeutic outcomes.

Keywords: Myofascial trigger points, Migraine, Nimesulide gel, Bupivacaine injection, Pain thresholds, Hyperalgesia

* Correspondence: gp@unich.it
†Francesco Cipollone and Maria Adele Giamberardino contributed equally to this work.
[1]Headache Center, Geriatrics Clinic, Department of Medicine and Science of Aging and Ce.S.I.-Met, G. D'Annunzio University of Chieti, 66100, Chieti, Italy
Full list of author information is available at the end of the article

Background

Migraine is a frequent and highly disabling pain condition; it is the 3rd most frequent disease in the world and is classified at the 6th place, when considered alone, and at the 3rd place, when also medication-overuse is included, in the list of the most invalidating diseases worldwilde, according to the World Health Organization [1–3]. In its typical expression migraine pain is unilateral and pulsating, very intense, accompanied by nausea and/or vomiting, phono and photophobia, aggravated by physical activity; during the attack the patient most often needs to stop any activity, lying in bed, avoiding any stimuli and contact with the environment. Furthermore, a number of studies have demonstrated that, especially when the mean number of montly attacks is high (e.g., > 7/month) or the condition is chronic (> 15 headache days/month), sensitization of somatic wall tissues (skin, subcutis and muscle) may occur in the site where migraine pain is perceived, proportional in extent to the frequency of the attacks, and persisting also in between the attacks [2].

Migraine is highly comorbid with other medical conditions, most of which painful, such as fibromyalgia, visceral pain/chronic pelvic pain, as well as myofascial pain syndromes (MPS) from trigger points (TrPs), i.e., sites of exquisite tenderness located in taut, palpable bands of muscle fibers, whose stimulation produces not only local pain but also pain referred to a distant area, called target [4–14]. TrPs are very frequent in the general population and in different patient groups [15–17], but in migraine patients their prevalence is indeed significantly higher than in healthy controls [18–24]. In addition, TrPs in cervical muscles of migraineurs most often present target areas coinciding with the sites of migraine pain [9]. This specific condition of comorbidity between migraine and cervical TrPs has been shown to be responsible not only for typical myofascial pain symptoms, but also for an increase in the number and intensity of migraine attacks [11, 25]. In these patients, the sensory evaluation at TrP and target level has furthermore evidenced a pain hypersensitivity (hyperalgesia, as revealed by a decrease in pain thresholds of the superficial and deep somatic tissues) which is increased with respect to that found in patients with MPS/TrPs only or migraine only [9, 26–31]. A previous study by this group showed that TrP injection (gold standard TrP therapy) with 0.5 ml bupivacaine (5 mg/ml) in repeated sessions (n. 5, within 2 months) not only determines TrP extinction, but also produces an improvement of migraine pain [11]. Patients undergoing this treatment, in fact, present, at the end of the therapeutic cycle, a significant reduction of the mean number of monthly migraine attacks and of their intensity, together with a significant improvement of the somatic hyperalgesia at TrP and target level.

Injection therapy of TrPs, however, though representing the gold standard treatment, is not deprived of undesirable effects, mostly pain during the procedure; in addition it necessarily requires the intervention of the physician who has to perform the injection periodically [32–34]. The possibility to treat the TrP topically, e.g., with application of a Non-Steroidal-Antiinflammatory-Drug (NSAID) on the overlying skin with the ischemic-compression technique, would have the advantage of avoiding the discomfort from the injection and any potential risk linked to this invasive procedure [32]. Furthermore the patient could be instructed to apply the product autonomously and therefore carry out the therapeutic cycle at home, without the intervention of the physician. Lastly, a topical treatment could be proposed also to patients who have needle phobia and refuse TrP injection for this reason [35].

Therefore if a topical NSAID treatment of the TrP proved equally effective as the TrP injection, but with lesser side effects/discomfort it would represent a valid alternative to the injection itself in TrP treatment. Nimesulide in gel formulation possesses antiinflammatory and analgesic properties; its use has already been approved for localized musculoskeletal pain conditions such as sprains, strains and tendinopathies [36–39]. Thanks to its characteristics of hydro and liposolubility, the gel formulation guarantees optimal penetration of the active molecule through the skin into the deep parietal tissues. In addition, after topical application of the gel, systemic levels of nimesulide have been shown to be 100 times lesser than those achieved after repeated oral administration [40, 41]. This preparation therefore presents adequate characteristics to be employed in the treatment of TrPs which are typically sites of localized inflammation in muscles [42].

On this basis, in migraine patients with a high frequency of attacks the aim of the study was to investigate if repeated applications of 3% nimesulide gel over cervical TrPs with target areas coinciding with the site of migraine pain are equally effective as the TrP anesthetic injections in extinguishing the TrPs and relieving migraine symptoms while producing lesser discomfort/side effects. The study was carried out by retrospectively analyzing records of patients with migraine plus cervical TrPs who underwent TrP injection or TrP topical treatment with nimesulide gel or no TrP treatment over the same time period.

Methods

Patients

Charts were retrospectively reviewed of consecutive patients referred for a first visit at the Headache Center, Department of Medicine and Science of Aging of the "G. D'Annunzio" University of Chieti in the period January 2012–December 2016, diagnosed with migraine without aura and myofascial trigger points of the cervical muscles with target areas coinciding with the site of migraine pain. Based on specific inclusion/exclusion criteria, patients were divided into three groups, i.e., patients who: received no TrP treatment (group 1), received TrP treatment with local anesthetic injection (group 2), received TrP treatment with 3% nimesulide gel (group 3).

Inclusion criteria for group 1 were as follows: both sexes, age 18–65 years, a diagnosis of migraine without aura performed according to the criteria established by the International Headache Society [2, 43] at least 1 year previously; number of monthly attacks: ≥ 7 in the past 2 months; presence of one ore more active myofascial trigger points in the cervical muscles, with target area coinciding with the site of migraine pain (diagnosis performed according to Travell and Simons criteria) [32–34]; exclusion of any other headache diagnosis except migraine without aura; a history of allergy and/or intolerance to NSAIDs and/or local anesthetics and/or phobia for the use of needles, preventing topical treatment or injection of the TrP; a negative clinical history for clinical conditions known to interfere with pain sensitivity in somatic tissues of the body wall (e.g., diabetes, hypertension, fibromyalgia) [4, 5, 8, 44, 45]; absence of neurological or neuropsychiatric diseases, or cognitive deficits potentially interfering with the correct execution of the evaluations routinely performed at the Center; no prophylaxis present at the moment of the first visit; start of standard prophylaxis with flunarizine 5 mg/day carried out for 3 months from the first visit; symptomatic therapy for the attacks with paracetamol 1 g (maximal dose: 3 g/day) or paracetamol + codeine (maximal dose: 2/day) and/or triptan (maximal dose: 2 administrations/day) [46–50]; for women in their fertile phase of life, negativity of pregnancy test and use, during the whole treatment period, of validated contraceptive methods; presence of the informed consent in the patients' records to undergo the standard evaluations and therapeutic protocols for their condition, routinely submitted to all patients at the first visit.

Inclusion criteria for patients of group 2 were the same as for group 1, except that they had a negative clinical history for intolerance to local anesthetics and presented no needle phobia, allowing local TrP treatment with anesthetic injections.

Inclusion criteria for patients of group 3 were the same as for group 1 except that they had a negative clinical history for allergy/intolerance to NSAIDs and had refused TrP injection due to either documented allergy/intolerance to local anesthetics or phobia for the use of needles, which had led to topical TrP treatment with 3% nimesulide gel.

The protocol was approved by the Institutional Review Board of the Department of Medicine and Science of Aging of the G D'Annunzio University of Chieti (Feb. 7, 2018; del. n. 90, Prot. N. 992/27.00 18, Tit III, CI 13).

Charts were reviewed consecutively, starting from December 2016 backwards, till reaching the number of 25 subjects per group.

A total of 757 charts had to be reviewed to select the 75 patients of the 3 groups.

Treatment groups

Group 1- no TrP treatment + migraine treatment. Patients did not receive TrP treatment, but only underwent migraine treatment (prophylaxis for 3 months, symptomatic on demand).

Group 2- TrP treatment with bupivacaine injection + migraine treatment. In addition to migraine treatment, patients received TrP treatment by the medical staff at the Center with n. 5 injections of the TrP with 0.5 ml of bupivacaine (5 mg/ml) over a period of 2 months (1 injection in basal conditions and then on the 3rd, 10th, 30th and 60th day after the first visit; injection was always performed after the sensory evaluation [see below]; in the case of multiple TrPs only the most active was treated) [11]. The injection was performed according to the internationally standardized technique [17].

Group 3 - TrP treatment with topical nimesulide + migraine treatment. In addition to migraine treatment, patients received TrP topical treament with nimesulide gel. The first application was carried out at the Center by the physician, then patients were instructed to treat their TrP at home, through massage/ischemic compression, with 1.5 g (corresponding to a 3 cm strip) of 3% nimesulide gel, over the TrP for further 14 consecutive days (15 application days overall). After 15 days of interruption they had to repeat the treatment cycle for further 15 days. The technique of massage/ischemic compression involves exact detection of the TrP, application of the gel on the overlying skin, and subsequent massage of the spot by applying a moderate compression so as to determine an ischemic condition of the microcirculation and, upon release, a reactive vasodilation, with washout of algogenic substances. The compression/release cycle has to be repeated 3–4 times in succession over several minutes [32–34].

This technique, in addition to promoting the wash-out of algogenic substances, promotes a better absorption of the gel.

Parameters examined

The following parameters are routinely evaluated at the Center in all patients with migraine at a high frequency of attacks plus cervical myofascial trigger points in basal conditions and after 30, 60 and 180 days from the start of treatment: (a) number of monthly migraine attacks through ad-hoc headache diary [10, 12, 51–54]; (b) intensity of headache attacks through numeric scale from 0 (no pain) to 10 (maximal imaginable pain) reported on the headache diary [55]; (c) monthly number of symptomatic drug consumption for the headache attacks through headache diary; (d) skin pain sensitivity through measurement of pain thresholds to electrical stimulation [EPTs] at TrP site and in the migraine pain area (target) according to a technique already described in detail elsewhere [4, 5, 10–12, 26, 35, 53, 54]; (e) muscle pain sensitivity through measurement of pain thresholds to pressure stimulation [PPTs] through Fischer's algometer at TrP site and in the migraine pain area [56]; (f) possible occurrence of adverse events.

Only in patients undergoing TrP therapy, at the end of the evaluation period the following parameters are assessed: (g) discomfort determined by the treatment procedure of the TrP, through numerical scale from 0 (absence of discomfort) to 10 (maximal discomfort); (h) acceptability of the treatment procedure through Visual Analogue Scale (VAS) from 0 (not acceptable) to 10 (totally acceptable); (i) availability to repetition of the treatment (YES or NO).

Technique for measurement of pain thresholds to electrical stimulation

A computerized constant current square wave electrical stimulator was used (R.S.D. stimulator, prototype, Florence 1997) [4, 5, 10, 11, 12, 26, 35, 53, 54]. The adopted stimuli were 18 msec trains of 0.5 ms square waves (internal frequency: 310 Hz), automatically delivered every 2 s.

To stimulate the skin, surface electrodes were used, constituted by 2 Ag/AgCl circular plates, 10 mm in diameter. The electrodes were positioned on the skin with interposition of a conductor paste, 1 cm apart in the longitudinal sense. Stimulation was initiated at low intensities of current (0.1 mA) and the intensity was automatically increased by the instrument, with every stimulus repeated at current increases of 0.1 mA until the subject reported a first tactile sensation and then continuing with the same rate of current increases until the subject reported a sensation of pricking pain.

Pain thresholds were measured with the method of the limits, i.e., the current value corresponding to the first report of the sensation of pricking pain was recorded and memorized by the computer, then the intensity of the stimulus was gradually decreased, always at the same rate (0.1 mA/sec), until the sensation disappeared (with recording of the corresponding current value). The intensity of the current was then again increased with recording of the corresponding value. The mean of these 3 values, automatically calculated by the stimulator computer, was considered as the final threshold for each examined site. The subject was instructed to signal the appearance/disappearance of the sensation by pressing a button connected to the stimulator. During the whole duration of the stimulation session the subject was lying comfortably on an adjustable

examination bed, in a quiet room, with the examinator close to the bed to place the electrodes and perform the test.

The subjects were informed that the evaluation test was not an endurance test for pain, that only a minimal sensation of pain had to be reported. They were further informed that they were free to interrupt the stimulation at any moment for any reason without any penalty.

Technique for pain threshold measurement to pressure stimulation

The evaluation was performed through Fischer's algometer (Great Neck, New York). The instrument is a pressure dynamometer with a rounded circular probe, 1 cm2 in diameter, with a 0-10 kg-f scale. The probe was perpendicularly positioned on the skin overlying the muscle area to be tested, and the pressure was gradually increased at a 0.1 kgf/sec rate until the subject reported a first sensation of discomfort. The corresponding kg-f value was recorded as pain threshold for that site [56].

Every subject was examined in a quiet room at constant temperature and humidity. The evaluations were always performed at the same time of day (h 9–14).

Statistical analysis

For each group, Means ± Standard Deviation (SD) were calculated for each parameter at every evaluation time. Within each group, the temporal trend of each variable was evaluated through Analysis of Variance (ANOVA) for repeated measures. The comparison among groups, for number and intensity of attacks, and consumption of symptomatics at every evaluation time was performed through 1-way ANOVA. The comparison between the two groups of patients undergoing active TrP treatment, regarding treatment discomfort and acceptability of treatment was performed via Student's t-test for independent data. The comparison between groups for the repeatability of treatment was performed via the chi-square test.

The level of significance was established at $p < 0.05$.

Results

In basal conditions, the three groups proved to be homogeneous regarding sex and age, i.e., group 1 (no TrP treatment): 19 women and 6 men, 30.76 ± 8.55 years (Mean ± SD); group 2 (TrP injection treatment): 19 women and 6 men, 33.6 ± 8.21 years; group 3 (TrP nimesulide gel treatment): 18 women and 7 men, 32.64 ± 7.40 years. There were furthermore no significant differences regarding all the evaluated parameters.

Patients of all groups were affected with unilateral frontal or temporal migraine without aura (with no alternation of side) and showed myofascial TrPs in the sternocleidomastoid, semispinalis cervicis or splenius cervicis with referred pain sites (targets) coinciding with the site of migraine pain (frontal and/or temporal region).

Migraine parameters and pain thresholds
Group 1 - no TrP treatment +migraine treatment
Number and intensity of migraine attacks progressively decreased during the treatment period (ANOVA: $p < 0.001$), but significant effects were only evident at 60 and 180 days from the start of treatment ($0.01 < p < 0.001$) (Fig. 1). Symptomatic drug consumption also progressively decreased (ANOVA: $p < 0.0001$), with significant effects at 60 and 180 days ($p < 0.001$) (Fig. 2).

Pain thresholds to electrical and pressure stimulation did not undergo any significant change (Figs. 3, 4).

None of the patients reported any improvement of other concurrent pre-existing painful conditions.

Group 2- TrP treatment with bupivacaine injection + migraine treatment
There was a significant trend for reduction of number and intensity of migraine attacks and, in parallel, also of symptomatic drug consumption (ANOVA: $p < 0.0001$) (Figs. 1, 2). The difference was already highly significant at day 30, becoming progressively more accentuated over the study period ($p < 0.001$ for all internal comparisons).

Pain thresholds to electrical and pressure stimulation at TrP and target significantly and progressively increased

with treatment (ANOVA: $p < 0.0001$), the difference was already highly significant at day 30, persisting so up to 180 days (Figs. 3, 4).

Lastly, n° 15 patients spontaneously reported an improvement of a concurrent cervicalgia/cervicobrachialgia.

Group 3 - TrP treatment with topical nimesulide + migraine treatment
There was a significant trend for reduction of number and intensity of migraine attacks and in parallel, also of symptomatic drug consumption (ANOVA: $p < 0.0001$) (Figs. 1, 2). The reduction was already significant at day 30 ($p < 0.05$ for number of attacks and drug consumption, $p < 0.01$ for intensity) and became progressively more accentuated over the evaluation period ($p < 0.001$ at 60 and 180 days). Pain thresholds to both electrical and pressure stimulation significantly increased with treatment in TrP and target (ANOVA: $p < 0.0001$), the difference was already significant at day 30 ($p < 0.01$) and became progressively more accentuated over the evaluation period ($p < 0.001$ at 60 and 180 days) (Figs. 3, 4).

Lastly, n. 12 patients spontaneously reported improvement of a concurrent cervicalgia/cervicobrachialgia.

Comparison among the three patient groups
The number of migraine attacks was significantly lower in the two groups undergoing active treatment of the

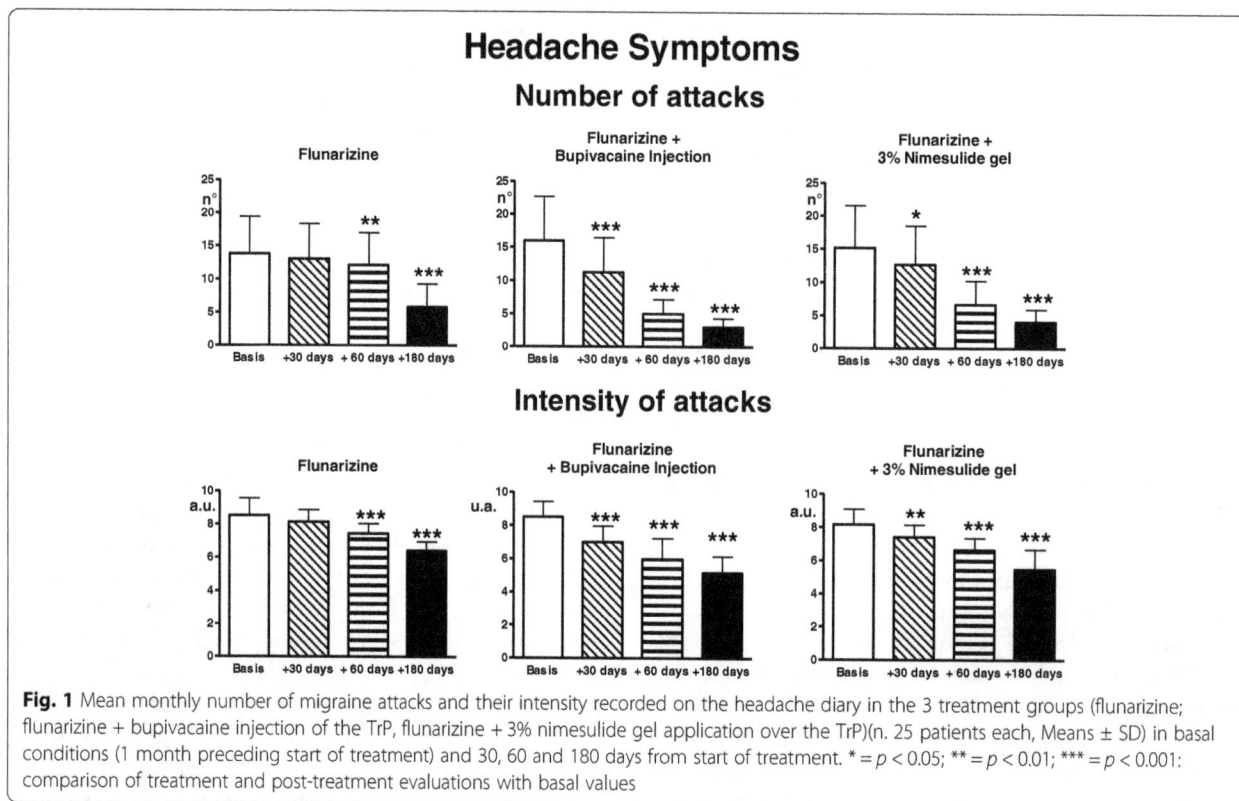

Fig. 1 Mean monthly number of migraine attacks and their intensity recorded on the headache diary in the 3 treatment groups (flunarizine; flunarizine + bupivacaine injection of the TrP, flunarizine + 3% nimesulide gel application over the TrP)(n. 25 patients each, Means ± SD) in basal conditions (1 month preceding start of treatment) and 30, 60 and 180 days from start of treatment. $* = p < 0.05$; $** = p < 0.01$; $*** = p < 0.001$: comparison of treatment and post-treatment evaluations with basal values

Symptomatic Drug Consumption

Fig. 2 Symptomatic drug consumption for migraine attacks. Legend as for Fig. 1

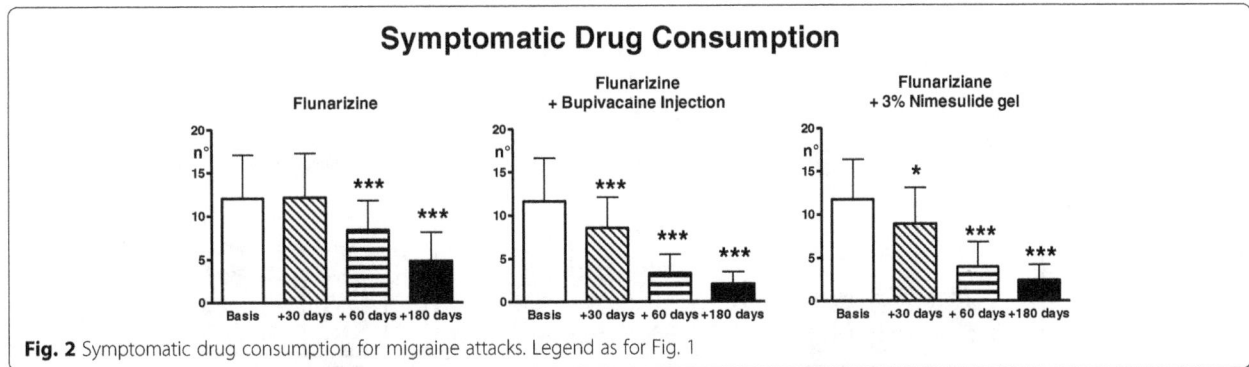

TrP with respect to the TrP-untreated group at 60 days (ANOVA: $p < 0.0001$, untreated vs injection and vs gel: $p < 0.001$) and 180 days (ANOVA: $p < 0.0004$, untreated vs injection: $p < 0.001$; untreated vs gel: $p < 0.05$)(Fig. 1).

The intensity of migraine attacks and the symptomatic drug consumption were significantly reduced in the two groups treated with bupivacaine injection and nimesulide gel with respect to the TrP-untreated group at 30, 60 and 180 days (for intensity at 30 days, ANOVA: $p < 0.0001$, untreated vs injection: $p < 0.001$; for intensity at 60 days, ANOVA: $p < 0.0001$, untreated vs injection: $p < 0.001$, untreated vs gel: $p < 0.01$; for intensity at 180 days, ANOVA $p < 0.0001$, untreated vs injection: $p < 0.001$; untreated vs gel: $p < 0.01$; for symptomatic drug consumption at 30 days, ANOVA: $p < 0.02$; untreated vs injection and vs gel: $p < 0.05$; at 60 days, ANOVA $p < 0.0001$, untreated vs injection and

vs gel: $p < 0.001$; at 180 days, ANOVA: $p < 0.0006$, untreated vs injection: $p < 0.001$, untreated vs gel: $p < 0.01$) (Figs. 1, 2).

The comparison among groups regarding skin EPTs in the trigger showed a significant trend at 30 days (ANOVA: $p < 0.0001$, untreated vs injection: $p < 0.001$; untreated vs gel: $p < 0.01$), 60 days (ANOVA: $p < 0.0001$; untreated vs injection and vs gel: $p < 0.001$), 180 days (ANOVA: $p < 0.0001$; untreated vs injection and vs gel: $p < 0.001$).

The comparison among groups regarding skin EPTs in the target showed a significant trend at 30 days (ANOVA: $p < 0.01$, untreated vs injection: $p < 0.05$), at 60 days (ANOVA: $p < 0.0001$, untreated vs injection and vs gel: $p < 0.001$) and 180 days (ANOVA: $p < 0.0001$; untreated vs injection and vs gel: $p < 0.001$).

The comparison among groups regarding PPTs at trigger level revealed a significant trend at 30 days

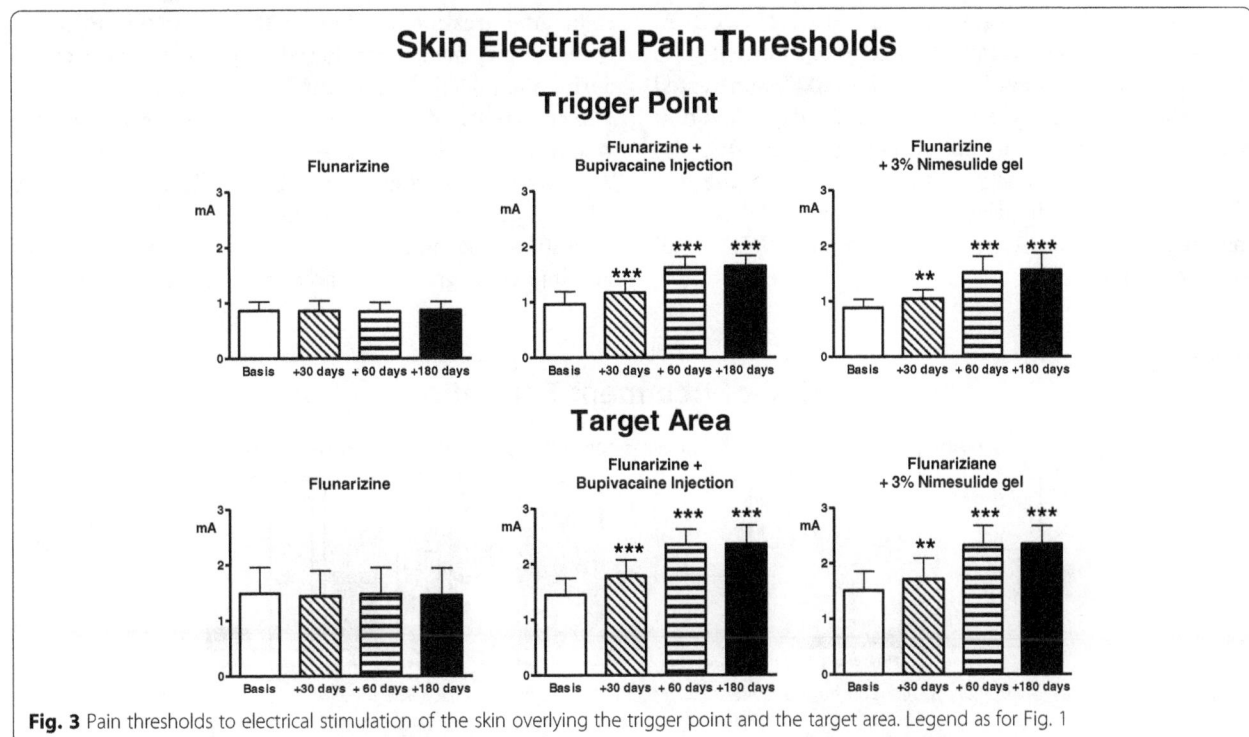

Skin Electrical Pain Thresholds

Trigger Point

Target Area

Fig. 3 Pain thresholds to electrical stimulation of the skin overlying the trigger point and the target area. Legend as for Fig. 1

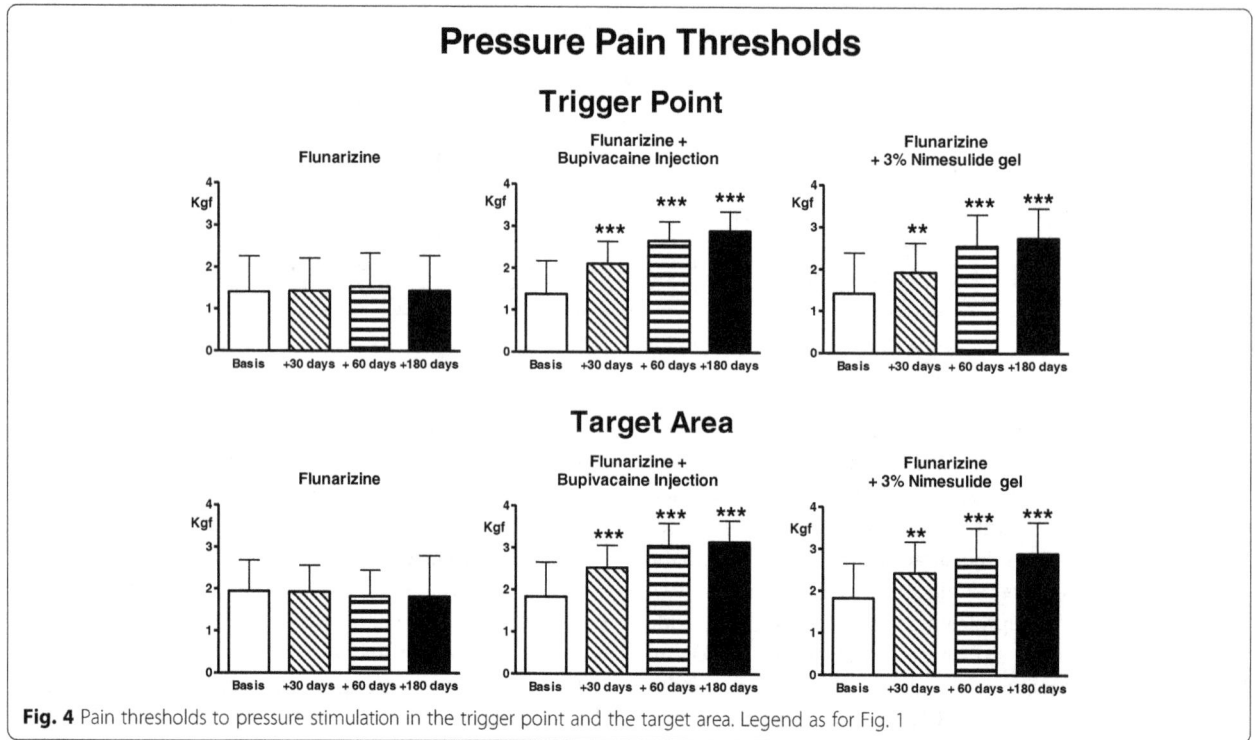

Fig. 4 Pain thresholds to pressure stimulation in the trigger point and the target area. Legend as for Fig. 1

(ANOVA: $p < 0.003$, untreated vs injection: $p < 0.01$, untreated vs gel: $p < 0.05$), at 60 days (ANOVA: $p < 0.0001$, untreated vs injection and vs gel: $p < 0.001$) and 180 days (ANOVA: $p < 0.0001$, untreated vs injection and vs gel: $p < 0.001$).

The comparison among groups regarding PPTs in the target showed a significant trend at 30 days (ANOVA: $p < 0.004$, untreated vs injection: $p < 0.01$, untreated vs gel: $p < 0.05$), at 60 days (ANOVA: $p < 0.0001$, untreated vs injection and vs gel: $p < 0.001$) and at 180 days (ANOVA: $p < 0.0001$, untreated vs injection and vs gel: $p < 0.001$).

There was no significant difference between the two TrP active groups (bupivacaine and nimesulide) regarding migraine parameters, skin EPTs and PPTs at all evaluation times.

End-of-study evaluation

No adverse event was recorded in any of the study groups.

The discomfort from treatment in the nimesulide group was significantly lower than that recorded in the injection group ($p < 0.0001$)(Fig. 5a). For nimesulide gel, the discomfort was attributed to the residual yellow color after treatment, while in the bupivacine injection group it was mainly attributed to the pain experienced during the injection procedure.

Acceptability of the treatment was significantly higher in the nimesulide gel-treated group compared with the bupivacaine-treated group ($p < 0.0001$)(Fig. 5b).

Lastly, as regards treatment repeatability, n° 22 patients of the nimesulide group and n° 14 patients of the injection group declared they were prepared to

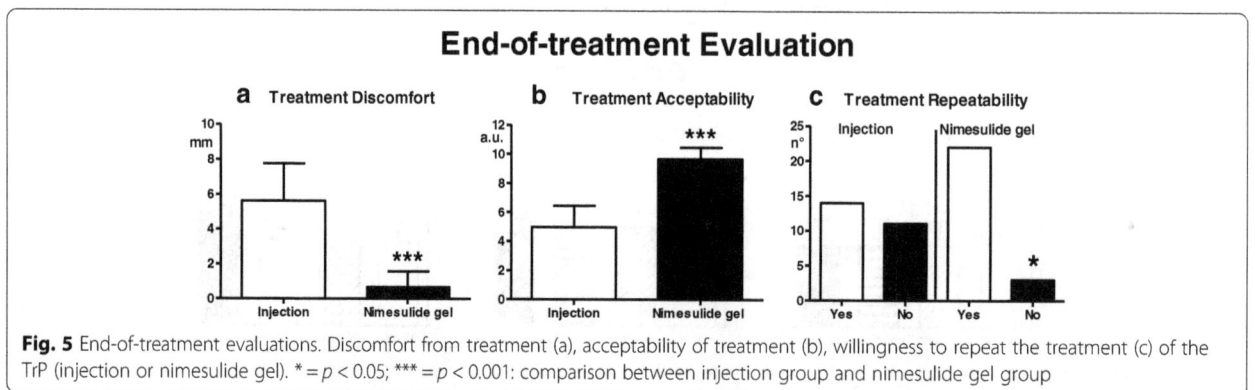

Fig. 5 End-of-treatment evaluations. Discomfort from treatment (a), acceptability of treatment (b), willingness to repeat the treatment (c) of the TrP (injection or nimesulide gel). * = $p < 0.05$; *** = $p < 0.001$: comparison between injection group and nimesulide gel group

repeat the treatment if necessary. The difference between the two groups was significant ($p < 0.05$)(Fig. 5c).

Discussion

In migraine patients with active cervical myofascial trigger points whose target area coincides with that of migraine pain, migraine prophylaxis with flunarizine for 3 months, not associated with TrP treatment, produces a significant improvement of migraine parameters (number and intensity of attacks, symptomatic drug consumption) from the 60th day after start of treatment, and continuing at 3 months after treatment suspension (180th day) but determines no improvement in specific myofascial pain symptoms related to TrPs, as shown by the lack of any change in sensory thresholds at both TrP and target area over the same time frame.

In M + TrPs patients in whom migraine prophylaxis with flunarizine is associated with TrP treatment, either with anesthetic injection or with topical 3% nimesulide gel, the improvement of migraine parameters occurs earlier (at the 30th day) and is significantly more pronounced than that occurring in M + TrPs patients receiving migraine prophylaxis only at all determination times, until the 180th day. In addition, both TrPs treatments produce a significant improvement of the sensory asset at TrP and target level, with reduction of superficial and deep somatic hyperalgesia, which is not observed in M + TrPs patients undergoing migraine prophylaxis only. Athough the injection procedure produces slightly better results than the topical treatment at 30 days for all parameters, the difference between the two active treatments is never significant.

No prominent side effects occur with either injection or topical TrP treatment, however the former procedure produces a much higher perceived discomfort than the latter (pain at injection vs a minimal discomfort from nimesulide due to cosmetic reasons, i.e., the residual yellow coloration), as a consequence the degree of acceptability of the therapy is significantly higher for the topical treatment than for the injection. The possibility of self-administration of nimesulide gel vs necessary medical intervention for the injection is also better perceived by the patients who are therefore willing to repeat the treatment, if necessary, in a significantly higher percentage than patients subjected to the injection.

The results of the present study firstly confirm the efficacy of local treatment of cervical TrPs on migraine symptoms already shown in a previous study with anesthetic injection [11]. The pathophysiology of this phenomenon remains to be elucidated in full, but a plausible hypothesis is that suppression of the afferent sensory signals towards the Central Nervous System from the TrPs, which are powerful sources of nociceptive inputs [42], reduces the level of central sensitization

of trigeminal neurons involved in migraine pain processing, thus decreasing migraine symptoms and somatic tissue hypersensitivity in the pain area [9, 11, 30].

The present study also shows for the first time that topical TrP treatment with a NSAID applied with massage/ischemic compression has similar efficacy as that of standard treatment modality with injection, but with the advantage of a better tolerability, easier modality of application and reduced costs for the health care system.

In a single Headache Center study in Italy, nimesulide orally administered was shown to represent the top preference NSAID in the treatment of acute migraine attacks [46]. Given the nonsignificant absorbtion in the general circulation of the molecule locally applied onto somatic tissues in gel formulation it is highly unlikely that the reduction of migraine symptoms in the present study, after TrP treatment with the gel, is due to a direct effect of nimesulide on the migraine condition. In addition, the duration of the benefits of the treatment goes far beyond a possible direct action of the molecule. Thus the only interpretation of migraine improvement with this treatment is an indirect action exerted by nimesulide gel onto the TrPs, similarly to what hypothesized for the effect of local anesthetic injection.

The present study has several limitations, firstly its retrospective nature, then the relatively short duration of the follow-up, and lastly the lack of a comparator group, i.e., massage/ischemic compression of the TrP without application of an active topical compound, to eliminate the confounding factor of the simple manoeuver of TrP release and separate the therapeutic effects of the manoeuver from those of the drug at local level. Further prospective studies will have to be conducted for confirmation.

In spite of these limitations, however, we believe that the results here presented have potential important therapeutic implications in migraine patients with the described characteristics.

Conclusion

In conclusion, in migraine patients with a high frequency of attacks plus cervical myofascial trigger points with target areas coinciding with the site of migraine pain, the combination of standard migraine prophylaxis with local TrP treatment provides better efficacy results than migraine prophylaxis only. TrP topical treatment with a NSAID, such as nimesulide gel, proves equally effective as the TrP anesthetic injection, but is better tolerated by the patients, with the further advantage of the possible self-administration. These results, though preliminary, are of relevance in routine medical practice, suggesting use of this topical treatment in addition to the standard migraine prevention measures, to help enhance the therapeutic outcome [47–50, 57].

Abbreviations

ANOVA: Analysis of Variance; EPTs: Electrical pain thresholds; M + cTrPs: Migraine patients with cervical myofascial trigger points whose target areas coincide with migraine sites; MPS: Myofascial pain syndromes; NSAID: Non Steroidal Antiinflammatory Drug; PPTs: Pressure pain thresholds; TrPs: Myofascial trigger points; VAS: Visual analogue scale

Acknowledgements

Not applicable.

Funding

No funding was received to carry out the present study.

Authors' contributions

GA conceived the protocol, participated in reviewing the patients' charts, data analysis, literature search and writing of the paper. RC participated in reviewing the patients' charts, data analysis, literature search and writing of the paper. CT, CS and DL participated in the analysis of data and literature searching. FC and MAG participated in the writing of the paper and its critical revision. All authors read and approved the final manuscript.

Competing interests

In the past 2 years: GA received personal fees for participation in Conferences from Epitech Group. MAG received research funding for topics unrelated to the present study from Epitech Group, and personal fees for participation in Conferences from IBSA Institute Biochimique, Helsinn Healthcare and Epitech Group. RC, CT, DL, CS and FC have no competing interests in relation to the present study.

Author details

[1]Headache Center, Geriatrics Clinic, Department of Medicine and Science of Aging and Ce.S.I.-Met, G. D'Annunzio University of Chieti, 66100, Chieti, Italy. [2]Institute of Surgical Pathology, G. D'Annunzio University of Chieti, Chieti, Italy. [3]Internal Medicine and Critical Subacute Care Unit, Medicine Geriatric-Rehabilitation Department, University-Hospital of Parma, Via Antonio Gramsci 14, 43126 Parma, Italy. [4]Department of Medicine and Science of Aging, G. D'Annunzio University of Chieti, Chieti, Italy. [5]Medical Clinic, G. D'Annunzio University of Chieti, Chieti, Italy.

References

1. Disease GBD, Injury I, Prevalence C (2017) Global, regional, and national incidence, prevalence, and years lived with disability for 328 diseases and injuries for 195 countries, 1990-2016: a systematic analysis for the global burden of disease study 2016. Lancet 390:1211–1259
2. Headache Classification of the International Headache Society (2013) The international classification of headache disorders, 3rd edition (beta version). Cephalalgia 33:627–808
3. Martelletti P (2018) Migraine disability complicated by medication overuse. Eur J Neurol 25(10):1193–1194
4. Costantini R, Affaitati G, Massimini F, Tana C, Innocenti P, Giamberardino MA (2016) Laparoscopic Cholecystectomy for Gallbladder Calculosis in Fibromyalgia Patients: Impact on Musculoskeletal Pain, Somatic Hyperalgesia and Central Sensitization. PLoS One 11(4):e0153408
5. Costantini R, Affaitati G, Wesselmann U, Czakanski P, Giamberardino MA (2017) Visceral pain as a triggering factor for fibromyalgia symptoms in comorbid patients. Pain 158(10):1925–1937
6. Costantini R, Di Bartolomeo N, Francomano F, Angelucci D, Innocenti P (2005) Epithelioid angiosarcoma of the gallbladder: case report. J Gastrointest Surg 9(6):822–825
7. Giamberardino MA, Affaitati G, Costantini R (2006) Chapter 24 referred pain from internal organs. Handb Clin Neurol 81:343–361
8. Giamberardino MA, Affaitati G, Fabrizio A, Costantini R (2011) Effects of treatment of myofascial trigger points on the pain of fibromyalgia. Curr Pain Headache Rep 15(5):393–399
9. Giamberardino MA, Affaitati G, Fabrizio A, Costantini R (2011) Myofascial pain syndromes and their evaluation. Best Pract Res Clin Rheumatol 25(2):185–198
10. Giamberardino MA, Affaitati G, Martelletti P, Tana C, Negro A, Lapenna D et al (2015) Impact of migraine on fibromyalgia symptoms. J Headache Pain. 17:28
11. Giamberardino MA, Tafuri E, Savini A, Fabrizio A, Affaitati G, Lerza R et al (2007) Contribution of myofascial trigger points to migraine symptoms. J Pain 8(11):869–878
12. Giamberardino MA, Tana C, Costantini R (2014) Pain thresholds in women with chronic pelvic pain. Curr Opin Obstet Gynecol 26(4):253–259
13. Giamberardino MA, Vecchiet L (1995) Visceral pain, referred hyperalgesia and outcome: new concepts. Eur J Anaesthesiol (Suppl) 10:61–66
14. Tana C, Tafuri E, Tana M, Martelletti P, Negro A, Affaitati G et al (2013) New insights into the cardiovascular risk of migraine and the role of white matter hyperintensities: is gold all that glitters? J Headache Pain 14:9
15. Costantini R, Sardellone A, Marino C, Giamberardino MA, Innocenti P, Napolitano AM (2005) Vacuum-assisted core biopsy (Mammotome) for the diagnosis of non-palpable breast lesions: four-year experience in an Italian center. Tumori 91(4):351–354
16. Ko EJ, Jeon JY, Kim W, Hong JY, Yi YG (2017) Referred symptom from myofascial pain syndrome: One of the most important causes of sensory disturbance in breast cancer patients using taxanes. Eur J Cancer Care (Engl) 26:6
17. Gerwin RD (2016) Myofascial trigger point pain syndromes. Semin Neurol 36(5):469–473
18. Calandre EP, Hidalgo J, García-Leiva JM, Rico-Villademoros F (2006) Trigger point evaluation in migraine patients: an indication of peripheral sensitization linked to migraine predisposition? Eur J Neurol 13(3):244–249
19. Cummings M, Baldry P (2007) Regional myofascial pain: diagnosis and management. Best Prac Res Clin Rheumatol 21:367–387
20. Do TP, Heldarskard GF, Kolding LT, Hvedstrup J, Schytz HW (2018) Myofascial trigger points in migraine and tension-type headache. J Headache Pain 19(1):84
21. Fernández-de-Las-Peñas C (2015) Myofascial head pain. Curr Pain Headache Rep 19(7):28
22. Fernández-de-Las-Peñas C, Cuadrado ML, Pareja JA (2006) Myofascial trigger points, neck mobility and forward head posture in unilateral migraine. Cephalalgia 26:1061–1070
23. Tali D, Menahem I, Vered E, Kalichman L (2014) Upper cervical mobility, posture and myofascial trigger points in subjects with episodic migraine: case-control study. J Bodyw Mov Ther 18:569–575
24. Vecchiet L, Giamberardino MA, Saggini R (1991) Myofascial pain syndromes: clinical and patophysiological aspects. Clin J Pain 7:16–22
25. Affaitati G, Giamberardino MA, Lapenna D, Costantini R (2018) Diclofenac epolamine topical patch for the treatment of pain. J Biol Regul Homeost Agents 32(3):435–441
26. Affaitati G, Fabrizio A, Savini A, Lerza R, Tafuri E, Costantini R et al (2009) A randomized, controlled study comparing a lidocaine patch, a placebo patch, and anesthetic injection for treatment of trigger points in patients with myofascial pain syndrome: evaluation of pain and somatic pain thresholds. Clin Ther 31(4):705–720
27. Buchgreitz L, Lyngberg AC, Bendtsen L, Jensen R (2008) Increased pain sensitivity is not a risk factor but a consequence of frequent headache: a population-based follow-up study. Pain 137(3):623–630
28. Burstein R, Yarnitsky D, Goor-Aryeh I, Ransil BJ, Bajwa ZH (2000) An association between migraine and cutaneous allodynia. Ann Neurol 47:614–624

29. Kitaj MB, Klink M (2005) Pain thresholds in daily transformed migraine versus episodic migraine headache patients. Headache 45:992–998

30. Lipton RB, Bigal ME, Ashina S, Burstein R, Silberstein S, Reed ML et al (2008) Cutaneous allodynia in the migraine population. Ann Neurol 63:148–158

31. Vecchiet L, Giamberardino MA, Dragani L, De Bigontina P, Albe-Fessard D (1990) Latent myofascial trigger points: changes in muscular and in subcutaneous pain thresholds at trigger point and target level. J Man Med 5:151–154

32. Simons DG (2008) New views of myofascial trigger points: etiology and diagnosis. Arch Phys Med Rehabil 89:157–159

33. Simons DG, Mense S (2003) Diagnosis and therapy of myofascial trigger points. Schmerz 17:419–424

34. Simons DG, Travell JG, Simons LS (1999) Travell & Simons' myofascial pain and dysfunction. In: The trigger point manual. Vol 1, upper half of body, 2nd edn. Williams & Wilkins, Baltimore

35. Affaitati G, Fabrizio A, Frangione V, Lanzarotti A, Lopopolo M, Tafuri E et al (2015) Effects of topical diclofenac plus heparin (DHEP+H plaster) on somatic pain sensitivity in healthy subjects with a latent algogenic condition of the lower limb. Pain Pract 15(1):58–67

36. Al-Abd AM, Al-Abbasi FA, Nofal SM, Khalifa AE, Williams RO, El-Eraky WI et al (2014) Nimesulide improves the symptomatic and disease modifying effects of leflunomide in collagen induced arthritis. PLoS One 9(11):e111843

37. Kress HG, Baltov A, Basiński A, Berghea F, Castellsague J, Codreanu C et al (2016) Acute pain: a multifaceted challenge - the role of nimesulide. Curr Med Res Opin 32(1):23–36

38. Rainsford KD (2006) Current status of the therapeutic uses and actions of the preferential cyclo-oxygenase-2 NSAID, nimesulide. Inflammopharmacology 14(3–4):120–137

39. Rainsford KD (2006) Nimesulide a multifactorial approach to inflammation and pain: scientific and clinical consensus. Curr Med Res Opin 22(6):1161–1170

40. Ergün H, Külcü D, Kutlay S, Bodur H, Tulunay FC (2007) Efficacy and safety of topical nimesulide in the treatment of knee osteoarthritis. Clin Rheumatol 13(5):251–255

41. Gupta SK, Ptrakash J, Awor L, Velpandian T, Sengupta S (1996) Anti-inflammatory activity of topical nimesulide gel in various experimental models. Inflamm Res 45(12):590–592

42. Shah JP, Phillips TM, Danoff JV, Gerber LH (2005) An in vivo microanalytical technique for measuring the local biochemical milieu of human skeletal muscle. J Appl Physiol 99:1977–1984

43. Headache Classification of the International Headache Society (2004) The International Classification of headache disorders, Cephalalgia, vol 24(1), 2nd edn, pp 1–151

44. Obrosova IG (2009) Diabetic painful and insensate neuropathy: pathogenesis and potential treatments. Neurotherapeutics 6:638–647

45. Viggiano A, Zagaria N, Passavanti MB, Pace MC, Paladini A, Aurilio C et al (2009) New and low-cost auto-algometry for screening hypertension-associated hypoalgesia. Pain Pract 9:260–265

46. Affaitati G, Martelletti P, Lopopolo M, Tana C, Massimini F, Cipollone F et al (2017) Use of nonsteroidal anti-inflammatory drugs for symptomatic treatment of episodic headache. Pain Pract 17(3):392–401

47. Bartolini M, Giamberardino MA, Lisotto C, Martelletti P, Moscato D, Panascia B et al (2011) A double-blind, randomized, multicenter, Italian study of frovatriptan versus almotriptan for the acute treatment of migraine. J Headache Pain 12(3):361–368

48. Karsan N, Palethorpe D, Rattanawong W, Marin JC, Bhola R, Goadsby PJ (2018) Flunarizine in migraine-related headache prevention: results from 200 patients treated in the UK. Eur J Neurol 25(6):811–817

49. Loder E, Rizzoli P (2018) Pharmacologic prevention of migraine: a narrative review of the state of the art in 2018. Headache. https://doi.org/10.1111/head.13375 [Epub ahead of print]

50. Pomes LM, Gentile G, Simmaco M, Borro M, Martelletti (2018) Tailoring Treatment in Polymorbid Migraine Patients through Personalized Medicine. CNS Drugs. https://doi.org/10.1007/s40263-018-0532-6 [Epub ahead of print]

51. Giamberardino MA, Affaitati G, Costantini R, Cipollone F, Martelletti P (2017) Calcitonin gene-related peptide receptor as a novel target for the management of people with eptisodic migraine: current evidence and safety profile of erenumab. J Pain Res 10:2751–2760

52. Giamberardino MA, Affaitati G, Curto M, Negro A, Costantini R, Martelletti P (2016) Anti-CGRP monoclonal antibodies in migraine: current perspectives. Intern Emerg Med 11(8):1045–1057

53. Giamberardino MA, Costantini R, Affaitati G, Fabrizio A, Lapenna D, Tafuri E et al (2010) Viscero-visceral hyperalgesia: characterization in different clinical models. Pain 151(2):307–322

54. Giamberardino MA, Affaitati G, Lerza R, Lapenna D, Costantini R, Vecchiet L (2005) Relationship between pain symptoms and referred sensory and trophic changes in patients with gallbladder pathology. Pain 114:239–249

55. Chapman CR, Syrjala KL (1990) Measurement of Pain. In: Bonica JJ (ed) The Management of Pain, 2nd edn. Lea & Febiger, Philadelphia, pp 580–594

56. Fischer AA (1998) Muscle pain syndromes and fibromyalgia. Pressure algometry for quantification of diagnosis and treatment outcome. J Musculoske Pain 1:6–152

57. Giamberardino MA, Costantini R (2017) Challenging chronic migraine: targeting the CGRP receptor. Lancet Neurol 16(6):410–411

8

Gender differences in functional connectivities between insular subdivisions and selective pain-related brain structures

Yu-Jie Dai[1,2,3†], Xin Zhang[1†], Yang Yang[1†], Hai-Yan Nan[1], Ying Yu[1], Qian Sun[1], Lin-Feng Yan[1], Bo Hu[1], Jin Zhang[1], Zi-Yu Qiu[4], Yi Gao[4], Guang-Bin Cui[1*], Bi-Liang Chen[2*] and Wen Wang[1*] (ID)

Abstract

Background: The incidence of pain disorders in women is higher than in men, making gender differences in pain a research focus. The human insular cortex is an important brain hub structure for pain processing and is divided into several subdivisions, serving different functions in pain perception. Here we aimed to examine the gender differences of the functional connectivities (FCs) between the twelve insular subdivisions and selected pain-related brain structures in healthy adults.

Methods: Twenty-six healthy males and 11 age-matched healthy females were recruited in this cross-sectional study. FCs between the 12 insular subdivisions (as 12 regions of interest (ROIs)) and the whole brain (ROI-whole brain level) or 64 selected pain-related brain regions (64 ROIs, ROI-ROI level) were measured between the males and females.

Results: Significant gender differences in the FCs of the insular subdivisions were revealed: (1) The FCs between the dorsal dysgranular insula (dId) and other brain regions were significantly increased in males using two different techniques (ROI-whole brain and ROI-ROI analyses); (2) Based on the ROI-whole brain analysis, the FC increases in 4 FC-pairs were observed in males, including the left dId - the right median cingulate and paracingulate/ right posterior cingulate gyrus/ right precuneus, the left dId - the right median cingulate and paracingulate, the left dId - the left angular as well as the left dId - the left middle frontal gyrus; (3) According to the ROI-ROI analysis, increased FC between the left dId and the right rostral anterior cingulate cortex was investigated in males.

Conclusion: In summary, the gender differences in the FCs of the insular subdivisions with pain-related brain regions were revealed in the current study, offering neuroimaging evidence for gender differences in pain processing.

Keywords: Gender differences, Insular subdivisions, Pain, Functional connectivity, Resting-state

* Correspondence: cgbtd@126.com; chenbiliang0728@126.com; wangwen@fmmu.edu.cn
Yu-Jie Dai, Xin Zhang and Yang Yang contributed equally to this work.
†Equal contributors
[1]Department of Radiology & Functional and Molecular Imaging Key Lab of Shaanxi Province, Tangdu Hospital, the Military Medical University of PLA Airforce (Fourth Military Medical University), 569 Xinsi Road, Xi'an, Shaanxi Province 710038, China
[2]Department of Obstetrics and Gynecology, Xijing Hospital, the Military Medical University of PLA Airforce (Fourth Military Medical University), 15 West Changle Road, Xi'an, Shaanxi Province 710032, China
Full list of author information is available at the end of the article

Background

Pain is one of the most common complaints making people seek medical attention, affecting over one-quarter of the global population, and its incidence increases with aging [1]. Besides aging, gender is another important factor affecting pain procession due to its high prevalence in women [2]. In a large scale study, women report higher pain intensity scores than men under the similar pain conditions [3]. Besides, females are more frequently suffered from pain disorders, such as migraine [4, 5], temporomandibular joint disorder [6], fibromyalgia [7, 8] as well as irritable bowel syndrome (IBS) [9, 10]. These findings suggest that there may be structural or functional gender differences in the brain matrix for pain processing in varied pain disorders [6]. Therefore, a thorough understanding of the central mechanisms underlying this gender differences in healthy people is pivotal for pain research.

Pain experience involves the interaction among sensory, emotional, cognitive, genetic and environmental factors [11] and pain processing is complicated, comprising a variety of brain regions working in concert. Functional magnetic resonance imaging (fMRI) technique has been performed to delineate a set of cortical and subcortical structures-the pain matrix-in pain perception [12, 13]. The classical pain matrix consists of three networks, i.e. the sensory, affective and cognitive networks [14–16]. The sensory network involves the lateral thalamus, primary (SI) and secondary (SII) somatic cortices, the insular cortex as well [17]. Among them, the insular cortex has been suggested to participate in both sensory-discriminative and affective-motivational aspects of pain processing [18]. The stronger pain activations of the somatosensory and the insular cortices in men while medial prefrontal cortex in women under pain challenging have been reported in the previous neuroimaging studies [19–21]. Furthermore, female IBS patients demonstrated significant functional alterations in the insular cortex than male patients [22]. Rather than evaluating evoked responses, it is possible to measure neural activity that is not linked to a specific stimulus or task. The most advanced approach is referred to as "functional connectivity (FC)" [23], which provides insight into how brain regions work together as network to produce pain and how these networks can become strengthened or weakened in pain disorders [24]. Due to the crucial role of insula in pain processing, its FCs with other pain-related brain regions may contribute to interpreting the above-mentioned gender differences. However, the insular cortex is functionally heterogeneous, consisting of multiple distinct subdivisions and the FCs between these subdivisions and other pain processing regions remain largely unknown.

In a recent study, insular cortex is divided into 6 subdivisions and the resting-state FCs between these 6 subdivisions and other 12 pain-related brain regions in both healthy men and women have been reported [25]. However, these subdivisions may not reflect the complexity of insular cortex. Recently, the insular cortex is divided into 12 subdivisions (http://atlas.brainnetome.org/) [26], but it has not been investigated the FCs between these 12 insular subdivisions and more pain-related brain structures, nor is it influenced by gender.

We thus designed the current study to compare the gender differences of FCs between 12 insular subdivisions and other pain-related brain regions by using 2 techniques: first, the gender differences of FCs between the 12 insular subdivisions and the whole brain (region of interest (ROI)-whole brain analysis); second, gender differences of FCs between the 12 insular subdivisions and the 64 selected pain-related brain regions (ROI-ROI analysis).

Methods

Participants

Thirty-seven healthy volunteers were recruited from the community participated in the trial, including 26 men (mean age, 49.46 ± 3.75 years) and 11 women (mean age, 52.09 ± 5.65 years). All subjects provided the written informed consent to the study prior to data collection. None participant possessed magnetic resonance imaging (MRI) examination contraindications. Exclusion criteria included neurological diseases or psychiatric disorders, severe internal disorders, concurrence of the cardiovascular system disease, pregnancy or lactation, and alcohol or tobacco dependence.

Clinical characteristics analysis

The statistical analysis was conducted by using of Statistical Program for Social Sciences (SPSS) 20.0 software. The demographic data of the two groups was compared using a two-sample t-test, and $p < 0.05$ was considered as statistical significance.

Resting-state functional data collection

Resting-state blood oxygenation level dependent (BOLD) images were acquired on GE Discovery MR750 3.0 T MR scanner with an eight-channel phased-array head coil at the Department of Radiology, Tangdu Hospital of the Fourth Military Medical University. Prior to scanning, the head of each subject was stabilized in order to minimize head motion. Moreover, the head position was monitored during the whole scanning. For each subject, structural T1 weighted imaging (T1WI) and T2 fluid attenuated inversion recovery (FLAIR) sequences were firstly employed to exclude apparent brain lesions. Resting-state BOLD images were collected utilizing an echo planar imaging (EPI) sequence. Through the scanning process, participants were placed in the supine position and informed to remain as motionless as possible, keep awake, relax their minds and think of nothing in particular. The EPI sequence scanning lasted for 6 min and 10 s. The scanning parameters were as the following:

T1WI:flip angle (FA) = 111°, echo time (TE) = 24 ms, number of echoes = 1, repetition time (TR) = 1750 ms, inversion time (TI) = 780 ms, receiver bandwidth = 41.67, field of view (FOV) = 24 mm², slice thickness = 5 mm, slice spacing = 1.5, number of slices = 20;

T2 FLAIR: TE = 145 ms, number of echoes = 1, TR = 8400 ms, TI = 2100 ms, receiver bandwidth = 83.33, FOV = 24 mm², slice thickness = 5 mm, slice spacing = 1.5, number of slices = 18;

BOLD: FA = 90°, TE = 30 ms, number of echoes = 1, TR = 2000 ms, number of shots = 1, FOV = 22 mm², slice thickness = 3 mm, slice spacing = 1.0, number of slices = 36, time points = 185.

Brain region masks
Masks for insular subdivisions
According to the published Brainnetome Atlas (http://atlas.brainnetome.org/download.html), the insular cortex is divided into 12 subdivisions, including the hypergranular (G), ventral agranular (vIa), dorsal agranular (dIa), ventral dysgranular and granular (vId/vIg), dorsal granular (dIg), dorsal dysgranular (dId) in left and right insular cortices [27]. The detailed information of the 12 insular subdivisions was presented in Table 1.

Masks for selected pain-related brain regions
Based on the neuroanatomical knowledge of brain as well as extensive literature reviewing, 64 pain-related brain regions were selected in the current fMRI study. The detailed information of these pain-related brain regions, including the location, label and Montreal Neurological Institute (MNI) coordinate, was shown in Table 2. Masks for most pain-related regions were selected from the Brainnetome Atlas, including ventral dorsolateral prefrontal cortex (vDLPFC), the opercular pars triangularis (oPT) and ventral pars triangularis (vPT), primary motor cortex (PMC), postcentral somatosensory association cortex (pSAC), the caudal supramarginal gyrus (cSG) and rostroventral supramarginal gyrus (rvSG), SI, the rostroventral ventral anterior cingulate cortex (rvVACC), caudal ventral anterior cingulate cortex (cvACC), pregenual dorsal anterior cingulate cortex (pdACC) and subgenual dorsal anterior cingulate cortex (sdACC), the dorsolateral putamen (dlPu), the medial prefrontal thalamus (mPFtha), premotor thalamus (mPMtha), posterior parietal thalamus (PPtha), caudal temporal thalamus (cTtha), and lateral prefrontal thalamus (lPFtha), the medial amygdala (mAmyg) and lateral amygdala (lAmyg), the rostral hippocampus (rHipp) and caudal hippocampus (cHipp). Besides, the mask for SII was chosen from the Juelich Histological Atlas, which was distributed with FMRIB Software Library (FSL) tool. In addition, the specific MNI coordinates of the rest pain-related regions were referred to the published studies, including rostral anterior cingulate cortex (rACC), ventrolateral prefrontal cortex (VLPFC), posterior midcingulate cortex (pMCC), orbitofrontal cortex (OFC) as well as the ventrolateral periaqueductal gray (vlPAG), lateral periaqueductal gray (lPAG), and dorsolateral periaqueductal gray (dlPAG) [28].

Table 1 MNI coordinates of the 12 insular subdivisions

Insular subdivision	Abbreviation	Left and right hemisphere	Label	MNI coordinate		
				X	Y	Z
Hypergranular insula	G	L	G_L	−36	−20	10
Hypergranular insula	G	R	G_R	37	−18	8
Ventral agranular insula	vIa	L	vIa_L	−32	14	−13
Ventral agranular insula	vIa	R	vIa_R	33	14	−13
Dorsal agranular insula	dIa	L	dIa_L	−34	18	1
Dorsal agranular insula	dIa	R	dIa_R	36	18	1
Ventral dysgranular and granular insula	vId/vIg	L	vId/vIg_L	−38	−4	−9
Ventral dysgranular and granular insula	vId/vIg	R	vId/vIg_R	39	−2	−9
Dorsal granular insula	dIg	L	dIg_L	−38	−8	8
Dorsal granular insula	dIg	R	dIg_R	39	−7	8
Dorsal dysgranular insula	dId	L	dId_L	−38	5	5
Dorsal dysgranular insula	dId	R	dId_R	38	5	5

L left, *R* right, *MNI* Montreal Neurological Institute

Table 2 MNI coordinates of the 64 selected pain-related brain regions

Location	Brain region	Abbreviation	Left and right hemisphere	Label	MNI coordinate		
					X	Y	Z
Middle frontal gyrus	ventral dorsolateral prefrontal cortex	vDLPFC	L	vDLPFC_L	−41	41	16
Middle frontal gyrus	ventral dorsolateral prefrontal cortex	vDLPFC	R	vDLPFC_R	42	44	14
Middle frontal gyrus	ventrolateral prefrontal cortex	VLPFC	L	VLPFC_L	−48	20	−8
Middle frontal gyrus	ventrolateral prefrontal cortex	VLPFC	R	VLPFC_R	48	20	−8
Inferior frontal gyrus	opercular pars triangularis	oPT	L	oPT_L	−39	23	4
Inferior frontal gyrus	opercular pars triangularis	oPT	R	oPT_R	42	22	3
Inferior frontal gyrus	ventral pars triangularis	vPT	L	vPT_L	−52	13	6
Inferior frontal gyrus	ventral pars triangularis	vPT	R	vPT_R	54	14	11
Frontal gyrus	orbitofrontal cortex	OFC	L	OFC_L	−24	34	−12
Frontal gyrus	orbitofrontal cortex	OFC	R	OFC_R	24	34	−12
Precentral gyrus	primary motor cortex	PMC	L	PMC_L	−52	0	8
Precentral gyrus	primary motor cortex	PMC	R	PMC_R	54	4	9
Superior parietal lobe	postcentral somatosensory association cortex	pSAC	L	pSAC_L	−22	−47	65
Superior parietal lobe	postcentral somatosensory association cortex	pSAC	R	pSAC_R	23	−43	67
Inferior parietal lobe	caudal supramarginal gyrus	cSG	L	cSG_L	−56	−49	38
Inferior parietal lobe	caudal supramarginal gyrus	cSG	R	cSG_R	57	−44	38
Inferior parietal lobe	rostroventral supramarginal gyrus	rvSG	L	rvSG_L	−53	−31	23
Inferior parietal lobe	rostroventral supramarginal gyrus	rvSG	R	rvSG_R	55	−26	26
Postcentral gyrus	primary somatosensory cortex (tongue and larynx region)	SI	L	SI_L	−56	−14	16
Postcentral gyrus	primary somatosensory cortex (tongue and larynx region)	SI	R	SI_R	56	−10	15
Postcentral gyrus	primary somatosensory cortex (trunk region)	SI	L	SI_L	−21	−35	68
Postcentral gyrus	primary somatosensory cortex (trunk region)	SI	R	SI_R	20	−33	69
Postcentral gyrus	secondary somatosensory cortex	SII	L	SII_L	−52	−26	22
Postcentral gyrus	secondary somatosensory cortex	SII	R	SII_R	56	−22	24
Cingulate gyrus	rostroventral ventral anterior cingulate cortex	rvVACC	L	rvVACC_L	−3	8	25
Cingulate gyrus	rostroventral ventral anterior cingulate cortex	rvVACC	R	rvVACC_R	5	22	12
Cingulate gyrus	caudal ventral anterior cingulate cortex	cvACC	L	cvACC_L	−5	7	37
Cingulate gyrus	caudal ventral anterior cingulate cortex	cvACC	R	cvACC_R	4	6	38
Cingulate gyrus	pregenual dorsal anterior cingulate cortex	pdACC	L	pdACC_L	−6	34	21
Cingulate gyrus	pregenual dorsal anterior cingulate cortex	pdACC	R	pdACC_R	5	28	27
Cingulate gyrus	subgenual dorsal anterior cingulate cortex	sdACC	L	sdACC_L	−4	39	−2
Cingulate gyrus	subgenual dorsal anterior cingulate cortex	sdACC	R	sdACC_R	5	41	6
Cingulate gyrus	rostral anterior cingulate cortex	rACC	L	rACC_L	−7	27	29
Cingulate gyrus	rostral anterior cingulate cortex	rACC	R	rACC_R	7	27	29
Cingulate gyrus	caudal ventral posterior cingulate cortex	cvPCC	L	cvPCC_L	−7	−23	41
Cingulate gyrus	caudal ventral posterior cingulate cortex	cvPCC	R	cvPCC_R	6	−20	40
Cingulate gyrus	posterior midcingulate cortex	pMCC	L	pMCC_L	−3	−21	51
Cingulate gyrus	posterior midcingulate cortex	pMCC	R	pMCC_R	3	−21	51
Basal ganglia	dorsolateral putamen	dlPu	L	dlPu_L	−28	−5	2
Basal ganglia	dorsolateral putamen	dlPu	R	dlPu_R	29	−3	1
Periaqueductal gray	ventrolateral periaqueductal gray	vlPAG	L	vlPAG_L	−3	−32	−12

Table 2 MNI coordinates of the 64 selected pain-related brain regions *(Continued)*

Location	Brain region	Abbreviation	Left and right hemisphere	Label	MNI coordinate		
					X	Y	Z
Periaqueductal gray	ventrolateral periaqueductal gray	vlPAG	R	vlPAG_R	3	−32	−12
Periaqueductal gray	lateral periaqueductal gray	lPAG	L	lPAG_L	−4	−31	−8
Periaqueductal gray	lateral periaqueductal gray	lPAG	R	lPAG_R	4	−31	−8
Periaqueductal gray	dorsolateral periaqueductal gray	dlPAG	L	dlPAG_L	−2	−32	−5
Periaqueductal gray	dorsolateral periaqueductal gray	dlPAG	R	dlPAG_R	2	−32	−5
Thalamus	medial prefrontal thalamus	mPFtha	L	mPFtha_L	−7	−12	5
Thalamus	medial prefrontal thalamus	mPFtha	R	mPFtha_R	7	−11	6
Thalamus	premotor thalamus	mPMtha	L	mPMtha_L	−18	−13	3
Thalamus	premotor thalamus	mPMtha	R	mPMtha_R	12	−14	1
Thalamus	posterior parietal thalamus	PPtha	L	PPtha_L	16	−24	6
Thalamus	posterior parietal thalamus	PPtha	R	PPtha_R	15	−25	6
Thalamus	caudal temporal thalamus	cTtha	L	cTtha_L	−12	−22	13
Thalamus	caudal temporal thalamus	cTtha	R	cTtha_R	10	−14	14
Thalamus	lateral prefrontal thalamus	lPFtha	L	lPFtha_L	−11	−14	2
Thalamus	lateral prefrontal thalamus	lPFtha	R	lPFtha_R	13	−16	7
Amygdala	medial amygdala	mAmyg	L	mAmyg_L	−19	−2	−20
Amygdala	medial amygdala	mAmyg	R	mAmyg_R	19	−2	−19
Amygdala	lateral amygdala	lAmyg	L	lAmyg_L	−27	−4	−20
Amygdala	lateral amygdala	lAmyg	R	lAmyg_R	28	−3	−20
Hippocampus	rostral hippocampus	rHipp	L	rHipp_L	−22	−14	−19
Hippocampus	rostral hippocampus	rHipp	R	rHipp_R	22	−12	−20
Hippocampus	caudal hippocampus	cHipp	L	cHipp_L	−28	−30	−10
Hippocampus	caudal hippocampus	cHipp	R	cHipp_R	29	−27	−10

L left, *R* right, *MNI* Montreal Neurological Institute

Processing of resting-state fMRI data

Data preprocessing

The preprocessing of the BOLD images was performed by using the Data Processing Assistant for Resting-State fMRI (DPARSF, Yan and Zang 2010, http://rfmri.org/DPARSF), which is based on Statistical Parametric Mapping (SPM8, http://www.fil.ion.ucl.ac.uk/spm) and the toolbox for Data Processing & Analysis of Brain Imaging (DPABI, Yan et al. 2016, http://rfmri.org/DPABI). Briefly, the first 10 volumes of each subject were discarded in order to reach the signal equilibration and allow the subjects to adapt to the scanning environment. The remained scans were corrected for acquisition time differences between different slices and next realigned to the middle time point to correct for head motion. Then the head motion parameters of the subject were obtained and assessed with a maximum rotation less than 1° or a maximum displacement less than 1 mm. Nuisance regression was applied on white matter and cerebrospinal fluid, separately. Then the motion-corrected BOLD images were spatially normalized by using EPI templates and resampled with a voxel size of

$3 \times 3 \times 3$ mm^3. After spatial normalization, the images were spatially smoothed with a Gaussian kernel of 4 mm full-width at half maximum (FWHM) to reduce spatial noise. In the end, a band-pass filter (0.01 Hz < f < 0.08 Hz) was utilized to remove the effects of low frequency physiological drift and high frequency noise. After performing these steps, a 4-dimensional residual time series dataset was set up for each subject in the standard MNI space.

FCs analysis between the 12 insular subdivisions and the whole brain

The ROI-whole brain analysis was conducted between the 12 insular subdivisions (a total of 12 ROIs) and the whole brain. The mean time series for each ROI were calculated and then correlated with the time courses of all other voxels in the brain for each subject. Pearson correlation coefficients were converted to normally distributed scores by use of the Fisher's r-to-z transformation [23]. Group-level analysis for the general linear model was performed applying two sample *t*-test between the z-scores of the male and female groups.

The reported results of the ROI-whole brain correlation analysis were carried out performing an uncorrected peak level of $p < 0.001$ to correct for false positive rates and a false discovery rate (FDR) correction by using SPM8 at cluster level for multiple comparisons with threshold of $p < 0.05$ [29, 30].

FCs analysis between the 12 insular subdivisions and the 64 selected pain-related regions

Next, 64 brain regions that were recognized to be associated with pain were selected to calculate the ROI-ROI level FCs with the 12 sub-insular divisions (a total of 12 ROIs). Similar to the above-mentioned ROI-whole brain level analysis, Fisher's r-to-z transformation was conducted to increase the normality of the fMRI data. Based on the 12×76 z-FC matrix, two-sample t-test was performed between the male group and the female group. FDR correction with threshold of $p < 0.05$ for multiple comparison was then employed using MATLAB 2012b and to identify the final FC pairs with significant difference attributed to the gender factor.

Results
Demographic data
The demographic data of the two groups were shown in Table 3. No significant differences were revealed between male and female groups in age, hand dominance as well as educational level.

Gender differences in ROI-whole brain level FCs
FCs between the 12 insular subdivisions and whole brain in male and female groups were first investigated. Male subjects showed significantly increased FCs between the left dId and other four brain regions, comprising the voxels containing the right median cingulate and paracingulate/ right posterior cingulate gyrus/ right precuneus, the right median cingulate and paracingulate, the left angular, and the left middle frontal gyrus (Table 4 and Fig. 1a). The surface visualization of these significantly increased clusters in males was presented in Fig. 1b.

Table 3 Demographic characteristics

	Male group (n = 26)	Female group (n = 11)	P
Age (years)	49.46 ± 3.75	52.09 ± 5.65	0.104
Hand dominance (L/R)	2/24	1/10	1.000
Education (years)	13.54 ± 3.27	12.18 ± 3.22	0.259

Continuous data were expressed as mean ± standard deviation (SD)
L left, R right

Gender differences in ROI-ROI level FCs
FCs between the insular subdivisions and selected pain-related brain regions in male and female groups were compared using ROI-ROI level analysis. In line with the above ROI-whole brain analysis, the significant gender differences of FCs were also investigated between the 12 insular subdivisions and the 64 selected pain-related brain regions. Only the FC between the left dId and the right rACC in the total 12×76 z-FC matrix was increased in the male subjects. The gender differences of 1 FC-pair with significance between the insular subdivisions and pain-related brain regions were shown in Fig. 2.

After merging the results of ROI-whole brain and ROI-ROI analyses, the dId in the left insular cortex was the primary insular subdivision that showed significantly increased FCs with the brain structures predominantly located in the right cingulate cortex in male subjects, shown in Fig. 3.

Discussion
In the current study, two analytical approaches were performed to explore the gender differences of FCs in insular subdivisions. Both ROI-whole brain and ROI-ROI analyses suggested that the FCs between left dId and right cingulate cortex were significantly increased in males. Our findings suggested that the increased FCs between left dId - right cingulate cortex in males played inhibiting role in the transmission and modulation of pain signals, thus decreased the pain intensity and incidence in male population.

According to the cytoarchitecture of the insular cortex, the dId locates in the posterior area of insula and participates in the sensory components of pain perception [27, 31]. In migraine patients, the dId was negatively connected to the median cingulate and paracingulate [25]. Female migraine patients also exhibited significantly decreased FCs between the posterior insula and the posterior cingulate cortex [5]. In addition to the above-mentioned gender differences in the clinical experience of migraine pain, healthy males in the current study showed statistically increased FCs between the insular subdivision and the cingulate cortex. Taking together the previous studies and our current one, the FCs between the insular and cingulate cortices were different between males and females, suggesting the functional distinctions in the brain matrix for pain processing among male and female populations.

Previous fMRI studies on gender differences in healthy subjects suggested that the male insular cortex is more activated under similar pain stimuli [19], however, without details of the activated subdivisions. Our study offered evidence that the male dorsal dysgranular area of the posterior insula was more spontaneously

Table 4 Significant FCs between the insular subdivision and the whole brain in males

Insular subdivision	Cluster index	Brain region	Cluster size	MNI coordinate			Peak T-value	FCs increased/ decreased
				X	Y	Z		
dId_L	1	Cingulum_Mid/Cingulum_Post/Precuneus_R	73	6	−45	39	4.82	Increased
	2	Cingulum_Mid_R	144	6	9	36	4.76	Increased
	3	Angular_L	71	−39	−72	48	4.96	Increased
	4	Frontal_Mid_L	56	−42	21	39	4.53	Increased

The threshold was set at uncorrected peak level of $p < 0.001$, FDR correction with threshold of $p < 0.05$, cluster size ≥ 50 voxels. T-values of significantly activated peak-voxels referred to MNI coordinates. Brain region labeling was performed using the AAL atlas. T statistics and MNI coordinates were reported for the peak voxel within each cluster. AAL, Automatic Anatomic Labeling; FCs, functional connectivities; L, left; R, right; MNI, Montreal Neurological Institute; dId, dorsal dysgranular insula; Cingulum_Mid, median cingulate and paracingulate gyrus; Cingulum_Post, posterior cingulate gyrus; Frontal_Mid, middle frontal gyrus

activated than females. Since the posterior insula primarily plays an important role in the sensory network of pain [32, 33], our data suggested the potential involvement of dorsal dysgranular area of the posterior insula in the different pain processing in males and females under pain disorders. Reduced activity in the posterior insula may contribute to increased pain thresholds [34], suggesting its role in inhibiting pain response. However, the detailed underlying mechanisms need to be further investigated.

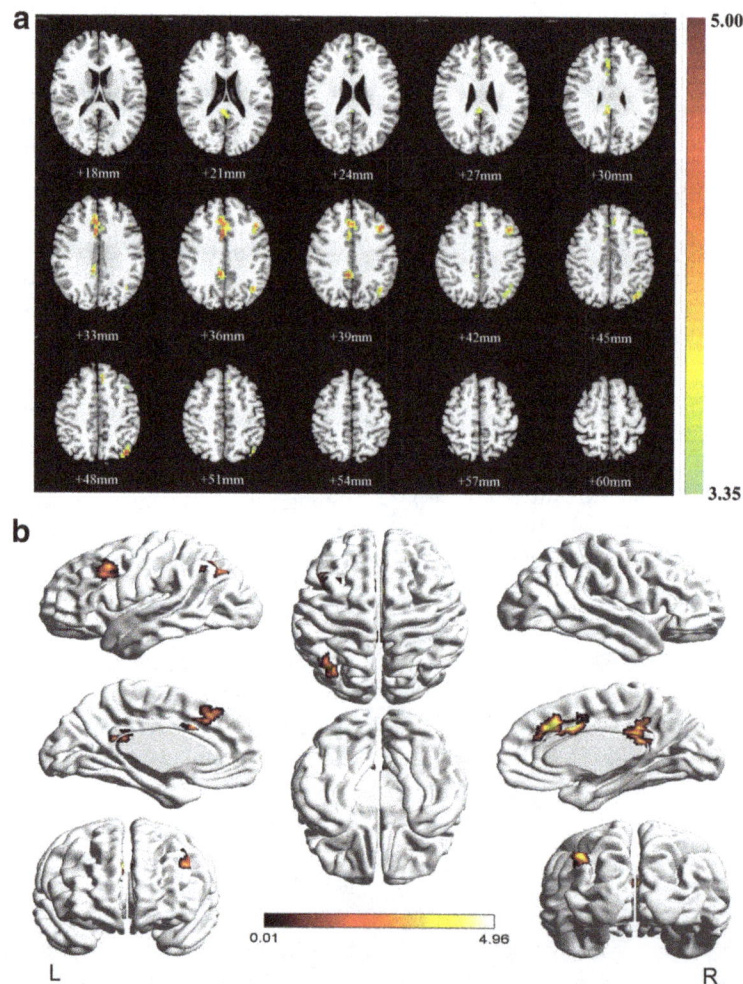

Fig. 1 ROI-whole brain analysis of FCs between the 12 insular subdivisions and the whole brain (visualization of the clusters on the brain surface). The warm color in the statistical differences map indicated the increased FCs between the dId_L and the whole brain in males. dId, dorsal dysgranular insula; L, left; R, right; FCs, functional connectivities; ROI, region of interest

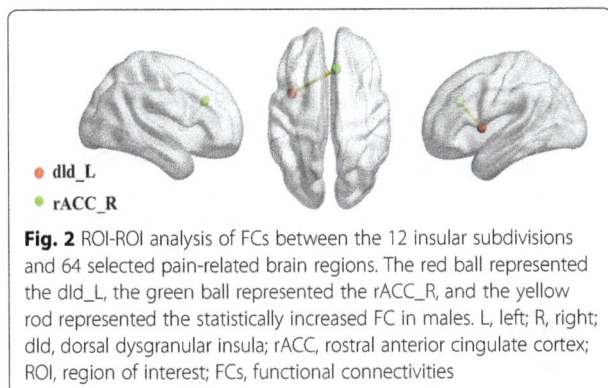

Fig. 2 ROI-ROI analysis of FCs between the 12 insular subdivisions and 64 selected pain-related brain regions. The red ball represented the dId_L, the green ball represented the rACC_R, and the yellow rod represented the statistically increased FC in males. L, left; R, right; dId, dorsal dysgranular insula; rACC, rostral anterior cingulate cortex; ROI, region of interest; FCs, functional connectivities

To our knowledge, information exchange between the insular and cingulate cortices has never been directly revealed. However, tracing studies in the monkey demonstrated that the posterior insula was connected to Brodmann areas 23 and 24 of the cingulate cortex [35], supporting our current findings. Based on the non-human primate functional neuroimaging studies, a co-activation of the insular and cingulate cortices was revealed in varied tasks [32, 36]. Furthermore, the posterior insular and the cingulate cortices were

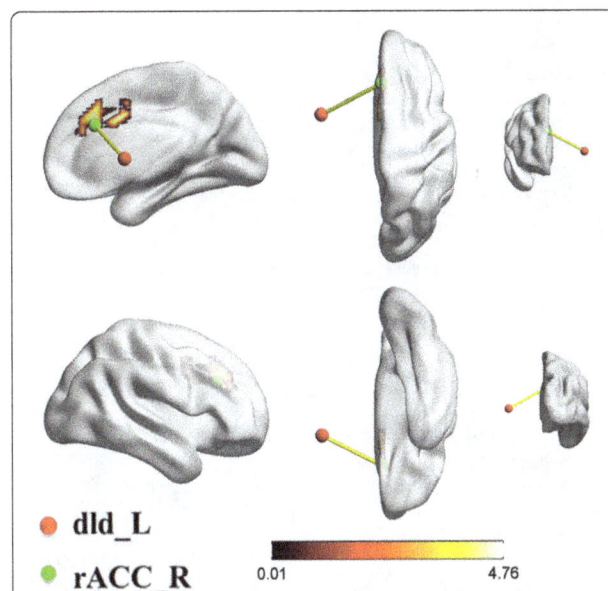

Fig. 3 Merging of ROI-whole brain and ROI-ROI analyses. The warm color in the statistical differences map exhibited the increased FCs between the dId_L and the whole brain in males (ROI-whole brain analysis). The red ball represented the dId_L, the green ball represented the rACC_R, and the yellow rod represented the statistically increased FC between the dId_L and the rACC_R in males (ROI-ROI analysis). L, left; R, right; dId, dorsal dysgranular insula; rACC, rostral anterior cingulate cortex; ROI, region of interest; FCs, functional connectivities

activated simultaneously in fibromyalgia patients [37]. Therefore, the distinct anatomical connections identified in the monkey combined with the evidence from functional imaging studies showing co-activation within specific areas of the insula and cingulate cortex, indicating multiple information processing pathways between the two brain structures [36]. Interestingly, the co-activation of the insular subdivision and the cingulate cortex also showed the gender differences in the current study. The FCs between the dId and cingulate cortex were significantly increased in male subjects. The FCs between insular subdivisions and other pain-related brain regions were also investigated in a recent study [25]. Despite the similar study design, there were apparent differences between their findings and ours. First, Wiech explored FCs between the insular subdivisions and other pain-related regions using the ROI-ROI method [25]. While we aimed to investigate that how the FCs between the insular subdivisions and other pain-relevant regions were influenced by gender difference (ROI-ROI analysis). In addition, we also identified the gender differences in FCs between the insular subdivisions and the whole brain (ROI-whole brain analysis). Second, the insular cortex was divided into 6 subdivisions in the previous study, while 12 subdivisions were utilized in the current study. Third, 12 pain-related brain regions were selected in Wiech's study, while 64 pain-related regions were selected in the present study based on an existing neuroanatomical knowledge and extensive literature review. Wiech revealed strongest FCs between the posterior insula and SII in 36 healthy adults (21 men and 15 women). Our study offered further information that the dId of the posterior insula is a major hub to cingulate cortex, performing pain inhibiting role.

There was limitation for our study. No pain-related psychological questionnaires were collected in the current study. Based on the existing evidence, healthy subjects also possess the pain-relevant psychological characteristics, such as pain vigilance and pain awareness [25]. The correlation analysis might reveal the potential relation between the FCs and the psychological traits of pain.

Conclusion

In conclusion, the present study identified the gender-relevant alterations in FCs of the insular subdivisions with other pain-related brain regions using two different methods. Specifically, men seem to have more access to a dId-mediated recruitment of the pain inhibition system than women. Given this, it is crucial for future study to take gender into account when probing the basic mechanisms of pain processing.

Abbreviations

AAL: Automatic anatomic labeling; BOLD: Blood oxygenation level dependent; DPABI: Data processing & analysis of brain imaging; DPARSF: Data processing assistant for resting-state fMRI; EPI: Echo planar imaging; FA: Flip angle; FC: Functional connectivity; FLAIR: Fluid attenuated inversion recovery; fMRI: Functional magnetic resonance imaging; FOV: Field of view; FSL: FMRIB software library; FWHM: Full-width at half maximum; IBS: IRRITABLE bowel syndrome; L: Left; MNI: Montreal neurological Institute; MRI: Magnetic resonance imaging; R: Right; ROI: Regions of interest; SD: Standard deviation; SI: Primary somatic cortices; SII: Secondary somatic cortices; SPM: Statistical parametric mapping; SPSS: Statistical program for social sciences; T1WI: T1 weighted imaging; TE: Echo time; TI: Inversion time; TR: Repetition time; VLPFC: Ventrolateral prefrontal cortex

Funding

This paper was sponsored by the National Natural Science Foundation of China (No. 81571656 and No. 61603399), the National Key Research and Development Program of China (No. 2016YFC0107105), the Innovation Foundation of Tangdu Hospital (No. 2016LCYJ011), and Key Project for Science Research and Development of Shaanxi Province (2017SF-012).

Authors' contributions

DYJ, ZX, YY and WW contributed to all stages, including data acquisition and analysis, drafting the manuscript and revising for important intellectual content, as well as final approval of the version to be submitted. WW, NHY, CGB, and CBL were integral to the conception and design of the study. YY, YLF, HB and ZJ were responsible to the analysis and interpretation of the imaging data. SQ, QZY, and GY assisted with data collection in addition to the drafting and revising of this article. All authors read and approved the final manuscript.

Competing interests

The authors declare that they have no competing interests.

Author details

[1]Department of Radiology & Functional and Molecular Imaging Key Lab of Shaanxi Province, Tangdu Hospital, the Military Medical University of PLA Airforce (Fourth Military Medical University), 569 Xinsi Road, Xi'an, Shaanxi Province 710038, China. [2]Department of Obstetrics and Gynecology, Xijing Hospital, the Military Medical University of PLA Airforce (Fourth Military Medical University), 15 West Changle Road, Xi'an, Shaanxi Province 710032, China. [3]Department of Clinical Nutrition, Xijing Hospital, the Military Medical University of PLA Airforce (Fourth Military Medical University), 15 West Changle Road, Xi'an, Shaanxi Province 710032, China. [4]Student Brigade, the Military Medical University of PLA Airforce (Fourth Military Medical University), 169 West Changle Road, Xi'an, Shaanxi Province 710032, China.

References

1. Mogil JS (2012) Sex differences in pain and pain inhibition: multiple explanations of a controversial phenomenon. Nat Rev Neurosci 13(12):859–866. https://doi.org/10.1038/nrn3360
2. Fillingim RB, King CD, Ribeiro-Dasilva MC, Rahim-Williams B, Riley JL 3rd (2009) Sex, gender, and pain: a review of recent clinical and experimental findings. J Pain 10(5):447–485. https://doi.org/10.1016/j.jpain.2008.12.001
3. Ruau D, Liu LY, Clark JD, Angst MS, Butte AJ (2012) Sex differences in reported pain across 11,000 patients captured in electronic medical records. J Pain 13(3):228–234. https://doi.org/10.1016/j.jpain.2011.11.002
4. Le H, Tfelt-Hansen P, Russell MB, Skytthe A, Kyvik KO, Olesen J (2011) Co-morbidity of migraine with somatic disease in a large population-based study. Cephalalgia 31(1):43–64. https://doi.org/10.1177/0333102410373159
5. Maleki N, Linnman C, Brawn J, Burstein R, Becerra L, Borsook D (2012) Her versus his migraine: multiple sex differences in brain function and structure. Brain 135(Pt 8):2546–2559. https://doi.org/10.1093/brain/aws175
6. Linnman C, Beucke JC, Jensen KB, Gollub RL, Kong J (2012) Sex similarities and differences in pain-related periaqueductal gray connectivity. Pain 153(2):444–454. https://doi.org/10.1016/j.pain.2011.11.006
7. Napadow V, Kim J, Clauw DJ, Harris RE (2012) Decreased intrinsic brain connectivity is associated with reduced clinical pain in fibromyalgia. Arthritis Rheum 64(7):2398–2403. https://doi.org/10.1002/art.34412
8. Napadow V, LaCount L, Park K, As-Sanie S, Clauw DJ, Harris RE (2010) Intrinsic brain connectivity in fibromyalgia is associated with chronic pain intensity. Arthritis Rheum 62(8):2545–2555. https://doi.org/10.1002/art.27497
9. Hong JY, Kilpatrick LA, Labus JS, Gupta A, Katibian D, Ashe-McNalley C, Stains J, Heendeniya N, Smith SR, Tillisch K, Naliboff B, Mayer EA (2014) Sex and disease-related alterations of anterior insula functional connectivity in chronic abdominal pain. J Neurosci 34(43):14252–14259. https://doi.org/10.1523/JNEUROSCI.1683-14.2014
10. Gupta A, Kilpatrick L, Labus J, Tillisch K, Braun A, Hong JY, Ashe-McNalley C, Naliboff B, Mayer EA (2014) Early adverse life events and resting state neural networks in patients with chronic abdominal pain: evidence for sex differences. Psychosom Med 76(6):404–412. https://doi.org/10.1097/PSY.0000000000000089
11. Rainville P (2002) Brain mechanisms of pain affect and pain modulation. Curr Opin Neurobiol 12(2):195–204
12. Bastuji H, Frot M, Perchet C, Magnin M, Garcia-Larrea L (2016) Pain networks from the inside: spatiotemporal analysis of brain responses leading from nociception to conscious perception. Hum Brain Mapp 37(12):4301–4315. https://doi.org/10.1002/hbm.23310
13. Garcia-Larrea L, Peyron R (2013) Pain matrices and neuropathic pain matrices: a review. Pain 154(Suppl 1):S29–S43. https://doi.org/10.1016/j.pain.2013.09.001
14. Apkarian AV, Bushnell MC, Treede RD, Zubieta JK (2005) Human brain mechanisms of pain perception and regulation in health and disease. Eur J Pain 9(4):463–484. https://doi.org/10.1016/j.ejpain.2004.11.001
15. Hofbauer RK, Rainville P, Duncan GH, Bushnell MC (2001) Cortical representation of the sensory dimension of pain. J Neurophysiol 86(1):402–411. https://doi.org/10.1152/jn.2001.86.1.402
16. Tracey I, Mantyh PW (2007) The cerebral signature for pain perception and its modulation. Neuron 55(3):377–391. https://doi.org/10.1016/j.neuron.2007.07.012
17. A CNC (2008) Pain perception and its genesis in the human brain. Sheng Li Xue Bao 60(5):677–685
18. Monroe TB, Fillingim RB, Bruehl SP, Rogers BP, Dietrich MS, Gore JC, Atalla SW, Cowan RL (2017) Sex differences in brain regions modulating pain among older adults: a cross-sectional resting state functional connectivity study. Pain Med. https://doi.org/10.1093/pm/pnx084
19. Kong J, Loggia ML, Zyloney C, Tu P, Laviolette P, Gollub RL (2010) Exploring the brain in pain: activations, deactivations and their relation. Pain 148(2):257–267. https://doi.org/10.1016/j.pain.2009.11.008
20. Moulton EA, Keaser ML, Gullapalli RP, Maitra R, Greenspan JD (2006) Sex differences in the cerebral BOLD signal response to painful heat stimuli. Am J Physiol Regul, Integrat Comp Physiol 291(2):R257–R267. https://doi.org/10.1152/ajpregu.00084.2006
21. Straube T, Schmidt S, Weiss T, Mentzel HJ, Miltner WH (2009) Sex differences in brain activation to anticipated and experienced pain in the medial prefrontal cortex. Hum Brain Mapp 30(2):689–698. https://doi.org/10.1002/hbm.20536
22. Hong JY, Kilpatrick LA, Labus J, Gupta A, Jiang Z, Ashe-McNalley C, Stains J, Heendeniya N, Ebrat B, Smith S, Tillisch K, Naliboff B, Mayer EA (2013) Patients with chronic visceral pain show sex-related alterations in intrinsic oscillations of the resting brain. J Neurosci 33(29):11994–12002. https://doi.org/10.1523/JNEUROSCI.5733-12.2013
23. Liu F, Wang Y, Li M, Wang W, Li R, Zhang Z, Lu G, Chen H (2017) Dynamic functional network connectivity in idiopathic generalized epilepsy with generalized tonic-clonic seizure. Hum Brain Mapp 38(2):957–973. https://doi.org/10.1002/hbm.23430
24. Davis KD, Moayedi M (2013) Central mechanisms of pain revealed through functional and structural MRI. J NeuroImmune Pharmacol 8(3):518–534. https://doi.org/10.1007/s11481-012-9386-8
25. Wiech K, Jbabdi S, Lin CS, Andersson J, Tracey I (2014) Differential structural and resting state connectivity between insular subdivisions and other pain-related brain regions. Pain 155(10):2047–2055. https://doi.org/10.1016/j.pain.2014.07.009

Gender differences in functional connectivities between insular subdivisions and selective pain-related brain...

79

26. Fan L, Li H, Zhuo J, Zhang Y, Wang J, Chen L, Yang Z, Chu C, Xie S, Laird AR, Fox PT, Eickhoff SB, Yu C, Jiang T (2016) The human Brainnetome atlas: a new brain atlas based on connectional architecture. Cereb Cortex 26(8): 3508–3526. https://doi.org/10.1093/cercor/bhw157

27. Yu ZB, Lv YB, Song LH, Liu DH, Huang XL, Hu XY, Zuo ZW, Wang Y, Yang Q, Peng J, Zhou ZH, Li HT (2017) Functional connectivity differences in the insular sub-regions in migraine without Aura: a resting-state functional magnetic resonance imaging study. Front Behav Neurosci 11:124. https://doi.org/10.3389/fnbeh.2017.00124

28. Coulombe MA, Erpelding N, Kucyi A, Davis KD (2016) Intrinsic functional connectivity of periaqueductal gray subregions in humans. Hum Brain Mapp 37(4):1514–1530. https://doi.org/10.1002/hbm.23117

29. Chumbley J, Worsley K, Flandin G, Friston K (2010) Topological FDR for neuroimaging. Neuro Image 49(4):3057–3064. https://doi.org/10.1016/j.neuroimage.2009.10.090

30. Liu F, Zhu C, Wang Y, Guo W, Li M, Wang W, Long Z, Meng Y, Cui Q, Zeng L, Gong Q, Zhang W, Chen H (2015) Disrupted cortical hubs in functional brain networks in social anxiety disorder. Clin Neurophysiol 126(9):1711–1716. https://doi.org/10.1016/j.clinph.2014.11.014

31. Kurth F, Zilles K, Fox PT, Laird AR, Eickhoff SB (2010) A link between the systems: functional differentiation and integration within the human insula revealed by meta-analysis. Brain Struct Funct 214(5–6):519–534. https://doi.org/10.1007/s00429-010-0255-z

32. Rance M, Ruttorf M, Nees F, Schad LR, Flor H (2014) Real time fMRI feedback of the anterior cingulate and posterior insular cortex in the processing of pain. Hum Brain Mapp 35(12):5784–5798. https://doi.org/10.1002/hbm.22585

33. Frot M, Magnin M, Mauguiere F, Garcia-Larrea L (2007) Human SII and posterior insula differently encode thermal laser stimuli. Cereb Cortex 17(3): 610–620. https://doi.org/10.1093/cercor/bhk007

34. Bar KJ, Berger S, Schwier C, Wutzler U, Beissner F (2013) Insular dysfunction and descending pain inhibition in anorexia nervosa. Acta Psychiatr Scand 127(4):269–278. https://doi.org/10.1111/j.1600-0447.2012.01896.x

35. Mesulam MM, Mufson EJ (1982) Insula of the old world monkey. III: efferent cortical output and comments on function. J Comp Neurol 212(1):38–52. https://doi.org/10.1002/cne.902120104

36. Taylor KS, Seminowicz DA, Davis KD (2009) Two systems of resting state connectivity between the insula and cingulate cortex. Hum Brain Mapp 30(9):2731–2745. https://doi.org/10.1002/hbm.20705

37. Ichesco E, Schmidt-Wilcke T, Bhavsar R, Clauw DJ, Peltier SJ, Kim J, Napadow V, Hampson JP, Kairys AE, Williams DA, Harris RE (2014) Altered resting state connectivity of the insular cortex in individuals with fibromyalgia. J Pain 15(8):815–826 e811. https://doi.org/10.1016/j.jpain.2014.04.007

9

Physiological, hematological and biochemical factors associated with high-altitude headache in young Chinese males following acute exposure at 3700 m

Kun Wang[1,3], Menghan Zhang[2,3], Yi Li[2,3,6], Weilin Pu[2], Yanyun Ma[2,3,6], Yi Wang[2,3], Xiaoyu Liu[2,3], Longli Kang[5], Xiaofeng Wang[1,3], Jiucun Wang[1,3,6], Bin Qiao[4] and Li Jin[1,3,6*]

Abstract

Background: High-altitude headache (HAH) is the most common sickness occurred in healthy people after rapid ascending to high altitude, and its risk factors were still not well understood. To investigate physiological, hematological and biochemical risk factors associated with high-altitude headache (HAH) after acute exposure to 3700 m, we conducted a two-stage, perspective observational study. In 72 h, total 318 young Han Chinese males ascended from sea level (altitude of 50 m) to altitude of 3700 m by train. Demographic data, physiological, hematological and biochemical parameters of all participants were collected within one week prior to the departure, and within 24 h after arrival.

Results: The incidence of HAH was 74.84%. For parameters measured at sea level, participants with HAH exhibited significantly higher age and lower BUN ($p < 0.05$). For parameters measured at 3700 m, participants with HAH exhibited significantly lower blood oxygen saturation (SpO_2), higher resting heart rate (HR), higher systolic blood pressure at resting (SBP) and lower blood urea nitrogen (BUN) (all $p < 0.05$). At 3700 m, the severity of HAH associated with SpO_2, HR and BUN significantly (all $p < 0.05$). Multivariate logistic regression revealed that for parameters at sea level, BUN was associated with HAH [BUN (OR:0.77, 95% CI:0.60–0.99)] and for parameters at 3700 m, SpO_2, HR and BUN were associated with HAH independently [SpO_2 (OR:0.84, 95% CI:0.76–0.93); HR (OR:1.03, 95% CI:1.00–1.07); BUN (OR:0.64, 95% CI:0.46–0.88)]. No association between hematological parameters and HAH was observed.

Conclusion: We confirmed that higher HR, lower SpO_2 are independent risk factors for HAH. Furthermore, we found that at both 50 m and 3700 m, lower BUN is a novel independent risk factor for HAH, providing new insights for understanding the pathological mechanisms.

Keywords: High-altitude headache, Hypoxia, Blood urea nitrogen, Oxygen saturation, Heart rate

* Correspondence: lijin@fudan.edu.cn
[1]State Key Laboratory of Genetic Engineering, Collaborative Innovation Center for Genetics and Development, School of Life Sciences, Fudan University, Shanghai 200438, China
[3]Human Phenome Institute, Fudan University, Shanghai 201203, China
Full list of author information is available at the end of the article

Background

For lowlanders who rapidly ascend to altitude above 2500 m, headache has been considered as the most frequent complaint [1, 2]. According to the most widely-accepted diagnose criteria, the Lake Louise Consensus scoring system identified headache as the cardinal symptom of acute mountain sickness (AMS) [3]. The International Headache Society defined high altitude headache (HAH) as a headache that develops within 24 h of ascent to high altitude and resolves within 8 h of descent [4, 5]. Previous studies have reported that the incidence of HAH is over 70% within 24 h after rapidly ascending above 2500 m [2].

Numerous studies have been emerged on epidemiology, clinical characteristics, pathophysiological mechanisms, treatment and risk factors of HAH [1, 6–8]. Recent studies suggested that the cause of HAH may be hypoxia-induced cerebral cytotoxic oedema, brain swelling and increased intracranial pressure [6]. In addition to oxygen inhalation, aspirin and acetaminophen were often used for HAH treatment, and the effect are contradictory [9, 10]. Several studies have demonstrated that young age, smoking history, higher body mass index history of migraine, high heart rate (HR) and low pulse oxygen saturation (SpO_2) are independent risk factors for HAH [1, 11–13]. Previously, Huang et al. performed the first investigation on the relationship between hematological parameters and HAH before and after rapid ascending at 3700 m with 45 subjects, and found that HAH is associated with sea-level reticulocyte and neutrophil counts [14]. Because erythrocytes are the principal carrier of oxygen in the circulatory system, the hematological parameters may provide useful information regarding HAH. Moreover, some studies demonstrated that fluid retention is an important feature of AMS, but other studies have demonstrated that low fluid intake is an independent risk factor of HAH, and glomerular filtration rate estimates increases with AMS severities after rapid ascent to high altitude [15–18]. Over all, most of the studies had small sample sizes, the results were contradictory, and no definitive clear answer is available.

The present study was based on the hypothesis that some hematological and biochemical parameters would be related with HAH. We aimed to explore the association between physiological, hematological, biochemical parameters (including renal function parameters) and the risk of HAH after a 3-days ascending to the altitude of 3700 m. We carried out a repeated measurement design based on two phases (50 m and 3700 m) before and after ascending at high altitude for 318 healthy young Han Chinese males. Physical, hematological and biochemical parameters were collected at each phase, respectively.

Methods

Participants

In total, 318 young Chinese males who lived at 50 m and ascended to Tibet for physical training were recruited in this study. All participants reported their disease history, medication history, smoking and drinking history in structured case report forms (CRFs). The inclusion criteria were healthy 18–35 year old Han Chinese men whose primary residence was at an altitude of ≤1000 m and had no high-altitude exposure in recent 2 years. The exclusion criteria were cardio-cerebrovascular diseases, neurological and psychiatric diseases, episodic or chronic migraine diseases or chronic headache symptoms (any headache occurring on more than 2 weeks/mouth), autoimmune diseases, respiratory diseases, malignancy, liver and kidney dysfunction, active infection or a bad cold. Participants who took acetazolamide, diuretics, steroids or nonsteroidal anti-inflammatory drugs during the ascending were excluded. Subjects who agreed to participate underwent a short instruction and explanation of the purpose of this study, and all participants have signed the informed consent before their first examinations. The study was approved by the Human Ethics Committee of Fudan University.

Study procedures and measurements

All participants ascended to altitude of 3700 m (Lhasa, Tibet) within 72 h by train from sea level (altitude of 50 m, Henan). The baseline physiological, hematological and biochemical measurements were performed in the morning, one week prior to the departure at 50 m. Within 24 h after their arrival at 3700 m, the participants underwent assessments of their physiological, hematological and biochemical parameters, as well as HAH. All participants were monitored by trained physicians for any signs of high-altitude cerebral or pulmonary edema, and immediate treatment will be addressed for emergent cases [19]. During the period of study, all participants maintained the same diet. Caffeine beverage consumption, alcohol consumption and medication use were prohibited, smoking and heavy exercises or physical labor were also avoided.

Structured case report forms (CRFs) were used to record the demographic data (age, body mass index (BMI), chest circumference, smoking and drinking history) and all measurements at sea level and 3700 m for each participants. After the acute exposure at 3700 m, the physicians scored HAH based on self-description of patients (0 = no headache; 1 = mild headache; 2 = moderate headache; 3 = severe headache) was recorded, and the time and place of headache onset was recorded retrospectively. We used a two-repeated measurement method to collect the heart rate at resting (HR, beats/min), systolic blood pressures at resting (SBP, mmHg), diastolic blood pressure at resting (DBP, mmHg) and Oxygen saturation (SpO$_2$, %), operated twice by two independent professional physicians and recorded the average value. SBP and DBP were measured using a standardized mercury sphygmomanometer, while SpO$_2$ was measured using Nellcor NPB-40 (USA).

Morning fasting venous blood (4 ml) was collected with EDTA-K2 at both sea level and 3700 m, and 2 ml of the samples were used to assay blood cell parameters by a hematology analyzer (Sysmex pocH-100i, Japan) within 2 h. The hematological parameters included red blood cell count (RBC, $\times 10^{12}$/L), hemoglobin (Hgb, g/L), hematocrit (Hct, %), mean corpuscular volume (MCV, fL), mean corpuscular hemoglobin (MCH, pg), white blood cell count (WBC, $\times 10^9$/L), lymphocyte percentage (LYM%), absolute lymphocyte count (LYM#), platelet count (PLT, $\times 10^9$/L) and mean platelet volume (MPV, fL). The rest 2 ml blood specimens were centrifuged 3000 r/min for 10 minus to separate plasma. Biochemical parameters including alanine aminotransferase (ALT, U/L), aspartate aminotransferase (AST, U/L), blood urea nitrogen (BUN, mmol/L), serum creatinine (CREA, umol/L), total serum bilirubin (T-BIL, umol/L), direct serum bilirubin (D-BIL, umol/L) and indirect serum bilirubin (I-BIL, umol/L) were measured using automatic biochemistry analyzer (TOSHIBA TBA-120FR).

The diagnosis of HAH was based on the International Classification of Headache Disorders 3β criteria [5], but not strictly (no test for descending), restricted by the complex situations of field study.

Statistical analyses

The normality of continuous data was assessed by Shapiro-Wilk's test. Normally distributed data were presented as the means±standard deviations (SD), non-normally distributed data were presented as median (interquartile range, IQR) and enumerated data were expressed as numbers (%). The differences of measurements between sea level and 3700 m were compared using paired-sample student's t-test for normally distributed data, and the comparisons of differences between HAH positive (HAH+) and HAH negative (HAH-) groups were analyzed by independent student's t-test. The non-normally data were compared using the Mann-Whitney U test. The spearman correlations between HAH score and the measurements at sea level and 3700 m were analyzed. Univariate logistic

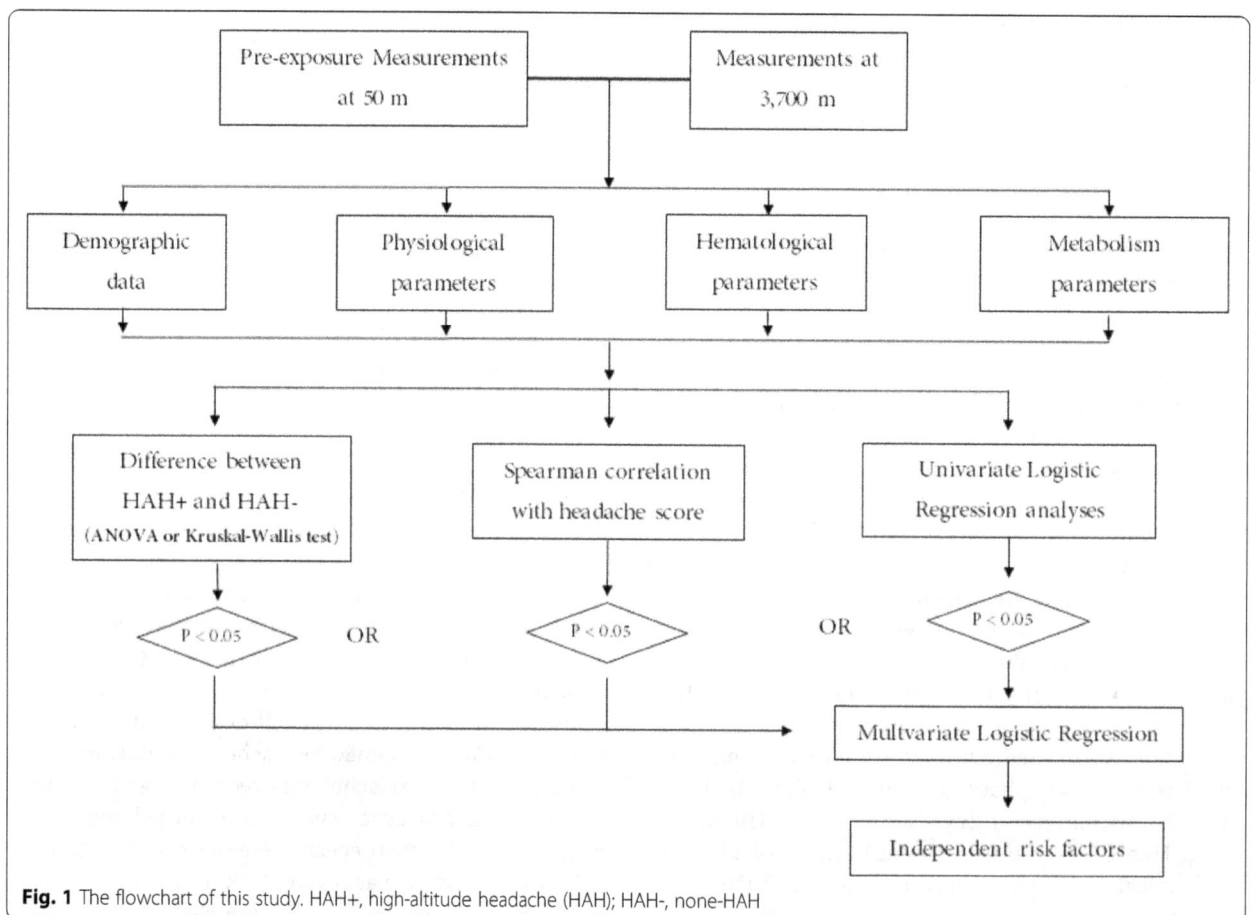

Fig. 1 The flowchart of this study. HAH+, high-altitude headache (HAH); HAH-, none-HAH

regression was performed to assess the relationships between each measurements and HAH at 3700 m. Significant variables in any of the above three analyses were included in forward stepwise multivariable logistic regression, and analyzed separately at sea level and 3700 m. The significant level of p-value is 0.05 (two-tailed). The analyses flowchart was shown in Fig. 1.

Results

Total 318 participants had complete CRFs, physiological, hematological and biochemical measurements

(Additional file 1). The mean age and BMI of the participants in this study were 21.87 ± 3.33 years and 22.06 ± 1.99 kg/m^2. The incidence of HAH after acute exposure to 3700 m is 74.84% (Additional files 2 and 3).

Alterations in physiological, hematological and biochemical measurements

Most of the physiological, hematological and biochemical parameters were dramatically altered after acute exposure to high altitude from sea level, beside of Hct, MCH and LYM%. For the physiological measurements, SpO$_2$

Table 1 Comparison of physiological, hematological and biochemical parameters between sea level and 3700 m ($N = 318$)

	Measurements at sea-level	Measurements at 3700 m	p
Demographic data			
Age, y	21.87 ± 3.33	the same as sea-level	–
BMI, kg/m^2	22.06 ± 1.99	the same as sea-level	–
chest circumstance, cm	86.11 ± 5.09	the same as sea-level	–
Smoking, yes(%)	102 (32.1)	the same as sea-level	–
Drinking, yes(%)	39 (12.3)	the same as sea-level	–
Physical parameters			
SpO$_2$, %	98.00 (98.00–98.20)	88.00 (85.10–90.20)	< 0.001**
HR, beats/min	67.49 ± 9.18	84.17 ± 12.15	< 0.001**
SBP, mmHg	111.22 ± 9.81	120.52 ± 12.8	< 0.001**
DBP, mmHg	71.85 ± 8.14	81.77 ± 9.56	< 0.001**
Hematological parameters			
RBC, *10^{12}	5.00 (4.80–5.20)	5.11 (4.82–5.49)	< 0.001**
Hgb, g/L	151.10 (144.00–157.00)	157.00 (147.00–169.30)	< 0.001**
Hct, %	44.49 ± 3.10	48.42 ± 6.08	< 0.001**
MCV, fL	92.20 (90.00–94.22)	86.50 (84.40–88.62)	< 0.001**
MCH, pg	30.59 (29.61–31.30)	30.90 (30.20–32.10)	< 0.001**
PLT, *10^9	206.79 ± 44.77	244.97 ± 69.80	< 0.001**
MPV, fL	10.50 (9.80–11.00)	10.60 (10.20–11.00)	0.006**
WBC, *10^9	6.10 (5.40–7.10)	7.90 (7.00–9.50)	< 0.001**
LYM%, %	36.23 ± 7.59	36.49 ± 9.06	0.833
LYM#, *10^9	2.20 (1.90–2.60)	2.95 (2.50–3.40)	< 0.001**
Biochemical parameters			
ALT, U/L	18.00 (15.00–23.00)	39.20 (30.40–48.50)	< 0.001**
AST, U/L	15.10 (12.30–18.50)	31.00 (25.50–40.60)	< 0.001**
BUN, mmol/L	4.45 (3.89–5.28)	4.60 (4.10–5.25)	0.109
CREA, umol/L	58.00 (49.00–68.10)	105.40 (98.60–114.00)	< 0.001**
TBIL, umol/L	12.60 (10.80–14.00)	12.30 (10.20–15.65)	0.023*
DBIL, umol/L	3.10 (2.30–3.50)	4.70 (3.90–5.80)	< 0.001**
IBIL, umol/L	9.70 (8.50–10.50)	7.70 (5.80–10.65)	< 0.001**

SpO$_2$ blood oxygen saturation, *HR* heart rate at resting, *SBP* systolic blood pressure, *DBP* diastolic blood pressure, *RBC* red blood cell count, *Hgb* hemoglobin, *Hct* hematocrit, *MCV* mean corpuscular volume, *MCH* mean corpuscular hemoglobin, *PLT* platelets count, *MPV* mean platelet volume, *WBC* white blood cell, *LYM%* lymphocyte rate, *LYM#* lymphocyte count, *ALT* alanine aminotransferase, *AST* aspartate aminotransferase, *BUN* blood urea nitrogen, *CREA* creatinine, *TBIL* total serum bilirubin, *DBIL* direct serum bilirubin, *IBIL* indirect serum bilirubin

Normally distributed variables were presented as mean ± SD, and compared using paired-sample T test; Non-normally distributed variables were presented as mean (interquartile range), and compared using Mann-Whitney U test

*p value indicates $p < 0.05$; **p value indicates $p < 0.01$

decreased from 98.00 (IQR, 98.00–98.20) to 88.00 (IQR, 85.10–90.20) ($p < 0.01$), while HR, SBP and DBP significantly increased from sea level to 3700 m. For the hematological measurements, RBC, Hgb, Hct, PLT, MCH, MPV, WBC and LYM# all significantly increased, while MCV showed significant decrease (all $p < 0.001$). However, the alteration of LYM% between sea level and 3700 m was not significant. For the biochemical measurements, ALT, AST, CREA, TBIL, DBIL and IBIL exhibited a significant increase, while BUN had no significant difference between sea level and 3700 m. (Table 1).

Comparison of physiological, hematological and biochemical parameters between the HAH+ and HAH- groups

Regarding the measurements at sea level, compared to the HAH- group, the HAH+ group had significant higher age

Table 2 Difference between HAH+ and HAH- subjects in demographics, physiological, hematological and biochemical parameters at sea level and 3700 m

	Measurements at sea level			Measurements at 3700 m		
	HAH+ ($n = 238$)	HAH- ($n = 80$)	p	HAH+ ($n = 238$)	HAH- ($n = 80$)	p
Demographic data						
Age (year)	22.05 ± 3.53	21.30 ± 2.69	0.046*	The same as sea-levels		
BMI (kg/m²)	22.08 ± 2.02	21.96 ± 1.86	0.662	The same as sea-levels		
Chest Circumstance (cm)	86.19 ± 5.30	86.04 ± 4.59	0.813	The same as sea-levels		
Smoking (yes, %)	73 (30.7)	29 (36.3)	0.417	The same as sea-levels		
Drinking (yes, %)	29 (12.2)	10 (12.5)	0.978	The same as sea-levels		
Physiological parameters						
SpO₂ (%)	98.00 (97.90–98.00)	98.00 (98.00–98.00)	0.171	88.00 (84.90–90.40)	90.00 (87.30–92.10)	< 0.001**
HR (beats/min)	67.72 ± 8.99	66.91 ± 9.86	0.522	85.30 ± 12.09	80.77 ± 11.75	< 0.001**
SBP (mmHg)	110.97 ± 10.09	111.98 ± 8.88	0.405	119.74 ± 13.10	123.41 ± 11.10	0.046*
DBP (mmHg)	71.69 ± 8.23	72.30 ± 7.91	0.569	81.42 ± 9.86	82.99 ± 8.39	0.251
Hematological parameters						
RBC (*10¹²)	5.00 (4.80–5.20)	5.00 (4.70–5.20)	0.559	5.10 (4.83–5.48)	5.11 (4.75–5.55)	0.955
Hgb (g/L)	151.30 (144.00–157.00)	150.00 (143.80–158.10)	0.945	157.00 (149.60–168.30)	157.00 (144.50–170.40)	0.641
Hct (%)	45.69 ± 2.46	45.70 ± 2.49	0.981	48.61 ± 5.95	47.83 ± 6.47	0.364
MCV (fL)	92.30 (90.00–94.75)	92.00 (90.20–94.10)	0.598	86.50 (84.40–88.92)	86.40 (84.30–87.75)	0.336
MCH (pg)	30.60 (29.59–31.36)	30.59 (29.73–31.02)	0.459	30.90 (29.95–32.10)	31.00 (30.18–31.75)	0.939
PLT (*10⁹)	207.95 ± 44.97	203.33 ± 44.27	0.438	244.8 ± 68.6	245.3 ± 73.8	0.960
MPV (fL)	10.50 (9.80–11.02)	10.40 (9.70–10.91)	0.326	10.60 (10.20–11.03)	10.60 (10.30–11.00)	0.965
WBC (*10⁹)	6.00 (5.40–7.00)	6.50 (5.50–7.35)	0.090	7.90 (7.10–9.50)	7.95 (6.98–9.38)	0.791
LYM rate (%)	36.60 ± 7.58	35.12 ± 7.56	0.144	36.53 ± 9.68	36.36 ± 6.89	0.871
LYM count (*10⁹)	2.20 (1.90–2.60)	2.15 (1.90–2.60)	0.703	3.00 (2.51–3.40)	2.95 (2.58–3.50)	0.910
Biochemical parameters						
ALT (U/L)	18.10 (15.00–24.10)	18.00 (14.00–21.00)	0.187	39.20 (28.50–49.30)	39.00 (29.30–46.80)	0.563
AST (U/L)	15.20 (12.00–20.00)	14.00 (12.10–17.75)	0.237	31.00 (25.00–40.25)	32.00 (27.20–38.50)	0.581
BUN (mmol/L)	4.38 (3.82–5.08)	4.69 (3.99–5.53)	0.029*	4.50 (4.02–5.20)	4.80 (4.40–5.40)	0.003**
CREA (umol/L)	58.00 (49.00–65.00)	59.00 (50.10–68.20)	0.082	105.30 (98.50–115.00)	106.80 (99.70–113.30)	0.811
TBIL (umol/L)	12.50 (10.80–14.00)	12.70 (10.85–14.00)	0.876	12.75 (10.20–15.75)	12.90 (10.20–15.50)	0.709
DBIL (umol/L)	3.10 (2.30–3.50)	3.10 (2.15–3.50)	0.553	4.85 (3.90–5.90)	4.60 (3.80–5.80)	0.274
IBIL (umol/L)	9.60 (8.50–10.43)	9.90 (8.50–10.55)	0.933	7.60 (5.80–10.70)	7.80 (6.00–10.40)	0.877

HAH high altitude headache, *HAH+* with high-altitude headache, *HAH-* without high-altitude headache, *SpO₂* blood oxygen saturation, *HR* heart rate at resting, *SBP* systolic blood pressure, *DBP* diastolic blood pressure, *RBC* red blood cell count, *Hgb* hemoglobin, *Hct* hematocrit, *MCV* mean corpuscular volume, *MCH* mean corpuscular hemoglobin, *PLT* platelets count, *MPV* mean platelet volume, *WBC* white blood cell, *LYM%* lymphocyte rate, *LYM#* lymphocyte count, *ALT* alanine aminotransferase, *AST* aspartate aminotransferase, *BUN* blood urea nitrogen, *CREA* creatinine, *TBIL* total serum bilirubin, *DBIL* direct serum bilirubin, *IBIL* indirect serum bilirubin

Normally distributed variables were presented as mean ± SD, and compared using student's t-test; Non-normally distributed variables were presented as mean (interquartile range), and compared using Mann-Whitney U test; Categorical variables were compared using fisher's exact test;

*p value indicates $p < 0.05$; **p value indicates $p < 0.01$

(HAH+: 22.05 ± 3.53 vs HAH-: 21.30 ± 2.69, $p = 0.046$) and significant lower BUN (HAH+: 4.38 (3.82–5.08) vs HAH-: 4.69 (3.99–5.53), $p = 0.029$). There were no significant differences in the physiological and hematological measurements at sea level (all $p > 0.05$, Table 2).

Regarding the measurements at 3700 m, compared with the HAH- group, the HAH+ group had significant lower SpO_2 (HAH+ 88.00 (84.90–90.40) vs HAH- 90.00 (87.30–92.10), $p < 0.001$), lower SBP (HAH+ 119.74 ± 13.10 vs HAH- 123.41 ± 11.10, $p = 0.046$) and lower BUN (HAH+ 4.50 (4.02–5.20) vs HAH- 4.80 (4.40–5.40), $p = 0.003$). The HAH+ group also had significant higher HR than HAH- group (HAH+ 85.30 ± 12.09 vs HAH- 80.77 ± 11.75, $p < 0.001$). The hematological measurements showed no significant differences between HAH+ and HAH- groups at 3700 m (all $p > 0.05$, Table 2).

Relationship between physiological, hematological and biochemical parameters and HAH

We further used Spearman's correlation analyses to explore the relationship between measurements and the HAH severity. For the measurements at sea level, no significant association was observed between demographic data or all measurements and HAH severity. For the measurements at 3700 m, HAH severity was significantly associated with SpO_2 ($r = -0.365$, $p < 0.001$), HR ($r = 0.249$, $p = 0.002$) and BUN ($r = -0.176$, $p = 0.006$). The hematological measurements showed no significant correlation with HAH severity (all $p > 0.05$, Table 3).

Risk factors for HAH at sea level and 3700 m

To discover risk factors for HAH, we performed univariate logistic regression for all parameters at sea level and at 3700 m. Among the sea level parameters, the univariate logistic regression revealed that only BUN associated with HAH significantly (OR:0.78, 95% CI:0.61–0.99, $p = 0.044$). Meanwhile, among the parameters at 3700 m, SpO_2 (OR:0.84, 95% CI:0.77–0.90, $p < 0.001$), HR (OR:1.03, 95% CI:1.01–1.06, $p = 0.004$) and BUN (OR:0.72, 95% CI:0.55–0.93, $p = 0.012$) exhibited significant association with HAH (Table 4).

Multivariate logistic regression was performed for parameters which showed significant associations with HAH in univariate logistic regression, correlated with headache score, or showed significant difference between HAH+ and HAH- groups. For parameters at sea level, only BUN showed significant protective effect on HAH (OR:0.77, 95% CI:0.60–0.99, $p = 0.040$), but for parameters at 3700 m, multivariate logistic regression revealed that SpO_2 (OR:0.84, 95% CI:0.76–0.93, $p < 0.001$), HR (OR:1.03, 95% CI:1.00–1.07, $p = 0.042$) and BUN (OR:0.64, 95% CI:0.46–0.88, $p = 0.007$) were all independent risk factors for HAH (Table 5).

Table 3 Relationships between HAH score and all the parameters at both sea level and 3700 m ($N = 318$)

	Measurements at sea-level		Measurements at 3700 m	
	With HAH score r	p	With HAH score r	p
Demographic data				
Age (y)	0.113	0.053	The same as sea-level	
BMI (kg/m²)	0.087	0.129	The same as sea-level	
Chest Circumference (cm)	0.079	0.187	The same as sea-level	
Physical parameters				
SpO_2 (%)	−0.085	0.168	−0.365	< 0.001**
HR (beats/min)	0.003	0.859	0.249	0.002**
SBP (mmHg)	−0.049	0.471	−0.050	0.518
DBP (mmHg)	−0.073	0.246	−0.008	0.865
Metabolic parameters				
RBC (*10¹²)	0.013	0.984	0.041	0.468
HGB (g/L)	0.008	0.910	0.046	0.358
HCT (%)	0.015	0.976	0.056	0.333
MCV (fL)	−0.012	0.927	−0.008	0.620
MCH (pg)	0.020	0.640	−0.042	0.941
PLT (*10⁹)	0.057	0.336	−0.021	0.420
MPV (fL)	0.077	0.428	−0.023	0.871
WBC (*10⁹)	−0.102	0.131	0.081	0.900
LYM% (%)	0.024	0.688	−0.061	0.341
LYM# (*10⁹)	0.035	0.687	0.017	0.278
Biochemical parameters				
ALT (U/L)	0.072	0.388	0.056	0.987
AST (U/L)	0.065	0.446	−0.051	0.100
BUN (mmol/L)	−0.071	0.211	−0.176	0.006**
CREA (umol/L)	−0.045	0.425	0.009	0.759
TBIL (umol/L)	−0.004	0.845	0.105	0.657
DBIL (umol/L)	0.037	0.581	0.034	0.672
IBIL (umol/L)	−0.027	0.539	0.106	0.583

HAH high altitude headache, SpO_2 blood oxygen saturation, HR heart rate at resting, SBP systolic blood pressure, DBP diastolic blood pressure, RBC red blood cell count, Hgb hemoglobin, Hct hematocrit, MCV mean corpuscular volume, MCH mean corpuscular hemoglobin, PLT platelets count, MPV mean platelet volume, WBC white blood cell, LYM% lymphocyte rate, LYM# lymphocyte count, ALT alanine aminotransferase, AST aspartate aminotransferase, BUN blood urea nitrogen, CREA creatinine, TBIL total serum bilirubin, DBIL direct serum bilirubin, IBIL indirect serum bilirubin
*p value indicates $p < 0.05$; **p value indicates $p < 0.01$

Discussion

Alterations in physiological, hematological and biochemical parameters

Our study identified alterations in physiological, hematological and biochemical parameters from sea level to altitude of 3700 m. High altitude hypoxia lead a reduction of SpO_2, which may result in a decrease in

Table 4 Univariate logistic regression for each measurements at sea level and 3700 m (N = 318)

	Measurements at sea level				Measurements at 3700 m			
	β-coefficient	OR	95% CI	p	β-coefficient	OR	95% CI	p
Demographic Data								
age (y)	0.076	1.08	0.99–1.19	0.090	The same as sea level			
BMI (kg/m2)	0.028	1.03	0.90–1.18	0.674	The same as sea level			
Chest (cm)	0.006	1.01	0.96–1.06	0.825	The same as sea level			
smoking	−0.249	0.76	0.42–1.33	0.453	The same as sea level			
drinking	−0.055	0.97	0.45–2.16	0.917	The same as sea level			
Physical parameters								
SpO₂ (%)	−0.058	0.94	0.75–1.12	0.555	− 0.176	0.84	0.77–0.90	< 0.001**
HR (beats/min)	0.010	1.01	0.98–1.04	0.501	0.032	1.03	1.01–1.06	0.004**
SBP (mmHg)	−0.010	0.99	0.96–1.02	0.433	−0.022	0.98	0.95–1.00	0.068
DBP (mmHg)	−0.009	0.99	0.96–1.02	0.576	−0.017	0.98	0.95–1.01	0.291
Hematological parameters								
RBC (*10¹²)	−0.197	0.82	0.39–1.76	0.605	0.072	1.07	0.75–1.55	0.696
HGB (g/L)	−0.002	1.00	0.97–1.03	0.906	0.004	1.00	0.99–1.02	0.460
HCT (%)	−0.001	1.00	0.90–1.11	0.981	0.022	1.02	0.98–1.07	0.341
MCV (fL)	0.014	1.01	0.96–1.06	0.580	0.020	1.02	0.98–1.07	0.356
MCH (pg)	0.023	1.02	0.89–1.16	0.718	0.015	1.02	0.92–1.13	0.770
PLT (*10⁹)	0.002	1.00	0.99–1.01	0.439	0.000	1.00	0.99–1.01	0.959
MPV (fL)	0.136	1.15	0.88–1.51	0.320	0.039	1.04	0.70–1.56	0.847
WBC (*10⁹)	−0.153	0.86	0.71–1.03	0.105	0.041	1.04	0.92–1.19	0.525
LYM% (%)	0.013	1.01	0.99–1.06	0.959	0.002	1.00	0.97–1.03	0.890
LYM# (*10⁹)	0.026	1.03	0.61–1.70	0.144	0.074	1.08	0.78–1.50	0.655
Biochemical parameters								
ALT (U/L)	0.027	1.03	0.99–1.07	0.119	0.014	1.01	0.97–1.07	0.561
AST (U/L)	0.030	1.03	0.99–1.08	0.180	0.005	1.00	0.98–1.03	0.670
BUN (mmol/L)	−0.252	0.78	0.61–0.99	0.044*	−0.330	0.72	0.55–0.93	0.012*
CREA (umol/L)	−0.021	0.98	0.95–1.00	0.096	0.003	1.00	0.98–1.03	0.823
TBIL (umol/L)	0.043	1.04	0.91–1.19	0.531	0.026	1.03	0.97–1.09	0.345
DBIL (umol/L)	0.161	1.17	0.79–1.75	0.427	0.137	1.15	0.97–1.37	0.117
IBIL (umol/L)	0.051	1.05	0.87–1.28	0.605	0.017	1.02	0.96–1.09	0.599

SpO₂ blood oxygen saturation, *HR* heart rate at resting, *SBP* systolic blood pressure, *DBP* diastolic blood pressure, *RBC* red blood cell count, *Hgb* hemoglobin, *Hct* hematocrit, *MCV* mean corpuscular volume, *MCH* mean corpuscular hemoglobin, *PLT* platelets count, *MPV* mean platelet volume, *WBC* white blood cell, *LYM%* lymphocyte rate, *LYM#* lymphocyte count, *ALT* alanine aminotransferase, *AST* aspartate aminotransferase, *BUN* blood urea nitrogen, *CREA* creatinine, *TBIL* total serum bilirubin, *DBIL* direct serum bilirubin, *IBIL* indirect serum bilirubin
*p value indicates $p < 0.05$; **p value indicates $p < 0.01$

the delivery of oxygen and energy to organs and tissues. Dropped blood oxygen level may stimulate carotid chemoreceptors and activate the autonomic nervous system, which results in the cardiac output improvement, finally leading to increased HR [20]. The observation of our study is in consistency with previous studies [1, 7, 13].

The low humidity, hypoxic tachypnea and reduced fluid intake can lead to insensible fluid lose at high altitude [15, 16]. In addition, within hours of exposure to high altitude hypoxia, hypoxic tachypnea may lead to respiratory alkalosis, increased natriuresis and diuresis, promoting fluid shift away from intravascular space, result in blood concentration, even hypovolemia [21]. Our study observed most hematological parameters (RBC, Hgb, Hct, MCH, PLT, WBC and LYM#) were elevated from sea-level to altitude of 3700 m within a 72 h ascending processes, which also in consistency with previous studies [14].

Our study also observed that serum creatinine increased dramatically after ascent from sea level to 3700 m, indicating a significantly decreased estimated glomerular filtration

Table 5 Forward stepwise multivariate logistic regression for HAH at sea level and 3700 m ($N = 318$)

	β-coefficient	OR	95% CI	p-value
Measurements at sea level (after variable selection)				
age	0.075	1.08	0.99–1.18	0.092
BUN	−0.259	0.77	0.60–0.99	0.040*
Measurements at 3700 m (after variable selection)				
age	0.090	1.09	0.98–1.23	0.110
SpO₂	−0.191	0.84	0.76–0.93	0.001**
HR	0.029	1.03	1.00–1.07	0.042*
SBP	−0.019	0.98	0.95–1.01	0.091
BUN	−0.452	0.64	0.46–0.88	0.007**

SpO_2 blood oxygen saturation, *HR* heart rate at resting, *SBP* systolic blood pressure, *BUN* blood urea nitrogen
*p value indicates $p < 0.05$; **p value indicates $p < 0.01$

rate (eGFR). Previous study has suggested that a linear decrease of eGFR with the increase of altitude, which may related to a reduction of renal plasma flow (secondary to the increased sympathetic activity) [18]. In addition, our study found that there was only little change of BUN from sea level to 3700 m, which is inconsistent with previous study [22]. Because both BUN and creatinine were commonly used as renal function markers, we draw a scatter plot to explore the change of the relationship between BUN and creatinine at 50 m and 3700 m (See fig. 2). This figure showed that there is a strong linear correlation between BUN and creatinine is at 50 m altitude, but no significant correlation after ascent to 3700 m. The BUN level represent the urea concentration of plasma, which can be reabsorbed in inner medullary collecting duct (IMCD), while creatinine can not be reabsorbed [23, 24]. Some studies indicated that urea generation in hepatocytes can be obstructed by insufficient adenosine triphosphate (ATP) supply and depressed

levels of arginine and citrulline after exposure to hypoxia, but the genesis of creatinine is relatively constant [25]. This may be an explanation to the change of relationship between BUN and creatinine after rapid ascending to high altitude.

The physiological risk factors for HAH at 3700 m
The elevation of altitude results in a lower partial pressure of oxygen in the inspired air, and SpO_2 is a direct parameter that reflect the oxygen delivery. Insufficient oxygen consumption of cerebral tissue leads to function disorder and cytotoxic oedema, which is the main cause of HAH [26]. In addition, increased HR reflect the activity of sympathetic nervous system, which can lead to higher cardiac output and vasoconstriction of viscera, promote the redistribution of blood (mostly into vital organs such as brain). The accumulation of fluid in the brain result in increased intracranial pressure (ICP), which is another crucial cause of HAH [6]. Multiple lines of studies have reported that reduced SpO_2 and increased HR are independent risk factors for HAH, which is supported by our findings [1, 7, 11].

Blood urea nitrogen is an independent risk factor for HAH at both sea level and 3700 m
Our results first found that BUN is an independent risk factor of HAH at both sea level and 3700 m, and the values of BUN at 3700 m positively associated with HAH severity. Although more evidence of this finding is lacking, there still can be some potential explanations.

The first possible explanation is that the urea concentration may reflect the oxygen supply and utilization in cells. As discussed above, the correlation between BUN and creatinine showed a good linearity at sea level but no correlation at 3700 m, suggest that the production of

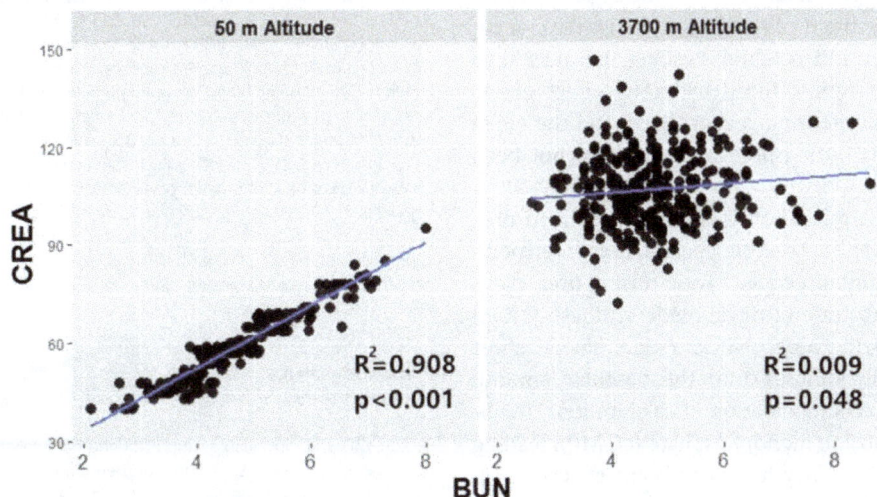

Fig. 2 the correlation between BUN and creatinine at 50 m and 3700 m. BUN, Blood urea nitrogen (mmol/L); CREA, creatinine (umol/L)

BUN may be affected by high altitude environment, and the concentration of BUN may partially reflect metabolism status and the oxygen utilization status of hepatocyte. Relative to BUN, other liver function parameters such as ALT, AST and bilirubin were aimed at substantial damage of liver and biliary tract. Some vitro experiments demonstrated that under hypobaric hypoxia, ATP was decreased in multiple cell lines, and as the oxygen concentration was decreased, production of both urea in isolated rat hepatocytes declined [25, 27, 28]. Study on the effect of acute hypoxic hypoxia on the profile of plasma amino acids in rats showed that after exposure to hypoxia for 5 h, the concentrations of arginine and citrulline (which are related to the urea cycle) were depressed [25]. These findings implicate that the BUN concentration in plasma may reflect the oxygen-driven catabolism, and higher BUN may indicate better oxygen supply and utilization of hepatocytes, even brain cells, which is the main cause of HAH.

The second potential explanation is that the hyperosmolar properties of urea may help with reducing intracranial pressure and brain volume [29]. Through brain imaging of patients with acute mountain sickness, some studies showed that intracellular and extracellular water accumulation influenced by increased permeability of the blood–brain barrier, resulted in cerebral swelling, sulci disappearing and changing of grey matter [6]. These verified that the inflation of brain volume and elevation of ICP is a vital sign of HAH. In 1960s, urea became the first widely used hyperosmolar compound in clinic for reducing ICP and alleviating cerebral swelling [30, 31]. The penetrability of urea from extracellular into brain tissue is 1/10 compared with the penetration into muscle, and its blood to brain transfer coefficient (a measurement of clearance) is 5×10^{-3} ml/g/min, a value that is 3 orders of magnitude lower than water [32]. Therefore, exogenous urea can maintain certain osmotic pressure inside and outside the brain cell and prevent excessive accumulation of liquids and cerebral swelling. Because urea undergoes renal excretion, the dehydrating effect of exogenous urea on parenchyma is short lived, and the effect of endogenous urea during brain oedema have not been studied.

Another possible explanation is the products from urea cycle, nitric oxide (NO). Arginine generated as intermediate products by argininosuccinate lyase during urea cycle, and is the basic substrate of nitric oxide synthase (NOS) for generating nitric oxide. Nitric oxide has a short half-life and rapidly diffuses into the vascular smooth muscle where it affects modulation of calcium ions, mediated by cyclic guanosine monophosphate (cGMP), leading to vasodilatation [33]. They have significant effects in relieving pulmonary hypertension, improve cardiac output and blood gas exchange [34]. However, relevant studies about the correlation between ICP, pulmonary hypertension and endogenic urea are still lacking.

Limitations

Limited by field study, the time of onset of headache of participants were recorded by memories, not precisely, which should be improved in future. After the onset of headache, participants have not descent to low altitude immediately, which not strictly satisfied the criteria of the International Classification of Headache Disorders. The sample size was small, and there are many other potential risk factors that can be considered in the study, such as nitric oxide and $PaCO_2$. The participants in our study were all young male individuals, which may limit extrapolation of our results.

Conclusions

Our study found the frequency of HAH was high (74.84%) after acute exposure to 3700 m. We confirmed that SpO_2 and HR at 3700 m are independent risk factors for HAH, and firstly identified the independent association between BUN and HAH at both sea level and 3700 m, which suggested that lower BUN may be a new independent risk factor for HAH.

Additional files

> **Additional file 1:** The distribution and QQ-norm plot of SpO2 at 50 m and 3700 m. (DOCX 168 kb)
>
> **Additional file 2:** The incidence of mild, moderate and severe headaches after ascent to 3700 m altitude. (DOCX 16 kb)
>
> **Additional file 3:** The Shapiro-Wilk normality test of parameters at 50 m and 3700 m. (DOCX 12 kb)

Abbreviations

ALT: alanine aminotransferase; AMS: acute mountain sickness; AST: aspartate aminotransferase; ATP: adenosine triphosphate; BMI: body mass index; BUN: blood urea nitrogen; cGMP: cyclic guanosine monophosphate; CREA: creatinine; CRFs: Structured case report forms; DBIL: direct serum bilirubin; DBP: diastolic blood pressure; eGFR: estimated glomerular filtration rate; HAH: high-altitude headache; Hct: hematocrit; Hgb: hemoglobin; HR: heart rate; IBIL: indirect serum bilirubin; ICP: intracranial pressure; IMCD: inner medullary collecting duct; IQR: interquartile range; LYM: absolute lymphocyte count; LYM%: lymphocyte percentage; MCH: mean corpuscular hemoglobin; MCV: mean corpuscular volume; MPV: mean platelet volume; NO: nitric oxide; NOS: nitric oxide synthase; OR: Odds ratio; PLT: platelet count; RBC: red blood cell count; SBP: systolic blood pressure; SD: standard deviations; SpO2: blood oxygen saturation; TBIL: total serum bilirubin; WBC: white blood cell count

Acknowledgements

The authors thank Wenyuan Duan, MD, Tongjian Wang, MD and Kai Dong, MM (Institute of Cardiovascular Disease, General Hospital of Jinan Military Region, China) for invaluable support during data collection. The authors also thank Yajun Yang, PhD, Dr. Xingdong Chen (Fudan University, China) and Ziyu Yan, Juan Zhang and Jiangli Xue (Fudan-Taizhou Institute of Health Sciences, China) for support with the data entry of this study. No one received compensation for his/her contribution.

Funding
This work was supported by the National Natural Science Foundation of China (31330038, 31521003, 31460286), Shanghai Municipal Science and Technology Major Project (2017SHZDZX01), Ministry of Science and Technology (2015FY1117000), Science and Technology Committee of Shanghai Municipality (16JC1400500), the 111 Project (B13016).

Authors' contributions
LJ were responsible for study supervision and contributed to the study concept and design, data collection, data analysis, drafting and revision of the manuscript. KW contributed to study supervision, and were responsible for data collection, data analysis, drafting and revision of the manuscript. XW, YM and YL contributed to study supervision and data collection. WP contributed to the revise of the manuscript. MZ, YW, YL and XL contributed to data analysis and interpretation, drafting and revision of the manuscript. JW contributed to study supervision, drafting and revision of the manuscript. LK contributed to the data collection. All authors read and approved the final manuscript.

Competing interests
The authors declare that they have no competing interests.

Author details
[1]State Key Laboratory of Genetic Engineering, Collaborative Innovation Center for Genetics and Development, School of Life Sciences, Fudan University, Shanghai 200438, China. [2]Ministry of Education Key Laboratory of Contemporary Anthropology, Department of Anthropology and Human Genetics, School of Life Sciences, Fudan University, Shanghai 200438, China. [3]Human Phenome Institute, Fudan University, Shanghai 201203, China. [4]Institute of Cardiovascular Disease, General Hospital of Jinan Military Region, Jinan 250022, Shandong, China. [5]Key Laboratory of High Altitude Environment and Genes Related to Diseases of Tibet Autonomous Region, School of Medicine, Xizang Minzu University, Xianyang 712082, China. [6]Six Industrial Research Institute, Fudan University, Shanghai 200433, China.

References
1. Burtscher M, Mairer K, Wille M, Broessner G (2011) Risk factors for high-altitude headache in mountaineers. Cephalalgia 31(6):706–711
2. Carod-Artal FJ (2014) High-altitude headache and acute mountain sickness. Neurologia 29(9):533–540
3. Roach RC, Bartsch P, Hackett P, Oelz O: The Lake Louise acute mountain sickness scoring system: the Lake Louise AMS scoring consensus committee; 1993
4. Headache Classification Subcommittee of the International Headache S (2004) The international classification of headache disorders: 2nd edition. Cephalalgia 24(Suppl 1):9–160
5. Bes A, Kunkel R, Lance JW, Nappi G, Pfaffenrath V, Rose FC, Schoenberg BS, Soyka D, Tfelt-Hansen P, Welch KMA et al (2013) The international classification of headache disorders, 3rd edition (beta version). Cephalalgia 33(9):629–808
6. Wilson MH, Newman S, Imray CH (2009) The cerebral effects of ascent to high altitudes. Lancet Neurol 8(2):175–191
7. Bian SZ, Zhang JH, Gao XB, Li M, Yu J, Liu X, Dong JQ, Chen GZ, Huang L (2013) Risk factors for high-altitude headache upon acute high-altitude exposure at 3700 m in young Chinese men: a cohort study. J Headache Pain 14:35
8. Bian SZ, Jin J, Li QN, Yu J, Tang CF, Rao RS, Yu SY, Zhao XH, Qin J, Huang L (2015) Hemodynamic characteristics of high-altitude headache following acute high altitude exposure at 3700 m in young Chinese men. J Headache Pain 16:527
9. Harris NS, Wenzel RP, Thomas SH (2003) High altitude headache: efficacy of acetaminophen vs. ibuprofen in a randomized, controlled trial. J Emerg Med 24(4):383–387
10. Mampreso E, Maggioni F, Viaro F, Disco C, Zanchin G (2009) Efficacy of oxygen inhalation in sumatriptan refractory "high altitude" cluster headache attacks. J Headache Pain 10(6):465–467

11. Lawley JS (2011) Identifying the possible risk factors for high-altitude headache in mountaineers. Cephalalgia 31(16):1677–1678
12. Sutherland AI, Morris DS, Owen CG, Bron AJ, Roach RC (2008) Optic nerve sheath diameter, intracranial pressure and acute mountain sickness on Mount Everest: a longitudinal cohort study. Br J Sports Med 42(3):183–188
13. Guo WY, Bian SZ, Zhang JH, Li QN, Yu J, Chen JF, Tang CF, Rao RS, Yu SY, Jin J et al (2017) Physiological and psychological factors associated with onset of high-altitude headache in Chinese men upon acute high-altitude exposure at 3700 m. Cephalalgia 37(4):336–347
14. Huang H, Liu B, Wu G, Xu G, Sun BD, Gao YQ (2017) Hematological risk factors for high-altitude headache in Chinese men following acute exposure at 3,700 m. Front Physiol 8:801
15. Jones RM, Terhaard C, Zullo J, Tenney SM (1981) Mechanism of reduced water intake in rats at high altitude. Am J Phys 240(3):R187–R191
16. Westerterp KR, Meijer EP, Rubbens M, Robach P, Richalet JP (2000) Operation Everest III: energy and water balance. Pflugers Archiv : European J Physiol 439(4):483–488
17. Bestle MH, Olsen NV, Poulsen TD, Roach R, Fogh-Andersen N, Bie P (2002) Prolonged hypobaric hypoxemia attenuates vasopressin secretion and renal response to osmostimulation in men. J Appl Physiol 92(5):1911–1922
18. Pichler J, Risch L, Hefti U, Merz TM, Turk AJ, Bloch KE, Maggiorini M, Hess T, Barthelmes D, Schoch OD et al (2008) Glomerular filtration rate estimates decrease during high altitude expedition but increase with Lake Louise acute mountain sickness scores. Acta Physiol 192(3):443–450
19. Hackett P, Rennie D (2002) High-altitude pulmonary edema. Jama 287(17): 2275–2278
20. Naeije R (2010) Physiological adaptation of the cardiovascular system to high altitude. Prog Cardiovasc Dis 52(6):456–466
21. Goldfarb-Rumyantzev AS, Alper SL (2014) Short-term responses of the kidney to high altitude in mountain climbers. Nephrol Dial Transplant 29(3):497–506
22. Shah MB, Braude D, Crandall CS, Kwack H, Rabinowitz L, Cumbo TA, Basnyat B, Bhasyal G (2006) Changes in metabolic and hematologic laboratory values with ascent to altitude and the development of acute mountain sickness in Nepalese pilgrims. Wilderness Environ Med 17(3):171–177
23. Muller F, Dommergues M, Bussieres L, LortatJacob S, Loirat C, Oury JF, Aigrain Y, Niaudet P, Aegerter P, Dumez Y (1996) Development of human renal function: reference intervals for 10 biochemical markers in fetal urine. Clin Chem 42(11):1855–1860
24. Deguchi E, Akuzawa M (1997) Renal clearance of endogenous creatinine, urea, sodium, and potassium in normal cats and cats with chronic renal failure. J Vet Med Sci 59(7):509–512
25. Kashiwagura T, Wilson DF, Erecinska M (1984) Oxygen dependence of cellular metabolism: the effect of O2 tension on gluconeogenesis and urea synthesis in isolated rat hepatocytes. J Cell Physiol 120(1):13–18
26. Kallenberg K, Bailey DM, Christ S, Mohr A, Roukens R, Menold E, Steiner T, Bartsch P, Knauth M (2007) Magnetic resonance imaging evidence of cytotoxic cerebral edema in acute mountain sickness. J Cereb Blood Flow Metab 27(5):1064–1071
27. Lipton P, Whittingham TS (1982) Reduced ATP concentration as a basis for synaptic transmission failure during hypoxia in the in vitro Guinea-pig hippocampus. J Physiol 325:51–65
28. Heerlein K, Schulze A, Hotz L, Bartsch P, Mairbaurl H (2005) Hypoxia decreases cellular ATP demand and inhibits mitochondrial respiration of a549 cells. Am J Respir Cell Mol Biol 32(1):44–51
29. Otvos B, Kshettry VR, Benzel EC (2014) The history of urea as a hyperosmolar agent to decrease brain swelling. Neurosurg Focus 36(4)
30. Stubbs J, Pennybacker J (1960) Reduction of intracranial pressure with hypertonic urea. Lancet 1(7134):1094–1097
31. Matson DD (1965) Treatment of cerebral swelling. N Engl J Med 272:626–628
32. Go KG, van Woudenberg F, Woldring MG, Ebels EJ, Beks JW, Smeets EH (1969) The penetration of 14C-urea and 3H-water into the rat brain with cold-induced cerebral oedema. Histological and autoradiographic study of the oedema. The effect of urovert. Acta Neurochir 21(2):97–122
33. Martinez-Romero R, Canuelo A, Siles E, Oliver FJ, Martinez-Lara E (2012) Nitric oxide modulates hypoxia-inducible factor-1 and poly(ADP-ribose) polymerase-1 cross talk in response to hypobaric hypoxia. J Appl Physiol 112(5):816–823
34. Pearson DL, Dawling S, Walsh WF, Haines JL, Christman BW, Bazyk A, Scott N, Summar ML (2001) Neonatal pulmonary hypertension–urea-cycle intermediates, nitric oxide production, and carbamoyl-phosphate synthetase function. N Engl J Med 344(24):1832–1838

10

Long-term study of the efficacy and safety of OnabotulinumtoxinA for the prevention of chronic migraine: COMPEL study

Andrew M. Blumenfeld[1*], Richard J. Stark[2], Marshall C. Freeman[3], Amelia Orejudos[4] and Aubrey Manack Adams[4]

Abstract

Background: OnabotulinumtoxinA is approved for the prevention of headache in those with chronic migraine (CM); however, more clinical data on the risk-benefit profile for treatment beyond one year is desirable.

Methods: The Chronic Migraine OnabotulinuMtoxinA Prolonged Efficacy open Label (COMPEL) Study (ClinicalTrials. gov, NCT01516892) is an international, multicenter, open-label long-term prospective study. Adults with CM received 155 U of onabotulinumtoxinA (31 sites in a fixed-site, fixed-dose paradigm across 7 head/neck muscles) every 12 weeks (±7 days) for 9 treatment cycles (108 weeks). The primary outcome was headache day reductions at 108 weeks; secondary outcomes were headache day reductions at 60 weeks and change in the 6-item Headache Impact Test (HIT-6) score. Safety and tolerability were assessed by reviewing the frequency and nature of adverse events (AEs). AEs were determined at each visit through patient self-report, general non-directed and, for specific AEs, directed questioning, and physical examination. Subgroup analyses for safety and efficacy included, but were not limited to, patients with/without concomitant oral preventive treatment and acute medication overuse at baseline.

Results: Enrolled patients ($N = 716$) were 18–73 years old and most were female ($n = 607$, 84.8%). At baseline, patients reported an average 22.0 (SD = 4.8) headache days per month. 52.1% of patients ($n = 373$) completed the study. By 60 and 108 weeks, a significant reduction in headache days ($- 9.2$ days and $- 10.7$ days, respectively, $P < 0.0001$) was observed. Significant improvements ($P < 0.0001$) in HIT-6 scores ($- 7.1$ point change at week 108) were also demonstrated. 131 patients (18.3%) reported ≥1 treatment-emergent adverse events; most frequently reported was neck pain ($n = 29$, 4.1%). One patient reported a serious treatment-related adverse event (rash). No deaths were reported.

Conclusions: The COMPEL Study provides additional clinical evidence for the consistency of the efficacy and for the long-term safety and tolerability of onabotulinumtoxinA for the prevention of headache in those with CM who have been treated with onabotulinumtoxinA every 12 weeks over 2 years (9 treatments) with the fixed-site, fixed-dose injection paradigm.

Keywords: OnabotulinumtoxinA, Efficacy, Safety, Long-term, Chronic migraine, Prophylaxis

* Correspondence: blumenfeld@neurocenter.com
[1]Headache Center of Southern California, The Neurology Center, 6010 Hidden Valley Road, Carlsbad, CA 92024, USA
Full list of author information is available at the end of the article

Background

Chronic migraine (CM) is a debilitating neurologic disease defined as headaches that occur on ≥15 days per month for > 3 months, with headaches having migraine features on ≥8 days per month [1]. CM affects approximately 1.4% to 2.2% of adults worldwide [2, 3] and has a substantial quality of life (QoL) and economic burden [4–9]. Both the frequency of attacks and the severity of the pain and associated symptoms have an impact on migraine-related disability [4]. Individuals with CM experience substantially greater headache-related disability [4, 10–12] than individuals with episodic migraine (EM).

High levels of headache-related disability reflect an unmet treatment need [4]. Despite the impact on QoL, < 50% of those with CM consistently take preventive medications [10, 13]. This is supported by large population-based longitudinal surveys which show that many people with CM do not receive adequate migraine treatment [13, 14].

OnabotulinumtoxinA is approved for prevention of headache in adults with CM. The Phase III REsearch Evaluating Migraine Prophylaxis Therapy (PREEMPT) clinical trials established the safety and efficacy of onabotulinumtoxinA for the treatment of CM [15–17]. OnabotulinumtoxinA reduced the frequency of headache days and of moderate or severe headache days and significantly improved health-related QoL at the end of the 24-week double-blind treatment period compared with placebo, [16] with a further reduction in the frequencies of headache days and moderate or severe headache days and improvement in health-related QoL at the end of the 32-week open-label phase (56-week total treatment period) [17].

The Chronic migraine OnabotulinuMtoxinA Prolonged Efficacy open Label (COMPEL; NCT01516892) Study was designed to expand on the current 56-week efficacy and safety data by evaluating the long-term efficacy and safety of onabotulinumtoxinA for prevention of headache in those with CM. Due to the extended duration of the study (108 weeks), and the established efficacy and safety of onabotulinumtoxinA in people with CM at 1 year, an open-label study was considered the optimal design. A randomized controlled trial would have led to a long period of exposure to placebo and possibly excessive discontinuation rates. It is likely that such an approach would not have been accepted by ethics committees. Alternatively, an observational study design and real-world data can be used to extend our knowledge of the safety and effectiveness profile of onabotulinumtoxinA when used in clinical practice. However, given that physicians often do not treat per label in practice, an observational design would not have evaluated the efficacy of onabotulinumtoxinA when used every 12 weeks with a fixed-site, fixed-dose injection paradigm, which was the primary research question evaluated by the COMPEL Study. Both real-world and open-label study data have considerable clinical utility because

the combination of data from such studies can help inform physicians on how to use onabotulinumtoxinA to optimally manage people with CM. The COMPEL Study also sought to evaluate outcomes in addition to the those related to reduction in headache days, including the effect of treatment on related comorbidities and quality-of-life measures. Herein, we report the primary and secondary outcomes for the COMPEL Study, as well as the subgroup analyses for these outcomes.

Methods
Study design

The COMPEL Study (clinicaltrials.gov identifier NCT0 1516892) was an international, multicenter, open-label long-term prospective study in adults with CM at 35 sites in the United States ($n = 24$), Australia ($n = 5$), and Korea ($n = 6$). The enrollment period was December 2011 to October 2013. The study design has been previously published [18]. The study duration was 112 weeks, including a 4-week baseline period and a 108-week, open-label treatment intervention phase (Fig. 1).

Demographics, medical history, physical exam, headache features, and headache treatment history were recorded at the baseline visit (week 0). Diary data (entered via interactive voice response system [IVRS]) for efficacy assessment were captured by the patient for the 28 days before the baseline visit, and then for the 28 days before week 24 (after treatment 2), week 60 (after treatment 5), week 84 (after treatment 7), and week 108 (after treatment 9).

OnabotulinumtoxinA (BOTOX®; Allergan plc, Dublin, Ireland) 155 U was administered every 12 weeks using the US Food and Drug Administration approved fixed-site, fixed-dose injection paradigm into 7 muscle areas and 31 sites [19].

The study received ethical approval from the Institutional Review Board or Independent Ethics Committee at each site, and written informed consent was obtained from patients before study enrollment.

Study participants

Adults aged ≥18 years with a diagnosis of CM, able to follow the study instructions, attend the treatment and follow-up visits, and with stable comorbidities were eligible for study inclusion. Physicians working in headache centers or tertiary institutions were responsible for ensuring patients met the criteria for CM, including having a diagnosis of migraine headache disease with headaches on ≥15 days per month lasting ≥4 h a day. Patients could take a single oral medication as headache prevention. The dose and regimen of the oral preventive treatment must have been stable for > 4 weeks before the first intervention visit (week 0, visit 2). The dose could then not be changed until at or after week 24. If a patient was not on any oral preventive treatment at week 0, they

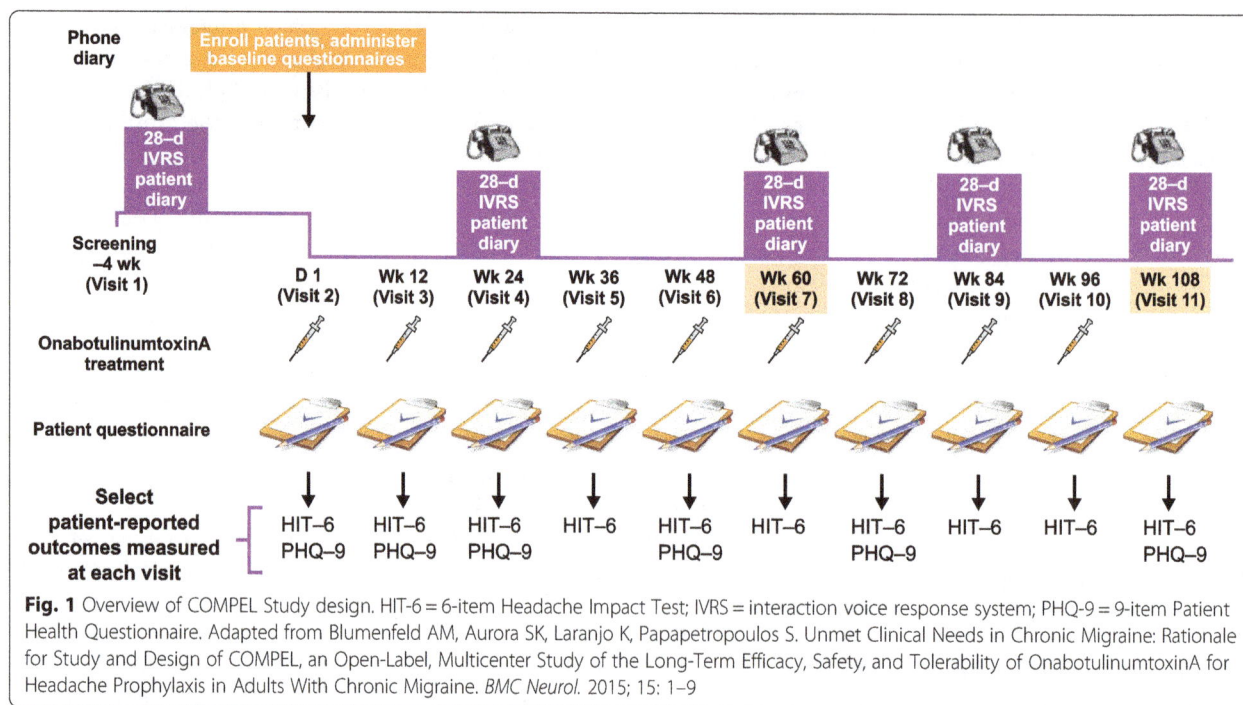

Fig. 1 Overview of COMPEL Study design. HIT-6 = 6-item Headache Impact Test; IVRS = interaction voice response system; PHQ-9 = 9-item Patient Health Questionnaire. Adapted from Blumenfeld AM, Aurora SK, Laranjo K, Papapetropoulos S. Unmet Clinical Needs in Chronic Migraine: Rationale for Study and Design of COMPEL, an Open-Label, Multicenter Study of the Long-Term Efficacy, Safety, and Tolerability of OnabotulinumtoxinA for Headache Prophylaxis in Adults With Chronic Migraine. *BMC Neurol.* 2015; 15: 1–9

must not have been on oral preventive treatment for the preceding 4 weeks and could only have an oral preventive treatment added after week 24.

Patients could take acute headache medication on an as-needed basis and were required to record the use of acute headache medication in their daily patient diary. At baseline, patients were defined as overusing acute headache medication if they were taking acute headache medication ≥2 times a week in any week with diary data on ≥5 days for the 4-week screening period. This differs from the definition of medication overuse adopted by the International Headache Society, which requires 3 months of medication overuse and has drug-specific treatment day minima [1].

Patients were excluded if they had previously received onabotulinumtoxinA for any reason, did not meet the study criteria for CM or had severe major depressive disorder or suicidal ideation [18].

Efficacy outcome measures

As recommended by the International Headache Society Clinical Trials Subcommittee Guidelines, [20] the primary efficacy measure was the number of headache days per 28-day period (headache frequency) immediately before week 108. Efficacy measures were based on daily diaries (recorded via IVRS).

Secondary efficacy measures included headache frequency at week 60, and change in 6-item Headache Impact Test (HIT-6) scores from baseline at weeks 60 and 108. HIT-6 is a 6-domain patient survey used to assess the impact of headaches. Each of the 6 questions was

scored and summed for a total possible score of 36 to 78, with higher scores indicating a greater adverse impact [21].

Exploratory efficacy measures included reduction in frequency of moderate or severe headache days.

A headache day was a day (00:00 to 23:59) for which the patient recorded ≥4 continuous hours of headache. Patients rated all headaches on a 4-point scale: 0 = none, 1 = mild, 2 = moderate, 3 = severe. A moderate or severe headache day was defined as a day with ≥4 continuous hours of headache that the patient had rated as moderate or severe [21].

Subgroup analysis

Subgroup analysis was undertaken based on race (Caucasian vs non-Caucasian), comorbid anxiety (none vs mild or moderate defined by Generalized Anxiety Disorder-7 score), comorbid depression (none vs mild or moderate defined by Patient Health Questionnaire-9 total score), body mass index (< 18.5 kg/m^2 vs 18.5 to < 25 kg/m^2 vs 25 to < 30 kg/m^2 vs ≥ 30 kg/m^2), history of acute headache medication overuse (yes vs no), age (18 to < 25 years vs 25 to ≤65 years vs > 65 years), use of oral preventive treatment for headache at baseline (yes vs no), previous use of preventive treatment for headache (yes vs no), and country (United States, Australia, and South Korea).

Safety and tolerability

Safety and tolerability were assessed by reviewing the frequency and nature of adverse events (AEs). AEs were determined at each visit through patient self-report, general non-directed questioning, direct questioning via the Columbia-Suicide Severity Rating Scale, and physical examinations. AEs were recorded starting at week 0 immediately after the first onabotulinumtoxinA treatment.

Patients were withdrawn from the study for safety reasons if they showed any signs of suicidal ideation or if they became pregnant [18]. They received no further protocol-related onabotulinumtoxinA treatment; however, these patients were included in the safety and tolerability analysis.

Statistical analysis

Based on the efficacy of onabotulinumtoxinA in the PREEMPT studies, assuming a standard deviation of 6.6, a sample size of 60 patients was considered sufficient to provide at least 80% power to detect between subgroup differences of ≥2.5 headache days reduction per 28-day period with a 95% significance level. Assuming that a subgroup was approximately 10% of the analysis population, an overall sample size of 600 patients was required to detect subgroup differences as outlined above. Subgroup analysis was only performed if it had sufficient individuals ($n \geq 60$) to detect significant differences.

For the primary efficacy endpoint, an intention-to-treat analysis was undertaken on all patients with ≥1 efficacy assessment. Missing headache days data were imputed using a modified last observation carried forward (mLOCF) methodology, with imputation applied chronologically. If a 28-day diary had 20 to 28 days of data, the measures of headache frequency and severity were prorated from the data recorded in the diary. If there were data for < 10 days in the diary, including for those who withdrew from the study, the number of headache days for the missing period was imputed by mLOCF based on the patient's previous 28-day diary period and adjusted by the mean change observed in all patients with diary records for the same periods. The intent was to preserve the patient's general position relative to the mean, using information from the patient and from the remaining patients. If there were data for 10 to 19 days, the number of headache days for the missing period was imputed by taking the average of the 2 estimates (the mLOCF estimate and the prorated estimate for the data recorded). For the secondary endpoint of HIT-6, for the baseline score if a patient answered < 50% of the questions on the HIT-6 survey, the HIT-6 score was set to missing; if ≥50% of the questions were answered, the total HIT-6 score was extrapolated from the mean score across all answered questions. For post-baseline visits, missing HIT-6 scores were imputed for all patients at each visit using mLOCF, based on the most recent results from a previous visit. For the subgroup analyses, missing headache days data and missing HIT-6 scores were imputed for all patients at each visit using a mLOCF.

Data from all investigative sites were pooled for the analyses. The analysis population included all enrolled patients who received ≥1 dose of onabotulinumtoxinA and ≥1 efficacy assessment. The safety population included all patients who received ≥1 dose of onabotulinumtoxinA.

A 2-sided paired t test was used to compare post-baseline efficacy outcomes with baseline efficacy outcomes, including testing the null hypothesis (that onabotulinumtoxinA treatment for 108 weeks caused no reduction in headache day frequency). A P value ≤0.05 was considered statistically significant. Similarly, a 2-sided group t test was used to assess differences between subgroups of two variables (ie, yes/no); one-way analysis of variance was used to test for differences between subgroups of three or more levels (eg, BMI).

Results

Patient disposition and demographics

A total of 716 patients were enrolled at 35 sites (United States, $n = 572$ [24 sites]; Korea, $n = 80$ [6 sites]; Australia, $n = 64$ [5 sites]). The intention-to-treat analysis population totaled 715 patients (United States, $n = 571$; Korea, $n = 80$; Australia, $n = 64$), and included 25 patients who reported < 15 headache days/month at baseline, despite having a diagnosis of CM. The safety population included all 716 enrolled patients who received ≥1 treatment with onabotulinumtoxinA.

All 9 study treatments were received by 402 patients (56.1%); 373 patients (52.1%) received all 9 study treatments and attended the final follow-up visit (ie, completed the study), and 343 patients (47.9%) withdrew from the study, primarily because of withdrawn consent ($n = 92$; 12.8%), being lost to follow-up ($n = 82$; 11.5%), or protocol violation ($n = 60$; 8.4%; Fig. 2). Suicidal ideation led to withdrawal from the study in 4 patients.

In the enrolled population, patients had a mean (SD) age of 43.0 (11.3) years and were predominantly female and Caucasian (Table 1). The mean (SD) age of onset of CM was 32.5 (13.7) years, patients had CM for a mean (SD) of 10.6 (11.0) years, and 62.7% of patients had a family history of migraine. Almost all patients (99.6%) reported headaches with moderate or severe pain and 68.2% of patients reported moderate or severe neck stiffness or pain.

At baseline, patients reported a mean (SD) of 22.0 (4.8) headache days per 28 days, with a mean (SD) of 18.0 (5.7) being moderate or severe. The majority of patients (89.2%) were using acute headache medications, and 63.7% were overusing their acute medication (Table 2). A total of 80.9% of patients had used oral preventive treatments in the past, with anticonvulsants (60.6%), antidepressants (45.1%), and beta blockers (29.5%) the most commonly used (Fig. 3). At baseline, 348 patients taking oral preventive treatments had a mean (SD) of 22.3 (4.8) headache days per 28 days; during the study 44 patients (6.1%) started taking an oral preventive treatments, most commonly topiramate ($n = 18$, 2.5%).

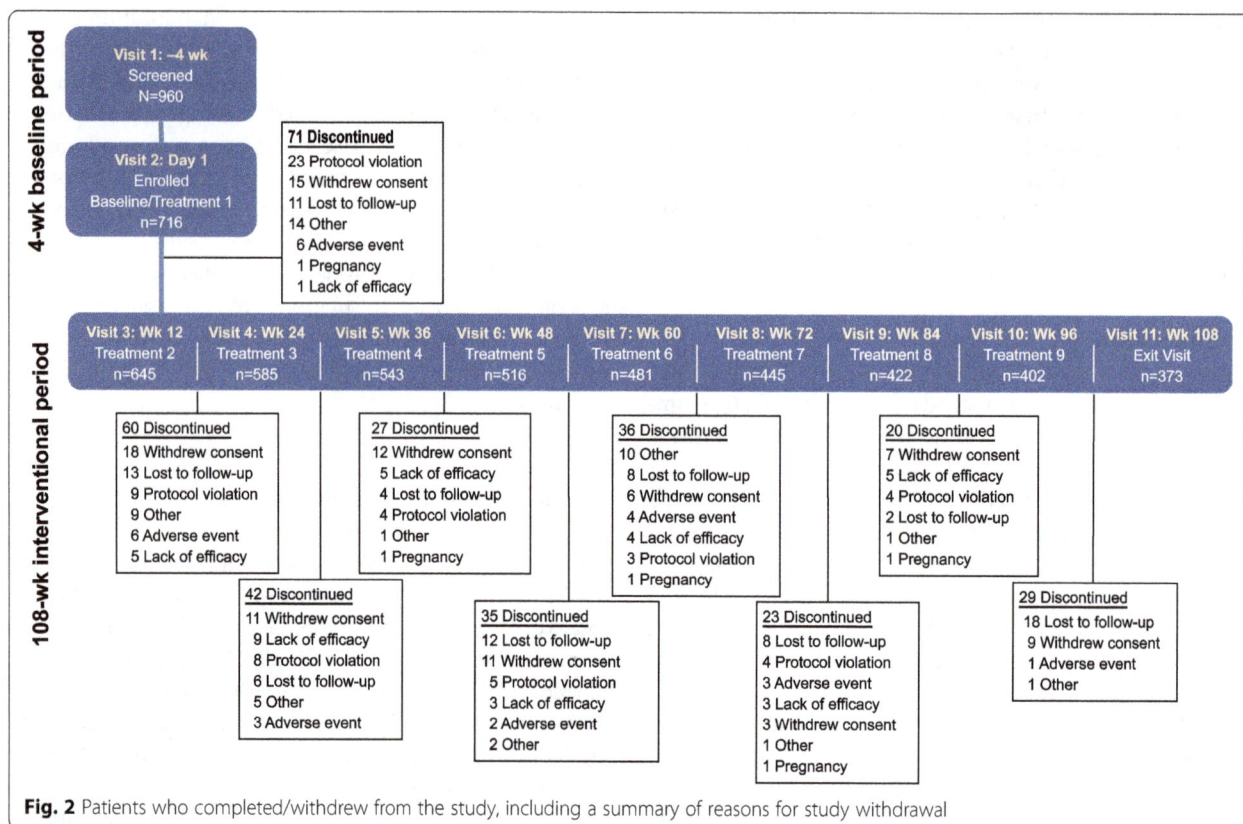

Fig. 2 Patients who completed/withdrew from the study, including a summary of reasons for study withdrawal

Efficacy outcomes

At week 108, onabotulinumtoxinA treatment reduced headache day frequency by 10.7 days from baseline, $P < 0.0001$ (Fig. 4a), with mean (SD) headache days reduced to 11.3 (7.4) days per 28-day period (from 22.0 [4.8] days at baseline; $P < 0.0001$).

Statistically significant reductions in headache day frequency were observed from the first assessment at week 24 (headache day frequency reduced by 7.4 days from baseline; $P < 0.0001$) and at all subsequent assessment points including week 60 (Fig. 4a). In a sensitivity analysis, similar reductions were observed at all time points using observed data without imputation (-7.9 days at week 24 to -11.6 days at week 108, all $P < 0.0001$). Based on observed data, the proportion of patients reporting a $\geq 50\%$ reduction in headache days from baseline increased over the duration of the study, from 39.5% (223 of 565 patients) at week 24 to 61.1% (193 of 316 patients) at week 108.

Baseline HIT-6 scores were available for 713 of 715 patients in the analysis population. Statistically significant improvements in total HIT-6 scores were observed at week 12 (HIT-6 score reduced by 4.4 points from baseline; $P < 0.0001$) and continued through to week 108 (-7.1 from baseline; $P < 0.0001$; Fig. 5b). A similar pattern was seen using observed data (week 12: -4.4 from baseline; week 108: -9.0 from baseline; both $P < 0.0001$).

At baseline, patients had a mean (SD) of 18.0 (5.7) moderate or severe headache days. The frequency of moderate or severe headache days was reduced from baseline by 6.5 days at week 24, a statistically significant change from baseline ($P < 0.0001$; Fig. 4b). The reduction in moderate or severe headache days remained significantly reduced compared with baseline at week 60 (-8.1 days; $P < 0.0001$) and at week 108 (-9.5 days; $P < 0.0001$).

Subgroup analysis

No statistically significant between-group differences were observed for the change from baseline in the number of headache days at week 108 for the subgroups of race, comorbid depression, comorbid anxiety, history of acute headache medication overuse, age, or BMI (Additional file 1: Figures S1–S6). Statistically significant between-group differences were observed for preventive treatment at baseline versus no preventive treatment at baseline. Patients with preventive treatment at baseline had a significantly smaller reduction in mean (SD) headache days from baseline at week 108 than patients without preventive treatment at baseline (-10.2 [6.3] vs -11.2 [6.5]; $P = 0.029$, Additional file 1: Figure S7). Similar results were observed for the between group differences for previous use of preventive treatment versus no previous use of preventive treatment (Additional file 1: Figure S8).

Table 1 Baseline Demographics and Clinical Features of CM

Variable	Enrolled Population N = 716
Mean (SD) age, y	43.0 (11.3)
Female, n (%)	607 (84.8)
Race, n (%)	
Caucasian	582 (81.3)
Asian	89 (12.4)
African American/black	41 (5.7)
Other	4 (0.6)
Mean (SD) height, cm	165.8 (8.7)
Mean (SD) weight, kg	75.6 (19.8)
Mean (SD) BMI, kg/m^2	27.4 (6.4)
Mean (SD) age of onset of CM, y	32.5 (13.7)
Mean (SD) time since onset of CM, y	10.6 (11.0)
Family history of migraine, yes, n (%)	449 (62.7)
Headache-related history,[a] n (%)	
Sleep disorder	210 (29.3)
Smoking	150 (20.9)
Head trauma	74 (10.3)
Childhood abuse/maltreatment	50 (7.0)
Severity of pain during headache, n (%)	
Mild	3 (0.4)
Moderate	296 (41.3)
Severe	417 (58.2)
Pain on one or both sides of head, n (%)	
One	382 (53.4)
Both	334 (46.6)
Type of head pain, n (%)	
Throbbing or pulsing	507 (70.8)
Pressing or squeezing	170 (23.7)
Neither throbbing, pulsing, pressing, squeezing	39 (5.4)
Severity of neck pain or stiffness, n (%)	
Mild	70 (9.8)
Moderate	331 (46.2)
Severe	157 (21.9)
None	158 (22.1)
Other headache features, n (%)	
Sensitivity to light	658 (91.9)
Physical activity worsens headache	642 (89.7)
Sensitivity to noise	639 (89.2)
Nausea with headache	583 (81.4)
Vomiting with headache	295 (41.2)
Cutaneous allodynia	290 (40.5)

Table 1 Baseline Demographics and Clinical Features of CM *(Continued)*

Variable	Enrolled Population N = 716
Mean (SD) headache days[b]	22.0 (4.8)
Mean (SD) moderate or severe headache days[b]	18.0 (5.7)
Mean (SD) HIT-6 total score[c]	64.7 (4.8)

CM chronic migraine, HIT-6 6-item Headache Impact Test
[a]Patients may be counted in > 1 category
[b]Headache days per 28 d in the analysis population (n = 715); includes 25 patients who reported < 15 headache days per 28 d at baseline
[c]In the analysis population (n = 715)

Similar reductions in headache day frequency were observed within each country subgroup; there were no statistically significant differences between countries (Fig. 6).

HIT-6 total score was significantly reduced from baseline in all subgroups at weeks 60 and 108. At week 108, the Korean subgroup had a significantly larger reduction in HIT-6 score compared with the US population (– 9.8 vs – 6.6; $P < 0.001$; Fig. 5b). In addition, non-Caucasian patients had a significantly greater reduction in HIT-6 score than Caucasian patients at week 108 (– 8.6 from baseline vs – 6.7 from baseline; $P = 0.005$; Additional file 1: Figure S1), as did the subgroup not on oral preventive treatment at baseline (– 7.4 from baseline vs – 6.1 from baseline for those on oral preventive treatment, at week 60 [$P = 0.012$]; – 8.0 vs – 6.1 at week 108 [$P < 0.001$]; Additional file 1: Figure S7). The outcomes for the subgroup on previous preventive treatment were almost identical (Additional file 1: Figure S8).

Safety and tolerability

At least 1 treatment-emergent adverse event (TEAE) was reported by 436 patients (60.9%; Table 3). Of these, serious

Table 2 Baseline Acute Headache Medication Use in Patients With CM[a]

Medication Use, n (%)	Enrolled Population N = 716
Acute headache medication use	639 (89.2)
Triptans	383 (53.5)
Simple analgesics	327 (45.7)
Combination analgesics	225 (31.4)
Opioids	117 (16.3)
Ergotamines	53 (7.4)
Acute headache medication overuse[b]	456 (63.7)
Triptans (≥10 d)	194 (27.1)
Combination analgesics (≥10 d)	88 (12.3)
Simple analgesics (≥15 d)	79 (11.0)
Opioids (≥10 d)	38 (5.3)
Ergotamines (≥10 d)	18 (2.5)

CM chronic migraine
[a]Data from patients with ≥20 d of data in their patient diary
[b]Definition of medication overuse is based on 4 wk. diary data

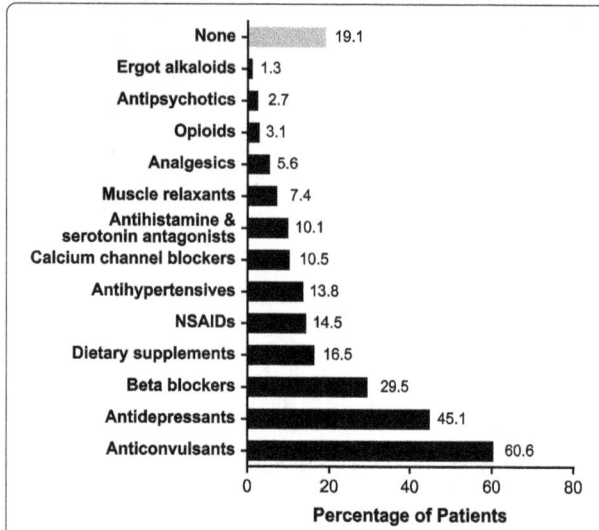

Fig. 3 Oral preventive treatments* currently or previously used by the enrolled population (N = 716). *Oral preventive treatments defined, for the purposes of this study, as any oral medication *specifically* prescribed for *daily use for prevention of headache*. NSAID = nonsteroidal anti-inflammatory drug

TEAEs occurred in 75 patients (10.5%). There were no deaths. TEAEs were reported in 32 patients (4.5%) who discontinued onabotulinumtoxinA. TEAEs that occurred in more than 2 patients who discontinued onabotulinumtoxinA were eyelid ptosis ($n = 3$, 0.4%), headache ($n = 3$, 0.4%), pregnancy ($n = 3$, 0.4%), suicidal ideation ($n = 4$, 0.6%) and rash ($n = 3$, 0.4%).

At least 1 treatment-related adverse event (TRAE) was reported in 131 patients (18.3%), with neck pain being the most commonly reported TRAE (Table 3). A TRAE was reported in 13 patients (1.8%) who discontinued onabotulinumtoxinA; with eyelid ptosis ($n = 3$, 0.4%) and rash ($n = 3$, 0.4%) being the most commonly reported TRAEs in patients who discontinued onabotulinumtoxinA. A serious TRAE of rash occurred in 1 patient (0.1%); onabotulinumtoxinA was discontinued in this patient.

Discussion

The COMPEL Study provides clinical evidence for consistency of the efficacy and long-term safety and tolerability for onabotulinumtoxinA for the prevention of headache in those with CM who have been treated every 12 weeks over 2 years (9 treatment cycles) with the fixed-site, fixed-dose injection paradigm. OnabotulinumtoxinA effectively reduced headache day frequency compared with

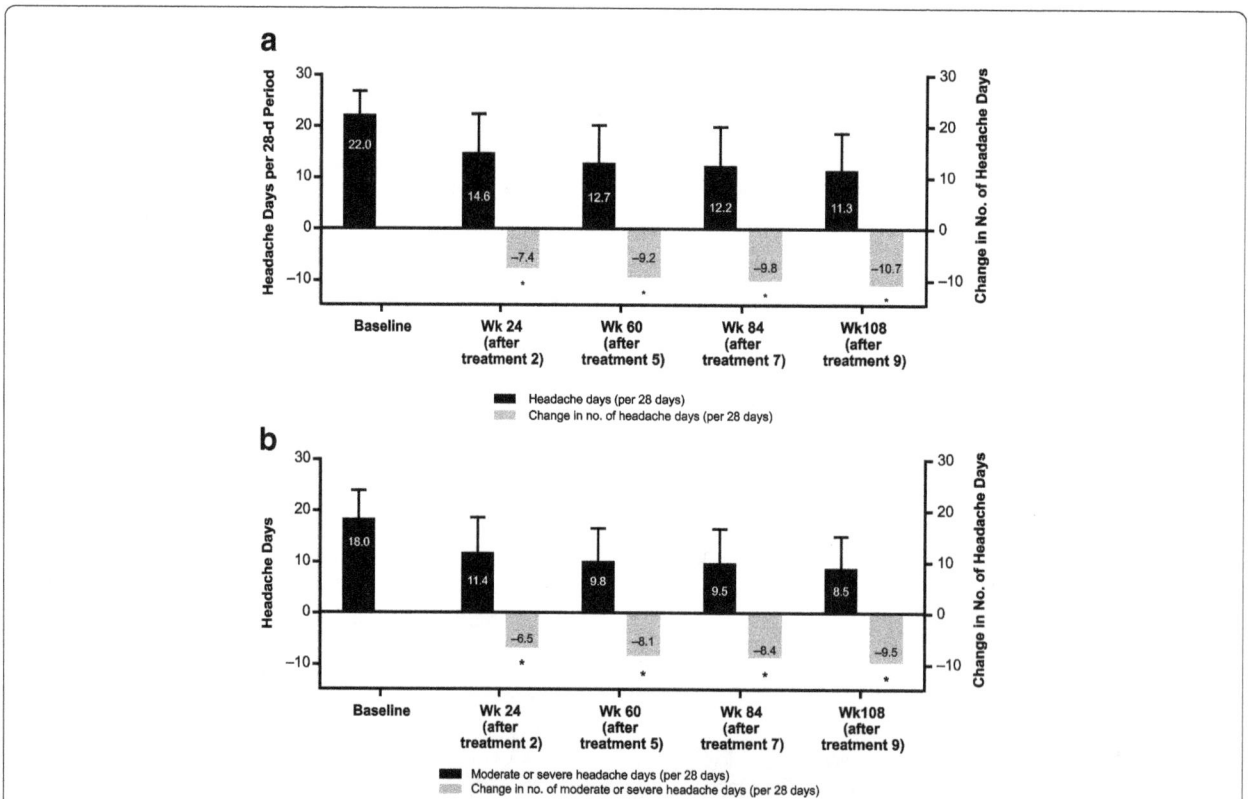

Fig. 4 Long-term effect of onabotulinumtoxinA on number of and change vs baseline. **a**) Number of headache days and **b**) number of moderate or severe headache days per 28-d period preceding the visit over 108 wk. (depicting the outcomes of treatment after 9 cycles). *$P < 0.0001$; paired *t*-test used to compare visit to baseline

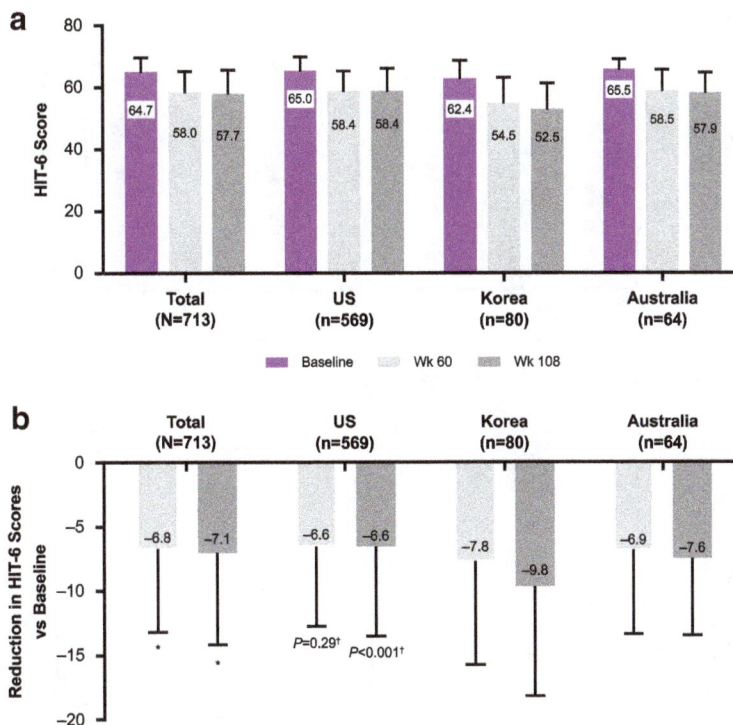

Fig. 5 Long-term effect of onabotulinumtoxinA by country. **a)** HIT-6 total score and **b)** change in HIT-6 total score vs baseline, depicting the outcomes after 5 (wk 60) and 9 (wk 180) treatments. HIT-6 = 6-item Headache Impact Test. *Indicates $P < 0.001$ vs baseline; paired t-test used to compare visit to baseline. †Indicates $P = 0.0008$ for comparison between subgroups; 1-way analysis of variance

baseline over 9 treatment cycles (108 weeks), improved HIT-6 scores and reduced moderate or severe headache day frequency. These outcomes align with and further expand on the results of the double-blind, placebo-controlled phase of the PREEMPT trials over 24 weeks [22]. The baseline demographics of our population were similar to those of the group randomized to receive onabotulinumtoxinA in the first 24 weeks of the PREEMPT trials, except that our population had a shorter time since the onset of CM (10.6 years vs 19.2 years in the PREEMPT population) despite having a similar mean age (43.0 years vs 41.3 years). Therefore, our patients appeared to have a considerably older age at onset of CM than those in the PREEMPT population (32.5 vs 21.5; Allergan plc, data on file).

The reduction in headache day frequency from baseline after 24 weeks was similar to that observed in the PREEMPT trials (– 7.4 vs – 8.4); [22] as was the reduction in headache frequency after 5 treatments (week 60) in our study compared with those achieved after 5 treatments in the open-label phase of PREEMPT [17]. Notably after 56 weeks (5 treatments), onabotulinumtoxinA treatment reduced the mean headache day frequency by 11.7 days in the PREEMPT studies versus a mean reduction of 9.2 days at week 60 in our study.

PREEMPT allowed for a "follow the pain strategy" in addition to the base fixed-site fixed-dose treatment,

allowing an additional 40 U of onabotulinumtoxinA to be administered at the clinician's discretion, which could account for these slightly improved outcomes at week 56. In a population consisting only of those with medication overuse CM, onabotulinumtoxinA 195 U (administered according to the fixed-dose, fixed-site and the follow-the-pain injection paradigm) was similarly found to have significantly better outcomes than onabotulinumtoxinA 155 U (fixed-dose, fixed-site) over a 2-year period [23].

The optimal injection paradigm for onabotulinumtoxinA remains to be established. Simpler injection paradigms into fewer injection sites have also had successful outcomes; [24] most recently, onabotulinumtoxinA 70 U to 150 U injection into corrugator, temporalis, with or without the trapezius muscles, resulted in 72% of patients in a small ($N = 63$) real-life study experiencing ≥50% decrease in headache day frequency after ≥2 consecutive sets of injections [25]. Interestingly, small doses of onabotulinumtoxinA injected via acupoint sites (2.5 U per site, 25 U per treatment) was found to reduce migraine frequency, intensity, and duration by approximately 75% in Chinese patients ($N = 102$) with chronic migraine [26].

Our study allowed the addition or modification of oral preventive treatment at 24 weeks, which occurred in 44 patients (6.1%). This change in concomitant oral preventive treatment may have had an effect on efficacy outcomes.

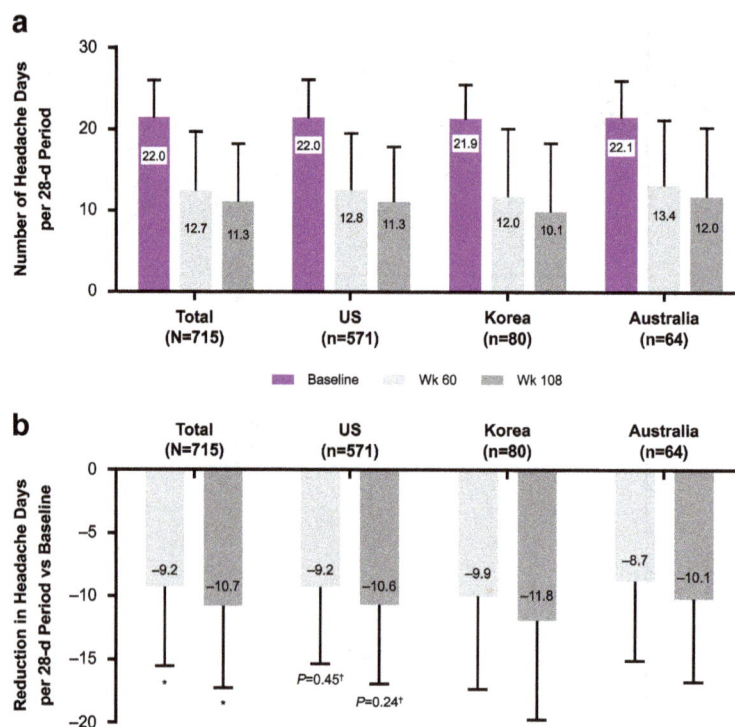

Fig. 6 Long-term effect of onabotulinumtoxinA by country. **a)** Number of headache days per 28-d period and **b)** change in number of headache days vs baseline, depicting the outcomes after 5 (wk 60) and 9 (wk 180) treatments. *$P < 0.001$; paired t-test used to compare visit to baseline. †P-value for comparing among subgroups is from one-way analysis of variance

Table 3 Summary of TEAEs and TRAEs in Patients Receiving ≥1 OnabotulinumtoxinA Treatment

Event, n (%)	Safety Population $N = 716$
TEAE	
≥ 1 TEAE	436 (60.9)
Serious TEAE	75 (10.5)
TEAE in those that discontinued treatment	32 (4.5)
TRAE	
≥ 1 TRAE	131 (18.3)
Serious TRAE	1 (0.1)
TRAE in those that discontinued treatment	13 (1.8)
TRAE with incidence ≥1%	
Neck pain	29 (4.1)
Eyelid ptosis	18 (2.5)
Musculoskeletal stiffness	17 (2.4)
Injection site pain	14 (2.0)
Headache	12 (1.7)
Muscular weakness	10 (1.4)
Facial paresis	9 (1.3)
Migraine	7 (1.0)
Skin tightness	7 (1.0)

TEAE treatment-emergent adverse event, *TRAE* treatment-related adverse event

The efficacy outcomes may also be influenced by the inclusion of patients on oral preventive treatment at baseline. Patients on oral preventive treatment at baseline ($n = 348$) had a slightly smaller reduction in headache day frequency (-10.2 from baseline vs -11.2 from baseline, $P = 0.029$) and a statistically smaller reduction in HIT-6 total score at week 108 than patients not receiving oral preventive treatment at baseline ($n = 367$; -6.1 from baseline vs -8.0 from baseline, $P < 0.001$) despite having similar baseline headache day frequency (22.3 and 21.7 headache days per month, respectively) and HIT-6 scores (64.8 and 64.6, respectively). This suggests that those who were receiving oral preventive treatment at baseline may have had more refractory CM. Nonetheless, onabotulinumtoxinA still significantly reduced both headache day frequency (-10.2 vs baseline, 95% CI -11.0 to -9.5) and HIT-6 score (-6.1 vs baseline, 95% CI -6.8 to -5.4) at week 108 in this population versus baseline.

Our results further demonstrate that treatment with onabotulinumtoxinA through to week 108 provides continued improvement over 2 years, complementing previous observations in a smaller ($N = 155$) single-center study in patients with CM attributable to medication overuse [27]. In that study also the reduction in frequency of headache days was most pronounced after the first few treatment cycles and continued to further decrease through the 8th treatment cycle. Historically, it is recommended that after 12 months of good headache control, oral preventive treatment is reduced or discontinued; the goal being to establish the minimum effective dose [28]. In contrast, some public health bodies recommend that when onabotulinumtoxinA is used for the prevention of headaches it is stopped when the number of headache days per month drops below 15 days per month for 3 consecutive months [29]. Based on our study results and those of others, [27, 30] we question whether it is appropriate to discontinue onabotulinumtoxinA after only 3 months of remission to EM. The incremental benefits observed over the course of the COMPEL Study and that of PREEMPT [30] and Negro and colleagues [27] suggest that continuing treatment for up to 12 months, as recommended for oral preventive treatment, may be more beneficial to people with CM than early treatment withdrawal.

Clinicians report a 30% to 50% reduction in headache day frequency as a good response to treatment [29]. However, in our experience the majority of people with CM are seeking to maximize treatment response and maintain the improvement in their headaches. Combination of oral preventive treatment with long-term onabotulinumtoxinA treatment may be helpful in supporting people with CM to achieve this goal. The COMPEL Study is one of the first clinical studies of onabotulinumtoxinA in CM to allow the concomitant use of oral preventive treatment.

Management of those overusing headache medications is challenging; typically preventive treatments are ineffective during the period of acute medication overuse [28]. Public health bodies have asked for randomized controlled trials to investigate the role of appropriate pharmacological preventive treatment during acute medication withdrawal [31]. OnabotulinumtoxinA could be a useful treatment for such investigations as our results demonstrated it reduced headache day frequency and HIT-6 scores in individuals with medication overuse at baseline. Similarly, Negro and colleagues reported onabotulinumtoxinA 155 U and 195 U both resulted in significant reduction in headache days, HIT-6 scores and medication intake days in individuals with medication overuse CM, [23, 27] again suggesting an important role for onabotulinumtoxinA in this difficult to treat group.

Further analysis of the COMPEL Study will help describe the use of oral preventive treatment across regions and comorbidities and determine the impact of onabotulinumtoxinA on several factors including the impact on sleep, fatigue, and anxiety/depression, QoL and healthcare resource utilization.

The incidence of TEAEs and TRAEs in our study were similar to the incidence reported in the PREEMPT studies, [17] and in individuals with medication overuse CM, [23] further supporting the long-term safety and tolerability of onabotulinumtoxinA. As observed over the 56-week study

period in the PREEMPT studies, neck pain (4.6%), eyelid ptosis (2.5%), muscular weakness (3.9%), injection site pain (2.0%), and muscle tightness (2.2%) were the most common TRAEs, closely matching the TRAEs reported over our 108-week study period. Our injectors were trained with insights gained from the PREEMPT Study, [32] supporting them to manage and avoid TRAEs such as eyelid ptosis and neck pain without reducing the dose or avoiding the injection site. Furthermore, by allowing the use of oral preventive treatment, the COMPEL Study data also provide some reassurance of the safety and tolerability of onabotulinumtoxinA in clinical practice. As the incidence of TEAEs and TRAEs in this current study were no worse than those reported in PREEMPT, the results of the COMPEL Study suggest that the addition of oral preventive treatment had no untoward impact on the safety profile of onabotulinumtoxinA.

As a large study in over 700 patients over 9 treatment cycles (108 weeks), the COMPEL Study has many strengths. In particular, the results help us to understand the ongoing efficacy and safety of onabotulinumtoxinA over prolonged treatment with the fixed-site and fixed-dose injection paradigm as well as in those taking concomitant oral preventive treatments and acute headache medications as they would in real-world conditions.

However, as a nonrandomized open-label study, our study is subject to inherent limitations particularly that there is no placebo or active comparator arm. An open label design is informative when the efficacy and safety profile of treatment is established, as it is with onabotulinumtoxinA for CM. However, open-label studies with long-term follow-up can be subject to unintentional bias, low persistency rates, and concomitant medication changes. Over a 2-year study, a relatively high level of discontinuation is to be expected; 56.1% (402/716) of patients received all 9 study treatments and 52.1% (373/716) received all study treatments and attended the final follow-up visit. The 2 primary reasons for discontinuation were withdrawn consent (12.8%) and lost to follow-up (11.5%). In the shorter PREEMPT studies, 72.6% of patients completed the 52-week study, with a lower proportion of patients (5.5%) lost to follow-up. Where patients referred to a single clinic for treatment of CM were enrolled in long-term studies of onabotulinumtoxinA, the withdrawal rates were substantially lower (14.8% and 16.9%), [23, 27] which is possibly more reflective of withdrawal rates in a real-world clinical setting.

Patients with no post baseline efficacy assessments were excluded from the analysis population; as only one patient was in this category, the impact on overall results would have been minimal. Because of the exclusion of patients with clinically significant conditions such as fibromyalgia, and those with severe depression and suicidal ideation, data from the patients who represent these or other populations who may be severely challenged may not have been captured [33]. Nonetheless, it is worth noting that that exploratory analyses of the COMPEL data demonstrated that concomitant mild or moderate anxiety or depression did not have a significant negative impact on outcomes. Efficacy results need to be interpreted with caution. The fixed-dose, fixed-site injection paradigm does not necessarily mirror real-world utilization and may underestimate real-world effectiveness, based on the slightly greater reduction in headache day frequency observed in the PREEMPT studies which included a follow-the-pain component to treatment. Conversely, the low persistency rates may overstate efficacy rates since those who do not experience benefit may not persist with treatment over the 108-week follow-up.

Conclusions

The results of this international, multicenter, open-label, long-term prospective study support the efficacy and safety of onabotulinumtoxinA for prevention of headaches in adults with CM for up to 9 treatment cycles (108 weeks). Data indicated that onabotulinumtoxinA was effective in reducing headache days throughout 9 cycles of treatment, reducing the impact of headache from the first assessment (week 24). OnabotulinumtoxinA appeared to be well tolerated over 108 weeks and 9 cycles of treatment, and no new safety concerns were identified.

Additional file

Additional file 1: Figure S1. Long-term effect of onabotulinumtoxinA on A) number of headache days per 28-d period, B)change in number of headache days vs baseline, C) HIT-6 score, and D) change in HIT-6 score vs baseline, depicting outcomes after 5 (wk 60) and 9 (wk 180) treatments, by race. **Figure S2.** Long-term effect of onabotulinumtoxinA on A) number of headache days per 28-d period, B) change in number of headache days, C) HIT-6 score, and D) change in HIT-6 score by comorbid anxiety group. **Figure S3.** Long-term effect of onabotulinumtoxinA on A) number of headache days per 28-d period, B) change in number of headache days, C) HIT-6 score, and D) change in HIT-6 score by comorbid depression group. **Figure S4.** Long-term effect of onabotulinumtoxinA on A) number of headache days per 28-d period, B) change in number of headache days, C) HIT-6 score, and D) change in HIT-6 score by BMI. **Figure S5.** Long-term effect of onabotulinumtoxinA on A) number of headache days per 28-d period, B) change in number of headache days, C) HIT-6 score, and D) change in HIT-6 score by history of acute medication overuse at baseline. **Figure S6.** Long-term effect of onabotulinumtoxinA on A) number of headache days per 28-d period, B) change in number of headache days, C) HIT-6 score, and D) change in HIT-6 score by age. **Figure S7.** Long-term effect of onabotulinumtoxinA on A) number of headache days per 28-d period, B) change in number of headache days, C) HIT-6 score, and D) change in HIT-6 score by use of oral preventive treatment at baseline. **Figure S8.** Long-term effect of onabotulinumtoxinA on A) number of headache days per 28-d period, B) change in number of headache days, C) HIT-6 score, and D) change in HIT-6 score by previous use of preventive treatment. (PDF 179 kb)

Abbreviations

AEs: adverse events; BMI: body mass index; CM: chronic migraine; COMPEL: Chronic migraine OnabotulinuMtoxinA Prolonged Efficacy open Label; EM: episodic migraine; HIT-6: 6-item Headache Impact Test; IVRS: interactive voice response system; mLOCF: modified last observation carried forward; PREEMPT: Phase III REsearch Evaluating Migraine Prophylaxis Therapy; QoL: quality of life; SD: standard deviation; TEAE: treatment-emergent adverse event; TRAE: treatment-related adverse event

Acknowledgements

This study was sponsored by Allergan plc (Dublin, Ireland). Writing and editorial assistance was provided to the authors by Lee B. Hohaia, PharmD, and Dana A. Franznick, PharmD, of Complete Healthcare Communications, LLC (West Chester, PA, USA), a CHC Group company, and funded by Allergan plc (Dublin, Ireland). All authors met the ICMJE authorship criteria. Neither honoraria nor payments were made for authorship.

Principal investigators for the COMPEL Study included: Lawrence D. Robbins, MD; Jan L. Brandes, MD; Tamara A. Miller, MD; Roger K. Cady, MD; Jo H. Bonner, MD; Paul K. Winner, DO, FAAN; Marshall C. Freeman, MD; Kathleen B. Mullin, MD; Andrew M. Blumenfeld, MD; Eric J. Eross, DO; Amy A. Gelfand, MD; Ejaz A. Shamim, MD; William B. Young Jr., MD; John F. Rothrock, MD; Stephen H. Landy, MD; J. Ivan Lopez, MD; George R. Nissan, DO; Soma Sahai-Srivastava, MD; Marcia Ribeiro, MD; Maria-Carmen Wilson, MD; Jose M. Casanova, MD, PhD; Laszlo L. Mechtler, MD; Richard J. Stark, MB BS, FRCAP; Andrew H. Evans, MD; John D. O'Sullivan, MD MBBS; Joseph Frasca, MBBS, FRACP; Min Kyung Chu, MD, PhD; Jeong-Wook Park, MD; ByungKun Kim, MD, PhD; Seong Taek Kim, DDS, MS, PhD; Kwang Soo Lee, MD, MS, PhD; Heui-Soo Moon, MD. The authors would also like to thank the patients for their participation in the study.

Funding

Allergan plc (Dublin, Ireland)

Authors' contributions

AB made substantial contributions to conception and design, and analysis and interpretation of data, drafting the manuscript and revising critically for important intellectual input; giving final approval for publication of manuscript and agrees to be accountable for all aspects of the work. RS and MF contributed to the analysis and interpretation of the data, drafting the manuscript and revising critically for important intellectual input; giving final approval for publication. AO and AMA made substantial contributions to conception and design, and analysis and interpretation of data, drafting the manuscript and revising critically for important intellectual input; giving final approval for publication of manuscript; and agree to be accountable for appropriate portions of the work.

Competing interests

Andrew M. Blumenfeld has served on advisory boards and/or has consulted for Allergan, Pernix, Teva, Avanir, Depomed, and Supernus, and has received funding for travel, speaking, and/or royalty payments from Allergan. Richard J. Stark has served on advisory boards and/or has consulted for Allergan, has served on advisory boards for Novartis and has received funding for travel and/or speaking payments from Allergan, MSD, AbbVie and SciGen, and from In Vivo Academy relating to a Pfizer-sponsored project. Marshall C. Freeman has served on advisory boards and/or has consulted or received research support from Alder, Allergan, Avani, Dr. Reddy's Laboratories, Eli Lilly, Scion, and Teva. Amelia Orejudos is an employee of Allergan plc. Aubrey Manack Adams is an employee of Allergan plc and owns stock in the company.

Author details

[1]Headache Center of Southern California, The Neurology Center, 6010 Hidden Valley Road, Carlsbad, CA 92024, USA. [2]Monash University and Alfred Hospital, Melbourne, VIC, Australia. [3]Headache Wellness Center, Greensboro, NC, USA. [4]Allergan plc, Irvine, CA, USA.

References

1. Headache Classification Committee of the International Headache Society (2013) The international classification of headache disorders, 3rd edition (beta version). Cephalalgia 33:629–808. https://doi.org/10.1177/0333102413485658

2. Manack AN, Buse DC, Lipton RB (2011) Chronic migraine: epidemiology and disease burden. Curr Pain Headache Rep 15:70–78. https://doi.org/10.1007/s11916-010-0157-z

3. Natoli JL, Manack A, Dean B, Butler Q, Turkel CC, Stovner L, Lipton RB (2010) Global prevalence of chronic migraine: a systematic review. Cephalalgia 30:599–609. https://doi.org/10.1111/j.1468-2982.2009.01941.x

4. Blumenfeld AM, Varon SF, Wilcox TK, Buse DC, Kawata AK, Manack A, Goadsby PJ, Lipton RB (2011) Disability, HRQoL and resource use among chronic and episodic migraineurs: results from the International Burden of Migraine Study (IBMS). Cephalalgia 31:301–315. https://doi.org/10.1177/0333102410381145

5. Buse DC, Manack AN, Serrano D, Reed ML, Varon S, Turkel CC, Lipton RB (2012) Headache impact of chronic and episodic migraine: results from the American Migraine Prevalence and Prevention Study. Headache 52:3–17. https://doi.org/10.1111/j.1526-4610.2011.02046.x

6. Buse DC, Manack Adams A, Serrano D, Turkel C, Lipton RB (2010) Sociodemographic and comorbidity profiles of chronic migraine and episodic migraine sufferers. J Neurol Neurosurg Psychiatry 81:428–432. https://doi.org/10.1136/jnnp.2009.192492

7. Chen YC, Tang CH, Ng K, Wang SJ (2012) Comorbidity profiles of chronic migraine sufferers in a national database in Taiwan. J Headache Pain 13:311-319. https://doi.org/10.1007/s10194-012-0447-4

8. Lipton RB, Varon SF, Grosberg B, McAllister PJ, Freitag F, Aurora SK, Dodick DW, Silberstein SD, Diener HC, DeGryse RE, Nolan ME, Turkel CC (2011) OnabotulinumtoxinA improves quality of life and reduces impact of chronic migraine. Neurology 77:1465–1472. https://doi.org/10.1212/WNL.0b013e318232ab65

9. Buse DC, Scher AI, Dodick DW, Reed ML, Fanning KM, Manack Adams A, Lipton RB (2016) Impact of migraine on the family: perspectives of people with migraine and their spouse/domestic partner in the CaMEO study. Mayo Clin Proc 91:596–611. https://doi.org/10.1016/j.mayocp.2016.02.013

10. Bigal ME, Serrano D, Reed M, Lipton RB (2008) Chronic migraine in the population: burden, diagnosis, and satisfaction with treatment. Neurology 71:559–566. https://doi.org/10.1212/01.wnl.0000323925.29520.e7

11. Buse DC, Manack AN, Fanning KM, Serrano D, Reed ML, Turkel CC, Lipton RB (2012) Chronic migraine prevalence, disability, and sociodemographic factors: results from the American Migraine Prevalence and Prevention Study. Headache 52:1456–1470. https://doi.org/10.1111/j.1526-4610.2012.02223.x

12. Bloudek LM, Stokes M, Buse DC, Wilcox TK, Lipton RB, Goadsby PJ, Varon SF, Blumenfeld AM, Katsarava Z, Pascual J, Lanteri-Minet M, Cortelli P, Martelletti P (2012) Cost of healthcare for patients with migraine in five European countries: results from the International Burden of Migraine Study (IBMS). J headache pain 13:361–378. https://doi.org/10.1007/s10194-012-0460-7

13. Dodick DW, Loder EW, Manack Adams A, Buse DC, Fanning KM, Reed ML, Lipton RB (2016) Assessing barriers to chronic migraine consultation, diagnosis, and treatment: results from the Chronic Migraine Epidemiology and Outcomes (CaMEO) study. Headache 56:821–834. https://doi.org/10.1111/head.12774

14. Serrano D, Buse DC, Manack Adams A, Reed ML, Lipton RB (2015) Acute treatment optimization in episodic and chronic migraine: results of the American Migraine Prevalence and Prevention (AMPP) study. Headache 55:502–518. https://doi.org/10.1111/head.12553

15. Diener HC, Dodick DW, Aurora SK, Turkel CC, DeGryse RE, Lipton RB, Silberstein SD, Brin MF (2010) OnabotulinumtoxinA for treatment of chronic migraine: results from the double-blind, randomized, placebo-controlled phase of the PREEMPT 2 trial. Cephalalgia 30:804-814. https://doi.org/10.1177/0333102410364677

16. Aurora SK, Dodick DW, Turkel CC, DeGryse RE, Silberstein SD, Lipton RB, Diener HC, Brin MF (2010) OnabotulinumtoxinA for treatment of chronic migraine: results from the double-blind, randomized, placebo-controlled

phase of the PREEMPT 1 trial. Cephalalgia 30:793-803. https://doi.org/10.1177/0333102410364676

17. Aurora SK, Winner P, Freeman MC, Spierings EL, Heiring JO, DeGryse RE, VanDenburgh AM, Nolan ME, Turkel CC (2011) OnabotulinumtoxinA for treatment of chronic migraine: pooled analyses of the 56-week PREEMPT clinical program. Headache 51:1358–1373. https://doi.org/10.1111/j.1526-4610.2011.01990.x

18. Blumenfeld AM, Aurora SK, Laranjo K, Papapetropoulos S (2015) Unmet clinical needs in chronic migraine: rationale for study and design of COMPEL, an open-label, multicenter study of the long-term efficacy, safety, and tolerability of onabotulinumtoxinA for headache prophylaxis in adults with chronic migraine. BMC Neurol 15:100. https://doi.org/10.1186/s12883-015-0353-x

19. BOTOX® for injection, for intramuscular, intradetrusor, or intradermal use (onabotulinumtoxinA). Full Prescribing Information, Allergan plc, Irvine, CA, 2016

20. Silberstein S, Tfelt-Hansen P, Dodick DW, Limmroth V, Lipton RB, Pascual J, Wang SJ (2008) Guidelines for controlled trials of prophylactic treatment of chronic migraine in adults. Cephalalgia 28:484–495. https://doi.org/10.1111/j.1468-2982.2008.01555.x

21. Rendas-Baum R, Yang M, Varon SF, Bloudek LM, DeGryse RE, Kosinski M (2014) Validation of the Headache Impact Test (HIT-6) in patients with chronic migraine. Health Qual Life Outcomes 12:117. https://doi.org/10.1186/s12955-014-0117-0

22. Dodick DW, Turkel CC, DeGryse RE, Aurora SK, Silberstein SD, Lipton RB, Diener HC, Brin MF (2010) OnabotulinumtoxinA for treatment of chronic migraine: pooled results from the double-blind, randomized, placebo-controlled phases of the PREEMPT clinical program. Headache 50:921–936. https://doi.org/10.1111/j.1526-4610.2010.01678.x

23. Negro A, Curto M, Lionetto L, Martelletti P (2016) A two years open-label prospective study of OnabotulinumtoxinA 195 U in medication overuse headache: a real-world experience. J Headache Pain 17:1. https://doi.org/10.1186/s10194-016-0591-3

24. Schaefer SM, Gottschalk CH, Jabbari B (2015) Treatment of chronic migraine with focus on botulinum neurotoxins. Toxins (Basel) 7:2615–2628. https://doi.org/10.3390/toxins7072615

25. Ranoux D, Martine G, Espagne-Dubreuilh G, Amilhaud-Bordier M, Caire F, Magy L (2017) OnabotulinumtoxinA injections in chronic migraine, targeted to sites of pericranial myofascial pain: an observational, open label, real-life cohort study. J Headache Pain 18:75. https://doi.org/10.1186/s10194-017-0781-7

26. Hou M, Xie JF, Kong XP, Zhang Y, Shao YF, Wang C, Ren WT, Cui GF, Xin L, Hou YP (2015) Acupoint injection of onabotulinumtoxin a for migraines. Toxins (Basel) 7:4442–4454. https://doi.org/10.3390/toxins7114442

27. Negro A, Curto M, Lionetto L, Crialesi D, Martelletti P (2015) OnabotulinumtoxinA 155 U in medication overuse headache: a two years prospective study. Spring erPlus 4:826. https://doi.org/10.1186/s40064-015-1636-9

28. Garza I, Swanson JW (2006) Prophylaxis of migraine. Neuropsychiatr Dis Treat 2:281–291

29. National Institute for Health and Care Excellence (2012) Botulinum toxin type A for the prevention of headaches in adults with chronic migraine. Available at: https://www.nice.org.uk/guidance/ta260/chapter/1-Guidance

30. Aurora SK, Dodick DW, Diener HC, DeGryse RE, Turkel CC, Lipton RB, Silberstein SD (2014) OnabotulinumtoxinA for chronic migraine: efficacy, safety, and tolerability in patients who received all five treatment cycles in the PREEMPT clinical program. Acta Neurol Scand 129:61–70. https://doi.org/10.1111/ane.12171

31. National Institute for Health and Care Excellence (2012) Headaches: diagnosis and management of headaches in young people and adults. Available at: https://www.nice.org.uk/guidance/cg150

32. Blumenfeld AM, Silberstein SD, Dodick DW, Aurora SK, Brin MF, Binder WJ (2017) Insights into the functional anatomy behind the PREEMPT injection paradigm: guidance on achieving optimal outcomes. Headache 57:766–777. https://doi.org/10.1111/head.13074

33. Lipton R, Chu MK, Seng EK, Reed ML, Fanning K, Adams A, Buse D (2016) The effect of psychiatric symptoms on headache-related disability in migraine: results from the Chronic Migraine Epidemiology and Outcomes (CaMEO) study. Paper presented at: 5th European headache and Migraine Trust International Congress (EHMTIC), Glasgow, Scotland, UK, 15-18 September 2016

11

The role of personality, disability and physical activity in the development of medication-overuse headache

Louise S. Mose[1,2]* ⓘ, Susanne S. Pedersen[3,4], Birgit Debrabant[5], Rigmor H. Jensen[6] and Bibi Gram[2]

Abstract

Background: Factors associated with development of medication-overuse headache (MOH) in migraine patients are not fully understood, but with respect to prevention, the ability to predict the onset of MOH is clinically important. The aims were to examine if personality characteristics, disability and physical activity level are associated with the onset of MOH in a group of migraine patients and explore to which extend these factors combined can predict the onset of MOH.

Methods: The study was a single-center prospective observational study of migraine patients. At inclusion, all patients completed questionnaires evaluating 1) personality (NEO Five-Factor Inventory), 2) disability (Migraine Disability Assessment), and 3) physical activity level (Physical Activity Scale 2.1). Diagnostic codes from patients' electronic health records confirmed if they had developed MOH during the study period of 20 months. Analyses of associations were performed and to identify which of the variables predict onset MOH, a multivariable least absolute shrinkage and selection operator (LASSO) logistic regression model was fitted to predict presence or absence of MOH.

Results: Out of 131 participants, 12 % (n=16) developed MOH. Migraine disability score (OR=1.02, 95 % CI: 1.00 to 1.04), intensity of headache (OR=1.49, 95 % CI: 1.03 to 2.15) and headache frequency (OR=1.02, 95 % CI: 1.00 to 1.04) were associated with the onset of MOH adjusting for age and gender. To identify which of the variables predict onset MOH, we used a LASSO regression model, and evaluating the predictive performance of the LASSO-mode (containing the predictors MIDAS score, MIDAS-intensity and –frequency, neuroticism score, time with moderate physical activity, educational level, hours of sleep daily and number of contacts to the headache clinic) in terms of area under the curve (AUC) was weak (apparent AUC=0.62, 95% CI: 0.41-0.82).

Conclusion: Disability, headache intensity and frequency were associated with the onset of MOH whereas personality and the level of physical activity were not. The multivariable LASSO model based on personality, disability and physical activity is applicable despite moderate study size, however it can be considered as a weak classifier for discriminating between absence and presence of MOH.

Keywords: Migraine, Medication-overuse headache, Personality, Disability, Physical activity

---

* Correspondence: Louise.schlosser@rsyd.dk
[1]Department of Neurology, Hospital Southwest Jutland, Esbjerg, Denmark
[2]The Research Unit of Health Science, Hospital of Southwest Jutland, Esbjerg and Department of Regional Health Research, University of Southern Denmark, Odense, Denmark
Full list of author information is available at the end of the article

Background

Migraine is a primary headache disorder characterized by recurring attacks, often described as a one-sided pulsating headache. The mean prevalence of current migraine in adults is around 15%, 8% in men versus 17.6 % in women in Europe [1]. Due to frequent pain-relieving medication intake, migraineurs are predisposed to develop medication-overuse headache (MOH) [2–5], which is defined as a chronic headache disorder developed as a consequence of regular overuse of acute or symptomatic headache medication [6]. Symptoms of MOH are often an aggravation and a chronification of the primary headache disorder [7]. Migraine is the primary headache for many MOH patients, however, not all migraine patients develop MOH. Clearly recognized predictors of developing MOH are unknown, but potential risk factors such as headache frequency, daily smoking, inactivity, comorbid pain conditions, anxiety and depression have all been discussed in literature [8]. Furthermore, also comorbidity with psychiatric conditions and psychological destress may negatively and significantly modify the outcome for migraine patients [9].

The psychological profile of migraine patients developing MOH is not fully understood, but the association between migraine and personality has been a topic of interest for many years [10, 11]. A common, well-established approach for describing personality traits is the Five Factor Model of personality [12, 13]. Theoretically, the Five Factor Model approaches personality as a hierarchical system of personality in terms of five basic independent domains: *Neuroticism, extroversion, openness to experience, agreeableness,* and *conscientiousness* [14]. Previous studies have demonstrated that a high score on the personality domain neuroticism is correlated with depression [13]. Both migraine (-MOH) and migraine patients (+MOH) have increased risk of developing depression, but migraine patients (+MOH) have a higher prevalence of depression compared to migraine patients (-MOH) [15]. Both the personality domain neuroticism and extraversion have been linked to general health [16] and a high score on neuroticism has been linked to migraine [17–19]. Additional research is needed to clarify the association between migraine and personality characteristics [10]. The Five Factor Model is commonly used to evaluate psychopathology, however, to the best of our knowledge only few studies have investigated personality characteristics of migraine patients using this framework [17, 20].

It is well-documented that headache patients in general experience decreased quality of life and disabilities [21, 22]. MOH patients frequently experience severe disability as compared to migraine patients without medication overuse [23, 24], but the role of disability in chronification is so far unknown. In the Global Burden of disease (GBD) study from 2016, migraine was estimated to be the main reason for years lived with disability in the age group 15-49, which represented a significant rise from the year before. The explanation was that MOH in GBD 2016 was attributed to the antecedent headache disorder instead of being reported separately [25, 26]. The 2016 GBD findings further underline the disabling role of migraine in general and in particular MOH as a sequela. Studies have shown that MOH patients have higher Migraine Disability Assessment Questionnaire scores (MIDAS) than migraine patients without medication overuse, indicating a higher degree of disability [21, 23, 24, 27]. Still, there is limited research on whether the MIDAS score in migraine patients correlates with the onset of MOH.

In a systematic review, Rhodes & Smith [28] concluded in correlation between personality characteristics and physical activity that neuroticism is negatively correlated with physical activity, while extraversion and conscientiousness have a positive correlation to physical activity [28]. A recent Danish cross-sectional study found an association between inactivity, daily smoking, obesity, and MOH [29]. Similarly, a population-based study investigating risk factors for a new onset of MOH in chronic headache patients found that physical inactivity and smoking were risk factors for developing MOH [8]. Evidence is lacking on the role of different intensity levels of physical activity in the development of MOH among migraine patients.

From a clinical point of view, knowledge of risk factors for the onset of MOH in patients with an established migraine diagnosis is paramount to prevent development of MOH. Factors such as personality, disability and physical activity level may be interesting as possible predictors of MOH, and at the same time, easy to establish and asses through the patients' medical history. Therefore, the aims of this study were firstly to investigate if personality, disability and physical activity level of migraine patients are associated with the development of MOH in a group of migraine patients who are in active treatment and secondly, to analyze to which extend these factors together can predict the onset of MOH. We hypothesized that personality, disability and level of physical activity varied between migraine patients (+MOH) and migraine patients (-MOH).

Methods
Design and participants

The design was a single-center prospective observational study of patients in active treatment recruited from the multidisciplinary Danish Headache Clinic, Hospital of Southwest Jutland in Denmark, between October 2015 and June 2017. Patients were eligible to participate, if they were between 18-65 years of age and had a primary diagnosis of migraine according to the diagnostic criteria from ICHD-III beta [6]. Exclusion criteria were presence of MOH based on diagnostic criteria of chronic migraine and MOH from ICHD-III beta [6] at inclusion. To minimize any errors and ambiguity in the personality data, we excluded patients with severe comorbid untreated depression or anxiety and patients diagnosed with personality disorders. All patients received standard treatment at the Headache Clinic, which included consultations with a neurologists or headache nurse every three months. As standard, patients were informed about the risk and criteria for MOH at the initial consultation. In between consultations, patients had the opportunity to contact a headache nurse by phone or mail.

Procedure

Patients were informed about the study by the neurologists at the consultations in the Headache Clinic. For logistic reasons, it was only possible to include patients two days a week and to extend the recruitment period to 20 months. Number of consultations in the clinic and years diagnosed with migraine varied, however all included patients were seen regularly in the clinic. Patients completed questionnaires regarding personality, extent of disabilities due to migraine, and physical activity level at the inclusion. Throughout the study period, patients' were followed regularly in the Headache clinic and during these consultations patients' self-reported headache diaries together with the physician's examination and assessment formed the basis of a confirmed diagnosis. Information about patients who developed MOH were obtained from the hospital electronic health records in June 2017 [6].

Ethics, consent and permissions

This study was part of a larger study that was approved by the Regional Committees on Health Research Ethics for Southern Denmark (ID S-20140114). It was conducted according to the Helsinki Declaration, meaning all patients were informed both orally and in writing prior to giving written informed consent. Permission was obtained from the Danish Data Protection Agency (2008-58-0035).

Measurements
NEO Five-Factor Inventory

We assessed personality with the Danish version of NEO Five-Factor Inventory questionnaire (NEO-FFI-3) [30]. The questionnaire consists of 60 items and is a brief version of the original NEO-PI-R [31]. For pragmatic reasons, the short version was chosen as it is less burdensome to patients as compared to the original version with 240 items. The questionnaire is designed as a hierarchical measure with personality seen as five well-established domains, which is also referred to as the Five Factor Model of personality. Each domain is assessed by means of 12 questions. The five domains are: (i)

Neuroticism (e.g. the tendency to experience negative emotions, such as anxiety, fear, and frustration); (ii) *Extraversion* (e.g. the tendency to be outgoing and talkative); (iii) *Openness to experience* (e.g. the tendency to be creative and imaginative); (iv) *Agreeableness* (e.g. the tendency to be empathic and altruistic); and (v) *Conscientiousness* (e.g. efficient, organized, and having self-control). All questions are answered on a five-point Likert scale from "totally disagree to "totally agree". For each domain a t-score is calculated as the sum of the 12 items' score ranging from 12-60 [30]. In the current study, the internal consistency of the domains ranged from 0.74-0.90, measured by Cronbach's alpha, which is considered satisfactory.

Migraine Disability Assessment

To quantify the extent of disability, the MIDAS questionnaire was used, which is one of the most frequently used measures to assess disability in migraine patients [32–34]. MIDAS consists of 5 items that captures information on disability on a four-point score. The grade of disability is scored as the sum of days with headache during the previous three months that prevented patients from or reduced productivity by at least 50% with respect to work/school, housework, and social/leisure activities. Furthermore, MIDAS consists of two additional questions on number of days with headache during the previous three months and intensity of headache measured on a numeric rating scale ranging from 0-10 where 0 is "no pain" and 10 is "worst imaginable pain".

Physical Activity Scale

To measure physical activity level, the questionnaire Physical Activity Scale 2.1 (PAS 2.1) was used [35]. In PAS 2.1, the patients were asked to specify number of hours and minutes in an average 24-hour day spent on physical activity categorized as i) sleeping, ii) work related sitting/standing/walking and heavy physical work, iii) transportation to or from work (walking/cycling to work), and iv) sedentary leisure time activities (e.g. TV-viewing). Additionally, PAS 2.1 provided estimates on hours and minutes on a weekly basis spent on physical activity at three different intensity levels: 'Light', 'moderate' and 'vigorous' physical activity.

Statistical analyses

The outcome of interest in this study was whether patients developed MOH during the study period or not. Baseline demographic characteristics comparing the two groups migraine (+MOH) and migraine (-MOH) were calculated using the chi-square test for larger samples and Fisher's exact for samples less than five categorical data and Mann-Whitney U test for data with skewed distribution and unpaired t-test for data following normal distribution. For hypothesis testing we used two-tailed test. P-values of < 0.05 were considered statistically significant.

Associations between development of MOH, personality, disability and physical activity

Using logistic regression, we investigated whether MOH onset was associated with personality characteristics, disabilities or physical activity level. Each of the following variables were tested in a separate regression model: Unemployment, neuroticism, extraversion, openness, agreeableness, conscientiousness, MIDAS score, MIDAS-intensity and MIDAS-frequency, and physical activity level divided into hours weekly on light, moderate or vigorous activity. All regression models were adjusted for age and gender to avoid confounding effects on both personality score and development of MOH [4, 30, 36–38].

Predicting presence or absence of MOH

To investigate the ability of our variables to jointly predict onset of MOH, we considered a multivariable prediction model obtained by least absolute shrinkage and selection operator (LASSO) regression. This penalized regression method allows for the integration of a large number of possible correlated predictors into one model and to select amongst these despite a small sample size. The following predictors were included: age, gender, civil status, educational level, primary diagnosis, contacts to the headache clinic, the five NEO-FFI-3 domains as separate variables, disability using MIDAS score, intensity and frequency, measurements from PAS 2.1 on times spent for sleeping, sedentary leisure time activities and times for light activities, moderate activities or vigorous activities and a binary variable indicating if patients were unemployed. Remaining variables from the PAS 2.1 assessing different activity levels during work times were not included, since they were not available for patients without employment. Educational level was included both as continuous and as categorical variable. We only used data from patients without missing data in any of the included covariates. Variable standardization prior to fitting was applied, but reported Odds ratios (OR) are returned on the original scale. Due to the LASSO penalty, ORs are biased towards one for the benefit of improved predictions. The tuning parameter controlling the strength of the penalty was chosen to maximize the goodness-of-fit in an 8-fold cross validation. Folds were chosen randomly, but each fold contained two (+MOH) patients. As goodness-of-fit-measure we used the area under the ROC curve (AUC). After the tuning parameter had been determined, we calculated the AUC in the complete dataset together with its 95% confidence interval. Because the AUC value of our prediction model for

new samples from the same population is expected to be below the calculated apparent AUC (especially because of the previous model selection incorporated in the LASSO approach), we applied bootstrap resampling as described in Steyerberg [39] to calculate an optimism-corrected AUC-value. We used 500 bootstrap samples, but discarded those for which the LASSO logistic regression failed to converge. At the same time and using the same approach, we calculated bootstrap based corrections for the lower and upper bound of the corresponding confidence interval.

Statistical analyses were performed with StatalC14 (StataCorp LP, College Station, Texas). We used the statistics software R (version 3.3.2) together with the packages glmnet version 2.0-10 [40], ROCR version 1.0-7 [41], pROC version 1.10.0 [42] and caret version 6.0-76 [43] to carry out the LASSO logistic regression model, calculate the AUC and its confidence intervals and to plot the ROC curve.

Results

A total of 156 patients were informed about the study and 131 accepted to participate. Two patients did not want to participate, as they felt uncomfortable about answering the questionnaires, while 23 patients failed to return the questionnaires. Of the 131 included patients, 119 (91%) received prophylactic treatment for migraine at inclusion and patients had a mean [range] follow-up time of 361[18-631] days. There were no statistically significant differences between non-responders and included patients regarding age, gender and primary headache diagnoses (all p-values > 0.05).

Clinical characteristics

Sixteen migraine patients (12%) developed MOH, while 88% (n=115) were still migraine patients without MOH at the end of the study period. The majority of migraine patients (-MOH) were women 87% (n=100) with a mean (SD) age of 39.2 (13) years. The distributions of primary headache diagnosis in the migraine (-MOH) group were 38 % (n=44) had tension-type headache (TTH) as co-morbidity, while 62% (n=71) had only migraine. Also in the migraine (+ MOH) group, women were predominant by 94 % (n=15) with a mean (SD) age of 37.3(13). In this group migraine was primary headache diagnosis for 50% (n=8) while 50 % (n=8) had comorbidity migraine and TTH. The migraine (+MOH) group had a significantly higher numbers of contacts to the Headache Clinic during the study period; median (IQR) contacts 8.5 (4 to 10) as compared to the migraine (-MOH) group with median (IQR) contacts 6 (3 to 7) (p= 0.028). No other statistically significant differences in demographic and headache characteristics were observed between the groups. Characteristics are summarized in Table 1.

Table 1 Patients' demographic and headache characteristics

	Migraine (-MOH) (n = 115)	Migraine (+ MOH) (n = 16)	All participants (n = 131)	P- value
Age (years)(mean±SD)	39.2±13	37.3±13	39.0±13	NS
Sex n (%)				
Female	100 (87)	15 (94)	115 (88)	NS
Male	15 (13)	1 (6)	16 (12)	
Civil status n (%)				
Single	25 (22)	3 (19)	28 (21)	NS
Cohabiting	90 (78)	13 (81)	103 (79)	
Educational level n (%)				
Primary/secondary school	16 (14)	5 (31)	21 (16)	NS
Vocational/High school	55 (48)	7 (44)	62 (47)	
Bachelor or higher degree	44 (38)	4 (25)	48 (37)	
Working status n (%)				
Employed/student	91 (79)	13 (81)	104 (82)	NS
Unemployed/sickness benefits/social welfare	24 (21)	3 (19)	27 (18)	
Sleep (hours daily) (mean±SD)	8±1	8±1	8±1	NS
Primary diagnosis n (%)				
Migraine	71 (62)	8 (50)	79 (60)	NS
Migraine + Tension Type Headache	44 (38)	8 (50)	52 (40)	
Contacts headache clinic median [IQR]	6 [3-7]	8.5 [4-10]	5 [3-8]	0.028

Differences between groups on normal distributed data were tested using unpaired t-test and Chi-square test for samples >5 and Fisher's exact for samples < 5. Data are presented as mean ± standard deviation (SD) or as numbers with percentages (%) in brackets. For skewed data Wilcoxon Mann-Whitney test were used and data were presented as median and interquartile range [IQR] in brackets. P-values < 0.05 were considered as statistically significant for all tests.

Comparison of personality characteristics between groups showed no statistical differences. Migraine (+MOH) had significantly higher headache intensity median (IQR) 7(6.5-8) as compared to the migraine (-MOH) group with median (IQR) of 6 (5-7), (*p*=0.041). Headache frequency for the previous three months, were also significantly higher among the migraine (+MOH) group with median (IQR) of 46 (28.5-87.5), compared to migraine (-MOH) with median (IQR) of 30 (15-54), (*p*=0.017) (Table 2). Overall, neither the migraineurs (-MOH) nor the migraineurs (+MOH) were physically active as they spent only few hours weekly on light physical activity, even fewer hours at moderate physical activity and almost no time on vigorous physical activity. No statistical significant differences were found between the groups regarding level of physical activity (Table 2).

Associations between development of MOH, personality, disability and physical activity

When adjusting for age and gender in the logistic regressions analysis for the onset of MOH, no significant differences in odds were found with respect to unemployment (OR=0.967, 95% CI: 0.24 to 3.77). The personality domains neuroticism (OR=1.06, 95 % CI: 0.99 to 1.13), extraversion (OR=0.96, 95 % CI: 0.88 to 1.04), openness (OR=0.99, 95 % CI: 0.91 to 1.08), agreeableness

(OR=1.00, 95 % CI: 0.93 to 1.08) and conscientiousness (OR=0.95, 95 % CI: 0.87 to 1.03) were not associated with onset of MOH in migraine patients.

Analyses on the relationship between MIDAS score and MOH demonstrated significant association between MIDAS score (OR=1.02, 95 % CI: 1.00 to 1.04) and intensity of headache (OR=1.49, 95 % CI: 1.03 to 2.15) and between MIIDAS score and headache frequency (OR=1.02, 95 % CI: 1.00 to 1.04).

The three variables describing levels of physical activity were not significantly associated with onset of MOH; light activity (OR=1.00, 95 % CI: 0.93 to 1.08), moderate activity (OR=0.87, 95 % CI: 0.70 to 1.07) and vigorous activity (OR=0.91, 95 % CI: 0.66 to 1.26). All association analyses using logistic regression are summarized in Table 3.

Predicting presence or absence of MOH

Two patients out of 131 were excluded from this analysis due to missing values. Table 4 illustrates our multivariable prediction model and shows the covariates selected by the multivariable LASSO logistic regression together with the estimated ORs.

The predicted odds for developing MOH increased by 21% (OR=1.210) by each unit of headache frequency reported. The predicted odds increased by 0.2% (OR=1.002)

Table 2 Comparison of personality, disability and physical activity levels between migraine (-MOH) and migraine (+MOH). All data are presented as medians [interquartile ranges]

	Migraine (-MOH) (n= 115)	Migraine (+MOH) (n= 16)	All participants (n=131)	P-value
Neuroticism (12-60)	35 [28-42]	38.5 [31- 46.5]	35 [28-42]	NS
Extraversion (12-60)	39 [34-44]	39 [30.5-41]	39 [33-44]	NS
Openness (12-60)	37 [33-42]	34.5 [34-43]	37 [33-42]	NS
Agreeableness (12-60)	44 [39- 48]	44.5 [39- 48.5]	44 [39- 48]	NS
Conscientiousness (12-60)	47 [43-51]	46.5 [39.5- 50]	47 [42-51]	NS
MIDAS score (0-270)	32 [16- 57]	42 [28- 94.5]	33 [17-58]	NS
MIDAS-frequency (days last 3 months)	30 [15-54]	46 [28.5-87.5]	30 [18- 63]	0.017
MIDAS-intensity (NRS 0-10)	6 [5-7]	7 [6.5-8]	7 [5-7]	0.041
Light physical activity (hours/week)	5.25 [3-10]	7 [4-13]	6 [3-10]	NS
Moderate physical activity(hours/week)	2.5 [1-5]	2 [0.5-4]	2.5 [0.5-5]	NS
Vigorous physical activity (hours/ week)	0 [0-2]	0 [0-1.5]	0 [0-2]	NS

Differences between groups were tested using Wilcoxon Mann-Whitney test. P-values< 0.05 were considered as statistically significant for all tests. NEO-FFI-3: NEO Five-Factor Inventory. MIDAS: Migraine disability assessment questionnaire. PAS 2.1: Physical Activity Scale questionnaire

for each additional MIDAS score point, and 0.6% (OR=0.006) for each unit of intensity of headache reported.

The predicted odds for experiencing MOH estimated by the LASSO model were 3.2% higher (OR=1.032) for each additional hour of sleep, and decreased by 1.7% (OR=0.983) for each hour spent on moderate physical activity. Regarding personality domains, an additional unit in the neuroticism score increased the odds by 1.7% (OR=1.017). Each additional level of education decreased the odds by 20.6% (OR=0.794) and each additional contact to the Headache clinic increased the odds by 1% (OR=1.010). Remaining covariates were not part of the selected model.

Evaluating the predictive performance of the LASSO-model, we obtained the ROC curve, shown in Fig. 1

Table 3 Associations between development of MOH and personality, disability and physical activity level

Covariates	OR	95% CI	P-value
Unemployment (n=131)	0.97	0.24-3.77	0.961
Light physical activity (hours/week)(n=130)	1.00	0.93-1.08	0.947
Moderate physical activity (hours/week)(n=130)	0.87	0.70-1.07	0.193
Vigorous physical activity (hours/week)(n=131)	0.91	0.66-1.26	0.588
MIDAS score (0-270)(n=131)	1.02	1.00-1.04	0.032
MIDAS-intensity (NRS 0-10) (n=131)	1.49	1.03-2.15	0.034
MIDAS-frequency (days last 3 months) (n=131)	1.02	1.00-1.04	0.032
Neuroticism score (12-60) (n=131)	1.06	0.99-1.13	0.069
Extraversion score (12-60) (n=131)	0.96	0.88-1.04	0.275
Openness score (12-60) (n=131)	0.99	0.91-1.08	0.763
Agreeableness score (12-60) (n=131)	1.00	0.93-1.08	0.970
Conscientiousness score (12-60) (n=131)	0.95	0.87-1.03	0.206

Values are adjusted odds ratio and their 95 % CI and P-values from multivariable regression model with age and gender as covariates. The results are obtained from 12 different regressions

together with an apparent area under the ROC curve (AUC) of 0.78 (95% CI: 0.65-0.91) in our sample. By obtaining the ROC curve we assess the ability of the predictors in the model to discriminate between absence and presence of MOH. The curve is obtained by the score divided from the LASSO logistic regression and based on the included predictors.

As the sample had already been used for model selection, this estimate of model performance is overly optimistic. During the following bootstrap procedure, 141 of the 500 bootstrap samples were discarded due to convergence problems during the estimation procedure. Using the remaining bootstrap samples, we obtained an optimism estimate of 0.16 resulting in a corrected AUC of 0.62. Similarly, the corrected 95% CI for the AUC was 0.41-0.82. The AUC presents a measurement of discrimination, that is, the ability of the model to correctly classify the onset of MOH. Given the fact that the corrected AUC is 0.62 (95% CI: 0.41-0.82), our model (containing the predictors MIDAS score, MIDAS-intensity and –frequency, neuroticism score, time with moderate physical activity, educational level, hours of sleep daily and number of contacts to the headache clinic)) the model can be considered as an weak classifier for discriminating between absence and presence of MOH.

Discussion

The main findings of the present study were that the logistic regressions indicated that the headache intensity and headache frequency were associated with onset of MOH and therefore could be factors to take into account to prevent the development of MOH. This could have important implications for clinicians and highlights that the intensity and frequency of headache may help

Table 4 Variables selected by the LASSO logistic regression

Covariates	OR (LASSO)	OR	95% CI (OR)
Sleep (hours daily)(n=129)	1.032	1.214	0.831-1.812
Moderate physical activity (hours/week) (n=129)	0.983	0.906	0.710-1.077
MIDAS score (n=129)	1.002	1.002	0.990-1.014
MIDAS-intensity (NRS 0-10) (n=129)	1.006	1.011	0.987-1.034
MIDAS-frequency (days last 3 months) (n=129)	1.210	1.564	1.042-2.517
Neuroticism score (12-60) (n=129)	1.017	1.052	0.981-1.133
Educational level (n=129)	0.794	0.586	0.233-1.396
Contacts headache clinic (n=129)	1.010	1.068	0.916-1.237

The table shows estimated (shrunken) odds ratio for the selected variables. These are complemented by odds ratios and their 95% CI afterwards obtained from an ordinary multivariable logistic regression model using the same variables. Odds ratios correspond to the variables' original scale

identify the sub group at risk of developing MOH. For this study, MIDAS questionnaire was chosen as an instrument, however other instruments measuring intensity and frequency (i.e. headache diary) could have been applicable. Furthermore, when comparing migraine patients (-MOH) and migraine patients (+MOH) , patients developing MOH reported higher intensity and frequency of headache using the MIDAS questionnaire as compared to the rest of the included migraine patients. This finding is consistent with a review that showed high headache frequency to be an important modifiable risk factor in migraine chronification progression [44] and with previous studies stating that headache frequency in particular may be a risk factor for onset MOH [8, 45]. Martelletti shows that MOH must be considered as sequela of chronic migraine and in light of that, it is

beneficial to focus on how to reduce headache frequency among migraine patients to avoid MOH as a consequence [46].

Bigal et al. [47] investigated psychological profiles including the role of personality characteristics in headache chronification and observed that episodic headache patients undergoing chronification had a different personality profile compared to patients with episodic headaches [47]. In contrast, when we compared personality characteristics between migraine (-MOH) and migraine (+MOH) patients, we were unable to detect any differences between the groups. This can be caused by the fact that all patients at starting point were migraine patients without MOH, and the two groups therefore remain very similar in personality characteristics, unaffected by the chronification process related to developing MOH.

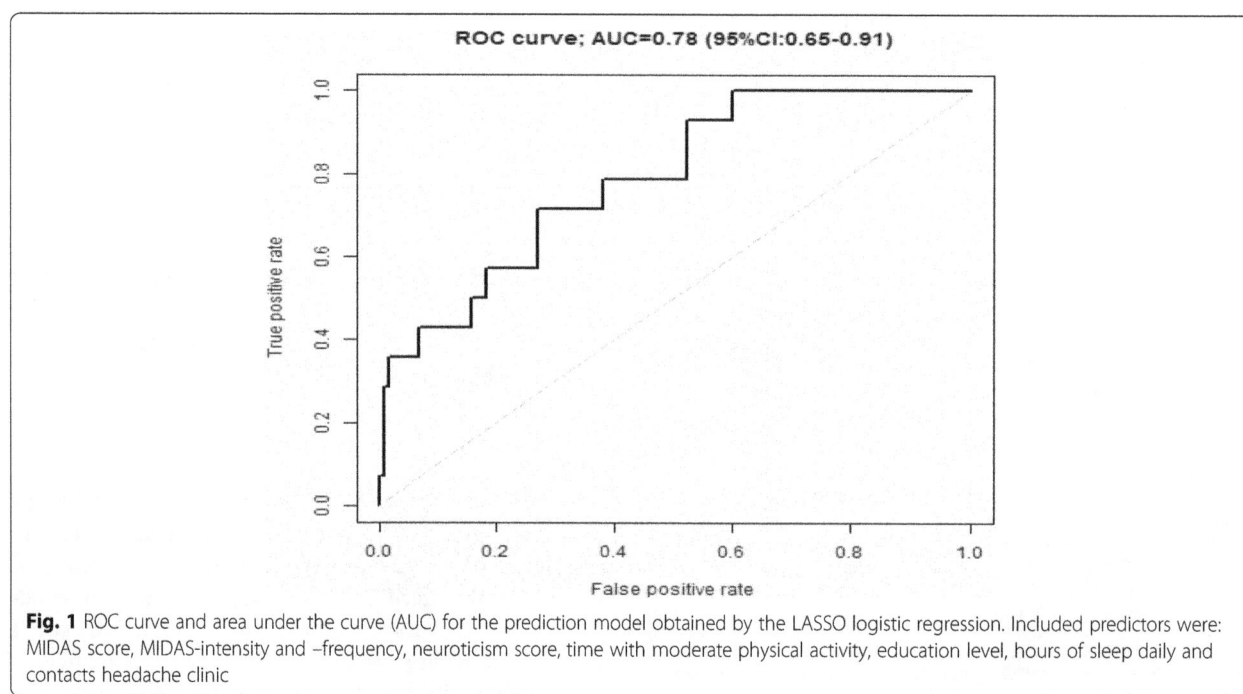

Fig. 1 ROC curve and area under the curve (AUC) for the prediction model obtained by the LASSO logistic regression. Included predictors were: MIDAS score, MIDAS-intensity and –frequency, neuroticism score, time with moderate physical activity, education level, hours of sleep daily and contacts headache clinic

Generally, few studies have investigated associations between different headache types and personality, and the results have been ambiguous [48]. Furthermore, different measurements of personality make studies difficult to compare. For this study we chose the NEO-FFI-3 which describes personality as five domains with 12 items each without the underlying in-depth facet score [31]. This facet scores could potentially increase the sensitivity of the personality evaluations, making it possible to detect subtle differences that our method could not. This could explain the insignificant differences between (+MOH) and (-MOH) in the current study.

MOH patients tend to be more physically inactive as compared to migraine patients [8]. According to Westergaard et al. the association between MOH and inactivity might be due to the fact that MOH patients have developed an inactive lifestyle in order to avoid triggering migraine attacks [29]. In this study, both patients with migraine (-MOH) and migraine (+MOH) spent very few hours on physical activities per week, which probably could be caused by headache burden. The difficulty of performing physical activity among migraine patients in association to development of MOH seems to be irrelevant as the odds for MOH only decreased by 1.7% (OR=0.983) for each hour spent on moderate physical activity. However, a study on physical activity and migraine treatment found that regular physical activity has beneficial effects on headache intensity and frequency, duration of headache attacks and patients well-being [49]. When MOH patients are physically inactive there could be a risk of maintaining MOH in an inappropriate circular process with inactivity, worsening in headache and increased medical intake.

This study is the first to investigate the predictive performance of models based on personality, disability and physical activity in predicting onset of MOH. It is challenging, but clinically relevant, to identify patients at risk of developing MOH and therefore studies developing predictive models of headache chronification are important [50]. In our prediction model we could not determine a strong causality between the included factors of personality, disability and physical activity level in the onset of MOH, however, we are not able to reject it either. Our findings substantiates that multiple factors potentially contributes to the onset of MOH, which is in line with another similar predictive study [20] were they found an AUC of 0.76 when including factors of personality, gene polymorphisms, headache characteristics and lifestyle. In both studies the AUC showed a weak model classifier for the onset of MOH.

As strength in this study the questionnaires used were not time consuming, which must be considered as an advantage, because it is easy to adopt in clinical practice. As a limitation we must consider the inclusion process since we only included patients two times per week. Therefore

we are fully aware that this study represents only a sample of a larger migraine patient flow in the clinic. However this study indicates how many migraine patients developed MOH during treatment at a headache clinic. Further we are limited by investigating patients who were seen and treated regularly and therefore, we are unable to assess how many patients would have developed MOH if they had no treatment options, and if this could have caused other predictive factors to emerge. Migraineurs with particularly high medication intake are at increased risk of developing MOH [51]. However, detailed knowledge about prophylactic and acute medical treatment is not part of the current study, since the patients' medical ordinations changed throughout the study. Overall, only 12% of the patients developed MOH during the study period and the small number of patients developing MOH is a limitation for immediate generalization of the results. This limits the power of the study and increases the risk for errors in both the estimated size as well as direction of effects. However, one way to handle these limitations is by looking at Gelman & Calin [52] who recommend a design calculation that provides a perspective on erroneous findings in small studies. The design calculation estimates the type S error, meaning the probability of an estimate being in the wrong direction, and type M errors being by which factor the magnitude of an effect is overestimated. Even though the dataset was small, we succeeded on characterizing the patients developing MOH and modeling our data via solid statistical methods highlighting important methods for assessing easy accessible clinical data in the prevention of MOH. The predictors included in the presented prediction model were those which best predicted presence or absence of MOH. Due to the small effective sample size of 16 cases of MOH in the dataset, the complexity of resulting models was a priori limited as larger models tend to be more prone to overfitting. Further, for penalized regression methods such as LASSO logistic regression, the number of selected predictors depends crucially on the chosen strength of the penalty. In this study, its choice was governed by cross-validation. Taking the variability incorporated in this procedure into account, a wider range of other prediction models including more or less predictors becomes plausible, see also Pfeiffer & Raymond [53] who estimated the rate of falsely included/excluded variables when applying LASSO logistic regression to a simulated dataset.

Conclusion

This study showed that the intensity and frequency of headache were associated with MOH onset, while there were no associations between personality and physical activity level and MOH onset, respectively. Our findings support that focus on headache frequency and intensity is essential for targeting a subgroup of migraine patients at risk of developing MOH.

The identification of predictors of MOH may have important clinical implications - specifically in relation to early detection of patients at risk of developing MOH and in the documentation of appropriate instruments for this detection.

Abbreviations

AUC: Area under the ROC curve is a measurement of discrimination, that is, the ability of the model to correctly classify the onset of medication-overuse headache; CI: Confidence Interval; LASSO: Least absolute shrinkage and selection operator; MIDAS: Migraine Disability Assessment Questionnaire; MOH: Medication-overuse headache defined according to the diagnostic criteria from ICHD-III beta; NEO-FFI-3: NEO Five-Factor Inventory questionnaire; NEO-PI-R: The revised NEO Personality Inventory is the longer version of NEO-FFI-3 containing 240 items.; OR: Odds Ratio; PAS 2.1: The Physical Activity Scale, which is a questionnaire.; ROC Curve: Receiver operating characteristic curve; TTH: Tension-type headache

Acknowledgements

The authors would like to thank the Neurology Department at Hospital Southwest Jutland for the collaboration and the staff of The Headache Clinic at the Hospital Southwest Jutland, Denmark for their support with inclusion, and of course all the participating patients.

Funding

Financial support with grants from TrygFonden, Carola Jørgensen Foundation and the Danish patient organization Migræne og Hovedpineforeningen.

Authors' contributions

LSM and BG conceived the idea for this article. LSM was project leader. BD and LSM performed the data analyses and data interpretations. LSM, BG, SSP, BD and RJ contributed with inputs to this article. The article was drafted by LSM and all authors reviewed and approved the final manuscript.

Competing interests

The authors declare that they have no competing interests.

Author details

[1]Department of Neurology, Hospital Southwest Jutland, Esbjerg, Denmark. [2]The Research Unit of Health Science, Hospital of Southwest Jutland, Esbjerg and Department of Regional Health Research, University of Southern Denmark, Odense, Denmark. [3]Department of Psychology, University of Southern Denmark, Odense, Denmark. [4]Department of Cardiology, Odense University Hospital, Odense, Denmark. [5]Epidemiology, Biostatistics and Biodemography Department of Public Health, University of Southern Denmark, Odense, Denmark. [6]Danish Headache Centre, Department of Neurology, Rigshospitalet-Glostrup, University of Copenhagen, Copenhagen, Denmark.

References

1. Stovner LJ, Andree C (2010) Prevalence of headache in Europe: a review for the Eurolight project. J Headache Pain 11:289–299. https://doi.org/10.1007/s10194-010-0217-0
2. Bigal ME, Lipton RB (2008) Excessive acute migraine medication use and migraine progression. Neurology 71:1821–1828. https://doi.org/10.1212/01.wnl.0000335946.53860.1d
3. Bigal ME, Serrano D, Buse D, Scher A, Stewart WF, Lipton RB (2008) Acute migraine medications and evolution from episodic to chronic migraine: a longitudinal population-based study. Headache 48:1157–1168. https://doi.org/10.1111/j.1526-4610.2008.01217.x
4. Evers S, Marziniak M (2010) Clinical features, pathophysiology, and treatment of medication-overuse headache. Lancet Neurol 9:391–401. https://doi.org/10.1016/s1474-4422(10)70008-9
5. Saper JR, Da Silva AN (2013) Medication overuse headache: history, features, prevention and management strategies. CNS drugs 27:867–877. https://doi.org/10.1007/s40263-013-0081-y
6. Headache Classification Committee of the International Headache Society (IHS) (2013) The International Classification of Headache Disorders, 3rd edition (beta version). Cephalalgia 33:629–808
7. Diener HC, Limmroth V (2004) Medication-overuse headache: a worldwide problem. Lancet Neurol 3:475–483. https://doi.org/10.1016/s1474-4422(04)00824-5
8. Hagen K, Linde M, Steiner TJ, Stovner LJ, Zwart JA (2012) Risk factors for medication-overuse headache: an 11-year follow-up study. The Nord-Trondelag Health Studies. Pain 153:56–61. https://doi.org/10.1016/j.pain.2011.08.018
9. Serafini G et al (2012) Gene variants with suicidal risk in a sample of subjects with chronic migraine and affective temperamental dysregulation. Eur Rev Med Pharmacol Sci 16:1389–1398
10. Davis RE, Smitherman TA, Baskin SM (2013) Personality traits, personality disorders, and migraine: a review. Neurol Sci 34(Suppl 1):S7–S10. https://doi.org/10.1007/s10072-013-1379-8
11. Silberstein SD, Lipton RB, Breslau N (1995) Migraine: association with personality characteristics and psychopathology. Cephalalgia 15:358–369; discussion 336. https://doi.org/10.1046/j.1468-2982.1995.1505358.x
12. Costa PT Jr, McCrae RR (1992) NEO PI-R:professional manual. Psychological Assesment Resources, Inc, Odessa
13. Costa PT Jr, McCrae RR (1995) Domains and facets: hierarchical personality assessment using the revised NEO personality inventory. J Pers Assess 64: 21–50. https://doi.org/10.1207/s15327752jpa6401_2
14. Mccrae RR, John OP (1992) An introduction to the five-factor model and its applications. J Pers 60:175–215
15. Lampl C et al (2016) Headache, depression and anxiety: associations in the Eurolight project. J Headache Pain 17:59. https://doi.org/10.1186/s10194-016-0649-2
16. Svedberg P, Bardage C, Sandin S, Pedersen NL (2006) A prospective study of health, life-style and psychosocial predictors of self-rated health. Eur J Epidemiol 21:767–776. https://doi.org/10.1007/s10654-006-9064-3
17. Cao M, Zhang S, Wang K, Wang Y, Wang W (2002) Personality traits in migraine and tension-type headaches: a five-factor model study. Psychopathology 35:254–258 63829
18. Merikangas KR, Stevens DE, Angst J (1993) Headache and personality: results of a community sample of young adults. J Psychiatr Res 27:187–196
19. Mongini F, Ibertis F, Barbalonga E, Raviola F (2000) MMPI-2 profiles in chronic daily headache and their relationship to anxiety levels and accompanying symptoms. Headache 40:466–472
20. Onaya T, Ishii M, Katoh H, Shimizu S, Kasai H, Kawamura M, Kiuchi Y (2013) Predictive index for the onset of medication overuse headache in migraine patients. Neurol Sci 34:85–92. https://doi.org/10.1007/s10072-012-0955-7
21. Lanteri-Minet M, Duru G, Mudge M, Cottrell S (2011) Quality of life impairment, disability and economic burden associated with chronic daily headache, focusing on chronic migraine with or without medication overuse: a systematic review. Cephalalgia 31:837–850. https://doi.org/10.1177/0333102411398400
22. Stovner L et al (2007) The global burden of headache: a documentation of headache prevalence and disability worldwide. Cephalalgia 27:193–210. https://doi.org/10.1111/j.1468-2982.2007.01288.x
23. Bendtsen L et al (2014) Disability, anxiety and depression associated with medication-overuse headache can be considerably reduced by detoxification and prophylactic treatment. Results from a multicentre, multinational study (COMOESTAS project). Cephalalgia 34:426–433. https://doi.org/10.1177/0333102413515338
24. Wallasch TM, Kropp P (2012) Multidisciplinary integrated headache care: a

prospective 12-month follow-up observational study. J Headache Pain 13: 521–529. https://doi.org/10.1007/s10194-012-0469-y

25. Steiner TJ, Stovner LJ, Vos T, Jensen R, Katsarava Z (2018) Migraine is first cause of disability in under 50s: will health politicians now take notice? J Headache Pain 19:17. https://doi.org/10.1186/s10194-018-0846-2

26. Vos T, Abajobir A, Abbafati C, Abbas K, Abate K, Abd-Allah F et al (2017) Global, regional, and national incidence, prevalence, and years lived with disability for 328 diseases and injuries for 195 countries, 1990-2016: a systematic analysis for the Global Burden of Disease Study 2016. Lancet 390: 1211–1259. https://doi.org/10.1016/s0140-6736(17)32154-2

27. Andrasik F, Grazzi L, Usai S, Kass S, Bussone G (2010) Disability in chronic migraine with medication overuse: treatment effects through 5 years. Cephalalgia 30:610–614. https://doi.org/10.1111/j.1468-2982.2009.01932.x

28. Rhodes RE, Smith NE (2006) Personality correlates of physical activity: a review and meta-analysis. Br J Sports Med 40:958–965. https://doi.org/10.1136/bjsm.2006.028860

29. Westergaard ML, Glumer C, Hansen EH, Jensen RH (2016) Medication overuse, healthy lifestyle behaviour and stress in chronic headache: Results from a population-based representative survey. Cephalalgia 36:15–28. https://doi.org/10.1177/0333102415578430

30. Costa PT, Jr., McCrae RR (eds) (2014) NEO-PI-3 vejledning klinisk. Hogrefe Psykologiske Forlag Frederiksberg Bogtrykkeri A/S

31. McCrae RR, Costa PT (2007) Brief Versions of the NEO-PI-3. J Individ Differ 28:116–128

32. Stewart WF, Lipton RB, Dowson AJ, Sawyer J (2001) Development and testing of the Migraine Disability Assessment (MIDAS) Questionnaire to assess headache-related disability. Neurology 56:S20–S28

33. Stewart WF, Lipton RB, Kolodner K, Liberman J, Sawyer J (1999a) Reliability of the migraine disability assessment score in a population-based sample of headache sufferers. Cephalalgia 19:107–114 discussion 174

34. Stewart WF, Lipton RB, Whyte J, Dowson A, Kolodner K, Liberman JN, Sawyer J (1999b) An international study to assess reliability of the Migraine Disability Assessment (MIDAS) score. Neurology 53:988–994

35. Andersen LG, Groenvold M, Jorgensen T, Aadahl M (2010) Construct validity of a revised Physical Activity Scale and testing by cognitive interviewing. Scan J Pub Health 38:707–714. https://doi.org/10.1177/1403494810380099

36. Costa PT Jr, McCrae RR (2009) The Five-Factor Model and the NEO Inventories. In: Butcher JN, editor. Oxford library of psychology. Oxford handbook of personality assessment (pp. 299-322). New York: Oxford University Press. https://doi.org/10.1093/oxfordhb/9780195366877.013.0016

37. Jensen R, Bendtsen L (2008) Medication overuse headache in Scandinavia. Cephalalgia 28:1237–1239. https://doi.org/10.1111/j.1468-2982.2008.01742.x

38. Westergaard ML, Hansen EH, Glumer C, Jensen RH (2015) Prescription pain medications and chronic headache in Denmark: implications for preventing medication overuse. Eur J Clin Pharmacol 71:851–860. https://doi.org/10.1007/s00228-015-1858-3

39. Steyerberg EW (2009) Clinical Prediction Models. Springer, New York

40. Frieman J, Hastie T, Tibshirani R (2010) Regularization Paths for Generalized Linear Models. J Stat Softw 33:1–22

41. Sing T, Sander O, Beerenwinkel N, Lengauer T (2005) ROCR: visualizing classifier performance in R. 21:Bioinformatics, 7881

42. Robin X, Turck N, Hainard A, Tiberti N, Lisacek F, Sanchez J-C, Müller M (2011) pROC: an open-source package for R and S+ to analyze and compare ROC curves. BMC Bioinformatics 12:77

43. Kuhn M (2008) Building Predictive Models in R Using the caret Package Journal of Statistical Software 28

44. Bigal ME, Lipton RB (2006) Modifiable risk factors for migraine progression. Headache 46:1334–1343. https://doi.org/10.1111/j.1526-4610.2006.00577.x

45. Katsarava Z et al (2004) Incidence and predictors for chronicity of headache in patients with episodic migraine. Neurology 62:788–790

46. Martelletti P (2018) The journey from genetic predisposition to medication overuse headache to its acquisition as sequela of chronic migraine. J Headache Pain 19:2. https://doi.org/10.1186/s10194-017-0830-2

47. Bigal ME, Sheftell FD, Rapoport AM, Tepper SJ, Weeks R, Baskin SM (2003) MMPI personality profiles in patients with primary chronic daily headache: a case-control study. Neurol Sci 24:103–110. https://doi.org/10.1007/s10072-003-0094-2

48. Luconi R, Bartolini M, Taffi R, Vignini A, Mazzanti L, Provinciali L, Silvestrini M (2007) Prognostic significance of personality profiles in patients with chronic migraine. Headache 47:1118–1124. https://doi.org/10.1111/j.1526-4610.2007.00807.x

49. Narin SO, Pinar L, Erbas D, Ozturk V, Idiman F (2003) The effects of exercise and exercise-related changes in blood nitric oxide level on migraine headache. Clin Rehabil 17:624–630. https://doi.org/10.1191/0269215503cr657oa

50. Katsarava Z, Jensen R (2007) Medication-overuse headache: where are we now? Curr Opin Neurol 20:326–330. https://doi.org/10.1097/WCO.0b013e328136c21c

51. Fritsche G, Frettloh J, Huppe M, Dlugaj M, Matatko N, Gaul C, Diener HC (2010) Prevention of medication overuse in patients with migraine. Pain 151:404–413. https://doi.org/10.1016/j.pain.2010.07.032

52. Gelman A, Carlin J (2014) Beyond Power Calculations: Assessing Type S (Sign) and Type M (Magnitude) Errors. Perspect Psychol Sci 9:641–651. https://doi.org/10.1177/1745691614551642

53. Pfeiffer RM, Redd A, Raymond CJ (2017) On the impact of model selection on predictor identification and parameter inference. Comput Stat 32:667–690

12

Dihydroergotamine inhibits the vasodepressor sensory CGRPergic outflow by prejunctional activation of α_2- adrenoceptors and 5-HT$_1$ receptors

Abimael González-Hernández[1,2], Jair Lozano-Cuenca[1], Bruno A. Marichal-Cancino[1,3], Antoinette MaassenVanDenBrink[4] and Carlos M. Villalón[1*] (iD)

Abstract

Background: Dihydroergotamine (DHE) is an antimigraine drug that produces cranial vasoconstriction and inhibits trigeminal CGRP release; furthermore, it inhibits the vasodepressor sensory CGRPergic outflow, but the receptors involved remain unknown. Prejunctional activation of $\alpha_{2A/2C}$-adrenergic, serotonin 5-HT$_{1B/1F}$, or dopamine D$_2$-like receptors results in inhibition of this CGRPergic outflow. Since DHE displays affinity for these receptors, this study investigated the pharmacological profile of DHE-induced inhibition of the vasodepressor sensory CGRPergic outflow.

Methods: Pithed rats were pretreated i.v. with hexamethonium (2 mg/kg·min) followed by continuous infusions of methoxamine (20 μg/kg·min) and DHE (3.1 μg/kg·min). Then, stimulus-response curves (spinal electrical stimulation; T$_9$-T$_{12}$) or dose-response curves (i.v. injections of α-CGRP) resulted in frequency-dependent or dose-dependent decreases in diastolic blood pressure.

Results: DHE inhibited the vasodepressor responses to electrical stimulation (0.56–5.6 Hz), without affecting those to i. v. α-CGRP (0.1–1 μg/kg). This inhibition by DHE (not produced by the methoxamine infusions): (i) was abolished by pretreatment with the combination of the antagonists rauwolscine (α_2-adrenoceptor; 310 μg/kg) plus GR127935 (5-HT$_{1B/1D}$; 31 μg/kg); and (ii) remained unaffected after rauwolscine (310 μg/kg), GR127935 (31 μg/kg) or haloperidol (D$_2$-like; 310 μg/kg) given alone, or after the combination of rauwolscine plus haloperidol or GR127935 plus haloperidol at the aforementioned doses.

Conclusion: DHE-induced inhibition of the vasodepressor sensory CGRPergic outflow is mainly mediated by prejunctional rauwolscine-sensitive α_2-adrenoceptors and GR127935-sensitive 5-HT$_{1B/1D}$ receptors, which correlate with $\alpha_{2A/2C}$-adrenoceptors and 5-HT$_{1B}$ receptors, respectively. These findings suggest that DHE-induced inhibition of the perivascular sensory CGRPergic outflow may facilitate DHE's vasoconstrictor properties resulting in an increased vascular resistance.

Keywords: CGRP, Dihydroergotamine, Pithed rat, Sensory neurons, Vasodepressor responses

* Correspondence: cvillalon@cinvestav.mx; http://farmacobiologia.cinvestav.
mx/Personal-Acad%C3%A9mico/Dr-Carlos-M-Villal%C3%B3n-Herrera
[1]Departamento de Farmacobiología, Cinvestav-Coapa, Tenorios 235, Col.
Granjas-Coapa, Deleg. Tlalpan, 14330 Ciudad de México, México
Full list of author information is available at the end of the article

Background

Dihydroergotamine (DHE) is a primary drug effective in the acute treatment of migraine [1–3] and its therapeutic effect may involve: (i) cranial vasoconstriction via vascular 5-HT$_{1B}$ and $\alpha_{2A/2C}$-adrenoceptors [4]; (ii) inhibition of neurogenic cranial vasodilatation produced by trigeminal release of calcitonin gene-related peptide (CGRP) [5, 6]; and probably (iii) inhibition of trigeminal nociceptive reflexes [7, 8]. More recently, DHE has been shown to increase diastolic blood pressure (an *index* of peripheral vascular resistance) by activation of vascular α_1 (α_{1A}, α_{1B} and α_{1D}) and α_2 (α_{2A}, α_{2B} and α_{2C})-adrenoceptors [9]. Interestingly, at peripheral level, CGRP released from primary sensory perivascular nerves induces vasodepressor responses [10–12], but this neuropeptide does not seem to be involved in the physiological regulation of blood pressure [13]. Notwithstanding, evidence is now growing suggesting that CGRP has a protective role in the generation of hypertension, which is most likely mediated via its effects at peripheral receptors [14]. Thus, the potential side-effects produced by DHE on the systemic CGRPergic transmission via its prejunctional interactions on perivascular sensory CGRPergic nerves deserve special attention [15]. Indeed, DHE is capable of inhibiting the vasodepressor responses induced by spinal stimulation of the perivascular sensory CGRPergic outflow in pithed rats [16]; however, the pharmacological profile of the receptors involved in this inhibitory action remains thus far unclear, probably because DHE displays complex pharmacological properties as it has affinity for an array of receptors [1–3, 17]. In this respect, by using selective agonists and antagonists, our group has previously shown that the rat vasodepressor sensory CGRPergic outflow (an *index* of sensory perivascular CGRP release in resistance blood vessels [12]) can be inhibited by prejunctional activation of receptors coupled to G$_{i/o}$ proteins, including: (i) α_2 (specifically $\alpha_{2A/2C}$)-adrenoceptors [18]; (ii) serotonin 5-HT$_{1B}$ [19] and 5-HT$_{1F}$ [20] receptors; and (iii) dopamine D$_2$-like receptors [21]. Since DHE displays affinity for these receptors (see Table 1), it is reasonable to hypothesize that

these receptors could be involved in DHE-induced inhibition of the vasodepressor sensory CGRPergic outflow. On this basis, the present study in pithed rats was designed to investigate: (a) whether DHE is capable of inhibiting the vasodepressor responses induced by either stimulation of the perivascular sensory CGRPergic outflow or i.v. bolus injections of exogenous α-CGRP; and (b) the pharmacological profile of the receptors involved in DHE-induced inhibition of the vasodepressor sensory CGRPergic outflow by analysing the effects of pre-treatment with the antagonists rauwolscine (α_2-adrenoceptors), GR127935 (5-HT$_{1B/1D}$) and haloperidol (D$_2$-like).

Methods

Animals

Male Wistar normotensive rats (300–350 g) were maintained at a 12/12-h light/dark cycle (with light beginning at 07:00 h) and housed in a special room at constant temperature (22 ± 2 °C) and humidity (50%), with food and water freely available in their home cages. All animal procedures, number of animals and the protocols of the present investigation were approved by our Institutional Ethics Committee on the use of animals in scientific experiments (CICUAL Cinvestav; protocol number 507–12), and followed the regulations established by the Mexican Official Norm (NOM-062-ZOO-1999), in accordance with ARRIVE (Animal Research: Reporting In Vivo Experiments) reporting guidelines for the care and use of laboratory animals.

General methods

Experiments were carried out in a total of 90 rats. After anaesthesia with ether and cannulation of the trachea, the rats were pithed by inserting a stainless-steel rod through the orbit and foramen magnum into the vertebral foramen [22]. Then, the animals were artificially ventilated with room air using a model 7025 Ugo Basile pump (56 strokes per min; stroke volume = 20 ml/kg), as established by Kleinman and Radford [23]. After bilateral vagotomy, catheters were placed in: (i) the left and right

Table 1 Binding affinity constants (pK$_i$) for the α_2-adrenergic, dopamine D$_2$-like or serotonin 5-HT$_1$ receptor families and their respective receptor subtypes for dihydroergotamine (DHE), rauwolscine, GR127935 and haloperidol for cloned human receptors (unless otherwise stated)

Receptors Ligands	pK$_i$ values										
	α_2-			D$_2$-like			5-HT$_1$				
	α_{2A}	α_{2B}	α_{2C}	D$_2$	D$_3$	D$_4$	1A[a]	1B	1D	1E	1F
DHE	8.7[a]	8.0[a]	9.0[a]	8.2[a]	8.2[a]	8.1[a]	9.3[a]	(r)7.8[a]	8.6[a]	6.2[a]	6.9[a]
Rauwolscine	8.9[b]	8.9[b]	9.3[b]	N.D.			N.D.	6.5[c]	7.8[c]	5.5[c]	N.D.
GR127935	< 6.0[d,*]			N.D.			7.2[e]	(r)8.8[f]	8.6[g]	5.4[g]	6.4[g]
Haloperidol	5.8[h,*]			9.4[i]	8.5[i]	8.8[i]	N.D.				

Data taken from: [a][33]; [b][34]; [c][35]; [d][36]; [e][37]; [f][38]; [g][39]; [h][40]; [i][41]. All data are given as pK$_i$ values at human recombinant receptors, except when stated otherwise: rodent (r) receptors; N.D., not determined; *These pK$_i$ values are referred for the respective family receptor

femoral and jugular veins, for the continuous infusions of agonists (methoxamine and DHE) and i.v. administration of the antagonists, respectively; and (ii) the left carotid artery, connected to a Grass pressure transducer (P23XL), for the recording of arterial blood pressure. Heart rate was measured with a tachograph (7P4, Grass Instrument Co., Quincy, MA, USA) triggered from the blood pressure signal. Both blood pressure and heart rate were recorded simultaneously by a model 7 Grass polygraph (Grass Instrument Co., Quincy, MA, USA). At this point, the 90 rats were divided into two main sets, so that the effects produced by the continuous infusions of methoxamine and DHE under different treatments could be evaluated on the vasodepressor responses induced by: (i) electrical stimulation of the vasodepressor sensory CGRPergic outflow (set 1; $n = 80$); and (ii) i.v. bolus injections of exogenous α-CGRP (set 2; $n = 10$). The vasodepressor stimulus-response curves and dose-response curves by electrical stimulation and exogenous α-CGRP, respectively, were elicited using a sequential schedule at 5–10 min intervals (see below) and were completed in about 50 min. Each response was elicited under unaltered values of resting blood pressure. The body temperature of each pithed rat was maintained at 37 °C by a lamp and monitored with a rectal thermometer.

Experimental protocols
After the animals ($n = 90$) had been in a stable haemodynamic condition for at least 15 min, baseline values of diastolic blood pressure (a more accurate indicator of peripheral vascular resistance, as previously established [12, 18–21]) and heart rate were determined.

Protocol 1. Electrical stimulation of the perivascular (vasodepressor) sensory outflow
In the first set of rats ($n = 80$), the pithing rod was replaced by an electrode enamelled except for 1.5 cm length 9 cm from the tip, so that the uncovered segment was situated at T_9-T_{12} of the spinal cord, and an indifferent electrode was placed dorsally [16, 18–22]. Before electrical stimulation, the animals received (i.v.): (i) a bolus injection of gallamine (25 mg/kg) to avoid electrically-induced muscular twitchings; (ii) ten min later, a continuous infusion of hexamethonium (2 mg/kg·min) to block the electrically-induced vasopressor responses that are produced by stimulation of the preganglionic sympathetic vasopressor outflow; and (iii) ten min later, a continuous infusion of methoxamine (20 µg/kg·min) to produce a sustained increase in diastolic blood pressure that allows us to produce the subsequent induction of vasodepressor responses, as previously described [16, 18–21]. Ten min later, this set of rats was divided into three groups.

The first group ($n = 10$) was subdivided into two subgroups ($n = 5$ each one) that received: (i) nothing (control experiment with no vehicles; see below); and (ii) an i.v. continuous infusion of DHE (3.1 µg/kg·min), a dose that has previously been shown to produce (amongst several doses) a maximal inhibition of the vasodepressor sensory CGRPergic outflow in pithed rats [16]. Twenty minutes later, diastolic blood pressure and heart rate were determined again, and then, the vasodepressor sensory CGRPergic outflow was electrically stimulated during the above treatments to elicit vasodepressor responses by applying 10-s trains of monophasic, rectangular pulses (2 msec, 50 V), at increasing frequencies of stimulation (0.56, 1, 1.8, 3.1 and 5.6 Hz). When diastolic blood pressure had returned to baseline levels, the next frequency was applied. This procedure was systematically performed until the stimulus-response curve had been completed.

The second group ($n = 35$) received an i.v. continuous infusion of 1% propylene glycol (PPG; vehicle for dissolving DHE) (0.02 ml/min). Ten min later, this group was subdivided into seven subgroups ($n = 5$ each) comprising i.v. bolus injections of, respectively: (i) saline (1 ml/kg); (ii) rauwolscine (310 µg/kg); (iii) GR127935 (31 µg/kg); (iv) haloperidol (310 µg/kg); (v) rauwolscine+GR127935 (310 and 31 µg/kg, respectively); (vi) rauwolscine+ haloperidol (310 µg/kg, each); and (vii) GR127935 + haloperidol (31 and 310 µg/kg, respectively). After 10 min, a stimulus-response curve was constructed as described above during the infusion of methoxamine to determine the effect of these antagonists per se.

The third group ($n = 35$) received an i.v. continuous infusion of DHE (3.1 µg/kg·min). Ten min later, this group was subdivided into seven subgroups ($n = 5$ each) comprising i.v. bolus injections of, respectively: (i) saline (1 ml/kg); (ii) rauwolscine (310 µg/kg); (iii) GR127935 (31 µg/kg); (iv) haloperidol (310 µg/kg); (v) rauwolscine +GR127935 (310 and 31 µg/kg, respectively); (vi) rauwolscine+haloperidol (310 µg/kg, each); and (vii) GR127935 + haloperidol (31 and 310 µg/kg, respectively). Ten minutes later, a stimulus-response curve was constructed as described above, during the infusion of DHE.

Protocol 2. Administration of exogenous α-CGRP
The second set of rats ($n = 10$) was prepared as describe above, but the pithing rod was left throughout the experiment and the administration of both gallamine and hexamethonium was omitted, as previously described [16, 18–21]. Then, this set received and i.v. continuous infusion of methoxamine (20 µg/kg·min); after 10 min, this set was divided into two groups ($n = 5$ each) that received, respectively: (i) nothing (control group); or (ii) an i.v. continuous infusion of DHE (3.1 µg/kg·min). Twenty min later, the values of diastolic blood pressure and

heart rate were determined again, and then, the vasodepressor responses elicited by i.v. bolus injections of exogenous α-CGRP (0.1, 0.18, 0.31, 0.56 and 1 µg/kg) were examined during the infusions of methoxamine and DHE.

Other procedures applying to protocols 1 and/or 2

The doses of hexamethonium, methoxamine and DHE were continuously infused at a rate of 0.02 ml/min by a WPI model sp100i pump (World Precision Instruments Inc., Sarasota, FL, USA). The dose of DHE was selected from a previous study [16]. The intervals between the different stimulation frequencies or doses of α-CGRP applied were dependent on the duration of the resulting vasodepressor responses (5–10 min), as we waited until diastolic blood pressure had returned to baseline values.

Drugs

Apart from the anaesthetic (diethyl ether), the compounds used in this study (obtained from the sources indicated) were: gallamine triethiodide, hexamethonium chloride, rat α-CGRP, methoxamine hydrochloride, rauwolscine hydrochloride, (Sigma Chemical Co., St Louis, MO, USA); N-[methoxy-3-(4-methyl-1-piperazinyl)phenyl]-2'-methyl-4'-(5-methyl-1,2,4-oxadiazol-3-yl)[1,1-biphenyl]-4-carboxamidehydrochloride (GR127935) (gift from GlaxoSmithKline, Stevenage, Hertfordshire, UK); and DHE tartrate (gift from Novartis Pharma A.G., Basel, Switzerland). All compounds were dissolved in saline, except: (i) DHE, which was dissolved in propylene glycol and gauged with saline to have a final solution of 1% PPG; and (ii) haloperidol, which was dissolved in some drops of 5% ascorbic acid and the resulting solution was finally diluted with saline. These vehicles had no effect on baseline diastolic blood pressure or heart rate (data not shown). Fresh solutions were prepared for each experiment. The doses of agonists refer to their respective salts, whereas those of the antagonists refer to their free base.

Data presentation and statistical evaluation

All data in the text, tables and figures, unless stated otherwise, are presented as mean ± standard error of the mean (S.E.M). The peak changes in diastolic blood pressure by electrical stimulation or exogenous α-CGRP were expressed as percent change from baseline, as previously reported [16, 18–21]. The difference in the absolute values of diastolic blood pressure and heart rate within one subgroup of animals before and during the continuous infusions of methoxamine (20 µg/kg·min) and DHE (3.1 µg/kg·min) were evaluated with paired Student's t-test. Moreover, a one-way analysis of variance was used to compare the absolute values of diastolic blood pressure and heart rate obtained during the continuous infusions of methoxamine

(20 µg/kg·min) and DHE (3.1 µg/kg·min) before, immediately after and 10 min after administration of saline or the antagonists used. Finally, the vasodepressor responses induced by electrical stimulation or exogenous α-CGRP in the different subgroups of animals were compared with a two-way analysis of variance. The one- and two-way analyses of variance were followed, if applicable, by the Student-Newman-Keuls' test. Statistical significance was accepted at $P < 0.05$. The statistical analysis was performed using the SigmaPlot software (V 12.0; Systat Software, Inc.), whereas the graphs were made with GraphPad Prism® software (V 6.01; GraphPad Software, Inc.).

Results

Systemic haemodynamic effects of the different treatments

The baseline values of diastolic blood pressure and heart rate in the 90 pithed rats were 57 ± 5 mmHg and 243 ± 8 beats per min, respectively; these variables remained unchanged after gallamine or hexamethonium. Twenty min after starting the i.v. continuous infusions of methoxamine, baseline values of diastolic blood pressure and heart rate were significantly ($P < 0.05$) increased in all animals (i.e. 140 ± 4 mmHg and 273 ± 4 beats per min, respectively). It is noteworthy that during the infusions of methoxamine and/or DHE a transient, but significant, decrease in diastolic blood pressure was produced immediately after administration of an i.v. bolus injections of rauwolscine, haloperidol or the combinations of these antagonists, but not with saline or GR127935 (see Table 2). However, the values of diastolic blood pressure in the different subgroups before and 10 min after administration of saline, or antagonists, were not significantly different ($P > 0.05$) (Table 2). Furthermore, the increase in diastolic blood pressure produced by the continuous infusion of methoxamine was sustained throughout the experiments, as illustrated in Fig. 1a.

Vasodepressor responses produced by electrical stimulation or exogenous α-CGRP

Figure 1a shows some representative experimental tracings illustrating that during the infusion of methoxamine the onset of the responses induced by electrical stimulation (0.56–5.6 Hz) of the vasodepressor sensory outflow (T_9-T_{12}) were immediate and resulted in frequency-dependent decreases in diastolic blood pressure. It must be emphasized that these vasodepressor responses were due to selective stimulation of the vasodepressor sensory CGRPergic outflow, since only negligible and inconsistent effects in heart rate were observed, as described earlier [16, 18–21]. In addition, as previously reported by Lozano-Cuenca et al. [16], stimulation of the vasodepressor sensory CGRPergic outflow also resulted in vasodepressor responses during the infusion of DHE (3.1 µg/kg·min), but the magnitude of these responses was

Table 2 Values of diastolic blood pressure and heart rate during the infusion of methoxamine (20 μg/kg·min): (i) before; (ii) immediately after (within 0–1 min after antagonist administration); and (iii) 10 min after i.v. administration of saline, rauwolscine, GR127935 and haloperidol given separately, as well as their respective combinations

Treatment	Dose (μg/kg)	n	Diastolic blood pressure (mm Hg)			Heart rate (beats per min)		
			Before	0–1 min after	10 min after	Before	0–1 min after	10 min after
Saline	1[a]	5	155 ± 9	158 ± 7	160 ± 13	260 ± 6	267 ± 3	259 ± 6
Rauwolscine (Rauw)	310	5	131 ± 5	105 ± 15*	134 ± 6	261 ± 6	257 ± 6	264 ± 5
GR127935 (GR)	31	5	137 ± 6	134 ± 7	140 ± 11	257 ± 4	251 ± 5	250 ± 5
Haloperidol (Halo)	310	5	124 ± 7	67 ± 4*	119 ± 7	234 ± 3	229 ± 3	230 ± 4
Rauw+GR	310, 31	5	168 ± 15	116 ± 13*	163 ± 11	264 ± 7	255 ± 8	271 ± 6
GR+ Halo	31, 310	5	149 ± 10	92 ± 15	119 ± 7	270 ± 10	259 ± 7	268 ± 9
Rauw+Halo	310, 310	5	123 ± 7	84 ± 6*	110 ± 3	298 ± 1	283 ± 3	300 ± 10

All values are expressed as mean ± S.E.M
[a]Saline was given at a dose of 1 ml/kg
*$P < 0.05$, significantly different from before. One-way analysis of variance

clearly smaller than those elicited during the infusion of methoxamine (20 μg/kg·min).

Moreover, during the methoxamine infusion (control; 20 μg/kg·min): (i) electrical stimulation of the perivascular sensory outflow resulted in frequency-dependent vasodepressor responses, which were inhibited during the infusion 3.1 μg/kg·min DHE (see Fig. 1b); and (ii) i.v. bolus injections of exogenous α-CGRP elicited dose-dependent vasodepressor responses, but these responses, unlike those by electrical stimulation, remained unchanged during the infusion of 3.1 μg/kg·min DHE Fig. 1c). In view that 3.1 μg/kg·min DHE inhibited the electrically-induced vasodepressor responses without affecting those by exogenous α-CGRP, we considered this infusion dose of DHE for further pharmacological analysis. In all cases, the vasodepressor responses to electrical stimulation or exogenous α-CGRP: (i) appeared about 10 s after starting each electrical stimulus or dose of α-CGRP, and reached a maximum 1 min after the stimulus had ended; and (ii) returned to baseline levels within 5–10 min after each stimulus/dose, as previously reported [18].

Effect per se of saline, rauwolscine, GR127935 or haloperidol (given separately or in combination) on the neurogenic vasodepressor responses during an infusion of methoxamine
During the methoxamine infusion (control; 20 μg/kg·min), the vasodepressor responses to electrical stimulation in control animals did not significantly differ from those elicited in animals pre-treated (see Additional file 1: Figure S1 [S1]) with an i.v. bolus injection of: (i) vehicle (1 ml/kg; Additional file 1: Figure S1a); (ii) rauwolscine (α2-drenoceptor antagonist, 310 μg/kg; Additional file 1: Figure S1b); (iii) GR127935 (5-HT_{1B/1D} receptor antagonist, 31 μg/kg; Additional file 1: Figure S1a); (iv) haloperidol (D2-like receptor antagonist, 310 μg/kg; Additional file 1: Figure S1d); (v) rauwolscine+GR127935 (310 and 31 μg/

kg respectively; Additional file 1: Figure S1e); (vi) rauwolscine+ haloperidol (310 μg/kg each; Additional file 1: Figure S1f); and (vii) GR127935+ haloperidol (31 and 310 μg/kg respectively; Additional file 1: Figure S1g). These results indicate that these compounds, at the doses used and under the present experimental conditions, were essentially devoid of any effect per se on the electrically-induced vasodepressor responses.

Effect of saline, rauwolscine, GR127935 or haloperidol (given separately or in combination) on DHE-induced inhibition of the neurogenic vasodepressor responses
Figure 2 shows that the inhibition induced by DHE (3.1 μg/kg·min) of the electrically-induced vasodepressor responses, which remained unaltered in animals pretreated with vehicle (1 ml/kg; Fig. 2a), was: (i) abolished in animals pretreated with rauwolscine+GR127935 (310 and 31 μg/kg respectively; Fig. 2e); and (ii) resistant to blockade in animals pretreated with rauwolscine (310 μg/kg; Fig. 2b); GR127935 (31 μg/kg; Fig. 2c); haloperidol (310 μg/kg; Fig. 2d); rauwolscine+haloperidol (310 and 310 μg/kg each; Fig. 2f); or GR127935+ haloperidol (31 and 310 μg/kg respectively; Fig. 2g).

Discussion
General
Apart from the implications discussed below, our study confirms that DHE can inhibit the vasodepressor sensory CGRPergic outflow in pithed rats by prejunctional mechanisms, as previously reported by Lozano-Cuenca et al. [16]. However, these authors made no attempt to identify the pharmacological profile of receptors involved in such inhibition by DHE. Hence, by using antagonists for α2-adrenoceptors (rauwolscine), 5-HT_{1B/1D} receptors (GR127935) and D2-like receptors (haloperidol) (since DHE displays affinity for these receptors; see Table 1), the present study suggests that α2-adrenoceptors and 5-HT_{1B/1D} receptors (but *not*

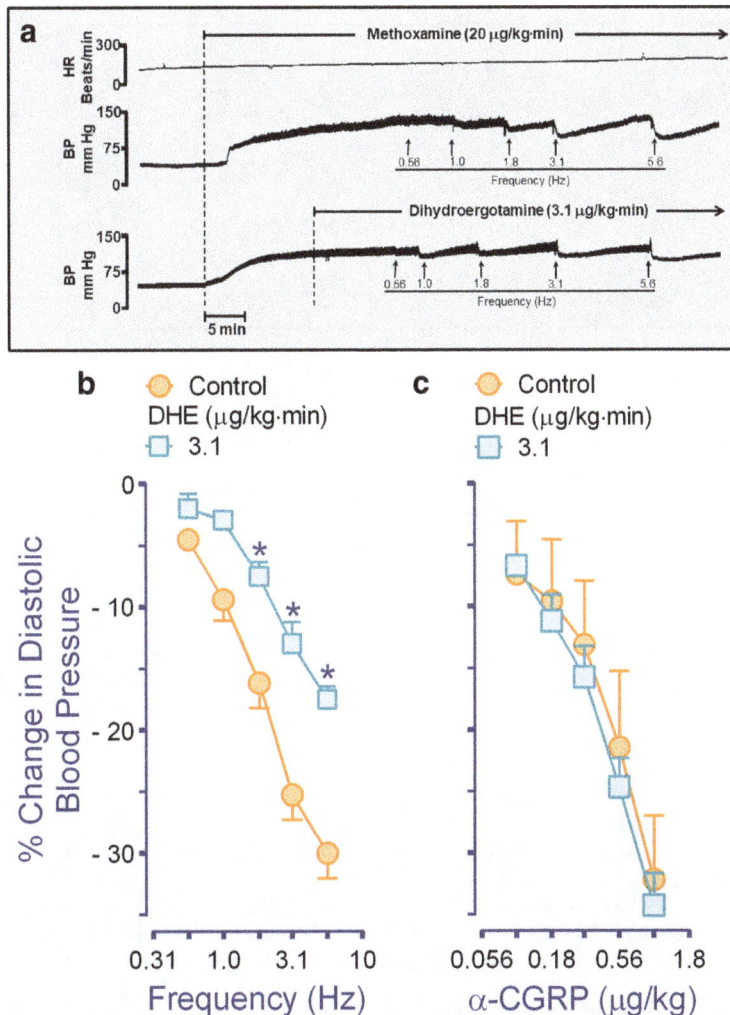

Fig. 1 Effect of dihydroergotamine (DHE) on the vasodepressor CGRPergic outflow in pithed rats. **a** Original experimental tracings illustrating the vasodepressor responses induced by electrical stimulation of the perivascular sensory CGRPergic outflow during continuous infusions of either methoxamine (control; above) or DHE (below). Note that during continuous infusions of DHE (3.1 µg/kg·min) the vasodepressor responses induced by electrical stimulation were attenuated versus control. In both cases, the vasodepressor responses were selective as no changes in heart rate were observed. Panels (**b**) and (**c**) show the vasodepressor responses by electrical stimulation or i.v. bolus injections of α-CGRP, respectively, induced during an i.v. continuous infusions of 3.1 µg/kg·min DHE ($n = 5$ each). For the sake of clarity, control responses (○) were induced during continuous infusions of methoxamine (20 µg/kg·min). * Significantly different responses ($P < 0.05$) vs. control. BP, blood pressure; HR, heart rate

D_2-like receptors) are involved in the prejunctional mechanisms by which DHE inhibits the vasodepressor sensory CGRPergic outflow in pithed rats.

Moreover, it is important to note that we did not measure sensory nerve activity directly, but the electrically-induced CGRP release in the systemic vasculature could be estimated indirectly by measurement of the evoked vasodepressor response, as previously established using the CGRP receptor antagonists $CGRP_{8-37}$ [12] and olcegepant [24]. Hence, the inhibition by DHE was considered sensory-inhibitory since this ergot inhibited the vasodepressor responses induced by spinal (T_9-T_{12}) stimulation of the vasodepressor sensory CGRPergic outflow (Fig. 1b), without affecting those by exogenous α-CGRP (Fig. 1c).

Systemic haemodynamic effects produced by methoxamine and DHE

As previously established in pithed rats [16, 18–21], the artificial and sustained increase in diastolic blood pressure (at around 140 mmHg) by a continuous infusion of the α_1-adrenoceptor agonist methoxamine (20 µg/kg·min; Fig. 1a) is a *conditio sine qua non* for inducing vasodepressor responses. Otherwise, the basal blood pressure in pithed rats is so low that there is no "window" for eliciting further decreases in this variable. The methoxamine-induced increase in diastolic blood pressure has been attributed to an increase in peripheral vascular resistance [25]. In addition, it is noteworthy that 3.1 µg/kg·min DHE can slightly increase diastolic blood pressure when the methoxamine

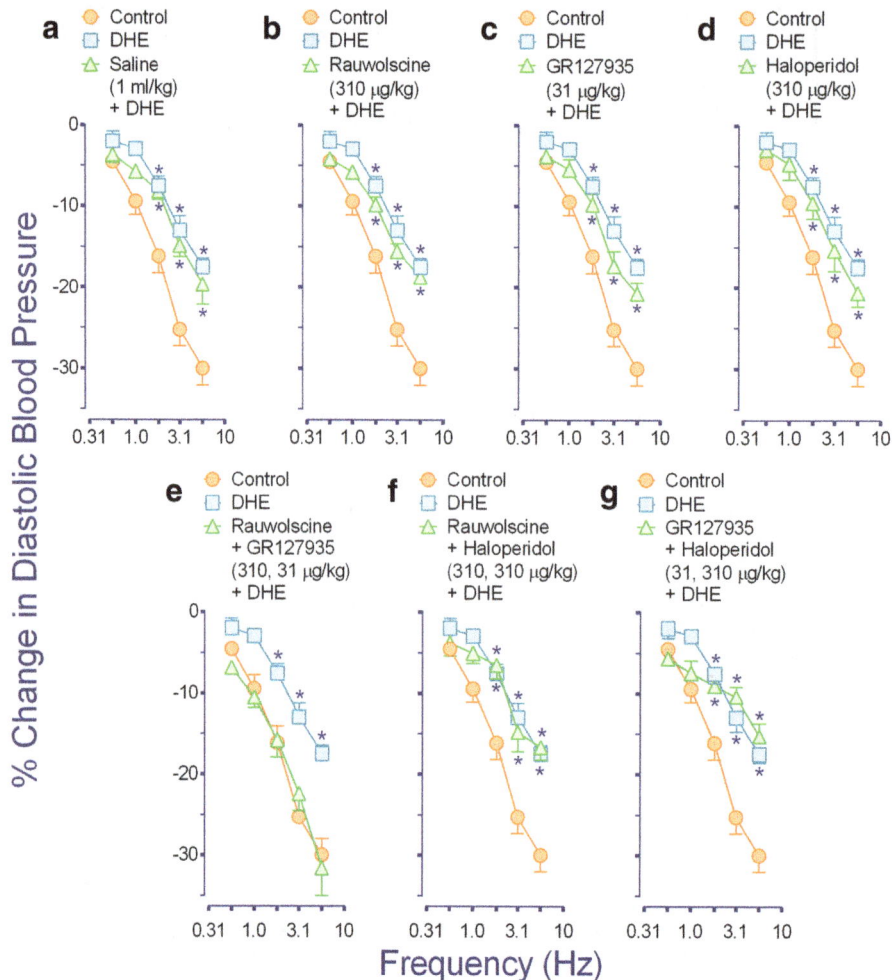

Fig. 2 Effect of i.v. bolus injections of: (**a**) saline (1 ml/kg); (**b**) rauwolscine (310 μg/kg); (**c**) GR127935 (31 μg/kg); or (**d**) haloperidol (310 μg/kg) given separately, as well as the combinations (**e**) rauwolscine plus GR127935 (310 and 31 μg/kg, respectively); (**f**) rauwolscine plus haloperidol (310 μg/kg each); or (**g**) GR127935 plus haloperidol (31 and 310 μg/kg, respectively) on the inhibition induced by dihydroergotamine (DHE; 3.1 μg/kg·min; □) of the electrically-induced vasodepressor responses. The control responses (o) represent that of animals receiving an i.v. continuous infusion of methoxamine (20 μg/kg·min) which is shown for comparison. * Significantly different responses ($P < 0.05$) vs. control

infusion is not given (i.e. when basal diastolic blood pressure is too low; data not shown). Accordingly, the methoxamine-induced increase in blood pressure, which is maximal [16, 18], could most probably have masked the slight effect of DHE on this variable. In fact, the pressor effect of DHE has been extensively described in humans [26, 27], and its pressor effect in pithed rats has recently been associated with vascular activation of α_1 (α_{1A}, α_{1B} and α_{1D}) and α_2 (α_{2A}, α_{2B} and α_{2C})-adrenoceptors [9].

Effects of several antagonists per se on systemic haemodynamic variables and on the sensory-induced vasodepressor responses

To identify the mechanisms involved in the prejunctional inhibition by DHE (Fig. 1b and c), we decided to evaluate the effect of several antagonists per se (Table 1) on systemic haemodynamic conditions and on the vasodepressor responses induced by electrical stimulation. A transient, but significant, decrease in diastolic blood pressure was observed when animals received a bolus injection of rauwolscine and/or haloperidol (Table 2). In the case of haloperidol, this effect could be explained by considering that this compound exhibits high affinity for α_1-adrenoceptors (pK_i: 8.0; see Table 1). Thus, it is tempting to suggest that haloperidol may have an antagonistic effect on methoxamine (α_1-adrenoceptor agonist)-induced increase in blood pressure. In contrast, we have no clear-cut explanation for the decreases in diastolic blood pressure induced by rauwolscine, which does not display affinity for α_1-adrenoceptors. Nevertheless, in all cases, 10 min after administration of antagonists the values of diastolic blood pressure had returned to baseline values (Table 2; before and 10 min after). These results, coupled to the lack of effect of the above antagonists (alone or in combination) on the electrically-induced vasodepressor responses (see Additional file 1: Figure S1) indicates that these compounds, at the doses used, were devoid of any effects per se on the above variables. Accordingly, these data suggest that any effect of a given antagonist on DHE-induced sensory inhibition is due to a direct interaction of the antagonist with its respective receptors. It must be emphasized that: (i) our suggestion supporting and/or excluding the role of α_2-adrenergic, 5-HT$_{1B/1D}$ or D$_2$-like receptors is based on the assumption that species differences between the binding of agonists and antagonists used do not play a major role (Table 1); and (ii) the doses of antagonists used were high enough to completely block prejunctional α_2-adrenoceptors (rauwolscine; [18]), 5-HT$_{1B/1D}$ receptors (GR127935; [19, 20, 28, 29]) and D$_2$-like receptors (haloperidol; [21]) mediating inhibition of neurogenic cardiovascular responses in pithed rats.

Role of α_2-adrenergic and 5-HT$_{1B/1D}$, but not D$_2$-like, receptors in the inhibition by DHE

As previously pointed out, DHE displays affinity for α_2-adrenergic, 5-HT$_1$ and D$_2$-like receptors (see Table 1). Activation of these receptors, which are coupled to G$_{i/o}$ proteins, may inhibit adenylyl cyclase activity, inactivate Ca^{2+} channels and/or activate inwardly rectifying K$^+$ channels [30, 31]. These are signal transduction systems usually associated with inhibition of neurotransmitter release [30, 31]. With this idea in mind and considering our results (Fig. 2), the simplest interpretation of these findings suggests that DHE-induced inhibition mainly involves the activation of prejunctional α_2-adrenergic and 5-HT$_{1B/1D}$ receptors, but not of D$_2$-like receptors since the DHE response was: (i) only abolished by rauwolscine plus GR127935 (Fig. 2e); and (ii) resistant to blockade by rauwolscine (Fig. 2b), GR127935 (Fig. 2c), haloperidol (Fig. 2d), rauwolscine plus haloperidol (Fig. 2f) or GR127935 plus haloperidol (Fig. 2g). However, the lack of blockade by some of the above treatments deserves further considerations. For example, the fact that rauwolscine or GR127935 alone failed to block DHE-induced inhibition may reflect the fact that a maximal dose of DHE was used [16]; accordingly, DHE could be stimulating α_2-adrenoceptors and 5-HT$_{1B/1D}$ receptors simultaneously; thus, when blocking only one of these receptors, the inhibition produced by the unblocked receptor will overshadow the antagonism produced on the other receptor. In addition, the involvement of D$_2$-like receptors seems unlikely based on the lack of effect of haloperidol, an antagonist with high affinity (pK_i) for the D$_2$-like receptors subtypes (D$_2$: 9.4; D$_3$: 8.5 and D$_4$: 8.8; see Table 1). This suggestion gains weight when considering that DHE-induced inhibition remained unaffected after rauwolscine plus haloperidol (Fig. 2f) or GR127935 plus haloperidol (Fig. 2g).

Having established the main involvement of rauwolscine-sensitive α_2-adrenoceptors and GR127935-sensitive 5-HT$_{1B/1D}$ receptors in DHE-induced inhibition, we have to recognize that no attempt was made here to further identify the specific subtypes of these main receptor families. The reason for this omission is based on the fact that we have previously shown (using selective agonists and antagonists) that these receptors correlate with the pharmacological profile of, respectively: (i) $\alpha_{2A/2C}$ (but not α_{2B})-adrenoceptor subtypes [18]; and (ii) 5-HT$_{1B}$ and 5-HT$_{1F}$ (but not 5-HT$_{1A}$ or 5-HT$_{1D}$) receptor subtypes [19, 20]. However, the fact that DHE-induced inhibition was abolished by the combination rauwolscine (310 μg/kg) + GR127935 (31 μg/kg), where the latter dose is not enough to block the prejunctional 5-HT$_{1F}$ receptors that inhibit the rat vasodepressor sensory CGRPergic outflow [20], makes the role of these subtypes rather unlikely. Finally, it is noteworthy that DHE also displays moderate affinity for other receptors, including the 5-ht$_{1E}$ (pK_i: 6.2) subtype (Table 1). However, the 5-ht$_{1E}$ retains its lower-case appellation as it is not a functional receptor [32].

Conclusion

The above results suggest that DHE-induced inhibition of the vasodepressor sensory CGRPergic outflow is mainly mediated by prejunctional activation of rauwolscine-sensitive α_2-adrenoceptors and GR127935-sensitive 5-HT$_{1B/1D}$ receptors which, most likely, correlate with $\alpha_{2A/2C}$-adrenoceptors [18] and 5-HT$_{1B}$ receptors [19], respectively. These findings may shed further light on the vascular side effects produced by DHE, namely: DHE-induced inhibition of the perivascular sensory CGRPergic outflow may facilitate DHE's vasoconstrictor properties resulting in an increased vascular resistance.

Additional file

Additional file 1: Figure S1. Effect per se of i.v. bolus injections of: (a) saline (1 ml/kg); (b) rauwolscine (310 μg/kg); (c) GR127935 (31 μg/kg); or (d) haloperidol (310 μg/kg) given separately; as well as the combinations (e) rauwolscine plus GR127935 (310 and 31 μg/kg, respectively); (f) rauwolscine plus haloperidol (310 μg/kg each); or (g) GR127935 plus haloperidol (31 and 310 μg/kg, respectively) on the electrically-induced vasodepressor responses produced during an i.v. continuous infusion of methoxamine (20 μg/kg. min) (n = 5 for each group). No significant effects were produced after administration of compounds (P > 0.05). (PDF 881 kb)

Abbreviations

ARRIVE: Animal Research: Reporting In Vivo Experiments; DHE: Dihydroergotamine; i.p.: Intraperitoneal; i.v.: Intravenous; PPG: Propylene glycol; α-CGRP: α-Calcitonin gene-related peptide

Acknowledgements

The authors would like to thank Mr. Arturo Contreras, Mr. Mauricio Villasana and Engr. José Rodolfo Fernández Calderón for their assistance. We are also indebted to the pharmaceutical companies for their generous gifts (see Drugs Section).

Funding

This work was sponsored by Consejo Nacional de Ciencia y Tecnología (CONACyT, Mexico City, Grant No. 219707 for CMV) and the Netherlands Organization for Scientific Research (NWO; VIDI 917.11.349 for AMVDB).

Authors' contributions

AGH – Performed the experiments, analysed the data and drafted the manuscript. JLC – Technical assistance during the experiments, analysed the data and drafted the manuscript. BAMC – Revised and approved the final manuscript. AMVDB – Revised and approved the final manuscript. CMV – Supervised the experiments and data analysis, drafted and revised the final manuscript. All authors read and approved the final manuscript.

Competing interests

The authors declare that they have no competing interests.

Author details

[1]Departamento de Farmacobiología, Cinvestav-Coapa, Tenorios 235, Col. Granjas-Coapa, Deleg. Tlalpan, 14330 Ciudad de México, México. [2]Departamento de Neurobiología del Desarrollo y Neurofisiología, Instituto de Neurobiología, Universidad Nacional Autónoma de México, Campus UNAM, Juriquilla, México. [3]Departamento de Fisiología y Farmacología, Centro de Ciencias Básicas, Universidad Autónoma de Aguascalientes, Ciudad Universitaria, 20131 Aguascalientes, Ags, México. [4]Division of Vascular Medicine and Pharmacology, Erasmus University Medical Center, P.O. Box 2040, 3000, CA, Rotterdam, The Netherlands.

References

1. Dahlöf C, MaassenVanDenBrink A (2012) Dihydroergotamine, ergotamine, methysergide and sumatriptan–basic science in relation to migraine treatment. Headache 52:707–714
2. Saper JR, Silberstein S (2006) Pharmacology of dihydroergotamine and evidence for efficacy and safety in migraine. Headache 46:S171–S181
3. Silberstein SD, McCrory DC (2003) Ergotamine and dihydroergotamine: history, pharmacology and efficacy. Headache 43:144–166
4. Villalón CM, Centurión D, Willems EW, Arulmani U, Saxena PR, Valdivia LF (2004) 5-HT$_{1B}$ receptors and alpha$_{2A/2C}$-adrenoceptors mediate external carotid vasoconstriction to dihydroergotamine. Eur J Pharmacol 484: 287–290
5. Buzzi MG, Carter WB, Shimizu T, Heath H III, Moskowitz MA (1991) Dihydroergotamine and sumatriptan attenuate levels of CGRP in plasma in rat superior sagital sinus during electrical stimulation of the trigeminal ganglion. Neuropharmacology 30:1193–1200
6. Goadsby PJ, Edvinsson L (1993) The trigeminovascular system and migraine: studies characterizing cerebrovascular and neuropeptide changes seen in humans and cats. Ann Neurol 33:48–56
7. Marichal-Cancino BA, González-Hernández A, Manrique-Maldonado G, Ruiz-Salinas II, Altamirano-Espinoza AH, MaassenVanDenBrink A, Villalon CM (2012) Intrathecal dihydroergotamine inhibits capsaicin-induced vasodilatation in the canine external carotid circulation via GR127935-and rauwolscine-sensitive receptors. Eur J Pharmacol 692:69–77
8. Price TJ, Hargreaves KM, Cervero F (2006) Protein expression and mRNA cellular distribution of the NKCC1 cotransporter in the dorsal root and trigeminal ganglia of the rat. Brain Res 1112:146–158
9. Rivera-Mancilla E, Avilés-Rosas VH, Manrique-Maldonado G, Altamirano-Espinoza AH, Villanueva-Castillo B, MaassenVanDenBrink A, Villalón CM (2017) The role of α$_1$- and α$_2$-adrenoceptor subtypes in the vasopressor responses induced by dihydroergotamine in ritanserin-pretreated pithed rats. J Headache Pain 18:104
10. Deng PY, Li YJ (2005) Calcitonin gene-related peptide and hypertension. Peptides 26:1676–1685
11. González-Hernández A, Marichal-Cancino BA, Lozano-Cuenca J, López-Canales JS, Muñoz-Islas E, Ramírez-Rosas MB, Villalón CM (2016) Heteroreceptors modulating CGRP release at neurovascular junction: potential therapeutic implications on some vascular related diseases. Biomed Res Int 2016:2056786
12. Taguchi T, Kawasaki H, Imamura T, Takasaki K (1992) Endogenous calcitonin gene-related peptide mediates nonadrenergic noncholinergic depressor response to spinal cord stimulation in the pithed rats. Circ Res 71:357–364
13. Smillie SJ, Brain SD (2011) Calcitonin gene-related peptide (CGRP) and its role in hypertension. Neuropeptides 45:93–104
14. Smillie SJ, King R, Kodji X, Outzen E, Pozsgai G, Fernandes E, Marshall N, De Winter P, Heads RJ, Dessapt-Baradez C, Gnudi L (2014) An ongoing role of α-calcitonin gene-related peptide as part of a protective network against hypertension, vascular hypertrophy, and oxidative stress. Hypertension 63:1056–1062
15. González-Hernández A, Marichal-Cancino BA, MaassenVanDenBrink A, Villalón CM (2018) Side effects associated with current and prospective antimigraine pharmacotherapies. Exp Opin Drug Metab Toxicol 14:25–41
16. Lozano-Cuenca J, González-Hernández A, Muñoz-Islas E, Sánchez-López A, Centurión D, Cobos-Puc LE, Villalón CM (2009) Effect of some acute and prophylactic antimigraine drugs on the vasodepressor sensory CGRPergic outflow in pithed rats. Life Sci 84:125–131
17. Sanders-Bush E, Mayer SE (2006) 5-hydroxytryptamine (serotonin): receptor agonists and antagonists. In: Brunton LL, Lazo JS, Parker KL (eds) Goodman & Gilman's the pharmacological basis of therapeutics, 11th edn. Mc Graw Hill, New York, pp 297–316
18. Villalón CM, Albarrán-Juárez JA, Lozano-Cuenca J, Pertz HH, Görnemann T, Centurión D (2008) Pharmacological profile of the clonidine-induced inhibition of vasodepressor sensory outflow in pithed rats: correlation with α2A/2C-adrenoceptors. Br J Pharmacol 154:51–59
19. González-Hernández A, Muñoz-Islas E, Lozano-Cuenca J, Ramírez-Rosas MB, Sánchez-López A, Centurión D, Ramírez-San Juan E, Villalón CM (2010) Activation of 5-HT1B receptors inhibits the vasodepressor sensory CGRPergic outflow in pithed rats. Eur J Pharmacol 637:131–137
20. González-Hernández A, Manrique-Maldonado G, Lozano-Cuenca J, Muñoz-Islas E, Centurión D, MaassenVanDenBrink A, Villalón CM (2011) The 5-HT$_1$ receptors inhibiting the rat vasodepressor sensory CGRPergic outflow: further involvement of 5-HT$_{1F}$, but not 5-HT$_{1A}$ or 5-HT$_{1D}$, subtypes. Eur J Pharmacol 659:233–243
21. Manrique-Maldonado G, González-Hernández A, Altamirano-Espinoza AH, Marichal-Cancino BA, Ruiz-Salinas I, Villalón CM (2014) The role of prejunctional D$_2$-like receptors mediating quinpirole-induced inhibition of the vasodepressor sensory CGRPergic out-flow in pithed rats. Basic Clin Pharmacol Toxicol 114:174–180
22. Gillespie JS, MacLaren A, Pollock D (1970) A method of stimulating different segments of the autonomic outflow from the spinal column to various organs in the pithed cat and rat. Br J Pharmacol 40:257–267
23. Kleinman L, Radford E (1964) Ventilation standards for small mammals. J Appl Physiol 19:360–362
24. Avilés-Rosas VH, Rivera-Mancilla E, Marichal-Cancino BA, Manrique-Maldonado G, Altamirano-Espinoza AH, MaassenVanDenBrink A, Villalón CM (2017) Olcegepant blocks neurogenic and non-neurogenic CGRPergic vasodepressor responses and facilitates noradrenergic vasopressor responses in pithed rats. Br J Pharmacol 174:2001–2014
25. Decker N, Ehrhardt JD, Leclerc G, Schwartz J (1984) Postjunctional α-adrenoceptors: α$_1$ and α$_2$ subtypes in rat vasculature in vitro and in vivo. Naunyn Schmiedeberg's Arch Pharmacol 326:1–6
26. Saxena PR, Den Boer MO (1991) Pharmacology of antimigraine drugs. J Neurol 238:S28–S35
27. Tfelt-Hansen PC, Koehler PJ (2008) History of the use of ergotamine and dihydroergotamine in migraine from 1906 and orward. Cephalalgia 28: 877–886
28. Cobos-Puc LE, Villalón CM, Sánchez-López A, Ramírez-Rosas MB, Lozano-Cuenca J, Pertz HH, Gömermann T, Centurión D (2009) Pharmacological characterization of ergotamine-induced inhibition of the cardioaccelerator sympathetic outflow in pithed rats. Naunyn Schmiedeberg's Arch Pharmacol 379:137–148
29. Sánchez-López A, Centurión D, Vázquez E, Arulmani U, Saxena PR, Villalón CM (2004) Further characterization of the 5-HT$_1$ receptors mediating cardiac sympatho-inhibition in pithed rats: pharmacological correlation with the 5-HT$_{1B}$ and 5-HT$_{1D}$ subtypes. Naunyn Schmiedeberg's Arch Pharmacol 369: 220–227

30. Boehm S, Kubista H (2002) Fine tuning of sympathetic transmitter release via ionotropic and metabotropic presynaptic receptors. Pharmacol Rev 54: 43–99

31. De Jong AP, Verhage M (2009) Presynaptic signal transduction pathways that modulate synaptic transmission. Curr Opin Neurobiol 19:245–253

32. Alexander SPH, Christopoulos A, Davenport AP, Kelly E, Marrion NV, Peters JA, Faccenda E, Harding SD, Pawson AJ, Sharman JL, Southan C, Davies JA (2017) CGTP collaborators - the concise guide to PHARMACOLOGY 2017/18: G protein-coupled receptors. Br J Pharmacol 174(S1):S17–S129

33. Leysen JE, Gommeren W, Heylen L, Luyten WH, Van de Weyer I, Vanhoenacker P, Schotte A, Van Gompel P, Wouters R, Lesage AS (1996) Alniditan, a new 5-hydroxytryptamine$_{1D}$ agonist and migraine-abortive agent: ligand-binding properties of human 5-hydroxytryptamine$_{1D}$ alpha, human 5-hydroxytryptamine$_{1D}$ beta, and calf 5-hydroxytryptamine$_{1D}$ receptors investigated with [^{3}H]5-hydroxytryptamine and [^{3}H]alniditan. Mol Pharmacol 50:1567–1580

34. Jasper JR, Lesnick JD, Chang LK, Yamanishi SS, Chang TK, Hsu SA, Daunt DA, Bonhaus DW, Eglen RM (1998) Ligand efficacy and potency at recombinant alpha$_2$ adrenergic receptors: agonist-mediated [^{35}S]GTPgammaS binding. Biochem Pharmacol 55:1035–1043

35. Uhlén S, Porter AC, Neubig RR (1994) The novel alpha-$_2$ adrenergic radioligand [^{3}H]-MK912 is α_{2C} selective among human α_{2A}, α_{2B} and α_{2C} adrenoceptors. J Pharmacol Exp Ther 271:1558–1565

36. Pauwels PJ (1996) Pharmacological properties of a putative 5-HT$_{1B/1D}$ receptor antagonist GR127935. CNS Drug Rev 2:415–428

37. Adham N, Kao HT, Schechter LE, Bard J, Olsen M, Urquhart D, Durkin M, Hartig PR, Weinshank RL, Branchek TA (1993) Cloning of another human serotonin receptor (5-HT$_{1F}$): a fifth 5-HT$_1$ receptor subtype coupled to the inhibition of adenylate cyclase. Proc Natl Acad Sci U S A 90:408–412

38. Beer MS, Heald MA, McAllister G, Stanton JA (1998) Pharmacological characterisation of a cloned dog 5-HT$_{1B}$ receptor cell line. Eur J Pharmacol 360:117–121

39. Price GW, Burton MJ, Collin LJ, Duckworth M, Gaster L, Göthert M, Jones BJ, Roberts C, Watson JM, Middlemiss DN (1997) SB-216641 and BRL-15572-compounds to pharmacologically discriminate h5-HT$_{1B}$ and h5-HT$_{1D}$ receptors. Naunyn Schmiedeberg's Arch Pharmacol 356:312–320

40. Arnt J, Skarsfeldt T (1998) Do novel antipsychotics have similar pharmacological characteristics? A review of the evidence. Neurophsychopharmacol 18:63–101

41. Millan MJ, Brocco M, Rivet JM, Audinot V, Newman-Tancredi A, Maiofiss L, Queriaux S, Despaux N, Peglion JL, Dekeyne A (2000) S18327 (1-[2-[4-(6-fluoro-1, 2-benzisoxazol-3-yl)piperid-1-yl]ethyl]3-phenyl imidazolin-2-one), a novel, potential antipsychotic displaying marked antagonist properties at α_1- and α_2-adrenergic receptors: II. Functional profile and a multiparametric comparison with haloperidol, clozapine, and 11 other antipsychotic agents. J Pharmacol Exp Ther 292:54–66

13

Patterns of medicinal cannabis use, strain analysis, and substitution effect among patients with migraine, headache, arthritis, and chronic pain in a medicinal cannabis cohort

Eric P. Baron[1]*, Philippe Lucas[2,3,4], Joshua Eades[2] and Olivia Hogue[5]

Abstract

Background: Medicinal cannabis registries typically report pain as the most common reason for use. It would be clinically useful to identify patterns of cannabis treatment in migraine and headache, as compared to arthritis and chronic pain, and to analyze preferred cannabis strains, biochemical profiles, and prescription medication substitutions with cannabis.

Methods: Via electronic survey in medicinal cannabis patients with headache, arthritis, and chronic pain, demographics and patterns of cannabis use including methods, frequency, quantity, preferred strains, cannabinoid and terpene profiles, and prescription substitutions were recorded. Cannabis use for migraine among headache patients was assessed via the ID Migraine™ questionnaire, a validated screen used to predict the probability of migraine.

Results: Of 2032 patients, 21 illnesses were treated with cannabis. Pain syndromes accounted for 42.4% ($n = 861$) overall; chronic pain 29.4% ($n = 598$;), arthritis 9.3% ($n = 188$), and headache 3.7% ($n = 75$;). Across all 21 illnesses, headache was a symptom treated with cannabis in 24.9% ($n = 505$). These patients were given the ID Migraine™ questionnaire, with 68% ($n = 343$) giving 3 "Yes" responses, 20% ($n = 102$) giving 2 "Yes" responses (97% and 93% probability of migraine, respectively). Therefore, 88% ($n = 445$) of headache patients were treating probable migraine with cannabis. Hybrid strains were most preferred across all pain subtypes, with "OG Shark" the most preferred strain in the ID Migraine™ and headache groups. Many pain patients substituted prescription medications with cannabis (41.2–59.5%), most commonly opiates/opioids (40.5–72.8%). Prescription substitution in headache patients included opiates/opioids (43.4%), anti-depressant/anti-anxiety (39%), NSAIDs (21%), triptans (8.1%), anti-convulsants (7.7%), muscle relaxers (7%), ergots (0.4%).

(Continued on next page)

* Correspondence: barone2@ccf.org
[1]Center for Neurological Restoration - Headache and Chronic Pain Medicine, Department of Neurology, Cleveland Clinic Neurological Institute, 10524 Euclid Avenue, C21, Cleveland, OH 44195, USA
Full list of author information is available at the end of the article

(Continued from previous page)

Conclusions: Chronic pain was the most common reason for cannabis use, consistent with most registries. The majority of headache patients treating with cannabis were positive for migraine. Hybrid strains were preferred in ID Migraine™, headache, and most pain groups, with "OG Shark", a high THC (Δ9-tetrahydrocannabinol)/THCA (tetrahydrocannabinolic acid), low CBD (cannabidiol)/CBDA (cannabidiolic acid), strain with predominant terpenes β-caryophyllene and β-myrcene, most preferred in the headache and ID Migraine™ groups. This could reflect the potent analgesic, anti-inflammatory, and anti-emetic properties of THC, with anti-inflammatory and analgesic properties of β-caryophyllene and β-myrcene. Opiates/opioids were most commonly substituted with cannabis. Prospective studies are needed, but results may provide early insight into optimizing crossbred cannabis strains, synergistic biochemical profiles, dosing, and patterns of use in the treatment of headache, migraine, and chronic pain syndromes.

Keywords: Cannabis, Cannabinoids, Marijuana, CBD, Cannabidiol, THC, $Δ^9$-tetrahydrocannabinol, Migraine, Headache, Terpenes, Arthritis, Pain

Background

The legal use of medicinal cannabis continues to increase globally, including the United States. At the time of this writing, there are currently 29 states which have legalized medicinal cannabis, 9 states and Washington DC which have legalized both medicinal and recreational cannabis use, and 18 states which have legalized cannabidiol (CBD)-only bills.

The use of medicinal cannabis for a multitude of health maladies, particularly chronic pain, has been well described through ancient, historical, and current times, and well supported through the medical literature [1–28]. In 2017, The National Academies of Sciences, Engineering, and Medicine published a statement that the use of cannabis for the treatment of pain is supported by well-controlled clinical trials and that there is substantial evidence that cannabis is an effective treatment for chronic pain in adults [24]. In 2014, the Canadian Pain Society revised their consensus statement to recommend cannabinoids as a third-level therapy for chronic neuropathic pain given the evidence of cannabinoid efficacy in the treatment of pain with a combined number needed to treat (NNT) of 3.4 [25]. Most medicinal cannabis registries report that chronic pain is the most common indication for use [29–39]. However, most of these registries do not further differentiate chronic pain into different pain subsets.

Supporting evidence also exists for cannabis/cannabinoids in the treatment of migraine and/or chronic migraine [1, 40–56], cluster headache [56–59], chronic headaches [13, 44, 60, 61], medication overuse headache [62], idiopathic intracranial hypertension [63], and multiple sclerosis associated trigeminal neuralgia [64]. Publications detailing this headache, migraine, and facial pain literature, as well as described mechanisms of pain relief with cannabis and cannabinoids are available and should be reviewed, but are beyond the scope of this paper [1, 2, 28, 51, 65]. At the time of this writing, the limited supporting headache literature

consists of one retrospective analysis, numerous case series, case studies, and case reports, clinical/anecdotal reports, and surveys. There are no placebo-controlled studies of cannabis for headache disorders, although a multicenter, double-blind, placebo-controlled study evaluating efficacy and safety of a synthetic $Δ^9$-tetrahydrocannabinol (THC), Dronabinol, in a metered dose inhaler for the treatment of migraine with and without aura has been completed, but results not available [66]. There are only two prospective trials containing a control group evaluating the use of cannabinoids in the treatment of headache disorders, specifically chronic migraine, cluster headache, and medication overuse headache [56, 62].

The first of these two prospective trials was a randomized, double-blind, active-controlled crossover trial with treatment refractory medication overuse headache (MOH) with daily analgesic intake for at least 5 years and several failed detoxification attempts. Patients completed a course of either Ibuprofen 400 mg or Nabilone 0.5 mg daily for 8 weeks, had a 1 week washout, then a second 8 weeks of the other medication. Results showed that Nabilone 0.5 mg daily, a synthetic cannabinoid, was superior in reducing daily analgesic intake, pain intensity, level of medication dependence, and improved quality of life in these patients [62].

The second prospective trial evaluated the use of cannabinoids as both a prophylaxis and acute treatment for both chronic migraine and chronic cluster headache [56]. Patients were given one of two compounds containing 19% THC or a combination of 0.4% THC + 9% CBD. In phase 1, dose finding observations to determine effective dosing was performed with a group of 48 chronic migraineurs. It was found that doses less than 100 mg produced no benefit, while an oral dose of 200 mg administered during a migraine attack decreased acute pain intensity by 55%, which was the dose used in phase 2. In phase 2, chronic migraine patients were assigned to 3 months prophylaxis treatment with either

25 mg per day of Amitriptyline or THC + CBD 200 mg per day. Chronic cluster headache patients were assigned to 1 month prophylaxis treatment with either Verapamil 480 mg per day or THC + CBD 200 mg per day. For acute pain attacks, additional dosing of THC + CBD 200 mg was allowed in both groups. In the migraine patients, the THC + CBD 200 mg prophylaxis provided a 40.4% improvement versus 40.1% with Amitriptyline. In the cluster headache patients, the THC + CBD 200 mg prophylaxis gave minimal to no benefit. Additional acute THC + CBD 200 mg dosing decreased pain intensity in migraine patients by 43.5%. This same result was seen in cluster headache patients, but only if they had a history of migraine in childhood. In cluster headache patients without a previous history of childhood migraine, the additional THC-CBD 200 mg abortive treatment provided no benefit as an acute treatment.

It is unclear whether certain types of pain may respond better to certain cannabis strains with specific combinations of cannabinoids, terpenes, or other biochemical properties. There have been a multitude of studies showing benefit in many forms of chronic pain, but there have been no studies attempting to differentiate which types and strains of cannabis along with associated compositions of cannabinoids and terpenes may be more effective for certain subsets of pain. This information would be of great clinical use in providing direction for treatment recommendations by healthcare providers.

Methods

Appropriate Investigational Review Boards approved the survey. A French and English electronic survey was sent to 16,675 Tilray medicinal cannabis patients. Tilray is a federally authorized medical cannabis production, distribution, and research company in Nanaimo, British Columbia. Data gathering was performed with REDCap (Research Electronic Data Capture), a HIPAA and PIPEDA compliant secure web application for building and managing online surveys and databases. A $10 account credit was offered to each patient completing the online survey, funded by Tilray. There was a response of 3405 (3390 English and 15 French), 2032 of which provided a verifiable Tilray patient number and were therefore included in the final analysis. The responses represent 12% of those reached. Recruitment was deliberately halted at 2000 (overlap with additional 32 subjects represents participants who were in the middle of completing the survey when it was halted). The survey launched at 9 AM PST on Monday January 9th 2017 and closed on Wednesday January 11th 2017 at 5 PM PST. The limit to responses was due to financial constraints, and patients were informed that the survey

would be available for a two-week period or until limit was reached, whichever came first.

An estimation of migraine prevalence among those surveyed was obtained by incorporating the ID Migraine™ questionnaire [67] into the survey, which is used to predict the probability of migraine. In the ID Migraine™ questionnaire, the patient is given 3 questions. If the patient answers "Yes" to 3 of these questions, there is a 97% chance they have migraine. If they answer "Yes" to 2 of these questions, there is a 93% chance they have migraine. The questions are: 1) Have your headaches interfered with your ability to work, study, or do what you needed to do? 2) Have you felt nauseated or sick to your stomach when you have a headache? 3) Does light bother you when you have a headache (a lot more than when you don't have a headache)?

Patients were asked a multitude of additional questions involving demographics, primary illnesses and symptoms treated with cannabis, frequency and quantity of use, favorite cannabis types and strains, methods of use, and prescription drugs substituted with cannabis.

Patients who reported headache as the primary illness were compared with each patient group reporting a diagnosis other than headache as the primary illness. Separately, patients who reported headache as the primary symptom (regardless of diagnosis) were compared with each patient group who both reported a diagnosis other than headache as the primary illness and also did not report headache as the primary symptom. Statistical methods were the same for each set of comparisons. Pearson chi-squared tests, or Fisher's exact tests where appropriate, were used to compare headache patients with each non-headache patient group, with regards to five cannabis strains: Hybrid, Indica, Sativa, 3:1 CBD: THC, and 1:1 CBD:THC. Significance for omnibus chi-squared tests was designated by $p < .05$. When omnibus chi-squared tests were found to be significant, pairwise comparisons were carried out using a Bonferroni correction. Given ten pairwise comparisons per omnibus test, significance for each pairwise comparison was indicated by $p < .005$. Methods chosen to control for multiple comparisons allow a moderately conservative level of control, and reflect the exploratory nature of the study. Analyses were two-tailed and performed using SAS Studio v 3.5.

Results

Of the 2032 patients included in the survey, 1271 (62.6%) were male, 758 (37.3%) were female, and 3 (0.15%) did not specify gender. Ages ranged from 9 to 85 years old, with an average age of 40. Reported ethnicities in the overall cohort revealed 1839 (90.5%) Caucasian, 62 (3.1%) Metis, 60 (3%) Aboriginal/First Nation, 39 (1.9%) Other, 37 (1.8%) South Asian (East Indian, Pakistani,

Sri Lankan, etc.), 35 (1.7%) Asian (Chinese, Japanese, Korean, Vietnamese, etc.), 25 (1.2%) Black (African, Caribbean, etc.), and 24 (1.2%) Hispanic (Mexican, Central American, South America, etc.), with some patients reporting more than one ethnicity. Relationship status showed 833 (41%) were married, 507 (25%) were single and never married, 274 (13.5%) were in a domestic partnership or civil union, 203 (10%) were single but cohabiting with a significant other, 132 (6.5%) were divorced, 64 (3.2%) were separated, and 19 (0.94%) were widowed. Habitation showed 883 (43.5%) to be living in an urban area, 795 (39.1%) in a suburban area, and 354 (17.4%) in a rural or remote area.

There were 21 primary illnesses that were reported as being treated with medicinal cannabis, as seen in Table 1. The subsets analyzed further were headache, chronic pain, and arthritis. Chronic pain was the most frequently reported primary illness for which medicinal cannabis was being used at 29.4% ($n = 598$), arthritis was 9.3% ($n = 188$), and headache was 3.7% ($n = 75$). Notably, when combined these three categories of pain syndromes accounted for 42.4% ($n = 861$) of the entire medicinal cannabis users.

Headache was then evaluated as a primary symptom being treated by medicinal cannabis across all primary illnesses (headache was the major symptom being treated with medicinal cannabis, among the primary illness categories), as seen in Table 2. There were 505 patients within the entire group surveyed (24.9%) who reported headache as a primary symptom for which they were using medicinal cannabis across all primary illness categories. Of these patients, 262 (51.9%) were male, 241 (47.7%) were female, and 2 (0.40%) did not specify gender. Ages ranged from 10 to 86 years old with an average age of 38. Reported ethnicities revealed 453 (89.7%) Caucasian, 23 (4.6%) Metis, 21 (4.2%) Aboriginal/First Nation, 12 (2.4%) Other, 11 (2.2%) Hispanic (Mexican, Central American, South America, etc.), 10 (2%) Asian (Chinese, Japanese, Korean, Vietnamese, etc.), 8 (1.6%) South Asian (East Indian, Pakistani, Sri Lankan, etc.), and 4 (0.8%) Black (African, Caribbean, etc.), with many patients reporting more than one ethnicity. Relationship status showed 181 (36%) were married, 125 (24.8%) were single and never married, 88 (17.4%) were in a domestic partnership or civil union, 62 (12.3%) were single but cohabiting with a significant other, 28 (5.5%) were divorced, 18 (3.6%) were separated, and 3 (0.6%) were

Table 1 Primary illness treated with medicinal cannabis

Primary Illness	Total	Male	Female	Unspecified
n	2032	1271 (62.6%)	758 (37.3%)	3 (0.15%)
Chronic Pain	598 (29.4%)	371 (62%)	227 (38%)	
Mental Health Condition	548 (27%)	319 (58.2%)	228 (41.6%)	1 (0.2%)
Insomnia/Sleep Disorder	198 (9.7%)	145 (73.2%)	53 (26.8%)	
Arthritis/Musculoskeletal	188 (9.3%)	112 (59.6%)	76 (40.4%)	
PTSD	93 (4.6%)	59 (63.4%)	33 (35.5%)	1 (1.1%)
Headache	75 (3.7%)	44 (58.7%)	31 (41.3)	
Gastrointestinal Disorder	62 (3.1%)	34 (54.8%)	28 (45.2%)	
Multiple sclerosis	45 (2.2%)	26 (57.8%)	19 (42.2%)	
Other	38 (1.9%)	23 (60.5%)	15 (39.5%)	
Cancer/Leukemia	35 (1.7%)	24 (68.6%)	11 (31.4%)	
Crohn's Disease	35 (1.7%)	27 (77.1%)	8 (22.9%)	
Brain Injury	24 (1.3%)	16 (66.7%)	8 (33.3%)	
Epilepsy/Seizure Disorder	21 (1.0%)	18 (85.7%)	3 (14.3%)	
Eating Disorder	20 (1.0%)	10 (50%)	10 (50%)	
Diabetes	16 (0.79%)	13 (81.3%)	3 (18.7%)	
Movement Disorder	10 (0.49%)	8 (80%)	1 (10%)	1 (10%)
AIDS/HIV	8 (0.39%)	7 (87.5%)	1 (12.5%)	
Hepatitis	6 (0.30%)	6 (100%)	0 (0%)	
Glaucoma	5 (0.25%)	5 (100%)	0 (0%)	
Osteoporosis	4 (0.20%)	3 (75%)	1 (25%)	
Skin Condition	3 (0.15%)	1 (33.3%)	2 (66.7%)	

Table 2 Headache as primary symptom treated with medicinal cannabis among various primary illnesses reported

Primary Illness	Total	Male	Female	Unspecified
n	505	262 (51.9%)	241 (47.7%)	2 (0.40%)
Chronic pain	148 (29.3%)	70 (47.3%)	78 (52.7%)	
Mental Health Condition	131 (25.9%)	65 (49.6%)	66 (50.4%)	
Headache	75 (14.9%)	44 (58.7%)	31 (41.3%)	
Insomnia	32 (6.3%)	25 (78.1%)	7 (21.9%)	
Arthritis/Musculoskeletal	29 (5.7%)	12 (41.4%)	17 (58.6%)	
PTSD	24 (4.8%)	9 (37.5%)	14 (58.3%)	1 (4.2%)
MS	13 (2.6%)	3 (23.1%)	10 (76.9%)	
Brain Injury	12 (2.4%)	8 (66.7%)	4 (33.3%)	
Gastrointestinal Disorder	11 (2.2%)	5 (45.5%)	6 (54.5%)	
Cancer/Leukemia	6 (1.2%)	3 (50%)	3 (50%)	
Movement Disorder	5 (1.0%)	4 (80%)	0 (0%)	1 (20%)
Other	4 (0.79%)	2 (50%)	2 (50%)	
Epilepsy/Seizure Disorder	3 (0.59%)	2 (66.7%)	1 (33.3%)	
Crohn's Disease	3 (0.59%)	3 (100%)	0 (0%)	
Diabetes	2 (0.40%)	1 (50%)	1 (50%)	
Glaucoma	2 (0.40%)	2 (100%)	0 (0%)	
Hepatitis	2 (0.40%)	2 (100%)	0 (0%)	
Eating Disorder	1 (0.20%)	1 (100%)	0 (0%)	
AIDS/HIV	1 (0.20%)	1 (100%)	0 (0%)	
Osteoporosis	1 (0.20%)	0 (0%)	1 (100%)	

widowed. Habitation showed 218 (43.2%) to be living in an urban area, 205 (40.6%) in a suburban area, and 82 (16.2%) in a rural or remote area. Chronic pain was the most common primary illness in which headache was reported to be a primary symptom being treated with medicinal cannabis (29.3%), followed by mental health condition (25.9%) and headache (14.9%).

The 505 patients who reported headache as a primary symptom being treated by medicinal cannabis were then analyzed to estimate how many of those patients had probable migraine, and thus, how many were using medicinal cannabis for probable migraine management. This data was obtained via responses to the ID Migraine™ questionnaire. There were 343 (68%) who gave 3 "Yes" responses, and 102 (20%) who gave 2 "Yes" responses. Based on these responses, 445 of these 505 patients (88%) had a very high probability between 93 and 97% that the headaches they were treating with medicinal cannabis represented migraine.

Data was collected among patients to determine the most commonly used and preferred types of cannabis, as well as preferred specific strains. The preferred types of cannabis included Indica, Sativa, Hybrid, 3:1 CBD:THC, or 1:1 CBD:THC. Indicas, Sativas and Hybrids were all high THC/low CBD strains or extracts, while 1:1 and 3:1 strains and extracts represent the CBD:THC ratio, and were considered high CBD strains. The Indica, Sativa,

and Hybrid types were further divided into specific strains within each of these cannabis types.

There were 42 different preferred treatment strains reported by patients and these included: Afghani, Afghani CBD, Alien OG, Barbara Bud, Black Tuna, Blueberry, Bubba Kush, Cannatonic, CBD House Blend, Cheese, Churchill, Dig Weed, Elwyn, Green Cush, Girl Scout Cookies (GSC), Harmony, Headband, Hybrid House Blend, Indica House Blend, Island Sweet Skunk, Jack Herer, Jean Guy, Lemon Sour Diesel, Limonene House Blend, Mango, Master Kush, Myrcene Blend, OG Kush, OG Shark, Pinene House Blend, Pink Kush, Purple Kush, Rockstar, Sativa House Blend, Sirius, Strawberry Cough (SBC), Skywalker OG, Sour Diesel, Sweet Skunk CBD, Warlock CBD, Watermelon, and White Widow.

Preferred cannabis types and strains were first analyzed between the headache as primary symptom, headache as primary illness, chronic pain as primary illness, and arthritis as primary illness groups. Hybrid strains were the most commonly preferred cannabis types across all pain groups. However, when patients with headache as a primary symptom were excluded from the groups, the arthritis group preferred Indica strains, while the others still preferred Hybrid strains. The top 15 preferred cannabis strains within each of these pain groups are seen in Tables 3 and 5. Preferred cannabis types and

Table 3 Preferred medicinal cannabis types and strains among headache patients and probable migraineurs based on "Yes" responses on ID Migraine™ questionnaire

	Headache as primary illness (75)	3 Yes[a] (343)	2 Yes[b] (102)	Headache as primary symptom (505)	3 + 2 Yes (445)
			Preferred Cannabis Type		
Hybrid	26 (34.7%)	118 (34.4%)	35 (34.3%)	165 (32.7%)	153 (34.4%)
Indica	19 (25.3%)	106 (30.9%)	20 (19.6%)	144 (28.5%)	126 (28.3%)
Sativa	20 (26.7%)	76 (22.2%)	36 (35.3%)	136 (26.9%)	112 (25.2%)
3:1 CBD:THC	5 (6.7%)	22 (6.4%)	7 (6.9%)	34 (6.7%)	29 (6.5%)
1:1 CBD:THC	5 (6.7%)	20 (5.8%)	4 (3.9%)	25 (5%)	24 (5.4%)
No response	0 (0%)	1 (0.3%)	0 (0%)	1 (0.2%)	1 (0.2%)

Headache as primary illness	3 Yes	2 Yes	Headache as primary symptom	3 + 2 Yes
		Preferred Cannabis Strains (Top 15)		
Skywalker OG (7; 10.6%)	OG Shark (20; 8.4%)	OG Shark (9; 11%)	OG Shark (34; 9.6%)	OG Shark (29; 8.9%)
Headband (5; 7.6%)	Afghani (19; 8.0%)	Skywalker OG (8; 9.8%)	Jean Guy (29; 8.2%)	Afghani (25; 7.7%)
Cannatonic (5; 7.6%)	Jack Herer (19; 8.0%)	White Widow (8; 9.8%)	Skywalker OG (28; 7.9%)	Skywalker OG (25; 7.7%)
Jack Herer (5; 7.6%)	Jean Guy (19; 8.0%)	Lemon Sour Diesel (7; 8.5%)	Lemon Sour Diesel (28; 7.9%)	Lemon Sour Diesel (25; 7.7%)
Afghani (4; 6.1%)	Lemon Sour Diesel (18; 7.6%)	Afghani (6; 7.3%)	Afghani (26; 7.4%)	Jack Herer (24; 7.3%)
Indica House Blend (4; 6.1%)	Skywalker OG (17; 7.1%)	Pink Kush (6; 7.3%)	White Widow (26; 7.4%)	Jean Guy (24; 7.3%)
Rock Star (4; 6.1%)	Master Kush (16; 6.7%)	Island Sweet Skunk (6; 7.3%)	Jack Herer (26; 7.4%)	White Widow (24; 7.3%)
Warlock CBD (3; 4.6%)	White Widow (16; 6.7%)	Jack Herer (5; 6.1%)	Pink Kush (22; 6.2%)	Pink Kush (21; 6.4%)
Sweet Skunk CBD (3; 4.6%)	Sweet Skunk CBD (15; 6.3%)	Jean Guy (5; 6.1%)	Sweet Skunk CBD (21; 5.9%)	Master Kush (20; 6.1%)
Jean Guy (3; 4.6%)	Pink Kush (15; 6.3%)	Headband (4; 4.9%)	Island Sweet Skunk (21; 5.9%)	Sweet Skunk CBD (18; 5.5%)
Girl Scout Cookies (GSC) (3; 4.6%)	Headband (13; 5.5%)	Master Kush (4; 4.9%)	Master Kush (21; 5.9%)	Headband (17; 5.2%)
OG Shark (2; 3%)	Cannatonic (13; 5.5%)	Sour Diesel (4; 4.9%)	Black Tuna (20; 5.7%)	Island Sweet Skunk (17; 5.2%)
Black Tuna (2; 3%)	Warlock CBD (13; 5.5%)	Black Tuna (4; 4.9%)	Headband (19; 5.4%)	Black Tuna (16; 4.9%)
Bubba Kush (2; 3%)	Blueberry (13; 5.5%)	Hybrid House Blend (3; 3.7%)	Cannatonic (18; 5.1%)	Warlock CBD (14; 4.3%)
CBD House Blend (2; 3%), Elwyn (2; 3%), Island Sweet Skunk (2; 3%), Mango (2; 3%), Master Kush (2; 3%), Blueberry (2; 3%), Pink Kush (2; 3%)	Black Tuna (12; 5.0%)	Sweet Skunk CBD (3; 3.7%)	Hybrid House Blend (15; 4.2%)	Cannatonic (14; 4.3%), Blueberry (14; 4.3%)

[a] 3 "Yes" responses = 97% probability of migraine
[b] 2 "Yes" responses = 93% probability of migraine

strains were then analyzed in the positive ID Migraine™ patients who answered 3 "Yes" responses (343), 2 "Yes" responses (102), or combined 3 + 2 "Yes" responses (445) to the ID Migraine™ questionnaire. Thus, they were the most probable group of headache patients who were treating migraine with medicinal cannabis. Hybrid strains were the most commonly preferred cannabis types across the positive ID Migraine™ groups with the exception that the 2 "Yes" group had a slight preference for Sativa, followed by Hybrid strains. The top 15 preferred cannabis strains within each positive ID Migraine™ group are seen in Table 3. "OG Shark" was the most commonly preferred strain across all of the positive ID Migraine™ and headache as primary symptom groups. Quantification and comparison of the cannabinoids and terpenes present in these top 15 preferred strains is seen in Table 4. The cannabinoids analyzed were Δ^9-tetrahydrocannabinol (THC), tetrahydrocannabinolic acid (THCA), cannabidiol (CBD), and cannabidiolic acid (CBDA). The terpenes analyzed were α-pinene, β-myrcene, D-limonene, linalool, β-caryophyllene, humulene, trans-nerolidol, and bisabolol. Notably, "OG Shark", a high THC/THCA, low CBD/CBDA strain with β-caryophyllene followed by β-myrcene as the predominant terpenes, was the most preferred strain in both the positive ID Migraine™ and headache as primary symptom groups.

For further comparison purposes, preferred cannabis types and strains were also analyzed for the three most common non-pain subsets of patients, which included

mental health condition/PTSD, insomnia/sleep disorder, gastrointestinal disorder/Crohn's Disease, and the overall patient cohort, as seen in Table 5. Indica strains were preferred in the insomnia/sleep disorders group, Sativa strains in the mental health condition/PTSD group, and Hybrid strains in the gastrointestinal disorder/Crohn's Disease group, regardless of whether patients with headache as a primary symptom were included or not. Table 6 shows these same groups, as well as the arthritis and chronic pain groups, with all groups excluding patients with headache as a primary symptom.

Statistical analysis was performed to determine if there were significant differences in preferred cannabis types reported by headache patients. The data were insufficient for statistical analysis of specific strain preferences. There were no statistically significant differences found between patients with headache as primary illness and those with chronic pain, arthritis, or mental health condition/PTSD. When compared to insomnia/sleep disorder patients, headache as primary illness patients were 7.7 times as likely to prefer 3:1 CBD:THC over Indica (OR 7.7, 95% CI 1.7-35.11, p = .003).

Patients with headache as primary symptom were 2.7 times as likely to prefer Sativa over 1:1 CBD:THC (OR 2.66, 95% CI 1.52-4.66, p < .001) when compared to chronic pain patients. When compared to arthritis patients, headache as primary symptom patients were 3.4 times as likely to prefer Sativa over 1:1: CBD:THC (OR 3.35, 95% CI 1.57-7.12, p = .001). When compared to insomnia patients, headache as primary symptom

Table 4 Terpenes and cannabinoids present in top 15 preferred medicinal cannabis strains in headache patients who replied with 3 or 2 "Yes" responses on ID Migraine™ questionnaire

Strain	Terpenes (%)								Cannabinoids (%)			
	α-Pinene	β-Myrcene	D-Limonene	Linalool	β-Caryophyllene	Humulene	Trans-nerolidol	Bisabolol	THCA	THC	CBDA	CBD
OG Shark	0.022	0.194	0.191	0.136	0.263	0.078	0.023	0.107	22.8	21.4	0.1	0
Afghani	0.024	0.101	0.036	0.033	0.132	0.055	0.032	0.066	16.9	15.6	0.1	0
Skywalker OG	0.037	0.217	0.208	0.159	0.319	0.149	0.024	0.110	24.2	22.9	0.2	0
Lemon Sour Diesel	0.127	0.235	0.037	0.026	0.169	0.067	0.022	0.026	19.9	18.3	0.1	0
Jack Herer	0.369	0.612	0.023	0.021	0.132	0.039	0.046	0.013	18.8	17.9	0.2	0
Jean Guy	0.031	0.066	0.069	0.063	0.156	0.047	0.050	0.052	18.1	17.3	0.1	0
White Widow	0.032	0.093	0.195	0.006	0.106	0.032	0.034	0.051	20.1	18.7	0.1	0
Pink Kush	0.019	0.187	0.178	0.148	0.317	0.093	0.058	0.124	27.7	25.8	0.1	0
Master Kush	0.045	0.168	0.192	0.203	0.353	0.169	0.039	0.130	28	25.6	0.1	0
Sweet Skunk CBD	0.054	0.162	0.042	0.014	0.051	0.019	0.015	0.028		9.1		11.2
Headband	0.028	0.238	0.230	0.138	0.318	0.094	0.065	0.124	25.1	23.4	0.1	0
Black Tuna	0.026	0.139	0.149	0.077	0.267	0.088	0.033	0.054	21.8	0.2	0.1	0
Warlock CBD	0.050	0.298	0.199	0.051	0.173	0.102	0.023	0.032	11.4	11	12.6	11.4
Cannatonic	0.059	0.152	0.038	0.022	0.099	0.032	0.015	0.035	10.9	9.4	7.6	7.5
Blueberry	0.000	0.333	0.000	0.052	0.324	0.089	0.021	0.023		21.7		0.1

Table 5 Preferred medicinal cannabis types and strains in all non-headache groups, including patients with headache as primary symptom

Preferred Cannabis Type

	Chronic pain as primary illness (598)	Arthritis as primary illness (188)	Mental Health Condition (548)/PTSD (93) = (641)	Insomnia/Sleep Disorder (198)	Gastrointestinal Disorder (62)/Crohn's Disease (35) = (97)	Overall Medicinal Cannabis Cohort (2032)
Hybrid	221 (37%)	57 (30.3%)	177 (27.6%)	61 (30.8%)	37 (38.1%)	651 (32%)
Indica	152 (25.4%)	56 (29.8%)	173 (27%)	88 (44.4%)	16 (16.5%)	569 (28%)
Sativa	121 (20.2%)	34 (18.1%)	207 (32.3%)	39 (19.7%)	23 (23.7%)	502 (24.7%)
3:1 CBD:THC	49 (8.2%)	22 (11.7%)	46 (7.2%)	3 (1.5%)	11 (11.3%)	154 (7.6%)
1:1 CBD:THC	52 (8.7%)	16 (8.5%)	35 (5.5%)	7 (3.5%)	10 (10.3%)	146 (7.2%)
No response	3 (0.5%)	3 (1.6%)	3 (0.5%)	0 (0%)	0 (0%)	10 (0.49%)

Preferred Cannabis Strains (top 15)

Chronic pain as primary illness	Arthritis as primary illness	Mental Health Condition/PTSD	Insomnia/Sleep Disorder	Gastrointestinal Disorder/Crohn's Disease	Overall Medicinal Cannabis Cohort
OG Shark (43; 10.5%)	Sweet Skunk CBD (13; 8.8%)	Jack Herer (52; 10.8%)	Lemon Sour Diesel (20; 13.8%)	Island Sweet Skunk (8; 9.8%)	OG Shark (120; 8.6%)
CBD House Blend (34; 8.3%)	OG Shark (12; 8.1%)	Island Sweet Skunk (50; 10.4%)	OG shark (15; 10.4%)	Jack Herer (8; 9.8%)	Jack Herer (119; 8.5%)
Pink Kush (34; 8.3%)	Cannatonic (11; 7.4%)	White Widow (46; 9.6%)	Skywalker OG (13; 9%)	Black Tuna (7; 8.5%)	White Widow (109; 7.8%)
Skywalker OG (29; 7.1%)	CBD House Blend (10; 6.8%)	Jean Guy (41; 8.5%)	Pink Kush (12; 8.3%)	Afghani (6; 7.3%)	Lemon Sour Diesel (109; 7.8%)
Master Kush (28; 6.8%)	Indica House Blend (9; 6.1%)	Lemon Sour Diesel (37; 7.7%)	Jack Herer (10; 6.9%)	Warlock CBD (6; 7.3%)	Pink Kush (109; 7.8%)
Warlock CBD (28; 6.8%)	Jack Herer (9; 6.1%)	Pink Kush (35; 7.3%)	White Widow (9; 6.2%)	White Widow (6; 7.3%)	Island Sweet Skunk (107; 7.6%)
Black Tuna (27; 6.6%)	Warlock CBD (8; 5.4%)	OG Shark (34; 7.1%)	Afghani (8; 5.5%)	CBD House Blend (5; 6.1%)	Jean Guy (95; 6.8%)
Jean Guy (26; 6.3%)	Lemon Sour Diesel (8; 5.4%)	Sweet Skunk CBD (30; 6.2%)	Indica House Blend (7; 4.8%)	Sweet Skunk CBD (5; 6.1%)	Skywalker OG (90; 6.4%)
Lemon Sour Diesel (26; 6.3%)	White Widow (8; 5.4%)	Afghani (28; 5.8%)	Sweet Skunk CBD (7; 4.8%)	Hybrid House Blend (5; 6.1%)	Afghani (87; 6.2%)
Jack Herer (25; 6.1%)	Island Sweet Skunk (8; 5.4%)	Skywalker OG (24; 5%)	Island Sweet Skunk (7; 4.8%)	Pink Kush (5; 6.1%)	Sweet Skunk CBD (81; 5.8%)
Cannatonic (24; 5.8%)	Hybrid House Blend (7; 4.7%)	Master Kush (24; 5%)	Black Tuna (7; 4.8%)	Cannatonic (4; 4.9%)	Cannatonic (77; 5.5%)
White Widow (24; 5.8%)	Master Kush (7; 4.7%)	Hybrid House Blend (23; 4.8%)	Jean Guy (6; 4.1%)	Lemon Sour Diesel (4; 4.9%)	Warlock CBD (77; 5.5%)

Table 5 Preferred medicinal cannabis types and strains in all non-headache groups, including patients with headache as primary symptom (*Continued*)

Island Sweet Skunk (22; 5.4%)	Pink Kush (7; 4.7%)	Warlock CBD (21; 4.4%)	Rock Star (6; 4.1%)	Headband (4; 4.9%)	CBD House Blend (76; 5.4%)
Sweet Skunk CBD (21; 5.1%)	Skywalker OG (7; 4.7%)	Cannatonic (20; 4.2%)	Sour Diesel (6; 4.1%)	OG Shark (3; 3.7%)	Master Kush (75; 5.4%)
Headband (20; 4.9%)	Afghani (6; 4.1%), Blueberry (6; 4.1%), Girl Scout Cookies (GSC) (6; 4.1%), Jean Guy (6; 4.1%)	Black Tuna (16; 3.3%)	Master Kush (6; 4.1%), Mango (6; 4.1%)	Jean Guy (3; 3.7%), Blueberry (3; 3.7%), Purple Kush (3; 3.7%)	Black Tuna (70; 5%)

Table 6 Preferred medicinal cannabis types and strains in all non-headache groups, excluding patients with headache as primary symptom

Preferred Cannabis Type

	Chronic pain as primary illness (450)	Arthritis as primary illness (159)	Mental Health Condition (417)/PTSD (69) = (486)	Insomnia/Sleep Disorder (166)	Gastrointestinal Disorder (51)/Crohn's Disease (32) = (83)	Overall Medicinal Cannabis Cohort (1527)
Hybrid	162 (36%)	46 (28.9%)	138 (28.4%)	52 (31.3%)	33 (39.8%)	486 (31.8%)
Indica	114 (25.3%)	51 (32.1%)	125 (25.7%)	74 (44.6%)	10 (12.1%)	426 (27.9%)
Sativa	88 (19.6%)	26 (16.4%)	154 (31.7%)	32 (19.3%)	20 (24.1%)	366 (24%)
3:1 CBD:THC	40 (8.9%)	17 (10.7%)	37 (7.6%)	2 (1.2%)	10 (12.1%)	120 (7.9%)
1:1 CBD:THC	43 (9.6%)	16 (10.1%)	30 (6.2%)	6 (3.6%)	10 (12.1%)	121 (7.9%)
No response	3 (0.7%)	3 (1.9%)	2 (0.4%)	0 (0%)	0 (0%)	8 (0.5%)

Preferred Cannabis Strains (top 15)

Chronic pain as primary illness	Arthritis as primary illness	Mental Health Condition + PTSD	Insomnia/Sleep Disorder	Gastrointestinal Disorder + Crohn's Disease	Overall Medicinal Cannabis Cohort
OG Shark (33; 10.5%)	OG Shark (11; 9.3%)	Jack Herer (42; 11.6%)	Lemon Sour Diesel (17; 14.4%)	Island Sweet Skunk (7; 10.6%)	Jack Herer (93; 8.9%)
Pink Kush (30; 9.6%)	Cannatonic (10; 8.5%)	Island Sweet Skunk (39; 10.7%)	OG shark (10; 8.5%)	Jack Herer (6; 9%)	Pink Kush (87; 8.3%)
CBD House Blend (29; 9.3%)	Sweet Skunk CBD (9; 7.6%)	White Widow (38; 10.5%)	Skywalker OG (10; 8.5%)	Warlock CBD (6; 9%)	OG Shark (86; 8.2%)
Skywalker OG (22; 7%)	CBD House Blend (9; 7.6%)	Jean Guy (28; 7.7%)	Pink Kush (10; 8.5%)	Sweet Skunk CBD (5; 7.6%)	Island Sweet Skunk (86; 8.2%)
Warlock CBD (21; 6.7%)	Jack Herer (9; 7.6%)	Pink Kush (27; 7.4%)	Jack Herer (9; 7.6%)	White Widow (5; 7.6%)	White Widow (83; 7.9%)
Jack Herer (20; 6.4%)	Indica House Blend (8; 6.8%)	Lemon Sour Diesel (26; 7.2%)	White Widow (9; 7.6%)	Hybrid House Blend (5; 7.6%)	Lemon Sour Diesel (81; 7.7%)
Master Kush (19; 6.1%)	Warlock CBD (7; 5.9%)	OG Shark (23; 6.3%)	Afghani (7; 5.9%)	Afghani (4; 6%)	Jean Guy (65; 6.2%)
Black Tuna (19; 6.1%)	Lemon Sour Diesel (7; 5.9%)	Sweet Skunk CBD (21; 5.8%)	Black Tuna (7; 5.9%)	Black Tuna (4; 6%)	Warlock CBD (63; 6%)
Afghani (18; 5.8%)	White Widow (7; 5.9%)	Afghani (20; 5.5%)	Sweet Skunk CBD (6; 5.1%)	Lemon Sour Diesel (4; 6%)	CBD House Blend (63; 6%)
Lemon Sour Diesel (18; 5.8%)	Pink Kush (7; 5.9%)	Warlock CBD (20; 5.5%)	Island Sweet Skunk (6; 5.1%)	Headband (4; 6%)	Skywalker OG (62; 5.9%)
Island Sweet Skunk (18; 5.8%)	Hybrid House Blend (6; 5.1%)	Cannatonic (18; 5%)	Indica House Blend (6; 5.1%)	Cannatonic (4; 6%)	Sweet Skunk CBD (60; 5.7%)
Sweet Skunk CBD (17; 5.4%)	Master Kush (6; 5.1%)	Master Kush (17; 4.7%)	Master Kush (6; 5.1%)		Afghani (59; 5.6%)

Table 6 Preferred medicinal cannabis types and strains in all non-headache groups, excluding patients with headache as primary symptom (*Continued*)

			CBD House Blend (3; 4.6%)	
Cannatonic (17; 5.4%)	Island Sweet Skunk (6; 5.1%)	Skywalker OG (16; 4.4%)	Jean Guy (5; 4.2%)	Purple Kush (3; 4.6%)	Cannatonic (59; 5.6%)
Jean Guy (17; 5.4%)	Girl Scout Cookies (GSC) (6; 5.1%)	Hybrid House Blend (15; 4.1%)	Blueberry (5; 4.2%)	Jean Guy (3; 4.6%)	Master Kush (54; 5.1%)
Girl Scout Cookies (GSC) (15; 4.8%)	Skywalker OG (5; 4.2%), Jean Guy (5; 4.2%)	Black Tuna (13; 3.6%)	Mango (5; 4.2%)	Pink Kush (3; 4.6%)	Black Tuna (50; 4.8%)

patients were over twice as likely to prefer Sativa over Indica (OR 2.18, 95% CI 1.36-3.52, $p = .001$) and 8.7 times as likely to prefer 3:1 CBD:THC over Indica (OR 8.74, 95% CI 2.04-37.37, $p < .001$). When compared to gastrointestinal disorder/Crohn's disease patients, headache as primary symptom patients were almost three times as likely to prefer Indica over Hybrid (OR 2.88, 95% CI 1.37-6.05, $p = .004$), 4.2 times as likely to prefer Indica over 3:1 CBD:THC (OR 4.24, 95% CI 1.63-10.98, $p = .002$), and 5.8 times as likely to prefer Indica over 1:1 THC:CBD (OR 5.76, 95% CI 2.17-15.26, $p < .001$). There were no statistically significant differences found between headache as primary symptom patients and mental health condition/PTSD patients, nor between all non-headache patients as a group.

A number of variables were assessed across all pain groups. These variables included primary method of cannabis use, prevalence of cannabis extract (drops, capsules) use and preferences, cannabis quantity and frequency of use, highest level of education completed, employment status, and prescription medications replaced with medicinal cannabis. The most common primary methods of use across all pain groups were vaporizing and joint use, although additional methods included waterpipe/bong, oral (edibles such as oil drops/extracts, baked goods, butter, tincture), pipe, juicing, tea, or topical use, as seen in Table 7. In the 505 patients with headache as a primary symptom, the most common primary methods

of use were joint in 170 (33.7%), and vaporizing in 162 (32.1%), and this pattern was similar in the positive ID Migraine™ groups. In general, primary methods of use were similar to the top non-pain related primary illnesses, and the overall patient cohort.

The majority of patients using cannabis extracts (drops, capsules) across pain groups preferred the 3:1 CBD:THC extract with the exception that the chronic pain group preferred 1:1 CBD:THC extract, the 3 "Yes" positive ID Migraine™ group preferred Indica extract, and the combined 3 + 2 "Yes" positive ID Migraine™ group equally preferred 3:1 CBD:THC and Indica extracts, as seen in Table 8. Overall, in the headache as primary symptom group, 195 (38.6%) were using cannabis extracts, and the 3:1 CBD:THC extract was most commonly used in 53 (27.2%) followed by the Indica extract in 51 (26.2%).

Quantity of cannabis used was estimated as one joint = 0.3-0.5 g, one eighth = 3.5 g, one quarter = 7 g, and one ounce = 28 g. The quantity and frequency of medicinal cannabis use across the groups ranged from 9.6-11.4 g/week, 1.4-1.7 g/day, 0.58-0.76 g/treatment, 5.9-6.5 days/week and 3.2-3.9 times/day. The quantity of medicinal cannabis use in the headache group averaged 11.4 g/week, 1.7 g/day, and 0.66 g/treatment, with a frequency of 6.4 days/week, and 3.9 times/day. The positive ID Migraine™ patients averaged similar patterns of use, although at the upper ranges of use. These results can all be seen in Table 9.

Table 7 Primary method of medicinal cannabis use among various pain syndromes, "Yes" responses on ID Migraine™ questionnaire, top non-pain related primary illnesses, and overall cohort

Primary method of use								
	Vaporizer	Pipe	Joint	Oral/ Edible	Waterpipe/ Bong	Juicing	Tea	Topical
Headache as primary symptom (505)	162 (32.1%)	50 (9.9%)	170 (33.7%)	58 (11.5%)	63 (12.5%)	1 (0.2%)	1 (0.2%)	
Headache as primary illness (75)	26 (34.7%)	8 (10.7%)	22 (29.3%)	9 (12%)	8 (10.7%)	1 (1.3%)	1 (1.3%)	
Chronic pain as primary illness (598)	179 (29.9%)	56 (9.4%)	183 (30.6%)	120 (20.1%)	56 (9.4%)	1 (0.17%)		3 (0.5%)
Arthritis as primary illness (188)	70 (37.2%)	16 (8.5%)	60 (31.9%)	36 (19.2%)	4 (2.1%)			2 (1.1%)
3 Yes (343)[a]	109 (31.8%)	37 (10.8%)	120 (35%)	37 (10.8%)	39 (11.4%)	1 (0.29%)		
2 Yes (102)[b]	34 (33.3%)	9 (8.8%)	29 (28.4%)	11 (10.8%)	19 (18.6%)			
3 + 2 Yes (445)	143 (32.1%)	46 (10.3%)	149 (33.5%)	48 (10.8%)	58 (13%)			
Mental Health Condition (548) + PTSD (93)	184 (28.7%)	89 (13.9%)	195 (30.4%)	74 (11.5%)	97 (15.1%)	1 (0.16%)	1 (0.16%)	
Insomnia/Sleep Disorder (198)	63 (31.8%)	19 (9.6%)	65 (32.8%)	30 (15.2%)	19 (9.6%)	1 (0.51%)		1 (0.51%)
Gastrointestinal Disorder (62) + Crohn's Disease (35)	34 (35.1%)	12 (12.4%)	26 (26.8%)	11 (11.3%)	14 (14.4%)			
Overall Medicinal Cannabis Cohort (2032)	632 (31.1%)	229 (11.3%)	617 (30.4%)	330 (16.2%)	212 (10.4%)	4 (0.20%)	2 (0.10%)	6 (0.30%)

[a]3 "Yes" responses = 97% probability of migraine
[b]2 "Yes" responses = 93% probability of migraine

Table 8 Medicinal cannabis extract use preferences among various pain syndromes and "Yes" responses on ID Migraine™ questionnaire

Cannabis extracts (drops, capsules)

	Total	Hybrid	Indica	Sativa	3:1 CBD:THC	1:1 CBD:THC
Headache as primary symptom (505)	195 (38.6%)	36 (18.5%)	51 (26.2%)	15 (7.7%)	53 (27.2%)	40 (20.5%)
Headache as primary illness (75)	26 (34.7%)	7 (26.9%)	5 (19.2%)	1 (3.9%)	9 (34.6%)	4 (15.4%)
Chronic pain as primary illness (598)	248 (41.5%)	44 (17.7%)	56 (22.6%)	18 (7.3%)	60 (24.2%)	66 (26.6%)
Arthritis as primary illness (188)	80 (42.6%)	14 (17.5%)	11 (13.8%)	5 (6.3%)	26 (32.5%)	24 (30%)
3 Yes (343)[a]	143 (41.7%)	25 (17.5%)	41 (28.7%)	6 (4.2%)	39 (27.3%)	32 (22.4%)
2 Yes (102)[b]	33 (32.4%)	6 (18.2%)	7 (21.2%)	5 (15.2%)	9 (27.3%)	6 (18.2%)
3 + 2 Yes (445)	176 (39.6%)	31 (17.6%)	48 (27.3%)	11 (6.3%)	48 (27.3%)	38 (21.6%)

[a]3 "Yes" responses = 97% probability of migraine
[b]2 "Yes" responses = 93% probability of migraine

The highest level of education completed across medicinal cannabis user groups can be seen in Table 10. Options included graduate degree, university degree (Bachelors' degree or equivalent), some college/university but no degree/certificate, technical/non-university degree, high school degree or equivalent (GED), and less than high school degree. The most common education level completed across all pain groups was technical/non-university degree, including the headache group, $n = 158$ (31.3%). The exception was in the 2 "Yes" positive ID Migraine™ group, which most commonly reported some college/university but no degree/certificate.

Employment status among medicinal cannabis users was assessed, and can be seen in Table 10. The options were employed working full-time, employed working part-time, retired, not employed looking for work, not employed not looking for work, and disabled not able to work. The vast majority of patients across all pain groups were employed working full time, including the headache group, $n = 268$ (53.1%).

Prescription medications that were replaced with medicinal cannabis were also recorded, as seen in Table 11, and included opiates/opioids, NSAIDs/analgesics, triptans, ergots, anti-depressant/anti-anxiety, anti-convulsant, and muscle relaxers. Many patients across all groups had replaced prescription medications with medicinal cannabis, including headache as primary symptom $n = 272$ (53.9%). Ranges of prescription medication replacement across pain groups varied between 41.2%-59.5% of patients. The most common prescription medications replaced by medicinal cannabis were opiates/opioids in every pain group, including headache as primary symptom $n = 118$ (43.4%). Ranges of opiate/opioid replacement across pain groups varied between 40.5%-72.8% of patients. Notably, additional prescription medications replaced by medicinal cannabis in headache patients included 106 (39%) anti-depressant/anti-anxiety, 57 (21%) NSAIDs, 22 (8.1%) triptans, 21 (7.7%) anticonvulsants, 19 (7%) muscle relaxers, and 1 (0.4%) ergots.

Discussion

The neurobiological pathways of cannabinoids and pain, including migraine and headache, have been detailed, summarized and should be reviewed [1, 2, 51, 65, 68–70]. Briefly, the endocannabinoid system is distributed throughout the central and peripheral nervous system, is involved

Table 9 Quantity and frequency of medicinal cannabis use among various pain syndromes and "Yes" responses on ID Migraine™ questionnaire

Cannabis quantity and frequency used

	Grams per week (Average)	Grams per day (Average)	Grams per treatment (Average)	Days used per week (Average)	Times used per day (Average)
Headache as primary symptom (505)	1 to > 28 (11.4)	≤0.25 to ≥4 (1.7)	≤0.25 to ≥4 (0.66)	1-7 (6.4)	1 to > 10 (3.9)
Headache as primary illness (75)	1 to > 28 (9.6)	≤0.25 to ≥4 (1.4)	≤0.25 to ≥4 (0.67)	1-7 (5.9)	1 to > 10 (3.3)
Chronic pain as primary illness (598)	1 to > 28 (10.8)	≤0.25 to ≥4 (1.6)	≤0.25 to ≥4 (0.68)	1-7 (6.2)	1 to > 10 (3.7)
Arthritis as primary illness (188)	1 to > 28 (9.8)	≤0.25 to ≥4 (1.4)	≤0.25 to ≥4 (0.58)	1-7 (6.1)	1 to > 10 (3.2)
3 Yes (343)[a]	1 to > 28 (11.2)	≤0.25 to ≥4 (1.7)	≤0.25 to ≥4 (0.63)	1-7 (6.4)	1 to > 10 (3.9)
2 Yes (102)[b]	1 to > 28 (11.3)	≤0.25 to ≥4 (1.7)	≤0.25 to ≥4 (0.76)	1-7 (6.5)	1 to > 10 (3.8)
3 + 2 Yes (445)	1 to > 28 (11.3)	≤0.25 to ≥4 (1.7)	≤0.25 to ≥4 (0.70)	1-7 (6.5)	1 to > 10 (3.9)

[a]3 "Yes" responses = 97% probability of migraine
[b]2 "Yes" responses = 93% probability of migraine

Table 10 Highest education level completed and employment status in medicinal cannabis users among various pain syndromes and "Yes" responses on ID Migraine™ questionnaire

	Highest level of education completed					
	Graduate degree	University degree (Bachelors' degree or equivalent)	Some college/ university, but no degree/certificate	Technical and non-university degree	High school degree or equivalent (GED)	Less than high school degree
All patients (2032)	122 (6%)	322 (15.9%)	432 (21.3%)	642 (31.6%)	375 (18.5%)	139 (6.8%)
Headache as primary symptom (505)	17 (3.4%)	81 (16%)	124 (24.6%)	158 (31.3%)	91 (18%)	34 (6.7%)
Headache as primary illness (75)	5 (6.7%)	18 (24%)	16 (21.3%)	22 (29.3%)	9 (12%)	5 (6.7%)
Chronic pain as primary illness (598)	39 (6.5%)	74 (12.4%)	131 (21.9%)	196 (32.8%)	107 (17.9%)	51 (8.5%)
Arthritis as primary illness (188)	10 (5.3%)	31 (16.5%)	36 (19.2%)	65 (34.6%)	38 (20.2%)	8 (4.3%)
3 Yes (343)[a]	10 (2.9%)	54 (15.7%)	87 (25.4%)	114 (33.2%)	53 (15.5%)	25 (7.3%)
2 Yes (102)[b]	4 (3.9%)	13 (12.8%)	30 (29.4%)	28 (27.5%)	21 (20.6%)	6 (5.9%)
3 + 2 Yes (445)	14 (3.2%)	67 (15.1%)	117 (26.3%)	142 (31.9%)	74 (16.6%)	31 (7.0%)

	Employment status					
	Employed, working full-time	Employed, working part-time	Retired	Not employed, looking for work	Not employed, not looking for work	Disabled, not able to work
All patients (2032)	1045 (51.4%)	231 (11.4%)	120 (5.9%)	164 (8.1%)	88 (4.3%)	384 (18.9%)
Headache as primary symptom (505)	268 (53.1%)	50 (9.9%)	10 (2%)	36 (7.1%)	30 (5.9%)	111 (22%)
Headache as primary illness (75)	56 (74.7%)	4 (5.3%)	1 (1.3%)	1 (1.3%)	5 (6.7%)	8 (10.7%)
Chronic pain as primary illness (598)	278 (46.5%)	64 (10.7%)	33 (5.5%)	30 (5%)	24 (4%)	169 (28.3%)
Arthritis as primary illness (188)	94 (50%)	18 (9.6%)	38 (20.2%)	13 (6.9%)	4 (2.1%)	21 (11.2%)
3 Yes (343)[a]	172 (50.2%)	31 (9%)	6 (1.8%)	24 (7%)	21 (6.1%)	89 (26%)
2 Yes (102)[b]	59 (57.8%)	12 (11.8%)	2 (2%)	9 (8.8%)	3 (2.9%)	17 (16.7%)
3 + 2 Yes (445)	231 (51.9%)	43 (9.7%)	8 (1.8%)	33 (7.4%)	24 (5.4%)	106 (23.8%)

[a] 3 "Yes" responses = 97% probability of migraine
[b] 2 "Yes" responses = 93% probability of migraine

in inflammatory and pain processing, and plays regulatory physiological roles across virtually every organ system [19, 46, 71–74]. The endocannabinoid system interacts within its own pathways, as well as within major endogenous pain pathways, including inflammatory, endorphin/enkephalin, vanilloid/transient receptor potential cation channel subfamily V (TRPV), subfamily M (TRPM), subfamily A (TRPA), and nuclear receptors/transcription factors called the peroxisome proliferator-activated receptors (PPAR) [75].

The activities of the endocannabinoid system are based on the pre-synaptic G protein-coupled cannabinoid 1 (CB1) and 2 (CB2) receptors [76]. There is also a presumed third cannabinoid receptor, G protein-coupled receptor 55 (GPR55), termed CB3 [77]. The primary endogenous cannabinoid receptor ligands (endogenous cannabinoids, or

endocannabinoids) are arachidonic acid derivatives, and they work via retrograde signaling receptor activation. The primary mediator of endocannabinoid signaling is N-arachidonoylethanolamine (anandamide, or AEA), and 2-arachidonoylglycerol (2-AG) is another primary endocannabinoid [71, 78–80]. Cannabis-based phytocannabinoids, as well as inherent endocannabinoids interact at the CB1 and CB2 receptors with variable affinities and actions [81–83].

The CB1 receptor is the most abundant G protein-coupled receptor in the brain and one of the most abundant in both the peripheral and central nervous system [81]. CB1 receptors are expressed primarily on presynaptic peripheral and central nerve terminals, and are found extensively through the anatomical pain pathways as well as many other neurological central and peripheral

Table 11 Medicinal cannabis reported as a substitute for prescription drugs among various pain syndromes and "Yes" responses on ID Migraine™ questionnaire

Prescription drugs replaced							
	Yes	Opiates, opioids	NSAIDs, Analgesics	Triptans/Ergots	Anti-depressant, Anti-anxiety	Anti-convulsant	Muscle Relaxers
Headache as primary symptom (505)	272 (53.9%)	118 (43.4%)	57 (21%)	22 (8.1%)/1 (0.4%)	106 (39%)	21 (7.7%)	19 (7%)
Headache as primary illness (75)	36 (48%)	19 (52.8%)	11 (30.6%)	14 (38.9%)	5 (13.9%)	1 (2.8%)	4 (11.1%)
Chronic pain as primary illness (598)	316 (52.8%)	230 (72.8%)	64 (20.3%)	3 (1%)	74 (23.4%)	41 (13%)	30 (9.5%)
Arthritis as primary illness (188)	90 (47.9%)	48 (53.3%)	37 (41.1%)	2 (2.2%)	15 (16.7%)	5 (5.6%)	7 (7.8%)
3 Yes (343)[a]	204 (59.5%)	92 (45.1%)	45 (22.1%)	20 (9.8%)/1 (0.5%)	84 (41%)	13 (6%)	15 (7.4%)
2 Yes (102)[b]	42 (41.2%)	17 (40.5%)	6 (14.3%)	2 (4.8%)	15 (35.7%)	6 (14.3%)	4 (9.5%)
3 + 2 Yes (445)	246 (55.3%)	109 (44.3%)	51 (20.7%)	22 (8.9%)/1 (0.4%)	99 (40.2%)	19 (7.7%)	19 (7.7%)

[a]3 "Yes" responses = 97% probability of migraine
[b]2 "Yes" responses = 93% probability of migraine

locations [19, 84–87]. CB1 receptors are associated with the "high" felt with some cannabis strains, activated by THC. Activation leads to hyperpolarization of the pre-synaptic terminal, closing of calcium channels with subsequent inhibition of released stored inhibitory and excitatory neurotransmitters, including glutamate, 5-hydroxytryptamine (5-HT; serotonin), gamma-aminobutyric acid (GABA), noradrenaline, dopamine, acetylcholine, D-aspartate, and cholecystokinin at inhibitory and excitatory synapses [19, 71, 73, 80, 86, 88–90], and can modulate pain pathways involving opioid, serotonin, and N-methyl-d-aspartate (NMDA) receptors through other indirect mechanisms [91].

The CB2 receptors are located primarily in the peripheral tissues and immune cells where they influence the release of cytokines, chemokines, and cell migration including neutrophils and macrophages, but do have some presence in the central nervous system [18, 86, 92–95], and may also contribute to pain relief by dopamine release modulation [96, 97].

Over 540 phytochemicals have been described in cannabis [98], 18 different chemical classes, and more than 100 different phytocannabinoids, although some are breakdown products [99, 100]. THC and CBD have been the most researched and are considered the major cannabinoids. There are many additional cannabinoids referred to as minor cannabinoids. The quantities of major and minor cannabinoids are widely variable between different types of cannabis strains. There is evidence for analgesic and anti-inflammatory effects in many of the cannabinoids, and this publication will focus primarily on these properties for the cannabinoids assessed in this study. However, a more extensive discussion and a comprehensive review of other medicinal properties of these, as well as many other cannabinoids, has been summarized and is available

[28]. The cannabinoids analyzed in this study were limited to THC, THCA, CBD, and CBDA.

THC is one of the most researched cannabinoids, and the cause of the psychoactive side effects of cannabis, suspected from modulation of glutamate and GABA systems [18, 83, 101–103]. It is a partial agonist at CB1 greater than CB2 receptors, which are its primary mechanisms of action. However, other mechanisms of action reflect its activity as an agonist at the PPAR-γ and TRPA1 receptors [83], a 5HT3A antagonist, a glycine receptor activation enhancer via allosteric modification, reduces elevated intracellular calcium levels from TRPM8 activity (cold and menthol receptor 1 (CMR1)), elevates calcium levels by TRPA1 or TRPV2, and stimulates G Protein Receptor 18 and other nuclear receptors [104–113]. It reduces NMDA responses by 30-40% [114–116], blocks capsaicin-induced hyperalgesia [117], inhibits CGRP activity [118], increases cerebral 5HT production, decreases 5HT reuptake, and inhibits 5HT release from platelets, all of which may influence trigeminovascular migraine circuitry [1, 68, 69, 119]. THC enhances analgesia from kappa opioid receptor agonist medications [120–123], stimulates production of beta-endorphin and increases proenkephalin mRNA levels in brainstem regions involved in pain processing [124–126], and intraventricular and intrathecal administration of THC produces analgesia similar to opioids [127].

THC is 20 times more anti-inflammatory than aspirin, twice as anti-inflammatory as hydrocortisone [128], and has well documented analgesic and anti-inflammatory benefits including arthritic and inflammatory conditions [83, 114, 127, 129–156]. There have been many positive studies across various chronic pain syndromes, showing benefit of THC in trials with smoked or vaporized cannabis comparing between different doses of THC, with benefit often noted at higher percentages [28, 47, 157–169]. However, compositions of other cannabinoids including CBD, minor cannabinoids, and other important compounds such as terpenes were not assessed in most of these trials. Given the entourage effects of cannabis [100, 170], where cannabinoids and terpenes influence activity of one another, resulting in strain-specific characteristics, effects and responses, it is often unclear if these studies showing positive (or negative) effects of cannabis are due to the THC alone, or due to synergy between undefined compositions of other cannabinoids and terpenes.

There have been a multitude of studies confirming benefit in various chronic pain syndromes with an oral-mucosal spray called Nabiximols (Sativex) [171–196], approved in 30 countries for various neurological symptoms. This is a tincture of cannabis made from cannabis plants [197]. Each spray delivers a standardized dose of 2.7 mg THC and 2.5 mg CBD, along with additional cannabinoids, flavonoids, and terpenes in unmeasured small amounts. Despite the standardized THC:CBD ratio, the actual concentrations of terpenes and other compounds are unknown. This again creates uncertainty as to what components are providing most of the benefit, although entourage effects are again suspected. There was also a study comparing between three varieties of this spray; 1:1 THC:CBD vs. THC alone vs. CBD alone and the sprays that contained THC showed the most pain benefit, over CBD alone [179]. Other cannabis extract studies of only THC and CBD in varying doses also showed pain benefit, although these did not evaluate each cannabinoid individually [187, 198].

The strong anti-emetic benefits of THC have also been well documented in adults [26, 83, 129, 130, 199–238] and children [235, 239–241], and migraine associated nausea and vomiting would certainly be another benefit of THC. In fact, the FDA has approved two synthetic forms of THC in the treatment of chemotherapy related nausea and vomiting; Dronabinol [242] and Nabilone [243]. Notably, these synthetic THC medications have also shown analgesic effects [55, 57, 62, 188, 244–256].

Besides THC, CBD is the other major cannabinoid. It has gained a lot of attention over the past several years due to its lack of any psychoactivity, as opposed to THC. In November 2017, The World Health Organization announced that in humans, CBD exhibits no evidence for abuse or dependence potential, and there is no evidence of public health related problems associated with the use of pure CBD [257]. In January 2018, the World Anti-Doping Agency (WADA) removed CBD from their prohibited list, no longer banning use by athletes [258]. CBD has powerful analgesic and anti-inflammatory effects [23, 83, 114, 129–131, 137–140, 149, 259–281] mediated by both cyclooxygenase and lipoxygenase

inhibition. Its anti-inflammatory effect is several hundred times more potent than aspirin [128, 282], although to date, there have been no clinical studies evaluating pure CBD in headache or chronic pain disorders. CBD has much lower affinity for CB1 or CB2 receptors, and acts as an antagonist of CB1 and CB2 agonists such as THC [276]. At low concentrations, its antagonism of CB1 underlies its neutralizing effects on the CB1 agonist THC side effects such as anxiety, tachycardia, and sedation [283–288]. CBD appears to attenuate some of these negative side effects of THC when the CBD:THC ratio is at least 8:1 (± 11.1), but may potentiate some of the THC side effects when the CBD:THC ratio is around 2:1 (± 1.4) [286, 288]. It is also an inverse agonist at the CB2 receptor, which may contribute to its anti-inflammatory effects [276].

CBD also interacts with a multitude of ion channels, enzymes, and other receptors [18, 83, 129, 130, 225, 259]. It acts as a TRPV1 agonist, similar to capsaicin, although without the noxious sides effects, and also inhibits AEA uptake and metabolism [108–110, 289, 290]. It acts as a positive allosteric modulator at $\alpha 1$ and $\alpha 1\beta$ glycine receptors [291], suggested to play a role in chronic pain after inflammation or nerve injury since glycine acts as an inhibitory postsynaptic neurotransmitter in the dorsal horn of the spinal cord. CBD acts as a μ opioid receptor ligand and a positive allosteric modulator at μ and δ opioid receptors suggesting that it may enhance opiate effects [83]. Additional mechanisms of action suggested to reflect its anti-inflammatory and analgesic effects, as well as other medicinal benefits, include TRPA1 agonist, TRPV1 agonist, TRPM8 antagonist [108–110], TRPV2 agonist in which it may mediate CGRP release from dorsal root ganglion neurons [292], T-type calcium^{2+} channel inhibitor [293], suppression of tryptophan degradation (precursor to 5HT) [294], phospholipase A2 modulator [295], 5-HT1A agonist [83, 296], regulator of intracellular calcium^{2+} [297, 298], fatty acid amide hydrolase (FAAH; breaks down AEA) inhibition [290], GPR55 antagonist [77], adenosine uptake competitive inhibitor [299], PPARγ agonist [300], 5-lipoxygenase and 15-lipoxygenase inhibitors [301], and antagonism of the abnormal-CBD receptor [83, 302].

Cannabinoid acids are the precursors to the cannabinoids in raw and live cannabis, and have no psychotropic qualities. They are decarboxylated by heat, UV exposure, and prolonged storage to form the active cannabinoids, although heat such as from smoking or vaporizing is the primary conversion factor. The two cannabinoid acids assessed in this study were THCA, which converts to THC, and CBDA, which converts to CBD.

THCA is a TRPA1 partial agonist [108], and TRPM8 antagonist [108] which may underlie a potential role in analgesia, and has been shown to have anti-inflammatory [140] and anti-nausea properties [303]. CBDA is often obtained through consumption of raw cannabis juice. It is a TRPA1 agonist [108], TRPV1 agonist [290], and TRPM8 antagonist [108] which may also reflect its potential as an analgesic. It is also anti-inflammatory [130, 140, 304] via selective COX2 inhibition, and has anti-nausea properties [237, 305].

The terpenes, or terpenoids, form the largest group of phytochemicals [99], and account for some pharmacological properties of cannabis, as well as many medicinal herbs, plants and essential oils. They are the source of flavors, aromas, and other characteristics that help differentiate cannabis strains. The terms terpenes and terpenoids are often used interchangeably in the literature, although technically, terpenes are basic hydrocarbons, while terpenoids contain extra functional groups of a wide range of chemical elements. Cannabis contains up to 200 different terpenes [100], and they are generally classified as primary and secondary terpenes, based on how frequent they occur in cannabis. They are lipophilic with wide ranging mechanisms of action sites including neurotransmitter receptors, G-protein receptors, muscle and neuronal ion channels, enzymes, cell membranes, and second messenger systems [100, 306, 307]. The terpenes work synergistically with the cannabinoids for a variety of therapeutic effects, and this phenomenon is known as the cannabis entourage effects [100, 170]. They have shown many medicinal benefits, including anti-inflammatory and analgesic properties [308]. This publication will focus primarily on the anti-inflammatory and analgesic evidence for the terpenes analyzed in this study, although a more extensive discussion and a comprehensive review of other medicinal properties of these, as well as many other terpenes has been summarized and is available [28]. The majority of this data comes from preclinical studies involving animal models or in vitro studies, and some of the reported benefits attributed to individual terpenes come from studies evaluating whole essential oils or plants in which the specified terpene may be a predominant constituent. However, therapeutic contribution from some of the other terpenes in some of these studies cannot be excluded. The terpenes analyzed in this study were limited to α-pinene, β-myrcene, D-limonene, linalool, β-caryophyllene, humulene, trans-nerolidol, and bisabolol.

Alpha-pinene (α-pinene) is the most commonly occurring terpene in nature [309], and accounts for the aroma of fresh sage, pine needles, and conifers, but is produced by many herbs such as basil, parsley, and dill as well. It has anti-inflammatory effects in human chondrocytes, suggesting anti-osteoarthritic activity [310, 311], anti-inflammatory effects by PGE-1 [312], and anti-nociception properties [313].

Beta-myrcene (β-myrcene), or myrcene, is common in lemongrass, basil, bay leaves, wild thyme, parsley, hops, and tropical fruits such as mango. It has potent anti-inflammatory, analgesic, and anxiolytic properties [314–316], and has benefit in muscle relaxation [317], and prominent sedation/hypnotic, helpful in sleep [317, 318]. Its analgesic effects were antagonized by naloxone suggesting an opioid-mediated mechanism [315, 316]. Its significant anti-inflammatory effects [319] occur via prostaglandin E2 [315] and it has anti-catabolic effects in human chondrocytes suggesting anti-osteoarthritic activity and the ability to halt or slow down cartilage destruction and osteoarthritis progression [320].

D-limonene (limonene) is prominent in the rinds of citrus fruits, and the second most commonly occurring terpene in nature [309]. It has analgesic [321], anti-inflammatory [320, 322–325], and antidepressant effects [321, 326]. It contributes to muscle relaxation and sleep [317], and is a powerful anxiolytic [327–330], which extended anxiolytic benefit to patients with chronic myeloid leukemia (CML) [331]. It increases the metabolic turnover of dopamine in the hippocampus and serotonin in the prefrontal cortex and striatum, suggesting that anxiolytic and antidepressant-like effects may occur by the suppression of dopamine activity related to enhanced serotonergic neurons, especially via 5-HT1A [332].

Linalool is found in flowers and spices including citrus, lavender, rosewood, birch trees, and coriander. It exhibits anti-inflammatory and analgesic activity [333–335] as well as anti-nociception via activation of opioidergic and cholinergic systems [333], anticonvulsant via anti-glutamatergic and GABA neurotransmitter systems [336–340], anti-anxiety/stress [341–344], sedation [343, 345–347], and anti-insomnia properties [100]. Its local anesthetic effects [348] were equivalent to procaine and menthol [349], and analgesic effects have been attributed to adenosine A_{2A} activity [350] and ionotropic glutamate receptors including AMPA, NMDA and kainate [351]. Morphine opioid usage in gastric banding surgical patients was significantly decreased following lavender inhalation vs. placebo, and this was attributed to the linalool concentration [352].

Beta-caryophyllene (β-caryophyllene) is found in spices and plants including cloves, cinnamon, black pepper, hops, rosemary, oregano, and basil. It has analgesic effects in inflammatory and neuropathic pain [353], and has potent anti-inflammatory effects [354–357], with local anesthetic properties [358]. Anti-inflammatory effects appear to occur via PGE-1 [359], with similar efficacy as indomethacin and etodolac [360, 361], and comparable to phenylbutazone [359, 360]. β-caryophyllene is a selective cannabinoid receptor 2 (CB2) agonist [362–364]. CB2 receptors have been implicated in anxiety and depression, and β-caryophyllene has shown anxiolytic and antidepressant effects [365].

Humulene (α-caryophyllene) is an isomer of β-caryophyllene and plays a role in many of the distinguishing characteristics between different cannabis strains. It is found in herbs and spices such as clove, basil, hops, sage, spearmint and ginseng, in addition to some vegetables and fruits. It has strong anti-inflammatory properties comparable to dexamethasone systemically, topically, and in allergic airway inflammation [354–356, 366, 367], as well as anti-nociceptive and analgesic properties [367].

Nerolidol (trans-nerolidol) is found in many herbs and spices including lavender, lemon grass, ginger, jasmine, tea tree, oranges, and present in orange and other citrus peels. It has anti-insomnia and sedative properties [368].

Alpha-bisabolol (α-bisabolol, bisabolol, levomenol) is produced by some flowers used in making tea, such as the chamomile flower. It has anti-inflammatory effects in the skin [369], as well as anti-nociceptive properties [370].

Cannabis sativa strains are generally described by patients as uplifting, energetic, creative, euphoria, spacey, cerebrally-focused effects, and better for day use, while *Cannabis indica* strains are typically described as calming, relaxing, sedative, full body effects such as "body buzz", and better for night use. Research suggests these effects are not likely due purely to CBD:THC ratios, as there are no significant differences in CBD:THC ratios between Sativa and Indica strains. Rather these different subjective effects are likely due to varying ratios of major cannabinoids as well as minor cannabinoids, terpenes and probably additional phytochemicals [100, 371–374]. High CBD strains are Sativa or Indica strains that have been crossed with high CBD hemp strains (1:1 CBD:THC up to approximately 5:1 CBD:THC), while pure CBD strains (ratios of > 10:1 CBD:THC, which can be up to approximately 50:1 CBD:THC) are considered hemp strains. Most strains utilized today are Hybrids designed with standardized ratios of CBD, THC, other cannabinoids, and other compounds such as terpenes and flavonoids, targeting specific symptoms, responses, and end user effects.

Although not of statistical significance, there were some pattern use trends noted. The majority of patients across all pain groups including the positive ID Migraine™, headache as primary symptom, chronic pain, and arthritis groups all preferred Hybrid cannabis strains followed by Indica, Sativa, and higher CBD strains (1:1 CBD:THC, 3:1 CBD:THC) when patients with headache as primary symptom were included. However, when these patients were excluded, the arthritis group preferred Indica strains. When comparing headache and migraine to non-headache groups, Indica strains were preferred in the insomnia/sleep disorders group, Sativa strains in the mental health condition/PTSD group, and Hybrid strains were still preferred in the gastrointestinal disorder/Crohn's Disease group. Perhaps the headache,

chronic pain, and gastrointestinal disorder/Crohn's groups preferred similar Hybrid strains due to underlying inflammatory pathophysiology. The positive ID Migraine™ and headache as primary symptom patients most commonly preferred the "OG Shark" Hybrid strain specifically, although this pattern was also noted in the chronic pain and arthritis groups, so was not unique to headache and migraine. This is a high THC/THCA, low CBD/CBDA strain with β-caryophyllene followed by β-myrcene as the predominant terpenes. This could reflect the potent analgesic, anti-inflammatory, and anti-emetic properties of THC, along with documented anti-inflammatory and analgesic properties of β-caryophyllene and β-myrcene. Given the prominent features of pain with nausea and vomiting in migraine headache, the fact that headache and migraine patients preferred a strain such as this, with its associated cannabinoid and terpene profile, would make sense given the known therapeutic effects of this cannabinoid and these terpenes. Furthermore, there were additional terpenes present in this strain of lower percentages, some of which also have analgesic and anti-inflammatory properties.

Substituting cannabis for alcohol, illicit drugs and/or prescription medications has been commonly observed in cross sectional surveys, suggesting a harm reduction role in the use of these substances, as well as implications for abstinence-based substance use treatment strategies [375–377]. The "opioid-sparing effect" of cannabinoids has been well described with extensive supporting evidence showing that combining cannabis with opiates decreases opiate dose requirements [166, 378]. CB1 receptors are 10 times more concentrated then mu-opioid receptors in the brain, and cannabinoid receptors co-localize with opioid receptors in many regions involved in pain pathways. This is suspected to contribute to synergistic augmentation of the analgesic opioid effects and decreased opioid dose requirements [8, 122–125, 166, 379–384], and studies have shown cannabis use did not affect blood levels of oxycodone or morphine [8, 166]. Cannabinoid receptor agonists increase endogenous opioid peptide release, and chronic THC use increases endogenous opioid precursor gene expression in supraspinal and spinal structures involved in pain perception [119, 126, 166, 379].

The synergistic effect of concomitant cannabis/cannabinoids and opioids in lowering both pain and opioid dose requirements without affecting serum opioid levels has been demonstrated prospectively [166]. A large meta-analysis showed that 17 of 19 pre-clinical studies provided good evidence of these synergistic effects from opioid and cannabinoid co-administration and that the median effective dose (ED50) of morphine administered with THC is 3.6 times lower than the ED50 of morphine alone, while the ED50 for codeine administered with THC was 9.5 times lower than the ED50 of codeine alone [378]. The combination of cannabis/cannabinoids and opioids appears to allow for opioid treatment at lower doses with fewer side effects, allowing easier detoxification and weaning due to lessening of tolerance and withdrawal from opiates, and rekindling of opiate analgesia after prior dosages have worn off [124]. Some pain specialists have suggested the use of medicinal cannabis treatment in addition to or in replacement of opiate treatments to help reduce overdose mortality and morbidity associated with opiate use [385]. Prospective studies have shown that chronic pain patients who use cannabis have improved pain and functional outcomes, and a significant reduction in opioid use [386], and medical cannabis use was associated with decreased opiate use, improvement in quality of life, and better side effect profile in a retrospective cross-sectional survey of chronic pain patients [387].

Notably, the most common prescription medications replaced by medicinal cannabis in this study were opiates/opioids in a large percentage within every pain group, up to 72.8% of patients in the chronic pain as primary illness group. Given the opioid epidemic, particularly in the United States, cannabis has been discussed as an option that may help in the opioid/opiate detoxification and weaning process and perhaps assist in combating the epidemic of opioid related death [377, 385, 388–390]. States with medicinal cannabis laws have been shown to have a 24.8% decreased annual opioid overdose mortality rate compared with states without medicinal cannabis laws. The association between medicinal cannabis law implementation and decrease in annual opioid overdose mortality strengthened over time to a decrease of 33.7% by year 5 [391].

The synergistic interactions between the phytocannabinoids, terpenes and other cannabis compounds resulting in various therapeutic benefits and responses have been termed the cannabis entourage effects [100, 170]. This synergy between the cannabinoids, terpenes, and other compounds leads to variable benefits, user effects, and strain characteristics. In addition, synergistic interactions between cannabis and opioid pathways may be a promising new weapon in the battle of the opioid epidemic. Further study is needed to determine optimal combinations for specific synergies and composition ratios of the cannabis constituents to best target different symptoms and diseases. Medicinal cannabis production has become a very sterile, scientific, standardized production process, and an emerging new industry. Similar to the broad category of anticonvulsants with many varieties targeting variable neurochemical pathways and channels with different responses and side effects, cannabis should also be thought of a broad category of

medicine, of which further therapeutic delineations and disease targeting differentiations between strains is necessary.

There are multiple limitations to this study beginning with its survey design and inherent limitations. Many of the patients who reported headache as a primary symptom for which they were treating with medicinal cannabis, had also reported other diseases or symptoms that they were using medicinal cannabis for. So, some of the answers provided may not have been specific for only headache treatment, but potentially other symptoms or a combination of symptoms including headache. This could also influence reported preferred strains being used since some strains are used more commonly for some symptoms, while other strains may be used for other symptoms. There may be some inaccuracy of patient numbers within the different pain groups of chronic pain, arthritis, and headache. For example, some patients who reported chronic pain as the primary illness for which they were using medicinal cannabis did not specify their type of chronic pain further. It is unknown if some of these patients may have been treating chronic pain of arthritis or headache types, but reporting it as chronic pain, and therefore some of these patients may have been more accurately listed in a different more specific category. Variability in patients' cannabis knowledge could potentially influence self-reporting accuracy. When documenting the preferred cannabis types and strains within each of the pain and non-pain groups, many patients did not provide an answer for their preferred type or strain. If a preferred cannabis type was not provided, but a preferred strain was provided, then their preferred type was presumed to correlate to their reported preferred strain, and counted as such. In addition, reported preferred cannabis types and strains sometimes did not correlate (reported strain did not fall under the correct reported type). Therefore, the preferred cannabis types and strains listed within each category, and their inferred potential benefits, may be inaccurate based on this inconsistent reporting by some patients, and the validity of the preferred cannabis type and strain data requires prospective validation.

Conclusions

Chronic pain was the most common reason for use of medicinal cannabis, consistent with the statistics of most registries. Identifying differences in use patterns between migraine, headache, arthritis, and chronic pain syndromes may be helpful in optimizing crossbred cannabis strains, synergistic biochemical profiles, or dosing differences between these pain subsets. The majority of patients treating headache with medicinal cannabis were positive for migraine (88%) according to the ID

Migraine™ questionnaire. This suggests that most headaches being treated with medicinal cannabis were likely of migrainous pathophysiology.

Hybrid cannabis strains were preferred across most pain groups. "OG Shark", a high THC/THCA, low CBD/CBDA strain with β-caryophyllene followed by β-myrcene as the predominant terpenes, was the most preferred strain in the positive ID Migraine™ and headache as primary symptom groups. This could reflect the potent analgesic, anti-inflammatory, and anti-emetic properties of THC, along with documented anti-inflammatory and analgesic properties of β-caryophyllene and β-myrcene. Since migraines also involve nausea and vomiting, the potent antiemetic properties of THC may be a reason for this preference. Vaporizing or joint use were the primary methods of use across all groups, including migraine and headache, likely reflecting the need for a quick acting inhaled or non-orally ingested therapy in migraine attacks before severe pain and nausea/vomiting become prominent.

Most patients in the pain groups reported replacing prescription medications with medicinal cannabis, the most common of which were opiates/opioids across all pain groups. This is notable given the well-described "opioid-sparing effect" of cannabinoids and growing abundance of literature suggesting that cannabis may help in weaning from these medications and perhaps providing a means of combating the opioid epidemic. There are several limitations to the data in this study, and these results require further confirmation with more sophisticated prospective study methods. However, these results may provide early insight and a framework for direction into optimizing crossbred cannabis strains, synergistic biochemical profiles, dosing, and patterns of use that may be of clinical benefit in the treatment of headache and migraine, as well as other chronic pain syndromes.

Abbreviations
2-AG: 2-arachidonoylglycerol; 5-HT: 5-hydroxytryptamine (serotonin); AEA: N-arachidonoylethanolamine (anandamide); AMPA: α-amino-3-hydroxy-5-methyl-4-isoxazolepropionic acid; CB1: Cannabinoid 1 receptor; CB2: Cannabinoid 2 receptor; CB3: Cannabinoid 3 receptor; CBD: Cannabidiol; CBDA: Cannabidiolic acid; CGRP: Calcitonin gene related peptide; CML: Chronic myeloid leukemia; CMR1: Cold and menthol receptor 1; COX2: Cyclooxygenase-2; ED50: Median effective dose; FAAH: Fatty acid amide hydrolase; FDA: Federal drug administration; GABA: Gamma-aminobutyric acid; GPR55: G protein-coupled receptor 55; NMDA: N-methyl-d-aspartate; NNT: Number needed to treat; NSAID: Non-steroidal anti-inflammatory drug; PGE-1: Prostaglandin E1; PPAR: Peroxisome proliferator-activated receptors; PTSD: Post-Traumatic Stress Disorder; THC: Δ9-Tetrahydrocannabinol; THCA: Tetrahydrocannabinolic acid; TRPA: Transient receptor potential cation channel, subfamily A; TRPM: Transient receptor potential cation channel, subfamily M; TRPV: Transient receptor potential cation channel subfamily V; WADA: World Anti-Doping Agency

Funding
A $10 patient account credit was offered to each patient completing the online survey, funded by Tilray ($20,000 budget).

Authors' contributions
EB is the primary author of the manuscript, helped incorporate the ID Migraine™ questionnaire into the survey, and analyzed/organized the survey data. PL designed the survey, coordinated its administration and data collection, and assisted in writing of the manuscript. JE conducted the biochemical analysis of cannabis strain cannabinoid and terpene compositions, and reviewed the manuscript. OH conducted the statistical analysis of the data and assisted with writing of the correlating statistical analysis data in the manuscript. All authors read and approved the final manuscript.

Competing interests
PL: Vice-President of Patient Research and Access for Tilray, ownership interest (stocks, stock options, or other ownership interest excluding diversified mutual funds), salary.
JE: Vice-President and Chief Science Officer for Tilray, ownership interest (stocks, stock options, or other ownership interest excluding diversified mutual funds), salary.

Author details
[1]Center for Neurological Restoration - Headache and Chronic Pain Medicine, Department of Neurology, Cleveland Clinic Neurological Institute, 10524 Euclid Avenue, C21, Cleveland, OH 44195, USA. [2]Tilray, 1100 Maughan Rd, Nanaimo, BC V9X 1J2, Canada. [3]Social Dimensions of Health, University of Victoria, 3800 Finnerty Rd, Victoria, BC V8P 5C2, Canada. [4]Canadian Institute for Substance Use Research, 2300 McKenzie Ave, Victoria, BC V8N 5M8, Canada. [5]Section of Biostatistics, Department of Quantitative Health Sciences, Cleveland Clinic Lerner Research Institute, 9500 Euclid Avenue, JJN3, Cleveland, OH 44195, USA.

References
1. Russo E (1998) Cannabis for migraine treatment: the once and future prescription? An historical and scientific review. Pain 76:3–8
2. Baron EP (2015) Comprehensive review of medicinal marijuana, cannabinoids, and therapeutic implications in medicine and headache: what a long strange trip it's been .... Headache 55:885–916
3. Brunner TF (1973) Marijuana in ancient Greece and Rome? The literary evidence. Bull Hist Med 47:344–355
4. Kuddus M, Ginawi IAM, Al-Hazimi A (2013) Cannabis sativa: an ancient wild edible plant of India. Emir J Food Agric 25:736–745
5. Mikuriya TH (1969) Marijuana in medicine: past, present and future. Calif Med 110:34–40
6. Mikuriya TH (1973) Marijuana: medical papers 1839-1972. Medi-Comp Press, Oakland
7. O'Shaughnessy WB (1843) On the preparations of the Indian hemp, or gunjah (cannabis indica): their effects on the animal system in health, and their utility in the treatment of tetanus and other convulsive diseases. Prov Med J Retrosp Med Sci 5:363–369
8. McGeeney BE (2013) Cannabinoids and hallucinogens for headache. Headache 53:447–458
9. McGeeney BE (2012) Hallucinogens and cannabinoids for headache. Headache 52(Suppl 2):94–97
10. Clendinning J (1843) Observations on the medical properties of the cannabis sativa of India. Med Chir Trans 26:188–210
11. Greene R (1872) Cannabis Indica in the treatment of migraine. Practitioner 41:267–270

12. Osler W, McCrae T (1915) The principles and practice of medicine. Appleton, New York

13. Mackenzie S (1887) Remarks on the value of Indian hemp in the treatment of a certain type of headache. Br Med J 1:97–98

14. Farlow JW (1889) On the use of belladonna and cannabis Indica by the rectum in gynecological practice. Boston Med Surg J 120:507–509

15. Reynolds JR (1890) On the therapeutic uses and toxic effects of cannabis Indica. Lancet 135:637–638

16. Fishbein M (1942) Migraine associated with menstruation. J Am Med Assoc 237:326

17. British Medical Association (1997) Therapeutic uses of Cannabis. Harwood Academic Publishers, Netherlands

18. Koppel BS, Brust JC, Fife T et al (2014) Systematic review: efficacy and safety of medical marijuana in selected neurologic disorders: report of the guideline development subcommittee of the American Academy of Neurology. Neurology 82:1556–1563

19. Aggarwal SK (2013) Cannabinergic pain medicine: a concise clinical primer and survey of randomized-controlled trial results. Clin J Pain 29:162–171

20. Lynch ME, Ware MA (2015) Cannabinoids for the treatment of chronic non-cancer pain: an updated systematic review of randomized controlled trials. J Neuroimmune Pharmacol 10:293–301

21. Lynch ME, Campbell F (2011) Cannabinoids for treatment of chronic non-cancer pain; a systematic review of randomized trials. Br J Clin Pharmacol 72:735–744

22. Whiting PF, Wolff RF, Deshpande S et al (2015) Cannabinoids for medical use: a systematic review and meta-analysis. JAMA 313:2456–2473

23. Boychuk DG, Goddard G, Mauro G, Orellana MF (2015) The effectiveness of cannabinoids in the management of chronic nonmalignant neuropathic pain: a systematic review. J Oral Facial Pain Headache 29:7–14

24. Committee of the Health Effects of Marijuana (2017) An evidence review and research agenda. The health effects of cannabis and cannabinoids. The current state of evidence and recommendations for research. The National Academies Press, Washington, DC

25. Moulin D, Boulanger A, Clark AJ et al (2014) Pharmacological management of chronic neuropathic pain: revised consensus statement from the Canadian Pain Society. Pain Res Manag 19:328–335

26. Gurley RJ, Aranow R, Katz M (1998) Medicinal marijuana: a comprehensive review. J Psychoactive Drugs 30:137–147

27. Zuardi AW (2006) History of cannabis as a medicine: a review. Rev Bras Psiquiatr 28:153–157

28. Baron EP (2018) Medicinal properties of cannabinoids, terpenes and flavonoids in cannabis, and potential roles in migraine, headache, and pain: an update on current evidence and cannabis science. Headache In Press

29. Ilgen MA, Bohnert K, Kleinberg F et al (2013) Characteristics of adults seeking medical marijuana certification. Drug Alcohol Depend 132:654–659

30. Hazekamp A, Heerdink ER (2013) The prevalence and incidence of medicinal cannabis on prescription in the Netherlands. Eur J Clin Pharmacol 69:1575–1580

31. Medical Marijuana Registry Statistics. Colorado Department of Health and Environment. https://www.colorado.gov/pacific/cdphe/medicalmarijuana. Accessed 1 Dec 2017

32. Medical Cannabis Registry. Minnesota Department of Health. http://www.health.state.mn.us/topics/cannabis/registry.html. Accessed 1 Dec 2017

33. Medical cannabis patient registry program. Illinois Department of Public Health. http://www.dph.illinois.gov/topics-services/prevention-wellness/medical-cannabis. Accessed 1 Dec 2017

34. Medical cannabis program. Hawaii Department of Health. http://health.hawaii.gov/medicalcannabis/. Accessed 1 Dec 2017

35. Oregon Medical Marijuana Program Statistics. Oregon Health Authority. http://www.oregon.gov/oha/PH/DISEASESCONDITIONS/CHRONICDISEASE/MEDICALMARIJUANAPROGRAM/Pages/data.aspx. Accessed 1 Dec 2017

36. Medicinal Marijuana Program. State of New Jersey Department of Health. http://www.nj.gov/health/medicalmarijuana/. Accessed 1 Dec 2017

37. Medical Marijuana-Reports. Arizona Department of Health Services. http://www.azdhs.gov/licensing/medical-marijuana/index.php#reports. Accessed 1 Dec 2017

38. Medical Marijuana Patient Cardholder Registry Monthly Reports. Nevada Division of Public and Behavioral Health (DPBH). http://dpbh.nv.gov/Reg/MM-Patient-Cardholder-Registry/MM_Patient_Cardholder_Registry_-_Home/. Accessed 1 Dec 2017

39. Michigan Medical Marihuana Act Statistical Reports. The Michigan Department of Licensing and Regulatory Affairs, Bureau of Medical Marihuana Regulation. http://www.michigan.gov/lara/0,4601,7-154-79571_82631-448788%2D-,00.html. Accessed 1 Dec 2017

40. el-Mallakh RS (1987) Marijuana and migraine. Headache 27:442–443

41. Grinspoon L, Bakalar JB (1993) Marihuana: the forbidden medicine. Yale University, New Haven

42. Volfe Z, Dvilansky A, Nathan I (1985) Cannabinoids block release of serotonin from platelets induced by plasma from migraine patients. Int J Clin Pharmacol Res 5:243–246

43. el-Mallakh RS (1989) Migraine headaches and drug abuse. South Med J 82:805

44. Schnelle M, Grotenhermen F, Reif M, Gorter RW (1999) Results of a standardized survey on the medical use of cannabis products in the German-speaking area. Forsch Komplementarmed 6(Suppl 3):28–36

45. Gorji A (2003) Pharmacological treatment of headache using traditional Persian medicine. Trends Pharmacol Sci 24:331–334

46. Greco R, Gasperi V, Maccarrone M, Tassorelli C (2010) The endocannabinoid system and migraine. Exp Neurol 224:85–91

47. Rhyne DN, Anderson SL, Gedde M, Borgelt LM (2016) Effects of medical marijuana on migraine headache frequency in an adult population. Pharmacotherapy 36:505–510

48. Donovan M (1845) On the physical and medicinal qualities of Indian hemp (Cannabis Indica); with observations on the best mode of administration, and cases illustrative of its powers. Dublin J Med Sci 26:368–461

49. Reynolds JR (1868) On some of the therapeutical uses of Indian hemp. Arch Med 2:154–160

50. Waring EJ (1874) Practical therapeutics. Lindsay & Blakiston, Philadelphia

51. Russo E (2001) Hemp for headache: an in-depth historical and scientific review of cannabis in migraine treatment. J Cannabis Ther 1:21–92

52. Ringer S (1886) A handbook of therapeutics. H.K. Lewis, London

53. Hare HA (1887) Clinical and physiological notes on the action of cannabis Indica. There Gaz 11:225–228

54. Suckling C (1891) On the therapeutic value of Indian hemp. Br Med J 2:11–12

55. Mikuriya TH (1991) Chronic migraine headache: five cases successfully treated with marinol and/or illicit cannabis. Schaffer Library of Drug Policy, Berkeley

56. Nicolodi M, Sandoval V, Terrine A. Therapeutic use of cannabinoids - dose finding, effects, and pilot data of effects in chronic migraine and cluster headache. Abstract presentation at 3rd congress of the European Academy of Neurology (EAN), Amsterdam, 2017

57. Robbins MS, Tarshish S, Solomon S, Grosberg BM (2009) Cluster attacks responsive to recreational cannabis and dronabinol. Headache 49:914–916

58. Leroux E, Taifas I, Valade D, Donnet A, Chagnon M, Ducros A (2013) Use of cannabis among 139 cluster headache sufferers. Cephalalgia 33:208–213

59. Donnet A, Lanteri-Minet M, Guegan-Massardier E et al (2007) Chronic cluster headache: a French clinical descriptive study. J Neurol Neurosurg Psychiatry 78:1354–1358

60. Noyes R Jr, Baram DA (1974) Cannabis analgesia. Compr Psychiatry 15:531–535

61. Nunberg H, Kilmer B, Pacula RL, Burgdorf J (2011) An analysis of applicants presenting to a medical marijuana specialty practice in California. J Drug Policy Anal 4(1):1-14

62. Pini LA, Guerzoni S, Cainazzo MM et al (2012) Nabilone for the treatment of medication overuse headache: results of a preliminary double-blind, active-controlled, randomized trial. J Headache Pain 13:677–684

63. Evans RW, Ramadan NM (2004) Are cannabis-based chemicals helpful in headache? Headache 44:726–727

64. Consroe P, Musty R, Rein J, Tillery W, Pertwee R (1997) The perceived effects of smoked cannabis on patients with multiple sclerosis. Eur Neurol 38:44–48

65. Lochte BC, Beletsky A, Samuel NK, Grant I (2017) The use of cannabis for headache disorders. Cannabis Cannabinoid Res 2:61–71

66. A Multicenter, Randomized, Double-blind, Parallel-group, Placebo-controlled, Efficacy, Safety and Tolerability Study of Dronabinol MDI in the Acute Treatment of Migraine Headache. ClinicalTrials.gov Identifier: NCT00123201. Global Clinical Director Solvay Pharmaceuticals. https://clinicaltrials.gov/ct2/show/study/NCT00123201. Accessed 15 Dec 2017

67. Lipton RB, Dodick D, Sadovsky R et al (2003) A self-administered screener for migraine in primary care: the ID migraine validation study. Neurology 61:375–382

68. Akerman S, Holland PR, Lasalandra MP, Goadsby PJ (2013) Endocannabinoids in the brainstem modulate dural trigeminovascular

nociceptive traffic via CB1 and "triptan" receptors: implications in migraine. J Neurosci 33:14869–14877

69. Akerman S, Holland PR, Goadsby PJ (2007) Cannabinoid (CB1) receptor activation inhibits trigeminovascular neurons. J Pharmacol Exp Ther 320:64–71

70. Akerman S, Kaube H, Goadsby PJ (2004) Anandamide is able to inhibit trigeminal neurons using an in vivo model of trigeminovascular-mediated nociception. J Pharmacol Exp Ther 309:56–63

71. Serrano A, Parsons LH (2011) Endocannabinoid influence in drug reinforcement, dependence and addiction-related behaviors. Pharmacol Ther 132:215–241

72. Rodriguez de Fonseca F, Del Arco I, Bermudez-Silva FJ, Bilbao A, Cippitelli A, Navarro M (2005) The endocannabinoid system: physiology and pharmacology. Alcohol Alcohol 40:2–14

73. Maccarrone M, Gasperi V, Catani MV et al (2010) The endocannabinoid system and its relevance for nutrition. Annu Rev Nutr 30:423–440

74. Howlett AC (2004) Efficacy in CB1 receptor-mediated signal transduction. Br J Pharmacol 142:1209–1218

75. Mallat A, Teixeira-Clerc F, Deveaux V, Manin S, Lotersztajn S (2011) The endocannabinoid system as a key mediator during liver diseases: new insights and therapeutic openings. Br J Pharmacol 163:1432–1440

76. Galve-Roperh I, Rueda D, Gomez del Pulgar T, Velasco G, Guzman M (2002) Mechanism of extracellular signal-regulated kinase activation by the CB(1) cannabinoid receptor. Mol Pharmacol 62:1385–1392

77. Ryberg E, Larsson N, Sjogren S et al (2007) The orphan receptor GPR55 is a novel cannabinoid receptor. Br J Pharmacol 152:1092–1101

78. De Petrocellis L, Di Marzo V (2009) An introduction to the endocannabinoid system: from the early to the latest concepts. Best Pract Res Clin Endocrinol Metab 23:1–15

79. Devane WA, Hanus L, Breuer A et al (1992) Isolation and structure of a brain constituent that binds to the cannabinoid receptor. Science 258:1946–1949

80. Battista N, Di Tommaso M, Bari M, Maccarrone M (2012) The endocannabinoid system: an overview. Front Behav Neurosci 6:9

81. Di Marzo V, Piscitelli F, Mechoulam R (2011) Cannabinoids and endocannabinoids in metabolic disorders with focus on diabetes. Handb Exp Pharmacol (203):75–104. https://doi.org/10.1007/978-3-642-17214-4_4

82. Di Marzo V, Petrocellis LD (2006) Plant, synthetic, and endogenous cannabinoids in medicine. Annu Rev Med 57:553–574

83. Pertwee RG (2008) The diverse CB1 and CB2 receptor pharmacology of three plant cannabinoids: delta9-tetrahydrocannabinol, cannabidiol and delta9-tetrahydrocannabivarin. Br J Pharmacol 153:199–215

84. Guindon J, Hohmann AG (2009) The endocannabinoid system and pain. CNS Neurol Disord Drug Targets 8:403–421

85. Guindon J, Beaulieu P (2009) The role of the endogenous cannabinoid system in peripheral analgesia. Curr Mol Pharmacol 2:134–139

86. Kraft B (2012) Is there any clinically relevant cannabinoid-induced analgesia? Pharmacology 89:237–246

87. Ramikie TS, Nyilas R, Bluett RJ et al (2014) Multiple mechanistically distinct modes of endocannabinoid mobilization at central amygdala glutamatergic synapses. Neuron 81:1111–1125

88. Grant I, Atkinson JH, Gouaux B, Wilsey B (2012) Medical marijuana: clearing away the smoke. Open Neurol J 6:18–25

89. Pertwee RG, Howlett AC, Abood ME et al (2010) International Union of Basic and Clinical Pharmacology. LXXIX. Cannabinoid receptors and their ligands: beyond CB(1) and CB(2). Pharmacol Rev 62:588–631

90. Katona I, Freund TF (2008) Endocannabinoid signaling as a synaptic circuit breaker in neurological disease. Nat Med 14:923–930

91. Raichlen DA, Foster AD, Gerdeman GL, Seillier A, Giuffrida A (2012) Wired to run: exercise-induced endocannabinoid signaling in humans and cursorial mammals with implications for the 'runner's high'. J Exp Biol 215:1331–1336

92. Iversen L (2003) Cannabis and the brain. Brain 126:1252–1270

93. Napchan U, Buse DC, Loder EW (2011) The use of marijuana or synthetic cannabinoids for the treatment of headache. Headache 51:502–505

94. Mackie K (2008) Signaling via CNS cannabinoid receptors. Mol Cell Endocrinol 286:S60–S65

95. Klein TW, Cabral GA (2006) Cannabinoid-induced immune suppression and modulation of antigen-presenting cells. J Neuroimmune Pharmacol 1:50–64

96. Zhang HY, Gao M, Liu QR et al (2014) Cannabinoid CB2 receptors modulate midbrain dopamine neuronal activity and dopamine-related behavior in mice. Proc Natl Acad Sci U S A 111:E5007–E5015

97. Zhang HY, Gao M, Shen H et al (2017) Expression of functional cannabinoid CB2 receptor in VTA dopamine neurons in rats. Addict Biol 22:752–765

98. Gould J (2015) The cannabis crop. Nature 525:S2–S3

99. Andre CM, Hausman JF, Guerriero G (2016) Cannabis sativa: the plant of the thousand and one molecules. Front Plant Sci 7:19

100. Russo EB (2011) Taming THC: potential cannabis synergy and phytocannabinoid-terpenoid entourage effects. Br J Pharmacol 163:1344–1364

101. Pertwee RG (2010) Receptors and channels targeted by synthetic cannabinoid receptor agonists and antagonists. Curr Med Chem 17:1360–1381

102. Hajos N, Ledent C, Freund TF (2001) Novel cannabinoid-sensitive receptor mediates inhibition of glutamatergic synaptic transmission in the hippocampus. Neuroscience 106:1–4

103. Govaerts SJ, Hermans E, Lambert DM (2004) Comparison of cannabinoid ligands affinities and efficacies in murine tissues and in transfected cells expressing human recombinant cannabinoid receptors. Eur J Pharm Sci 23:233–243

104. Marcu JP (2016) An overview of major and minor phytocannabinoids. In: Preedy V (ed) Neuropathology of drug addictions and substance misuse, Volume 1: foundations of understanding, tobacco, alcohol, cannabinoids and opioids. Academic Press, London, pp 672–678

105. O'Sullivan SE, Kendall DA, Randall MD (2009) Time-dependent vascular effects of endocannabinoids mediated by peroxisome proliferator-activated receptor gamma (PPARgamma). PPAR Res 2009:425289

106. O'Sullivan SE, Kendall DA (2010) Cannabinoid activation of peroxisome proliferator-activated receptors: potential for modulation of inflammatory disease. Immunobiology 215:611–616

107. De Petrocellis L, Orlando P, Moriello AS et al (2012) Cannabinoid actions at TRPV channels: effects on TRPV3 and TRPV4 and their potential relevance to gastrointestinal inflammation. Acta Physiol (Oxf) 204:255–266

108. De Petrocellis L, Vellani V, Schiano-Moriello A et al (2008) Plant-derived cannabinoids modulate the activity of transient receptor potential channels of ankyrin type-1 and melastatin type-8. J Pharmacol Exp Ther 325:1007–1015

109. De Petrocellis L, Di Marzo V (2010) Non-CB1, non-CB2 receptors for endocannabinoids, plant cannabinoids, and synthetic cannabimimetics: focus on G-protein-coupled receptors and transient receptor potential channels. J Neuroimmune Pharmacol 5:103–121

110. De Petrocellis L, Ligresti A, Moriello AS et al (2011) Effects of cannabinoids and cannabinoid-enriched Cannabis extracts on TRP channels and endocannabinoid metabolic enzymes. Br J Pharmacol 163:1479–1494

111. Barann M, Molderings G, Bruss M, Bonisch H, Urban BW, Gothert M (2002) Direct inhibition by cannabinoids of human 5-HT3A receptors: probable involvement of an allosteric modulatory site. Br J Pharmacol 137:589–596

112. Hejazi N, Zhou C, Oz M, Sun H, Ye JH, Zhang L (2006) Delta9-tetrahydrocannabinol and endogenous cannabinoid anandamide directly potentiate the function of glycine receptors. Mol Pharmacol 69:991–997

113. McHugh D, Page J, Dunn E, Bradshaw HB (2012) Delta(9)-tetrahydrocannabinol and N-arachidonyl glycine are full agonists at GPR18 receptors and induce migration in human endometrial HEC-1B cells. Br J Pharmacol 165:2414–2424

114. Hampson AJ, Grimaldi M, Axelrod J, Wink D (1998) Cannabidiol and (–)Delta9-tetrahydrocannabinol are neuroprotective antioxidants. Proc Natl Acad Sci U S A 95:8268–8273

115. Hampson AJ, Bornheim LM, Scanziani M et al (1998) Dual effects of anandamide on NMDA receptor-mediated responses and neurotransmission. J Neurochem 70:671–676

116. Hampson AJ, Grimaldi M, Lolic M, Wink D, Rosenthal R, Axelrod J (2000) Neuroprotective antioxidants from marijuana. Ann N Y Acad Sci 899:274–282

117. Li J, Daughters RS, Bullis C et al (1999) The cannabinoid receptor agonist WIN 55,212-2 mesylate blocks the development of hyperalgesia produced by capsaicin in rats. Pain 81:25–33

118. Russo EB, Jiang HE, Li X et al (2008) Phytochemical and genetic analyses of ancient cannabis from Central Asia. J Exp Bot 59:4171–4182

119. Russo EB (2008) Cannabinoids in the management of difficult to treat pain. Ther Clin Risk Manag 4:245–259

120. Fine PG, Rosenfeld MJ (2013) The endocannabinoid system, cannabinoids, and pain. Rambam Maimonides Med J 4:e0022

121. Welch SP (1993) Blockade of cannabinoid-induced antinociception by norbinaltorphimine, but not N,N-diallyl-tyrosine-Aib-phenylalanine-leucine, ICI 174,864 or naloxone in mice. J Pharmacol Exp Ther 265:633–640

122. Smith FL, Cichewicz D, Martin ZL, Welch SP (1998) The enhancement of morphine antinociception in mice by delta9-tetrahydrocannabinol. Pharmacol Biochem Behav 60:559–566

123. Smith PA, Selley DE, Sim-Selley LJ, Welch SP (2007) Low dose combination of morphine and delta9-tetrahydrocannabinol circumvents antinociceptive tolerance and apparent desensitization of receptors. Eur J Pharmacol 571:129–137

124. Cichewicz DL, McCarthy EA (2003) Antinociceptive synergy between delta(9)-tetrahydrocannabinol and opioids after oral administration. J Pharmacol Exp Ther 304:1010–1015

125. Cichewicz DL (2004) Synergistic interactions between cannabinoid and opioid analgesics. Life Sci 74:1317–1324

126. Manzanares J, Corchero J, Romero J, Fernandez-Ruiz JJ, Ramos JA, Fuentes JA (1998) Chronic administration of cannabinoids regulates proenkephalin mRNA levels in selected regions of the rat brain. Brain Res Mol Brain Res 55: 126–132

127. Manzanares J, Julian M, Carrascosa A (2006) Role of the cannabinoid system in pain control and therapeutic implications for the management of acute and chronic pain episodes. Curr Neuropharmacol 4:239–257

128. Evans FJ (1991) Cannabinoids: the separation of central from peripheral effects on a structural basis. Planta Med 57:S60–S67

129. Brown AJ (2007) Novel cannabinoid receptors. Br J Pharmacol 152:567–575

130. Izzo AA, Borrelli F, Capasso R, Di Marzo V, Mechoulam R (2009) Non-psychotropic plant cannabinoids: new therapeutic opportunities from an ancient herb. Trends Pharmacol Sci 30:515–527

131. Rahn EJ, Hohmann AG (2009) Cannabinoids as pharmacotherapies for neuropathic pain: from the bench to the bedside. Neurotherapeutics 6:713–737

132. Pacher P, Batkai S, Kunos G (2006) The endocannabinoid system as an emerging target of pharmacotherapy. Pharmacol Rev 58:389–462

133. Noyes R Jr, Brunk SF, Avery DA, Canter AC (1975) The analgesic properties of delta-9-tetrahydrocannabinol and codeine. Clin Pharmacol Ther 18:84–89

134. Noyes R Jr, Brunk SF, Baram DA, Canter A (1975) Analgesic effect of delta-9-tetrahydrocannabinol. J Clin Pharmacol 15:139–143

135. Schley M, Legler A, Skopp G, Schmelz M, Konrad C, Rukwied R (2006) Delta-9-THC based monotherapy in fibromyalgia patients on experimentally induced pain, axon reflex flare, and pain relief. Curr Med Res Opin 22:1269–1276

136. Maurer M, Henn V, Dittrich A, Hofmann A (1990) Delta-9-tetrahydrocannabinol shows antispastic and analgesic effects in a single case double-blind trial. Eur Arch Psychiatry Clin Neurosci 240:1–4

137. Srivastava MD, Srivastava BI, Brouhard B (1998) Delta9 tetrahydrocannabinol and cannabidiol alter cytokine production by human immune cells. Immunopharmacology 40:179–185

138. Kozela E, Pietr M, Juknat A, Rimmerman N, Levy R, Vogel Z (2010) Cannabinoids Delta(9)-tetrahydrocannabinol and cannabidiol differentially inhibit the lipopolysaccharide-activated NF-kappaB and interferon-beta/STAT proinflammatory pathways in BV-2 microglial cells. J Biol Chem 285:1616–1626

139. Barrie N, Manolios N (2017) The endocannabinoid system in pain and inflammation: its relevance to rheumatic disease. Eur J Rheumatol 4: 210–218

140. Ruhaak LR, Felth J, Karlsson PC, Rafter JJ, Verpoorte R, Bohlin L (2011) Evaluation of the cyclooxygenase inhibiting effects of six major cannabinoids isolated from cannabis sativa. Biol Pharm Bull 34:774–778

141. Martin BR, Compton DR, Thomas BF et al (1991) Behavioral, biochemical, and molecular modeling evaluations of cannabinoid analogs. Pharmacol Biochem Behav 40:471–478

142. Martin BR, Lichtman AH (1998) Cannabinoid transmission and pain perception. Neurobiol Dis 5:447–461

143. DeLong GT, Wolf CE, Poklis A, Lichtman AH (2010) Pharmacological evaluation of the natural constituent of cannabis sativa, cannabichromene and its modulation by Delta(9)-tetrahydrocannabinol. Drug Alcohol Depend 112:126–133

144. Zygmunt PM, Andersson DA, Hogestatt ED (2002) Delta 9-tetrahydrocannabinol and cannabinol activate capsaicin-sensitive sensory nerves via a CB1 and CB2 cannabinoid receptor-independent mechanism. J Neurosci 22:4720–4727

145. Burston JJ, Sagar DR, Shao P et al (2013) Cannabinoid CB2 receptors regulate central sensitization and pain responses associated with osteoarthritis of the knee joint. PLoS One 8:e80440

146. Gui H, Liu X, Wang ZW, He DY, Su DF, Dai SM (2014) Expression of cannabinoid receptor 2 and its inhibitory effects on synovial fibroblasts in rheumatoid arthritis. Rheumatology (Oxford) 53:802–809

147. Clayton N, Marshall FH, Bountra C, O'Shaughnessy CT (2002) CB1 and CB2 cannabinoid receptors are implicated in inflammatory pain. Pain 96:253–260

148. Nagarkatti P, Pandey R, Rieder SA, Hegde VL, Nagarkatti M (2009) Cannabinoids as novel anti-inflammatory drugs. Future Med Chem 1:1333–1349

149. Jensen B, Chen J, Furnish T, Wallace M (2015) Medical marijuana and chronic pain: a review of basic science and clinical evidence. Curr Pain Headache Rep 19:50

150. Weber J, Schley M, Casutt M et al (2009) Tetrahydrocannabinol (Delta 9-THC) treatment in chronic central neuropathic pain and fibromyalgia patients: results of a multicenter survey. Anesthesiol Res Pract 2009. https://doi.org/10.1155/2009/827290 Epub 2009 Oct 25

151. Weber M, Goldman B, Truniger S (2010) Tetrahydrocannabinol (THC) for cramps in amyotrophic lateral sclerosis: a randomised, double-blind crossover trial. J Neurol Neurosurg Psychiatry 81:1135–1140

152. Smith PB, Martin BR (1992) Spinal mechanisms of delta 9-tetrahydrocannabinol-induced analgesia. Brain Res 578:8–12

153. Smith FL, Fujimori K, Lowe J, Welch SP (1998) Characterization of delta9-tetrahydrocannabinol and anandamide antinociception in nonarthritic and arthritic rats. Pharmacol Biochem Behav 60:183–191

154. Walker JM, Huang SM (2002) Cannabinoid analgesia. Pharmacol Ther 95:127–135

155. Walker JM, Strangman NM, Huang SM (2001) Cannabinoids and pain. Pain Res Manag 6:74–79

156. Walker JM, Hohmann AG, Martin WJ, Strangman NM, Huang SM, Tsou K (1999) The neurobiology of cannabinoid analgesia. Life Sci 65:665–673

157. Ware MA, Wang T, Shapiro S et al (2010) Smoked cannabis for chronic neuropathic pain: a randomized controlled trial. CMAJ 182:E694–E701

158. Wilsey B, Marcotte T, Deutsch R, Gouaux B, Sakai S, Donaghe H (2013) Low-dose vaporized cannabis significantly improves neuropathic pain. J Pain 14: 136–148

159. Wilsey B, Marcotte T, Tsodikov A et al (2008) A randomized, placebo-controlled, crossover trial of cannabis cigarettes in neuropathic pain. J Pain 9:506–521

160. Ellis RJ, Toperoff W, Vaida F et al (2009) Smoked medicinal cannabis for neuropathic pain in HIV: a randomized, crossover clinical trial. Neuropsychopharmacology 34:672–680

161. Abrams DI, Jay CA, Shade SB et al (2007) Cannabis in painful HIV-associated sensory neuropathy: a randomized placebo-controlled trial. Neurology 68: 515–521

162. Corey-Bloom J, Wolfson T, Gamst A et al (2012) Smoked cannabis for spasticity in multiple sclerosis: a randomized, placebo-controlled trial. CMAJ 184:1143–1150

163. Wallace MS, Marcotte TD, Umlauf A, Gouaux B, Atkinson JH (2015) Efficacy of inhaled cannabis on painful diabetic neuropathy. J Pain 16:616–627

164. Wallace M, Schulteis G, Atkinson JH et al (2007) Dose-dependent effects of smoked cannabis on capsaicin-induced pain and hyperalgesia in healthy volunteers. Anesthesiology 107:785–796

165. Greenwald MK, Stitzer ML (2000) Antinociceptive, subjective and behavioral effects of smoked marijuana in humans. Drug Alcohol Depend 59:261–275

166. Abrams DI, Couey P, Shade SB, Kelly ME, Benowitz NL (2011) Cannabinoid-opioid interaction in chronic pain. Clin Pharmacol Ther 90:844–851

167. Eisenberg E, Ogintz M, Almog S (2014) The pharmacokinetics, efficacy, safety, and ease of use of a novel portable metered-dose cannabis inhaler in patients with chronic neuropathic pain: a phase 1a study. J Pain Palliat Care Pharmacother 28:216–225

168. Ware MA, Wang T, Shapiro S, Collet JP (2015) COMPASS study team. Cannabis for the Management of Pain: Assessment of Safety Study (COMPASS). J Pain 16:1233–1242

169. Fiz J, Duran M, Capella D, Carbonell J, Farre M (2011) Cannabis use in patients with fibromyalgia: effect on symptoms relief and health-related quality of life. PLoS One 6:e18440

170. Ben-Shabat S, Fride E, Sheskin T et al (1998) An entourage effect: inactive endogenous fatty acid glycerol esters enhance 2-arachidonoyl-glycerol cannabinoid activity. Eur J Pharmacol 353:23–31

171. Nurmikko TJ, Serpell MG, Hoggart B, Toomey PJ, Morlion BJ, Haines D (2007) Sativex successfully treats neuropathic pain characterised by allodynia: a randomised, double-blind, placebo-controlled clinical trial. Pain 133:210–220

172. Rog DJ, Nurmikko TJ, Young CA (2007) Oromucosal delta9-tetrahydrocannabinol/cannabidiol for neuropathic pain associated with multiple sclerosis: an uncontrolled, open-label, 2-year extension trial. Clin Ther 29:2068–2079

173. Rog DJ, Nurmikko TJ, Friede T, Young CA (2005) Randomized, controlled trial of cannabis-based medicine in central pain in multiple sclerosis. Neurology 65:812–819

174. Blake DR, Robson P, Ho M, Jubb RW, McCabe CS (2006) Preliminary assessment of the efficacy, tolerability and safety of a cannabis-based medicine (Sativex) in the treatment of pain caused by rheumatoid arthritis. Rheumatology (Oxford) 45:50–52

175. Serpell MG, Notcutt W, Collin C (2013) Sativex long-term use: an open-label trial in patients with spasticity due to multiple sclerosis. J Neurol 260:285–295

176. Wade DT, Makela PM, House H, Bateman C, Robson P (2006) Long-term use of a cannabis-based medicine in the treatment of spasticity and other symptoms in multiple sclerosis. Mult Scler 12:639–645

177. Portenoy RK, Ganae-Motan ED, Allende S et al (2012) Nabiximols for opioid-treated cancer patients with poorly-controlled chronic pain: a randomized, placebo-controlled, graded-dose trial. J Pain 13:438–449

178. Wade DT, Robson P, House H, Makela P, Aram J (2003) A preliminary controlled study to determine whether whole-plant cannabis extracts can improve intractable neurogenic symptoms. Clin Rehabil 17:21–29

179. Notcutt W, Price M, Miller R et al (2004) Initial experiences with medicinal extracts of cannabis for chronic pain: results from 34 'N of 1' studies. Anaesthesia 59:440–452

180. Notcutt W, Langford R, Davies P, Ratcliffe S, Potts R (2012) A placebo-controlled, parallel-group, randomized withdrawal study of subjects with symptoms of spasticity due to multiple sclerosis who are receiving long-term Sativex(R) (nabiximols). Mult Scler 18:219–228

181. Berman JS, Symonds C, Birch R (2004) Efficacy of two cannabis based medicinal extracts for relief of central neuropathic pain from brachial plexus avulsion: results of a randomised controlled trial. Pain 112:299–306

182. Langford RM, Mares J, Novotna A et al (2013) A double-blind, randomized, placebo-controlled, parallel-group study of THC/CBD oromucosal spray in combination with the existing treatment regimen, in the relief of central neuropathic pain in patients with multiple sclerosis. J Neurol 260:984–997

183. Johnson JR, Burnell-Nugent M, Lossignol D, Ganae-Motan ED, Potts R, Fallon MT (2010) Multicenter, double-blind, randomized, placebo-controlled, parallel-group study of the efficacy, safety, and tolerability of THC:CBD extract and THC extract in patients with intractable cancer-related pain. J Pain Symptom Manag 39:167–179

184. Johnson JR, Lossignol D, Burnell-Nugent M, Fallon MT (2013) An open-label extension study to investigate the long-term safety and tolerability of THC/CBD oromucosal spray and oromucosal THC spray in patients with terminal cancer-related pain refractory to strong opioid analgesics. J Pain Symptom Manag 46:207–218

185. Zajicek JP, Sanders HP, Wright DE et al (2005) Cannabinoids in multiple sclerosis (CAMS) study: safety and efficacy data for 12 months follow up. J Neurol Neurosurg Psychiatry 76:1664–1669

186. Zajicek JP, Apostu VI (2011) Role of cannabinoids in multiple sclerosis. CNS Drugs 25:187–201

187. Zajicek JP, Hobart JC, Slade A, Barnes D, Mattison PG, MUSEC Research Group (2012) Multiple sclerosis and extract of cannabis: results of the MUSEC trial. J Neurol Neurosurg Psychiatry 83:1125–1132

188. Zajicek J, Fox P, Sanders H et al (2003) Cannabinoids for treatment of spasticity and other symptoms related to multiple sclerosis (CAMS study): multicentre randomised placebo-controlled trial. Lancet 362:1517–1526

189. Vaney C, Heinzel-Gutenbrunner M, Jobin P et al (2004) Efficacy, safety and tolerability of an orally administered cannabis extract in the treatment of spasticity in patients with multiple sclerosis: a randomized, double-blind, placebo-controlled, crossover study. Mult Scler 10:417–424

190. Collin C, Davies P, Mutiboko IK, Ratcliffe S, Sativex Spasticity in MS Study Group (2007) Randomized controlled trial of cannabis-based medicine in spasticity caused by multiple sclerosis. Eur J Neurol 14:290–296

191. Collin C, Ehler E, Waberzinek G et al (2010) A double-blind, randomized, placebo-controlled, parallel-group study of Sativex, in subjects with symptoms of spasticity due to multiple sclerosis. Neurol Res 32:451–459

192. Wade DT, Makela P, Robson P, House H, Bateman C (2004) Do cannabis-based medicinal extracts have general or specific effects on symptoms in multiple sclerosis? A double-blind, randomized, placebo-controlled study on 160 patients. Mult Scler 10:434–441

193. Serpell M, Ratcliffe S, Hovorka J et al (2014) A double-blind, randomized, placebo-controlled, parallel group study of THC/CBD spray in peripheral neuropathic pain treatment. Eur J Pain 18:999–1012

194. Syed YY, McKeage K, Scott LJ (2014) Delta-9-tetrahydrocannabinol/cannabidiol (Sativex(R)): a review of its use in patients with moderate to severe spasticity due to multiple sclerosis. Drugs 74:563–578

195. Lakhan SE, Rowland M (2009) Whole plant cannabis extracts in the treatment of spasticity in multiple sclerosis: a systematic review. BMC Neurol 9:59

196. Barnes MP (2006) Sativex: clinical efficacy and tolerability in the treatment of symptoms of multiple sclerosis and neuropathic pain. Expert Opin Pharmacother 7:607–615

197. GW Pharmaceuticals. Sativex product monograph., 2010

198. Holdcroft A, Maze M, Dore C, Tebbs S, Thompson S (2006) A multicenter dose-escalation study of the analgesic and adverse effects of an oral cannabis extract (Cannador) for postoperative pain management. Anesthesiology 104:1040–1046

199. Sallan SE, Zinberg NE, Frei E 3rd (1975) Antiemetic effect of delta-9-tetrahydrocannabinol in patients receiving cancer chemotherapy. N Engl J Med 293:795–797

200. Sallan SE, Cronin C, Zelen M, Zinberg NE (1980) Antiemetics in patients receiving chemotherapy for cancer: a randomized comparison of delta-9-tetrahydrocannabinol and prochlorperazine. N Engl J Med 302:135–138

201. Vinciguerra V, Moore T, Brennan E (1988) Inhalation marijuana as an antiemetic for cancer chemotherapy. N Y State J Med 88:525–527

202. Carey MP, Burish TG, Brenner DE (1983) Delta-9-tetrahydrocannabinol in cancer chemotherapy: research problems and issues. Ann Intern Med 99:106–114

203. Lucas VS Jr, Laszlo J (1980) delta 9-tetrahydrocannabinol for refractory vomiting induced by cancer chemotherapy. JAMA 243:1241–1243

204. Frytak S, Moertel CG, O'Fallon JR et al (1979) Delta-9-tetrahydrocannabinol as an antiemetic for patients receiving cancer chemotherapy. A comparison with prochlorperazine and a placebo. Ann Intern Med 91:825–830

205. Ungerleider JT, Andrysiak T, Fairbanks L, Goodnight J, Sarna G, Jamison K (1982) Cannabis and cancer chemotherapy: a comparison of oral delta-9-THC and prochlorperazine. Cancer 50:636–645

206. Orr LE, McKernan JF, Bloome B (1980) Antiemetic effect of tetrahydrocannabinol. Compared with placebo and prochlorperazine in chemotherapy-associated nausea and emesis. Arch Intern Med 140:1431–1433

207. Orr LE, McKernan JF (1981) Antiemetic effect of delta 9-tetrahydrocannabinol in chemotherapy-associated nausea and emesis as compared to placebo and compazine. J Clin Pharmacol 21:76S–80S

208. Levitt M, Wilson A, Bowman D et al (1981) Physiologic observations in a controlled clinical trial of the antiemetic effectiveness of 5, 10, and 15 mg of delta 9-tetrahydrocannabinol in cancer chemotherapy. Ophthalmologic implications. J Clin Pharmacol 21:103S–109S

209. McCabe M, Smith FP, Macdonald JS, Woolley PV, Goldberg D, Schein PS (1988) Efficacy of tetrahydrocannabinol in patients refractory to standard antiemetic therapy. Investig New Drugs 6:243–246

210. Niiranen A, Mattson K (1985) A cross-over comparison of nabilone and prochlorperazine for emesis induced by cancer chemotherapy. Am J Clin Oncol 8:336–340

211. Herman TS, Einhorn LH, Jones SE et al (1979) Superiority of nabilone over prochlorperazine as an antiemetic in patients receiving cancer chemotherapy. N Engl J Med 300:1295–1297

212. Vincent BJ, McQuiston DJ, Einhorn LH, Nagy CM, Brames MJ (1983) Review of cannabinoids and their antiemetic effectiveness. Drugs 25(Suppl 1):52–62

213. Einhorn L (1982) Nabilone: an effective antiemetic agent in patients receiving cancer chemotherapy. Cancer Treat Rev 9(Suppl B):55–61

214. Einhorn LH, Nagy C, Furnas B, Williams SD (1981) Nabilone: an effective antiemetic in patients receiving cancer chemotherapy. J Clin Pharmacol 21:64S–69S

215. Ahmedzai S, Carlyle DL, Calder IT, Moran F (1983) Anti-emetic efficacy and toxicity of nabilone, a synthetic cannabinoid, in lung cancer chemotherapy. Br J Cancer 48:657–663

216. Garb S, Beers AL, Bograd M et al (1980) Two-pronged study of tetrahydrocannabinol (THC) prevention of vomiting for cancer chemotherapy. IRCS Med Sci 8:203–204

217. Lane M, Smith FE, Sullivan RA, Plasse TF (1990) Dronabinol and prochlorperazine alone and in combination as antiemetic agents for cancer chemotherapy. Am J Clin Oncol 13:480–484

218. Lane M, Vogel CL, Ferguson J et al (1991) Dronabinol and prochlorperazine in combination for treatment of cancer chemotherapy-induced nausea and vomiting. J Pain Symptom Manag 6:352–359

219. Plasse TF, Gorter RW, Krasnow SH, Lane M, Shepard KV, Wadleigh RG (1991) Recent clinical experience with dronabinol. Pharmacol Biochem Behav 40:695–700

220. Cunningham D, Forrest GJ, Soukop M, Gilchrist NL, Calder IT, McArdle CS (1985) Nabilone and prochlorperazine: a useful combination for emesis induced by cytotoxic drugs. Br Med J (Clin Res Ed) 291:864–865

221. Gonzalez-Rosales F, Walsh D (1997) Intractable nausea and vomiting due to gastrointestinal mucosal metastases relieved by tetrahydrocannabinol (dronabinol). J Pain Symptom Manag 14:311–314

222. Chang AE, Shiling DJ, Stillman RC et al (1979) Delata-9-tetrahydrocannabinol as an antiemetic in cancer patients receiving high-dose methotrexate. A prospective, randomized evaluation. Ann Intern Med 91:819–824

223. Staquet M, Bron D, Rozencweig M, Kenis Y (1981) Clinical studies with a THC analog (BRL-4664) in the prevention of cisplatin-induced vomiting. J Clin Pharmacol 21:60S–63S

224. Sharkey KA, Darmani NA, Parker LA (2014) Regulation of nausea and vomiting by cannabinoids and the endocannabinoid system. Eur J Pharmacol 722:134–146

225. Parker LA, Rock EM, Limebeer CL (2011) Regulation of nausea and vomiting by cannabinoids. Br J Pharmacol 163:1411–1422

226. Tramer MR, Carroll D, Campbell FA, Reynolds DJ, Moore RA, McQuay HJ (2001) Cannabinoids for control of chemotherapy induced nausea and vomiting: quantitative systematic review. BMJ 323:16–21

227. Sutton IR, Daeninck P (2006) Cannabinoids in the management of intractable chemotherapy-induced nausea and vomiting and cancer-related pain. J Support Oncol 4:531–535

228. Pisanti S, Malfitano AM, Grimaldi C et al (2009) Use of cannabinoid receptor agonists in cancer therapy as palliative and curative agents. Best Pract Res Clin Endocrinol Metab 23:117–131

229. Tortorice PV, O'Connell MB (1990) Management of chemotherapy-induced nausea and vomiting. Pharmacotherapy 10:129–145

230. Cunningham D, Bradley J, Forrest GJ et al (1988) A randomized trial of oral nabilone and prochlorperazine compared to intravenous metoclopramide and dexamethasone in the treatment of nausea and vomiting induced by chemotherapy regimens containing cisplatin or cisplatin analogues. Eur J Cancer Clin Oncol 24:685–689

231. Soderpalm AH, Schuster A, de Wit H (2001) Antiemetic efficacy of smoked marijuana: subjective and behavioral effects on nausea induced by syrup of ipecac. Pharmacol Biochem Behav 69:343–350

232. Machado Rocha FC, Stefano SC, De Cassia Haiek R, Rosa Oliveira LM, Da Silveira DX (2008) Therapeutic use of cannabis sativa on chemotherapy-induced nausea and vomiting among cancer patients: systematic review and meta-analysis. Eur J Cancer Care (Engl) 17:431–443

233. Musty R, Rossi R (2001) Effects of smoked cannabis and oral delta-9-tetrahydrocannabinol on nausea and emesis after cancer chemotherapy: a review of state clinical trials. J Cannabis Ther 1:29–42

234. Meiri E, Jhangiani H, Vredenburgh JJ et al (2007) Efficacy of dronabinol alone and in combination with ondansetron versus ondansetron alone for delayed chemotherapy-induced nausea and vomiting. Curr Med Res Opin 23:533–543

235. Ekert H, Waters KD, Jurk IH, Mobilia J, Loughnan P (1979) Amelioration of cancer chemotherapy-induced nausea and vomiting by delta-9-tetrahydrocannabinol. Med J Aust 2:657–659

236. Pertwee RG (2012) Targeting the endocannabinoid system with cannabinoid receptor agonists: pharmacological strategies and therapeutic possibilities. Philos Trans R Soc Lond Ser B Biol Sci 367:3353–3363

237. Rock EM, Connolly C, Limebeer CL, Parker LA (2016) Effect of combined oral doses of Delta(9)-tetrahydrocannabinol (THC) and cannabidiolic acid (CBDA) on acute and anticipatory nausea in rat models. Psychopharmacology 233:3353–3360

238. Green ST, Nathwani D, Goldberg DJ, Kennedy DH (1989) Nabilone as effective therapy for intractable nausea and vomiting in AIDS. Br J Clin Pharmacol 28:494–495

239. Chan HS, Correia JA, MacLeod SM (1987) Nabilone versus prochlorperazine for control of cancer chemotherapy-induced emesis in children: a double-blind, crossover trial. Pediatrics 79:946–952

240. Dalzell AM, Bartlett H, Lilleyman JS (1986) Nabilone: an alternative antiemetic for cancer chemotherapy. Arch Dis Child 61:502–505

241. Abrahamov A, Abrahamov A, Mechoulam R (1995) An efficient new cannabinoid antiemetic in pediatric oncology. Life Sci 56:2097–2102

242. Abbott Products Inc. Marinol product monograph., 2010

243. Valeant Canada. Cesamet product monograph., 2009

244. Narang S, Gibson D, Wasan AD et al (2008) Efficacy of dronabinol as an adjuvant treatment for chronic pain patients on opioid therapy. J Pain 9:254–264

245. Svendsen KB, Jensen TS, Bach FW (2005) Effect of the synthetic cannabinoid dronabinol on central pain in patients with multiple sclerosis–secondary publication. Ugeskr Laeger 167:2772–2774

246. Svendsen KB, Jensen TS, Bach FW (2004) Does the cannabinoid dronabinol reduce central pain in multiple sclerosis? Randomised double blind placebo controlled crossover trial. BMJ 329:253

247. Skrabek RQ, Galimova L, Ethans K, Perry D (2008) Nabilone for the treatment of pain in fibromyalgia. J Pain 9:164–173

248. Naef M, Curatolo M, Petersen-Felix S, Arendt-Nielsen L, Zbinden A, Brenneisen R (2003) The analgesic effect of oral delta-9-tetrahydrocannabinol (THC), morphine, and a THC-morphine combination in healthy subjects under experimental pain conditions. Pain 105:79–88

249. Pinsger M, Schimetta W, Volc D, Hiermann E, Riederer F, Polz W (2006) Benefits of an add-on treatment with the synthetic cannabinomimetic nabilone on patients with chronic pain–a randomized controlled trial. Wien Klin Wochenschr 118:327–335

250. Wissel J, Haydn T, Muller J et al (2006) Low dose treatment with the synthetic cannabinoid Nabilone significantly reduces spasticity-related pain : a double-blind placebo-controlled cross-over trial. J Neurol 253:1337–1341

251. Toth C, Mawani S, Brady S et al (2012) An enriched-enrolment, randomized withdrawal, flexible-dose, double-blind, placebo-controlled, parallel assignment efficacy study of nabilone as adjuvant in the treatment of diabetic peripheral neuropathic pain. Pain 153:2073–2082

252. Turcotte D, Doupe M, Torabi M et al (2015) Nabilone as an adjunctive to gabapentin for multiple sclerosis-induced neuropathic pain: a randomized controlled trial. Pain Med 16:149–159

253. Notcutt WG, Price M, Chapman G (1997) Clinical experience with nabilone for chronic pain. Pharm Sci 3:551–555

254. Hamann W, di Vadi PP (1999) Analgesic effect of the cannabinoid analogue nabilone is not mediated by opioid receptors. Lancet 353:560

255. Berlach DM, Shir Y, Ware MA (2006) Experience with the synthetic cannabinoid nabilone in chronic noncancer pain. Pain Med 7:25–29

256. Martyn CN, Illis LS, Thom J (1995) Nabilone in the treatment of multiple sclerosis. Lancet 345:579

257. Cannabidiol (CBD) Pre-Review Report. World Health Organization: Expert Committee on Drug Dependence. http://www.who.int/medicines/access/controlled-substances/5.2_CBD.pdf. Accessed 20 Dec 2017

258. "Prohibited List: January 2018". The World Anti-Doping Code International Standard. World Anti-Doping Agency (WADA). https://www.wada-ama.org/sites/default/files/prohibited_list_2018_en.pdf. Accessed 23 Apr 2018

259. Zuardi AW (2008) Cannabidiol: from an inactive cannabinoid to a drug with wide spectrum of action. Rev Bras Psiquiatr 30:271–280

260. Mechoulam R, Parker LA, Gallily R (2002) Cannabidiol: an overview of some pharmacological aspects. J Clin Pharmacol 42:11S–19S

261. Pagano E, Capasso R, Piscitelli F et al (2016) An orally active Cannabis extract with high content in cannabidiol attenuates chemically-induced intestinal inflammation and hypermotility in the mouse. Front Pharmacol 7:341

262. Mechoulam R, Peters M, Murillo-Rodriguez E, Hanus LO (2007) Cannabidiol–recent advances. Chem Biodivers 4:1678–1692

263. Malfait AM, Gallily R, Sumariwalla PF et al (2000) The nonpsychoactive cannabis constituent cannabidiol is an oral anti-arthritic therapeutic in murine collagen-induced arthritis. Proc Natl Acad Sci U S A 97:9561–9566

264. Formukong EA, Evans AT, Evans FJ (1988) Analgesic and antiinflammatory activity of constituents of cannabis sativa L. Inflammation 12:361–371

265. Formukong EA, Evans AT, Evans FJ (1989) The medicinal uses of cannabis and its constituents. Phytother Res 3:219–231

266. Costa B, Trovato AE, Comelli F, Giagnoni G, Colleoni M (2007) The non-psychoactive cannabis constituent cannabidiol is an orally effective therapeutic agent in rat chronic inflammatory and neuropathic pain. Eur J Pharmacol 556:75–83

267. Costa B, Colleoni M, Conti S et al (2004) Oral anti-inflammatory activity of cannabidiol, a non-psychoactive constituent of cannabis, in acute carrageenan-induced inflammation in the rat paw. Naunyn Schmiedeberg's Arch Pharmacol 369:294–299

268. Booz GW (2011) Cannabidiol as an emergent therapeutic strategy for lessening the impact of inflammation on oxidative stress. Free Radic Biol Med 51:1054–1061

269. McHugh D, Tanner C, Mechoulam R, Pertwee RG, Ross RA (2008) Inhibition of human neutrophil chemotaxis by endogenous cannabinoids and phytocannabinoids: evidence for a site distinct from CB1 and CB2. Mol Pharmacol 73:441–450

270. Zhornitsky S, Potvin S (2012) Cannabidiol in humans-the quest for therapeutic targets. Pharmaceuticals (Basel) 5:529–552

271. Ribeiro A, Almeida VI, Costola-de-Souza C et al (2015) Cannabidiol improves lung function and inflammation in mice submitted to LPS-induced acute lung injury. Immunopharmacol Immunotoxicol 37:35–41

272. Ribeiro A, Ferraz-de-Paula V, Pinheiro ML et al (2012) Cannabidiol, a non-psychotropic plant-derived cannabinoid, decreases inflammation in a murine model of acute lung injury: role for the adenosine A(2A) receptor. Eur J Pharmacol 678:78–85

273. Kozela E, Lev N, Kaushansky N et al (2011) Cannabidiol inhibits pathogenic T cells, decreases spinal microglial activation and ameliorates multiple sclerosis-like disease in C57BL/6 mice. Br J Pharmacol 163:1507–1519

274. Mecha M, Feliu A, Inigo PM, Mestre L, Carrillo-Salinas FJ, Guaza C (2013) Cannabidiol provides long-lasting protection against the deleterious effects of inflammation in a viral model of multiple sclerosis: a role for A2A receptors. Neurobiol Dis 59:141–150

275. Mecha M, Torrao AS, Mestre L, Carrillo-Salinas FJ, Mechoulam R, Guaza C (2012) Cannabidiol protects oligodendrocyte progenitor cells from inflammation-induced apoptosis by attenuating endoplasmic reticulum stress. Cell Death Dis 3:e331

276. Thomas A, Baillie GL, Phillips AM, Razdan RK, Ross RA, Pertwee RG (2007) Cannabidiol displays unexpectedly high potency as an antagonist of CB1 and CB2 receptor agonists in vitro. Br J Pharmacol 150:613–623

277. Comelli F, Bettoni I, Colleoni M, Giagnoni G, Costa B (2009) Beneficial effects of a cannabis sativa extract treatment on diabetes-induced neuropathy and oxidative stress. Phytother Res 23:1678–1684

278. Comelli F, Giagnoni G, Bettoni I, Colleoni M, Costa B (2008) Antihyperalgesic effect of a cannabis sativa extract in a rat model of neuropathic pain: mechanisms involved. Phytother Res 22:1017–1024

279. Kohli DR, Li Y, Khasabov SG et al (2010) Pain-related behaviors and neurochemical alterations in mice expressing sickle hemoglobin: modulation by cannabinoids. Blood 116:456–465

280. Howard J, Anie KA, Holdcroft A, Korn S, Davies SC (2005) Cannabis use in sickle cell disease: a questionnaire study. Br J Haematol 131:123–128

281. Maione S, Piscitelli F, Gatta L et al (2011) Non-psychoactive cannabinoids modulate the descending pathway of antinociception in anaesthetized rats through several mechanisms of action. Br J Pharmacol 162:584–596

282. Williamson EM, Evans FJ (2000) Cannabinoids in clinical practice. Drugs 60:1303–1314

283. Russo E, Guy GW (2006) A tale of two cannabinoids: the therapeutic rationale for combining tetrahydrocannabinol and cannabidiol. Med Hypotheses 66:234–246

284. Murillo-Rodriguez E, Millan-Aldaco D, Palomero-Rivero M, Mechoulam R, Drucker-Colin R (2006) Cannabidiol, a constituent of cannabis sativa, modulates sleep in rats. FEBS Lett 580:4337–4345

285. Nicholson AN, Turner C, Stone BM, Robson PJ (2004) Effect of Delta-9-tetrahydrocannabinol and cannabidiol on nocturnal sleep and early-morning behavior in young adults. J Clin Psychopharmacol 24:305–313

286. Zuardi AW, Hallak JE, Crippa JA (2012) Interaction between cannabidiol (CBD) and (9)-tetrahydrocannabinol (THC): influence of administration interval and dose ratio between the cannabinoids. Psychopharmacology 219:247–249

287. Zuardi AW, Shirakawa I, Finkelfarb E, Karniol IG (1982) Action of cannabidiol on the anxiety and other effects produced by delta 9-THC in normal subjects. Psychopharmacology 76:245–250

288. Zuardi AW, Finkelfarb E, Bueno OF, Musty RE, Karniol IG (1981) Characteristics of the stimulus produced by the mixture of cannabidiol with delta 9-tetrahydrocannabinol. Arch Int Pharmacodyn Ther 249:137–146

289. Bisogno T, Hanus L, De Petrocellis L et al (2001) Molecular targets for cannabidiol and its synthetic analogues: effect on vanilloid VR1 receptors and on the cellular uptake and enzymatic hydrolysis of anandamide. Br J Pharmacol 134:845–852

290. Ligresti A, Moriello AS, Starowicz K et al (2006) Antitumor activity of plant cannabinoids with emphasis on the effect of cannabidiol on human breast carcinoma. J Pharmacol Exp Ther 318:1375–1387

291. Ahrens J, Demir R, Leuwer M et al (2009) The nonpsychotropic cannabinoid cannabidiol modulates and directly activates alpha-1 and alpha-1-Beta glycine receptor function. Pharmacology 83:217–222

292. Qin N, Neeper MP, Liu Y, Hutchinson TL, Lubin ML, Flores CM (2008) TRPV2 is activated by cannabidiol and mediates CGRP release in cultured rat dorsal root ganglion neurons. J Neurosci 28:6231–6238

293. Ross HR, Napier I, Connor M (2008) Inhibition of recombinant human T-type calcium channels by Delta9-tetrahydrocannabinol and cannabidiol. J Biol Chem 283:16124–16134

294. Jenny M, Santer E, Pirich E, Schennach H, Fuchs D (2009) Delta9-tetrahydrocannabinol and cannabidiol modulate mitogen-induced tryptophan degradation and neopterin formation in peripheral blood mononuclear cells in vitro. J Neuroimmunol 207:75–82

295. Evans AT, Formukong E, Evans FJ (1987) Activation of phospholipase A2 by cannabinoids. Lack of correlation with CNS effects. FEBS Lett 211:119–122

296. Russo EB, Burnett A, Hall B, Parker KK (2005) Agonistic properties of cannabidiol at 5-HT1a receptors. Neurochem Res 30:1037–1043

297. Drysdale AJ, Ryan D, Pertwee RG, Platt B (2006) Cannabidiol-induced intracellular Ca2+ elevations in hippocampal cells. Neuropharmacology 50:621–631

298. Ryan D, Drysdale AJ, Lafourcade C, Pertwee RG, Platt B (2009) Cannabidiol targets mitochondria to regulate intracellular Ca2+ levels. J Neurosci 29:2053–2063

299. Carrier EJ, Auchampach JA, Hillard CJ (2006) Inhibition of an equilibrative nucleoside transporter by cannabidiol: a mechanism of cannabinoid immunosuppression. Proc Natl Acad Sci U S A 103:7895–7900

300. O'Sullivan SE, Sun Y, Bennett AJ, Randall MD, Kendall DA (2009) Time-dependent vascular actions of cannabidiol in the rat aorta. Eur J Pharmacol 612:61–68

301. Takeda S, Usami N, Yamamoto I, Watanabe K (2009) Cannabidiol-2′,6′-dimethyl ether, a cannabidiol derivative, is a highly potent and selective 15-lipoxygenase inhibitor. Drug Metab Dispos 37:1733–1737

302. Walter L, Franklin A, Witting A et al (2003) Nonpsychotropic cannabinoid receptors regulate microglial cell migration. J Neurosci 23:1398–1405

303. Rock EM, Kopstick RL, Limebeer CL, Parker LA (2013) Tetrahydrocannabinolic acid reduces nausea-induced conditioned gaping in rats and vomiting in Suncus murinus. Br J Pharmacol 170:641–648

304. Takeda S, Misawa K, Yamamoto I, Watanabe K (2008) Cannabidiolic acid as a selective cyclooxygenase-2 inhibitory component in cannabis. Drug Metab Dispos 36:1917–1921

305. Bolognini D, Rock EM, Cluny NL et al (2013) Cannabidiolic acid prevents vomiting in Suncus murinus and nausea-induced behaviour in rats by enhancing 5-HT1A receptor activation. Br J Pharmacol 168:1456–1470

306. Buchbauer G, Bohusch R (2015) Biological activities of essential oils: an update. In: Husnu Can Baser K, Buchbauer G (eds) Handbook of essential oils: science, technology, and applications, 2nd edn. CRC Press, Boca Raton, pp 281–322

307. Bowles EJ (2004) The chemistry of aromatherapeutic oils. Allen & Unwin, Crows Nest

308. Paduch R, Kandefer-Szerszen M, Trytek M, Fiedurek J (2007) Terpenes: substances useful in human healthcare. Arch Immunol Ther Exp 55:315–327

309. Noma Y, Asakawa Y (2010) Biotransformation of monoterpenoids by microorganisms, insects, and mammals. In: Baser KHC, Buchbauer G (eds) Handbook of essential oils: science, technology, and applications. CRC Press, Boca Raton, pp 585–736

310. Rufino AT, Ribeiro M, Judas F et al (2014) Anti-inflammatory and chondroprotective activity of (+)-alpha-pinene: structural and enantiomeric selectivity. J Nat Prod 77:264–269

311. Neves A, Rosa S, Goncalves J et al (2010) Screening of five essential oils for identification of potential inhibitors of IL-1-induced Nf-kappaB activation and NO production in human chondrocytes: characterization of the inhibitory activity of alpha-pinene. Planta Med 76:303–308

312. Gil ML, Jimenez J, Ocete MA, Zarzuelo A, Cabo MM (1989) Comparative study of different essential oils of bupleurum gibraltaricum lamarck. Pharmazie 44:284–287

313. Him A, Ozbek H, Turel I, Oner AC (2008) Antinociceptive activity of α-pinene and fenchone. Pharmacol Online 3:363–369

314. Van Cleemput M, Cattoor K, De Bosscher K, Haegeman G, De Keukeleire D, Heyerick A (2009) Hop (Humulus lupulus)-derived bitter acids as multipotent bioactive compounds. J Nat Prod 72:1220–1230

315. Lorenzetti BB, Souza GE, Sarti SJ, Santos Filho D, Ferreira SH (1991) Myrcene mimics the peripheral analgesic activity of lemongrass tea. J Ethnopharmacol 34:43–48

316. Rao VS, Menezes AM, Viana GS (1990) Effect of myrcene on nociception in mice. J Pharm Pharmacol 42:877–878

317. do Vale TG, Furtado EC, Santos JG Jr, Viana GS (2002) Central effects of citral, myrcene and limonene, constituents of essential oil chemotypes from lippia alba (Mill.) n.e. brown. Phytomedicine 9:709–714

318. Bisset NG, Wichtl M (2004) Herbal drugs and phytopharmaceuticals: a handbook for practice on a scientific basis, 3rd edn. Medpharm Scientific Publishers: Stuttgart; CRC Press, Boca Raton

319. Souza MC, Siani AC, Ramos MF, Menezes-de-Lima OJ, Henriques MG (2003) Evaluation of anti-inflammatory activity of essential oils from two Asteraceae species. Pharmazie 58:582–586

320. Rufino AT, Ribeiro M, Sousa C et al (2015) Evaluation of the anti-inflammatory, anti-catabolic and pro-anabolic effects of E-caryophyllene, myrcene and limonene in a cell model of osteoarthritis. Eur J Pharmacol 750:141–150

321. Piccinelli AC, Santos JA, Konkiewitz EC et al (2015) Antihyperalgesic and antidepressive actions of (R)-(+)-limonene, alpha-phellandrene, and essential oil from Schinus terebinthifolius fruits in a neuropathic pain model. Nutr Neurosci 18:217–224

322. Hirota R, Roger NN, Nakamura H, Song HS, Sawamura M, Suganuma N (2010) Anti-inflammatory effects of limonene from yuzu (Citrus junos Tanaka) essential oil on eosinophils. J Food Sci 75:H87–H92

323. Chaudhary SC, Siddiqui MS, Athar M, Alam MS (2012) D-limonene modulates inflammation, oxidative stress and Ras-ERK pathway to inhibit murine skin tumorigenesis. Hum Exp Toxicol 31:798–811

324. d'Alessio PA, Ostan R, Bisson JF, Schulzke JD, Ursini MV, Bene MC (2013) Oral administration of d-limonene controls inflammation in rat colitis and displays anti-inflammatory properties as diet supplementation in humans. Life Sci 92:1151–1156

325. Kim MJ, Yang KW, Kim SS et al (2014) Chemical composition and anti-inflammation activity of essential oils from citrus unshiu flower. Nat Prod Commun 9:727–730

326. Komori T, Fujiwara R, Tanida M, Nomura J, Yokoyama MM (1995) Effects of citrus fragrance on immune function and depressive states. Neuroimmunomodulation 2:174–180

327. de Almeida AA, Costa JP, de Carvalho RB, de Sousa DP, de Freitas RM (2012) Evaluation of acute toxicity of a natural compound (+)-limonene epoxide and its anxiolytic-like action. Brain Res 1448:56–62

328. Carvalho-Freitas MI, Costa M (2002) Anxiolytic and sedative effects of extracts and essential oil from citrus aurantium L. Biol Pharm Bull 25:1629–1633

329. Pultrini Ade M, Galindo LA, Costa M (2006) Effects of the essential oil from citrus aurantium L. in experimental anxiety models in mice. Life Sci 78:1720–1725

330. Saiyudthong S, Marsden CA (2011) Acute effects of bergamot oil on anxiety-related behaviour and corticosterone level in rats. Phytother Res 25: 858–862

331. Pimenta FC, Alves MF, Pimenta MB et al (2016) Anxiolytic effect of citrus aurantium L. on patients with chronic myeloid leukemia. Phytother Res 30: 613–617

332. Komiya M, Takeuchi T, Harada E (2006) Lemon oil vapor causes an anti-stress effect via modulating the 5-HT and DA activities in mice. Behav Brain Res 172:240–249

333. Peana AT, D'Aquila PS, Chessa ML, Moretti MD, Serra G, Pippia P (2003) (−)-linalool produces antinociception in two experimental models of pain. Eur J Pharmacol 460:37–41

334. Peana AT, D'Aquila PS, Panin F, Serra G, Pippia P, Moretti MD (2002) Anti-inflammatory activity of linalool and linalyl acetate constituents of essential oils. Phytomedicine 9:721–726

335. Peana AT, Marzocco S, Popolo A, Pinto A (2006) (−)-linalool inhibits in vitro NO formation: probable involvement in the antinociceptive activity of this monoterpene compound. Life Sci 78:719–723

336. de Sousa DP, Nobrega FF, Santos CC, de Almeida RN (2010) Anticonvulsant activity of the linalool enantiomers and racemate: investigation of chiral influence. Nat Prod Commun 5:1847–1851

337. Elisabetsky E, Marschner J, Souza DO (1995) Effects of linalool on glutamatergic system in the rat cerebral cortex. Neurochem Res 20:461–465

338. Ismail M (2006) Central properties and chemical composition of Ocimum basilicum essential oil. Pharm Biol 44:619–626

339. Silva Brum LF, Emanuelli T, Souza DO, Elisabetsky E (2001) Effects of linalool on glutamate release and uptake in mouse cortical synaptosomes. Neurochem Res 26:191–194

340. Nunes DS, Linck VM, da Silva AL, Figueiro M, Elisabetsky E (2010) Psychopharmacology of essential oils. In: Baser KHC, Buchbauer G (eds) Handbook of essential oils: science, technology, and applications. CRC Press, Boca Raton, pp 297–314

341. Nakamura A, Fujiwara S, Matsumoto I, Abe K (2009) Stress repression in restrained rats by (R)-(−)-linalool inhalation and gene expression profiling of their whole blood cells. J Agric Food Chem 57:5480–5485

342. Russo EB (2001) Handbook of psychotropic herbs: a scientific analysis of herbal remedies for psychiatric conditions. Haworth Press, Binghamton

343. Cline M, Taylor JE, Flores J, Bracken S, McCall S, Ceremuga TE (2008) Investigation of the anxiolytic effects of linalool, a lavender extract, in the male Sprague-Dawley rat. AANA J 76:47–52

344. Cheng BH, Sheen LY, Chang ST (2014) Evaluation of anxiolytic potency of essential oil and S-(+)-linalool from Cinnamomum osmophloeum ct. linalool leaves in mice. J Tradit Complement Med 5:27–34

345. Buchbauer G, Jirovetz L, Jager W, Dietrich H, Plank C (1991) Aromatherapy: evidence for sedative effects of the essential oil of lavender after inhalation. Z Naturforsch C 46:1067–1072

346. Jirovetz L, Buchbauer G, Jager W, Woidich A, Nikiforov A (1992) Analysis of fragrance compounds in blood samples of mice by gas chromatography, mass spectrometry, GC/FTIR and GC/AES after inhalation of sandalwood oil. Biomed Chromatogr 6:133–134

347. Buchbauer G, Jirovetz L, Jager W, Plank C, Dietrich H (1993) Fragrance compounds and essential oils with sedative effects upon inhalation. J Pharm Sci 82:660–664

348. Re L, Barocci S, Sonnino S et al (2000) Linalool modifies the nicotinic receptor-ion channel kinetics at the mouse neuromuscular junction. Pharmacol Res 42:177–182

349. Ghelardini C, Galeotti N, Salvatore G, Mazzanti G (1999) Local anaesthetic activity of the essential oil of lavandula angustifolia. Planta Med 65:700–703

350. Peana AT, Rubattu P, Piga GG et al (2006) Involvement of adenosine A1 and A2A receptors in (−)-linalool-induced antinociception. Life Sci 78:2471–2474

351. Batista PA, Werner MF, Oliveira EC et al (2008) Evidence for the involvement of ionotropic glutamatergic receptors on the antinociceptive effect of (−)-linalool in mice. Neurosci Lett 440:299–303

352. Kim JT, Ren CJ, Fielding GA et al (2007) Treatment with lavender aromatherapy in the post-anesthesia care unit reduces opioid requirements of morbidly obese patients undergoing laparoscopic adjustable gastric banding. Obes Surg 17:920–925

353. Klauke AL, Racz I, Pradier B et al (2014) The cannabinoid CB(2) receptor-selective phytocannabinoid beta-caryophyllene exerts analgesic effects in mouse models of inflammatory and neuropathic pain. Eur Neuropsychopharmacol 24:608–620

354. Passos GF, Fernandes ES, da Cunha FM et al (2007) Anti-inflammatory and anti-allergic properties of the essential oil and active compounds from Cordia verbenacea. J Ethnopharmacol 110:323–333

355. Rogerio AP, Andrade EL, Leite DF, Figueiredo CP, Calixto JB (2009) Preventive and therapeutic anti-inflammatory properties of the sesquiterpene alpha-humulene in experimental airways allergic inflammation. Br J Pharmacol 158:1074–1087

356. Medeiros R, Passos GF, Vitor CE et al (2007) Effect of two active compounds obtained from the essential oil of cordia verbenacea on the acute inflammatory responses elicited by LPS in the rat paw. Br J Pharmacol 151: 618–627

357. Horvath B, Mukhopadhyay P, Kechrid M et al (2012) beta-caryophyllene ameliorates cisplatin-induced nephrotoxicity in a cannabinoid 2 receptor-dependent manner. Free Radic Biol Med 52:1325–1333

358. Ghelardini C, Galeotti N, Di Cesare Mannelli L, Mazzanti G, Bartolini A (2001) Local anaesthetic activity of beta-caryophyllene. Farmaco 56:387–389

359. Basile AC, Sertie JA, Freitas PC, Zanini AC (1988) Anti-inflammatory activity of oleoresin from Brazilian Copaifera. J Ethnopharmacol 22:101–109

360. Ozturk A, Ozbek H (2005) The anti-inflammatory activity of Eugenia caryophyllata essential oil: an animal model of anti-inflammatory activity. Eur J Gen Med 2:159–163

361. Apel MA, Lima ME, Sobral M et al (2010) Anti-inflammatory activity of essential oil from leaves of Myrciaria tenella and Calycorectes sellowianus. Pharm Biol 48:433–438

362. Al Mansouri S, Ojha S, Al Maamari E, Al Ameri M, Nurulain SM, Bahi A (2014) The cannabinoid receptor 2 agonist, beta-caryophyllene, reduced voluntary alcohol intake and attenuated ethanol-induced place preference and sensitivity in mice. Pharmacol Biochem Behav 124:260–268

363. Gertsch J (2008) Anti-inflammatory cannabinoids in diet: towards a better understanding of CB(2) receptor action? Commun Integr Biol 1:26–28

364. Gertsch J, Leonti M, Raduner S et al (2008) Beta-caryophyllene is a dietary cannabinoid. Proc Natl Acad Sci U S A 105:9099–9104

365. Bahi A, Al Mansouri S, Al Memari E, Al Ameri M, Nurulain SM, Ojha S (2014) beta-caryophyllene, a CB2 receptor agonist produces multiple behavioral changes relevant to anxiety and depression in mice. Physiol Behav 135:119–124

366. Fernandes ES, Passos GF, Medeiros R et al (2007) Anti-inflammatory effects of compounds alpha-humulene and (–)-trans-caryophyllene isolated from the essential oil of Cordia verbenacea. Eur J Pharmacol 569:228–236

367. Chaves JS, Leal PC, Pianowisky L, Calixto JB (2008) Pharmacokinetics and tissue distribution of the sesquiterpene alpha-humulene in mice. Planta Med 74:1678–1683

368. Binet L, Binet P, Miocque M, Roux M, Bernier A (1972) Reserches sur les proprietes pharmcodynamiques (action sedative et action spasmolytique) de quelques alcools terpeniques aliphatiques. Ann Pharm Fr 30:611–616

369. Maurya AK, Singh M, Dubey V, Srivastava S, Luqman S, Bawankule DU (2014) Alpha-(–)-Bisabolol reduces pro-inflammatory cytokine production and ameliorates skin inflammation. Curr Pharm Biotechnol 15:173–181

370. Nurulain S, Prytkova T, Sultan AM et al (2015) Inhibitory actions of bisabolol on alpha7-nicotinic acetylcholine receptors. Neuroscience 306:91–99

371. Fischedick JT, Hazekamp A, Erkelens T, Choi YH, Verpoorte R (2010) Metabolic fingerprinting of cannabis sativa L., cannabinoids and terpenoids for chemotaxonomic and drug standardization purposes. Phytochemistry 71:2058–2073

372. Hillig KW (2004) A chemotaxonomic analysis of terpenoid variation in Cannabis. Biochem Syst Ecol 32:875–891

373. Hillig KW, Mahlberg PG (2004) A chemotaxonomic analysis of cannabinoid variation in cannabis (Cannabaceae). Am J Bot 91:966–975

374. Sawler J, Stout JM, Gardner KM et al (2015) The genetic structure of marijuana and hemp. PLoS One 10:e0133292

375. Lucas P, Walsh Z (2017) Medical cannabis access, use, and substitution for prescription opioids and other substances: a survey of authorized medical cannabis patients. Int J Drug Policy 42:30–35

376. Lucas P, Walsh Z, Crosby K et al (2016) Substituting cannabis for prescription drugs, alcohol and other substances among medical cannabis patients: the impact of contextual factors. Drug Alcohol Rev 35:326–333

377. Lucas P (2017) Rationale for cannabis-based interventions in the opioid overdose crisis. Harm Reduct J 14:58. https://doi.org/10.1186/s12954-017-0183-9

378. Nielsen S, Sabioni P, Trigo JM et al (2017) Opioid-sparing effect of cannabinoids: a systematic review and meta-analysis. Neuropsychopharmacology 42:1752–1765

379. Bushlin I, Rozenfeld R, Devi LA (2010) Cannabinoid-opioid interactions during neuropathic pain and analgesia. Curr Opin Pharmacol 10:80–86

380. Parolaro D, Rubino T, Vigano D, Massi P, Guidali C, Realini N (2010) Cellular mechanisms underlying the interaction between cannabinoid and opioid system. Curr Drug Targets 11:393–405

381. Welch SP, Stevens DL (1992) Antinociceptive activity of intrathecally administered cannabinoids alone, and in combination with morphine, in mice. J Pharmacol Exp Ther 262:10–18

382. Pugh G Jr, Smith PB, Dombrowski DS, Welch SP (1996) The role of endogenous opioids in enhancing the antinociception produced by the combination of delta 9-tetrahydrocannabinol and morphine in the spinal cord. J Pharmacol Exp Ther 279:608–616

383. Cichewicz DL, Welch SP, Smith FL (2005) Enhancement of transdermal fentanyl and buprenorphine antinociception by transdermal delta9-tetrahydrocannabinol. Eur J Pharmacol 525:74–82

384. Cichewicz DL, Martin ZL, Smith FL, Welch SP (1999) Enhancement mu opioid antinociception by oral delta9-tetrahydrocannabinol: dose-response analysis and receptor identification. J Pharmacol Exp Ther 289:859–867

385. Collen M (2012) Prescribing cannabis for harm reduction. Harm Reduct J 9:1

386. Haroutounian S, Ratz Y, Ginosar Y et al (2016) The effect of medicinal cannabis on pain and quality-of-life outcomes in chronic pain: a prospective open-label study. Clin J Pain 32:1036–1043

387. Boehnke KF, Litinas E, Clauw DJ (2016) Medical cannabis use is associated with decreased opiate medication use in a retrospective cross-sectional survey of patients with chronic pain. J Pain 17:739–744

388. Livingston MD, Barnett TE, Delcher C, Wagenaar AC (2017) Recreational cannabis legalization and opioid-related deaths in Colorado, 2000-2015. Am J Public Health 107:1827–1829

389. Scavone JL, Sterling RC, Weinstein SP, Van Bockstaele EJ (2013) Impact of cannabis use during stabilization on methadone maintenance treatment. Am J Addict 22:344–351

390. Raby WN, Carpenter KM, Rothenberg J et al (2009) Intermittent marijuana use is associated with improved retention in naltrexone treatment for opiate-dependence. Am J Addict 18:301–308

391. Bachhuber MA, Saloner B, Cunningham CO, Barry CL (2014) Medical cannabis laws and opioid analgesic overdose mortality in the United States, 1999-2010. JAMA Intern Med 174:1668–1673

14

Factors associated with acute medication overuse in people with migraine: results from the 2017 migraine in America symptoms and treatment (MAST) study

Todd J. Schwedt[1*], Aftab Alam[2], Michael L. Reed[3], Kristina M. Fanning[3], Sagar Munjal[2], Dawn C. Buse[4], David W. Dodick[1] and Richard B. Lipton[5]

Abstract

Background: The MAST Study is a longitudinal, cross-sectional survey study of US adults with migraine. These analyses were conducted to estimate rates of acute medication overuse (AMO) and determine associations of AMO with individual and headache characteristics.

Methods: Eligible respondents had ICHD-3-beta migraine, reported ≥3 monthly headache days (MHDs) in the past 3 months, ≥1 MHD in the past 30 days, and currently took acute headache medication. AMO was defined according to ICHD-3-beta thresholds for monthly days of medication taking when diagnosing medication overuse headache.

Results: Eligible respondents ($N = 13,649$) had a mean age of 43.4 ± 13.6 years; most were female (72.9%) and Caucasian (81.9%). Altogether, 15.4% of respondents met criteria for AMO. Compared with those not overusing medications, respondents with AMO were significantly more likely to be taking triptans (31.3% vs 14.2%), opioids (23.8% vs 8.0%), barbiturates (7.8% vs 2.7%), and ergot alkaloids (3.1% vs 0.6%) and significantly less likely to be taking NSAIDs (63.3% vs 69.8%) ($p < 0.001$ for all comparisons). Respondents with AMO had significantly more MHDs (12.9 ± 8.6 vs 4.3 ± 4.3, $p < 0.001$); higher migraine symptom severity (17.8 ± 2.7 vs 16.4 ± 3.0, $p < 0.001$), higher pain intensity scores (7.4 vs 6.5, $p < 0.001$); and higher rates of cutaneous allodynia (53.7% vs 37.5%, $p < 0.001$). Adjusted for MHDs, the odds of AMO were increased by each additional year of age (OR 1.02, 95% CI 1.02, 1.03); being married (OR 1.19, 95% CI 1.06, 1.34); smoking (OR 1.54, 95% CI 1.31, 1.81); having psychological symptoms (OR 1.62, 95% CI 1.43, 1.83) or cutaneous allodynia (OR 1.22, 95% CI 1.08, 1.37); and greater migraine symptom severity (OR 1.06, 95% CI 1.04, 1.09) and pain intensity (OR 1.27, 95% CI 1.22, 1.32). Cutaneous allodynia increased the risk of AMO by 61% in males (OR 1.61, 95% CI 1.28, 2.03) but did not increase risk in females (OR 1.08, 95% CI 0.94, 1.25).

Conclusions: AMO was present in 15% of respondents with migraine. AMO was associated with higher symptom severity scores, pain intensity, and rates of cutaneous allodynia. AMO was more likely in triptan, opioid, and barbiturate users but less likely in NSAID users. Cutaneous allodynia was associated with AMO in men but not women. This gender difference merits additional exploration.

Keywords: Migraine, Medication overuse headache, Epidemiology, Adults, Allodynia

* Correspondence: schwedt.todd@mayo.edu
[1]Mayo Clinic, 5777 East Mayo Boulevard, Phoenix, AZ 85054, USA
Full list of author information is available at the end of the article

Background

Excessive use of acute therapies by individuals with headache has been recognized as a problem in the management of migraine for nearly 70 years [1]. According to the International Classification of Headache Disorders, Third Edition (ICHD-3), acute medication overuse (AMO) can accompany and complicate primary and secondary headaches, including migraine, tension-type headache, new daily persistent headache and posttraumatic headache, among others [2]. Although this state of using acute migraine medications too frequently is most commonly referred to as "medication overuse", the term "acute medication overuse" is used within this manuscript since this terminology more specifically describes the condition. Overuse of drugs within certain medication classes has been associated with an increased risk of transformation from episodic to chronic migraine [3–7]. AMO is associated with greater pain intensity and disability and worse 24 h pain relief outcomes in patients with chronic migraine [8, 9], as well as the development of a secondary headache disorder known as medication-overuse headache (MOH) — at least 15 monthly headache days (MHDs) in patients with a pre-existing primary headache and developing as a consequence of regular overuse of acute headache medication for more than 3 months [2]. The term MOH implies that the overused medication is the cause of the headaches. Herein, we use AMO to describe the behavior of medication taking above a certain threshold without assumptions about causing headaches.

In the general population, about 2% of people are believed to have AMO, but headache clinics report that 50% to 70% of their patients overuse medication [5, 10–14]. Previous research has identified a number of risk factors for AMO or MOH. These include being female [15, 16], having frequent headache attacks, smoking, physical inactivity, comorbid mental health conditions and low socioeconomic status among other factors [17–24]. Many acute headache medications have been associated with AMO and MOH [2], but the highest risks are seen with barbiturate containing combination analgesics and opioids [25, 26].

Previous analyses from the 2017 MAST Study estimated that that about 35% of US adults with migraine consider their usual acute treatment to be poor or very poor (unpublished). One quarter (23.6%) never/rarely become pain-free within 2 h of taking medication, and nearly one fifth (18%) get no relief from their usual acute medication (unpublished).

The objective of the current MAST Study analysis was to estimate rates of AMO in a nonclinic sample of people with migraine and to determine associations of AMO with demographic features, migraine characteristics, and comorbidities. In prior research [9], females were at significantly greater risk than males for allodynia, and

individuals with allodynia were at greater risk for AMO. Thus, we hypothesized that females would have greater odds of AMO.

Methods

Ethics

The information and consent form, as well as the MAST survey instrument, were reviewed by Ethical and Independent Review Services (Independence, MO), which granted an exemption under (45 CFR 46.101 [2]) and certified the exemption status of the MAST Study (#16106–01) on 31 August 2016. Before initiating the survey, respondents read a description of the study, confirmed that they understood the purpose and conduct of the study, and electronically signed informed consent to participate.

Study design

Details about the methodology of the MAST Study have been previously published [27]. In brief, the MAST Study is a longitudinal and cross-sectional survey study of US adults 18 years or older with migraine. The baseline assessment included sociodemographics and a battery of questions about headache features, medication use, unmet treatment needs, diagnosis and consultation, and treatment response. The follow up 6- and 12-month assessments will re-evaluate these same variables in baseline cohorts to measure headache symptom and frequency changes over time.

Stratified sampling methods were used to establish a sample of respondents representative of the US adult population in sex, age, household income, race, marital status, and US Census region. Respondent demographics were maintained within 5% of 2015 US Census data.

Recruiting and inclusion criteria

Study respondents were members of an internet research panel (Research Now, Plano, TX), which has 2.4 million active US members, that is generally representative of US demography. Panel members were invited to participate in a survey about health, and after consenting, they were asked to complete an initial screening survey that included demographics and a checklist of health conditions. Persons endorsing headache or migraine on the screening survey were evaluated with a symptom screening module that used ICHD-3 beta criteria for migraine. The symptom screening module, employed previously in the American Migraine Study (AMS) and the American Migraine Prevalence and Prevention Study (AMPP), is based on lifetime recall of symptoms associated with respondents' most severe headaches. The AMS/AMPP module captures pain characteristics (unilateral location, pulsating/throbbing quality, moderate to severe intensity); exacerbation by routine activity; and associated symptoms (nausea, phonophobia, and photophobia), and it has a sensitivity of 100% and specificity of 82% for episodic migraine diagnosis and sensitivity of 91% and specificity of 80% for chronic migraine diagnosis [28]. Respondents meeting AMS/AMPP symptom criteria for migraine were assessed for headache frequency, and those reporting 3 or more monthly headache days (MHDs) in the past 3 months and at least 1 MHD in the past 30 days satisfied frequency criteria, completed screening, and qualified for inclusion in the study.

Only respondents currently taking medication to treat their headaches who provided self-reported monthly treatment day frequency were included in these analyses. Respondents not using medications to treat headaches and those who did not know number of days per month medication was used were excluded from the analyses.

Assessments

The MAST Study baseline assessment used validated instruments where available. The main outcome, medication usage, was assessed by asking respondents if they were currently using prescription or nonprescription medication to treat headaches. Medications of interest for this study included simple analgesics, combination analgesics, triptans, nonsteroidal anti-inflammatory drugs (NSAIDs), barbiturates, opioids, isometheptene, and ergot alkaloids. AMO was defined according to medication use thresholds included in ICHD-3 beta diagnostic criteria for MOH [29]. AMO was considered present if a respondent reported using a triptan, opioid, barbiturate, isometheptene, ergot alkaloid medication, or combination analgesic on at least 10 days per month or an NSAID or simple analgesic on at least 15 days per month.

Covariates were obtained from single survey items and included sex (male or female); age (years); married (yes or no); education (< 4-year college degree or ≥ 4-year college degree); race (Caucasian or non-Caucasian); health insurance (yes or no); and total annual household income (<$25,000; $25,000–$49,999; $50,000–$74,999; $75,000–$99,999; and ≥ $100,000). Current tobacco use was assessed by asking respondents if they had smoked at least 100 cigarettes (lifetime recall) and if they currently smoked. Body mass index (BMI) was calculated by dividing weight in pounds by height in inches squared and multiplying by a conversion factor of 703; it is represented as a continuous variable and was used to categorize respondents as underweight (< 18.5), normal weight (18.5–24.9), overweight (25.0–29.9), and obese (≥ 30.0). Psychological symptoms (depression and/or anxiety) were based on 2-week recall and measured with the Patient Health Questionnaire for Depression and Anxiety (PHQ-4) [30].

MHD frequency was derived by asking about the number of headache days over the past 3 months (affected by headache for any part or the whole of the day), and dividing this number by 3. The MHD variable differentiated respondents using modified diagnostic criteria for episodic and chronic migraine (headache frequency of ≥ 15 MHDs for chronic and < 15 MHDs for episodic over the preceding 3 months). Chronic migraine was defined according to ICHD-3 beta criteria, but the requirement that 8 MHDs be migraine was excluded because participants would need to keep diaries and be individually interviewed, which is impractical in large population studies.

The presence of ictal cutaneous allodynia was assessed using the 12-item Allodynia Symptom Checklist (ASC-12) [31]. Migraine symptoms were measured with the Migraine Symptom Severity Scale (MSSS), a composite index that incorporates information about 7 headache features (unilateral pain, pulsatile pain, moderate or severe pain intensity, routine activities worsen pain, nausea, photophobia, phonophobia). The overall MSSS score ranges from 0 to 21 and was calculated by adding scores ranging from 0 to 3 for each of the 7 headache features assessed. Headache pain intensity was reported using a 0 to 10 scale, where 0 was no pain and 10 was the worst pain.

Statistical analysis

Data were from the MAST baseline survey. The objective of these analyses was to provide data on respondent populations with and without AMO. Differences in sociodemographics and headache features among those with AMO versus those without AMO were of interest. Percentages were used to report dichotomous variables, including sex, marital status, education, race, health insurance status, psychological symptoms, employment, current smoking status, and cutaneous allodynia. Percentages were used to report categorical variables, including age group, BMI category, household income, and MHDs. The chi-square test was used to identify statistically significant medication overuse differences for dichotomous or categorical variables. Mean ± SD was used to report continuous variables, including age, BMI, MSSS, and pain intensity. Independent-group t tests were used to evaluate significant differences for continuous variables.

Six binary logistic models were run, with AMO as the outcome. The first model included the sociodemographic variables sex, age, marital status, race, household income, education, BMI, health insurance status, and smoking status. Race, household income, and health insurance status produced nonsignificant p-values and were excluded from subsequent analyses. In the refined models, psychological symptomology (depression and/or anxiety) and headache features (pain intensity, MSSS, cutaneous allodynia, and MHDs) were added. Additional models explored the relationship of sex and the presence of cutaneous allodynia on medication overuse. To this end, a model was run including a sex-by-allodynia interaction and 2 separate models fully adjusted for sex. Odds ratios (OR) and 95% confidence intervals (CI) are shown. P-values less than 0.05 were considered statistically significant, and all statistical tests were two-tailed. To control for familywise error in the multiple comparisons on sociodemographics, we applied the conservative Bonferroni adjustment (alpha 0.05/number of statistical tests). All analyses were performed in IBM SPSS Statistics, version 20.0 (IBM, Armonk, NY; 2011).

Results

Analysis sample

MAST Study baseline data collection started in October 2016 and ended in January 2017. Of fielded surveys, 95,821 provided usable data, 18,363 respondents met symptom criteria for migraine, and 15,133 satisfied headache frequency criteria. In total, 13,649 respondents were taking medication to treat headaches and reported monthly frequency of treatment.

Sociodemographic characteristics

The sociodemographic profile of study respondents who met study criteria is shown in Table 1. Overall, the sample had a mean age of 43.4 ± 13.6 years and was predominantly comprised of females (72.9%) and Caucasians (81.9%). AMO criteria were met by 15.4% of the population. Respondents in the AMO group were significantly more likely than those who were not overusing medications to be taking every acute headache medication class with the exception of NSAIDs. NSAID use was less likely in persons with AMO (Fig. 1, $P < 0.001$ for all comparisons). Compared with respondents who did not overuse their headache medication, those in the AMO group were significantly older (45.8 ± 13.2 vs 43.0 ± 13.6 years, $p < 0.001$) and more likely to be male (29.5% vs 26.6%, $p < 0.01$), had higher BMI (28.9 ± 8.5 vs 28.1 ± 7.4, $p < 0.001$) and were more likely to be married (58.6% vs 54.3%, $p < 0.001$). Most respondents (58.8%) had at least a 4-year college degree, but persons in the AMO group were significantly less likely than those not overusing medications to have at least a 4-year college degree (51.7% vs 60.0%, $p < .001$). While only 11.3% of the sample smoked cigarettes, individuals reporting AMO were significantly more likely to be smokers than those not overusing medications (18.5% vs 10.0%, $p < 0.001$). As shown in Table 1, psychological symptoms affected 23.2% of respondents, and those in the AMO group were significantly more likely to have symptoms of depression and/or anxiety than respondents in the group not overusing medications (39.5% vs 20.2%, $p < 0.001$).

Headache features

Table 2 shows that respondents in the AMO group reported significantly more MHDs than those not overusing medications (12.9 ± 8.6 vs 4.3 ± 4.3, $p < 0.001$). The mean MSSS score of the total sample was 16.6 ± 3.0, and MSSS scores were significantly higher among those in the AMO group than in those not overusing medications (17.8 ± 2.7 vs 16.4 ± 3.0, $p < 0.001$). Allodynia was present in 40.0% of the total sample, and those in the AMO group were significantly more likely to be allodynic than individuals not overusing medications (53.7% vs 37.5%, $p < 0.001$). Pain intensity scores were significantly higher in the AMO group than in those not overusing medications (7.4 vs 6.5, $p < 0.001$), as shown in Table 2. After application of the Bonferroni adjustment, AMO differences on each of the 11 sociodemographic parameters and the 4 headache features remained statistically significant ($p < 0.003$ for all parameters).

Logistic regression

Covariates were entered sequentially to an initial model predicting AMO as a dichotomous outcome. The initial sociodemographic model (Table 3, column 1) showed that AMO was associated with increases in age and BMI, being married, and currently smoking, whereas having at least a 4-year college degree was protective of AMO. Race, household income, and having health insurance did not significantly contribute and were trimmed from subsequent analyses. Respondents' sex, while not significantly associated with AMO, was included in all models.

Adding psychological symptoms from the PHQ-4 to the adjusted sociodemographic model (Table 3, column 2) showed that the presence of depression and/or anxiety increased the odds of AMO by 2.6 times relative to those without psychological symptoms. In the fully adjusted model — sociodemographics plus psychological symptoms and headache features (Table 3, column 3) — the risk of AMO was increased versus the lowest MHD category (0 to 4) among those with 5 to 9 MHDs, 10 to 14 MHDs, and at least 15 MHDs. After adjusting for MHDs, the odds of being in the AMO group were increased by additional years of age, marriage, smoking, psychological symptoms, cutaneous allodynia, additional MSSS points, and greater pain intensity. Education and BMI were not associated with AMO in the fully adjusted model.

Although we predicted that females would have greater odds of AMO, the fully adjusted model revealed that relative to women, males had an increased likelihood of being in the AMO group (OR 1.32, CI 1.16, 1.50). To explore this unexpected finding, a final model included a sex-by-allodynia interaction (Table 3, column 4). Because the interaction was significant (OR 1.53, 95% CI 1.18, 1.97), we ran separate models for men and women to explore the relationship more completely. As shown in Table

Table 1 Sociodemographics of Survey Respondents with Migraine According to Medication Overuse[a]

	Not Overusing Medication $n = 11,542$	Overusing Medication $n = 2107$	Total Sample $n = 13,649$	Chi	P-value
Sex					
Men	3074 (26.6)	621 (29.5)	3695 (27.1)	7.136	0.008
Women	8468 (73.4)	1486 (70.5)	9954 (72.9)		
Age[b], years (mean ± SD)	43.0 ± 13.6	45.8 ± 13.2	43.41 ± 13.62	8.891	< 0.001
Age group, years					
18–24	899 (7.8)	80 (3.8)	979 (7.2)	96.346	< 0.001
25–34	2831 (24.5)	409 (19.4)	3240 (23.7)		
35–44	2775 (24.0)	518 (24.6)	3293 (24.1)		
45–54	2566 (22.2)	546 (25.9)	3112 (22.8)		
55–64	1572 (13.6)	348 (16.5)	1920 (14.1)		
65–74	815 (7.1)	184 (8.7)	999 (7.3)		
75+	84 (0.7)	22 (1.0)	106 (0.8)		
Married					
No	5261 (45.7)	867 (41.4)	6128 (45.1)	13.436	< 0.001
Yes	6245 (54.3)	1229 (58.6)	7474 (54.9)		
Race					
Non-Caucasian	2091 (18.2)	361 (17.2)	2452 (18.1)	1.166	0.280
Caucasian	9379 (81.8)	1736 (82.8)	11,115 (81.9)		
Household income, $					
< 25,000	1254 (11.2)	292 (14.2)	1546 (11.6)	17.025	0.002
25,000–49,999	2422 (21.6)	444 (21.6)	2866 (21.6)		
50,000–74,999	2493 (22.2)	437 (21.3)	2930 (22.1)		
75,000–99,999	1986 (17.7)	363 (17.7)	2349 (17.7)		
≥ 100,000	3070 (27.3)	516 (25.1)	3586 (27.0)		
Education, ≥4-year college degree					
No	4612 (40.0)	1018 (48.3)	5630 (41.2)	51.000	< 0.001
Yes	6930 (60.0)	1089 (51.7)	8019 (58.8)		
BMI[b], kg/m^2 (mean ± SD)	28.1 ± 7.4	28.9 ± 8.5	28.3 ± 7.6	4.380	< 0.001
BMI category					
Underweight	329 (2.9)	94 (4.5)	423 (3.1)	44.240	< 0.001
Normal	4154 (36.0)	645 (30.6)	4799 (35.2)		
Overweight	3387 (29.3)	588 (27.9)	3975 (29.1)		
Obese	3672 (31.8)	780 (37.0)	4452 (32.6)		
Health insurance					
No	945 (8.2)	184 (8.7)	1129 (8.3)	0.628	0.428
Yes	10,597 (91.8)	1923 (91.3)	12,520 (91.7)		
Psychological symptoms[c]					
No	9210 (79.8)	1275 (60.5)	10,485 (76.8)	370.957	< 0.001
Yes	2332 (20.2)	832 (39.5)	3164 (23.2)		
Current smoker					
No	10,387 (90.0)	1718 (81.5)	12,105 (88.7)	126.127	< 0.001
Yes	1155 (10.0)	389 (18.5)	1544 (11.3)		

SD standard deviation, *BMI* body mass index
[a]Values are n (%) unless otherwise indicated
[b]Determined by *t* test
[c]Anxiety and/or depression, as determined by the Patient Health Questionnaire for Depression and Anxiety (PHQ-4)

Factors associated with acute medication overuse in people with migraine: results from the 2017 migraine...

155

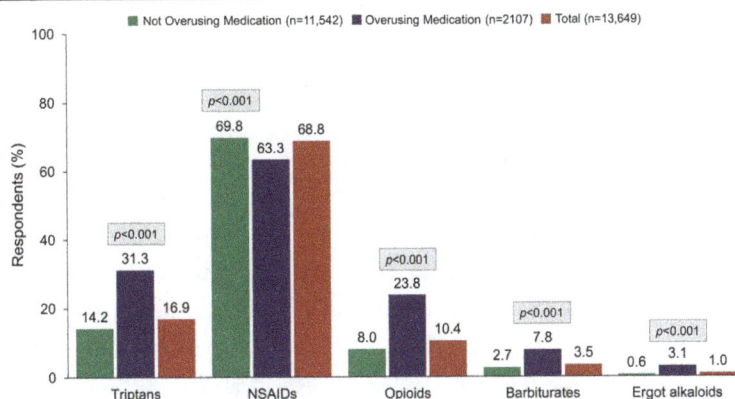

Fig. 1 Medication Overuse by Drug Class Among Respondents with Migraine Currently Using Acute Medication for Headache. Legend: NSAID, nonsteroidal anti-inflammatory drug

3, columns 5 and 6, men with cutaneous allodynia were at higher odds for the development of AMO (61%) compared to women with cutaneous allodynia (8%).

Discussion

This analysis of MAST Study data was conducted to estimate rates of AMO in a representative sample of people with migraine and to determine associations of AMO with individual and migraine characteristics. Overall, 15.4% of MAST respondents met criteria for AMO. Compared with respondents who were not overusing acute medications, those who were overusing acute medications were less likely to be using NSAIDs, but they were more than twice as likely to be using triptans and nearly 3 times as likely to be using barbiturates or opioids. Though persons with AMO were 5 times more likely to be using ergot alkaloids, ergot use was rare. The likelihood of AMO was significantly increased among respondents who were male, older, married, less educated, smokers, and in a higher BMI category, as well as those who had symptoms of

anxiety or depression, cutaneous allodynia, greater severity of migraine symptoms, and greater pain intensity. Race, household income, and health insurance status had no effect on the incidence of AMO. Although AMO should be discussed with all patients who have frequent headaches who use acute medications, identification of factors that are associated with AMO can help clinicians determine with which patients the risk of AMO should be an area of greater focus. Furthermore, although cause-and-effect relationships cannot be determined from this cross-sectional analysis, it is possible that intervening on certain factors, like anxiety and severe migraine attack symptoms, could reduce the likelihood of developing AMO.

Some of the most important MAST Study findings align with earlier work. The overall rate of AMO in the MAST Study is similar to the results of previous studies reporting that 17% to 18% of adults with migraine met criteria for AMO [32, 33]. The results for individual agents are also compatible with prior research showing that migraine progression and AMO are positively

Table 2 Headache Features and Characteristics of Respondents with Migraine According to Medication Overuse

	Not Overusing Medication $n = 11,542$	Overusing Medication $n = 2107$	Total Sample $n = 13,649$	Chi	P-value
MHDs[a] (mean ± SD)	4.3 ± 4.3	12.9 ± 8.6	5.6 ± 6.0	69.7	< 0.001
MHD category, n (%)					
0–4	8054 (69.8)	451 (21.4)	8505 (62.3)	2830.498	< 0.001
5–9	2351 (20.4)	380 (18.0)	2731 (20.0)		
10–14	656 (5.7)	417 (19.8)	1073 (7.9)		
≥ 15	481 (4.2)	859 (40.8)	1340 (9.8)		
Cutaneous allodynia, n (%)					
No	7208 (62.5)	976 (46.3)	8184 (60.0)	192.380	< 0.001
Yes	4334 (37.5)	1131 (53.7)	5465 (40.0)		
MSSS[a] (scale of 0–21)	16.4 ± 3.0	17.8 ± 2.7	16.6 ± 3.0	19.433	< 0.001
Pain intensity[a] (scale of 0–10)	6.5 ± 1.6	7.4 ± 1.6	6.7 ± 1.6	22.7	< 0.001

MHD monthly headache day, *SD* standard deviation, *MSSS* Migraine Symptom Severity Score
[a]Determined by independent-group *t* test

Table 3 Risk (odds ratios [95% CI]) of Medication Overuse Among Respondents with Migraine Currently Using Acute Medication for Headache (N = 13,649)

	Model					
	1	2	3	4	5	6
	Sociodemographics	Psychological symptoms[a]	Headache characteristics	Sex-by-allodynia interaction	Men	Women
Male	1.05 (0.95, 1.17)	1.01 (0.91, 1.13)	1.32 (1.16, 1.50)	1.10 (0.93, 1.31)	–	–
Age	1.01 (1.01, 1.02)	1.02 (1.01, 1.02)	1.02 (1.02, 1.03)	1.02 (1.02, 1.03)	1.02 (1.01, 1.03)	1.02 (1.02, 1.03)
Married	1.12 (1.02, 1.24)	1.19 (1.07, 1.31)	1.19 (1.06, 1.34)	1.18 (1.05, 1.33)	1.44 (1.14, 1.83)	1.10 (0.95, 1.26)
< 4-year college degree	0.80 (0.72, 0.88)	0.85 (0.77, 0.94)	0.99 (0.88, 1.12)	0.99 (0.88, 1.11)	1.13 (0.90, 1.41)	0.93 (0.81, 1.07)
BMI	1.01 (1.01, 1.02)	1.01 (1.00, 1.01)	1.00 (1.00, 1.01)	1.00 (1.00, 1.01)	1.44 (1.14, 1.83)	1.00 (1.00, 1.01)
Psychological symptoms[a]	–	2.61 (2.36, 2.89)	1.62 (1.43, 1.83)	1.60 (1.41, 1.81)	1.94 (1.54, 2.45)	1.48 (1.28, 1.72)
Current smoker	2.05 (1.80, 2.33)	1.78 (1.56, 2.03)	1.54 (1.31, 1.81)	1.52 (1.30, 1.79)	1.65 (1.25, 2.16)	1.42 (1.16, 1.74)
Cutaneous allodynia	–	–	1.22 (1.08, 1.37)	1.09 (0.95, 1.25)	1.61 (1.28, 2.03)	1.08 (0.94, 1.25)
MHDs (vs 0–4, reference)			1.0			
5–9	–	–	2.50 (2.15, 2.90)	2.50 (2.15, 2.90)	2.46 (1.89, 3.20)	2.52 (2.10, 3.01)
10–14	–	–	9.73 (8.27, 11.45)	9.75 (8.28, 11.47)	8.20 (6.03, 11.16)	10.44 (8.60, 12.67)
≥ 15	–	–	27.34 (23.43, 31.89)	27.45 (23.53, 32.04)	21.01 (15.64, 28.21)	30.25 (25.20, 36.30)
MSSS	–	–	1.06 (1.04, 1.09)	1.06 (1.04, 1.09)	1.06 (1.02, 1.10)	1.06 (1.03, 1.09)
Pain intensity	–	–	1.27 (1.22, 1.32)	1.27 (1.22, 1.32)	1.21 (1.13, 1.31)	1.28 (1.22, 1.35)
Sex-by-allodynia interaction	–	–	–	1.53 (1.18, 1.97)	–	–

MHD monthly headache day, *MSSS* Migraine Symptom Severity Scale
[a]Anxiety and/or depression, as determined by the Patient Health Questionnaire for Depression and Anxiety (PHQ-4)

associated with the use of triptans, opioids, and ergot alkaloids [5, 7, 26] and negatively associated with NSAIDs [26]. The finding that AMO was more likely among MAST Study respondents in higher BMI categories and who currently smoke confirms previous research showing a higher prevalence of MOH among individuals with a BMI of at least 30 [16] and smokers [34].

Other MAST Study results differ from those previously reported. For example, the rate of allodynia in the total sample (~ 40.0%) is similar to some previous studies [35] but lower than the 50% to 80% found in other studies [31, 36–41]. We are not sure what accounts for the variation in rates of allodynia among studies using the ASC-12. However, the greater risk for AMO among men with allodynia versus women with allodynia observed in this study is a new finding. The odds of being in the AMO group were elevated among men, and the presence of allodynia increased the likelihood of AMO in men by more than 60%. Reasons for the sex differences in the frequency of AMO and in the association of allodynia with AMO are unknown. Possibilities include: 1) biologic differences in the way that men and women experience allodynia; 2) variations in how men and women report symptoms of allodynia, including how they respond to questions on the ASC-12; 3) differential effects of having allodynia on the decision to take acute migraine medications; and 4) differential effects of AMO on the

development of allodynia. Future studies are needed to test these different theories.

We expected that AMO would be associated with attack frequency in MAST Study respondents. However, after adjusting for MHDs, pain intensity, and sociodemographics, those with AMO were still significantly more likely to have symptoms of depression and/or anxiety than respondents who were not overusing medications, and individuals with psychological symptoms were almost 3 times as likely to be overusing medication as those who were not overusing medication. Future studies are needed to determine if reductions in anxiety and/or depression correlate with reductions in the frequency of taking acute migraine medications.

Strengths of the study include its use of a large and well-defined sample that was generally representative of current US demography, and the inclusion of validated assessments of symptoms of other relevant respondent characteristics. Limitations of the study include the inability of cross-sectional population-based study to record data that would establish a causal relationship between AMO and increasing MHDs [2]. We also did not assess risk of AMO by individual medication class (ie, MAST drug class usage categories are not mutually exclusive), information that might have helped to guide drug choices and targeted educational efforts in clinical practice.

Conclusions

Approximately 15% of persons with migraine met criteria for AMO. As expected, people with frequent attacks were more likely to have AMO than those with less frequent attacks. After adjusting for headache frequency, the odds of being in the AMO group increased with each additional year of age, each 1-point increase in BMI, being married, smoking, psychological symptoms, cutaneous allodynia, each additional MSSS point, and with greater pain intensity. Of note, males with allodynia were more likely to meet criteria for AMO than females with allodynia. Although this cross-sectional study cannot determine temporal sequence or causality for these associations, treating modifiable predictors of AMO is good clinical practice.

Abbreviations

AMPP: American Migraine Prevalence and Prevention Study; AMS: American Migraine Study; ASC-12: Allodynia Symptom Checklist; ICHD: International Classification of Headache Disorders; MAST: Migraine in America Symptoms and Treatment; MHD: Monthly headache day; MIDAS: Migraine Disability Assessment Scale; MSSS: Migraine Symptom Severity Score; NSAID: Nonsteroidal anti-inflammatory drug; OTC: Over-the-counter; PHQ-4: Patient Health Questionnaire for Depression and Anxiety; SD: Standard deviation

Acknowledgements

The authors wish to thank Valerie Marske for assistance with survey instrument development and data collection and Ryan Bostic for assistance with data processing and analysis. Medical writing services were provided by Christopher Caiazza. DRL Publication #831.

Funding

This study was sponsored by Promius Pharma, a subsidiary of Dr. Reddy's Laboratories, Princeton, NJ, USA, which develops and markets acute medications for migraine.

Authors' contributions

All authors conceived and designed the study. MLR and KF managed data collection. All authors contributed to data analysis and interpretation, wrote the paper, and revised and approved the final manuscript.

Competing interests

Todd Schwedt owns stock options from Nocira and Second Opinion and receives royalties from UpToDate. He receives grant support from the National Institutes of Health, the US Department of Defense, the Patient Centered Outcomes Research Institute, the American Migraine Foundation, Arizona State University, and the Mayo Clinic. He serves as a consultant, advisory board member, or has received honoraria from Alder, Allergan, Amgen, American Headache Society, Autonomic Technologies, Avanir, Dr. Reddy's Laboratories/ Promius Pharma, Eli Lilly and Company, Ipsen Biosciences, Nocira, Novartis, and Teva.

Aftab Alam is an employee of Dr. Reddy's Laboratories and owns stock in the company.

Michael Reed receives support from Allergan, Dr. Reddy's Laboratories/Promius Pharma, Eli Lilly and Conpamy, GlaxoSmithKline, Merck & Co., Inc., NuPathe, Novartis, and Ortho-McNeil, via grants to the National Headache Foundation.

Kristina Fanning receives support from Allergan, Dr. Reddy's Laboratories/ Promius Pharma, Eli Lilly and Company, GlaxoSmithKline, Merck & Co., Inc., NuPathe, Novartis, and Ortho-McNeil, via grants to the National Headache Foundation.

Sagar Munjal is an employee of Dr. Reddy's Laboratories and owns stock in the company.

Dawn Buse receives grant support and honoraria from Allergan, Avanir, Dr. Reddy's Laboratories/Promius Pharma, and Eli Lilly and Company. She is an employee of Montefiore Medical Center, which has received research support funded by Allergan, CoLucid, Endo Pharmaceuticals, GlaxoSmithKline, MAP Pharmaceuticals, Merck, NuPathe, Novartis, Ortho-McNeil, and Zogenix, via grants to the National Headache Foundation. She serves on the editorial boards of the Current Pain and Headache Reports, Journal of Headache and Pain, Pain Medicine News, and Pain Pathways magazine.

Dr. Dodick has received compensation from serving on advisory boards and/ or consulting within the past 5 years for: Allergan, Amgen, Novartis, Alder, Arteaus, Pfizer, Colucid, Merck, NuPathe, Eli Lilly and Company, Autonomic Technologies, Ethicon J&J, Zogenix, Supernus, Labrys, Boston Scientific, Medtronic, St Jude, Bristol-Myers Squibb, Lundbeck, Impax, MAP, Electrocore, Tonix, Novartis, Teva, Alcobra, Zosano, Insys, Ipsen, GBS/Nocira, Acorda, eNeura, Charleston Laboratories, Gore, Biohaven, Biocentric, Magellan, Theranica, Xenon, Dr. Reddy's/Promius Pharma, Electrocore. Dr. Dodick owns equity in Epien, GBS/Nocira, Second Opinion, Healint, and Theranica. Dr. Dodick has received funding for travel, speaking, editorial activities, or royalty payments from IntraMed, SAGE Publishing, Sun Pharma, Allergan, Oxford University Press, American Academy of Neurology, American Headache Society, West Virginia University Foundation, Canadian Headache Society, Healthlogix, Universal Meeting Management, WebMD, UptoDate, Medscape, Oregon Health Science Center, Albert Einstein University, University of Toronto, Starr Clinical, Decision Resources, Synergy, MedNet LLC, Peer View Institute for Medical Education, Medicom, Chameleon Communications, Academy for Continued Healthcare Learning, Haymarket Medical Education, Global Scientific Communications, HealthLogix, Miller Medical, MeetingLogiX, Wiley Blackwell. Dr. Dodick, through his employer, has consulting use agreements with NeuroAssessment Systems and Myndshft. He holds board of director positions with King-Devick Technologies, and Epien Inc. He holds the following Patent 17,189,376.1–1466:vTitle: Botulinum Toxin Dosage Regimen for Chronic Migraine Prophylaxis (no compensation).

Richard Lipton receives grant support from the National Institutes of Health, the National Headache Foundation, and the Migraine Research Fund and serves as consultant, serves as an advisory board member, or has received honoraria from Alder, Allergan, American Headache Society, Autonomic Technologies, Boston Scientific, Bristol Myers Squibb, Cognimed, CoLucid, Dr. Reddy's Laboratories/Promius Pharma, Eli Lilly and Company, eNeura Therapeutics, Merck, Novartis, Pfizer, and Teva, Inc. He receives royalties from Wolff's Headache, 8th Edition (Oxford University Press, 2009).

Author details

[1]Mayo Clinic, 5777 East Mayo Boulevard, Phoenix, AZ 85054, USA. [2]Promius Pharma, 107 College Rd East, Princeton, NJ 08540, USA. [3]Vedanta Research, 23 Tanyard Ct, Chapel Hill, NC 27517, USA. [4]Albert Einstein College of Medicine, 1250 Waters Place, 8th Floor, Bronx, NY 10461, USA. [5]Montefiore Medical Center, The Saul R. Korey Department of Neurology, Albert Einstein College of Medicine, 1165 Morris Park Avenue, Rousso Building, Room 332, Bronx, NY 10461, USA.

References

1. Peters GA, Horton BT (1950) Headache; With special reference to the excessive use of ergotamine tartrate and dihydroergotamine. J Lab Clin Med 36:972–973

2. Headache Classification Committee of the International Headache Society (IHS) (2018) The International Classification of Headache Disorders, 3rd edition. Cephalalgia. 38(1):–211

3. Bigal ME, Serrano D, Buse D, Scher A, Stewart WF, Lipton RB (2008) Acute migraine medications and evolution from episodic to chronic migraine: a longitudinal population-based study. Headache 48:1157–1168

4. Krymchantowski AV (2003) Overuse of symptomatic medications among chronic (transformed) migraine patients: profile of drug consumption. Arq Neuropsiquiatr 61:43–47

5. Bigal ME, Rapoport AM, Sheftell FD, Tepper SJ, Lipton RB (2004) Transformed migraine and medication overuse in a tertiary headache Centre–clinical characteristics and treatment outcomes. Cephalalgia 24:483–490

6. Bahra A, Walsh M, Menon S, Goadsby PJ (2003) Does chronic daily headache arise de novo in association with regular use of analgesics? Headache 43:179–190

7. Lipton RB, Serrano D, Nicholson RA, Buse DC, Runken MC, Reed ML (2013) Impact of NSAID and Triptan use on developing chronic migraine: results from the American migraine prevalence and prevention (AMPP) study. Headache 53:1548–1563

8. Suh GI, Park JW, Shin HE (2012) Differences in clinical features and disability according to the frequency of medication use in patients with chronic migraine. J Clin Neurol 8:198–203

9. Lipton RB, Munjal S, Buse DC, Fanning KM, Bennett A, Reed ML (2016) Predicting inadequate response to acute migraine medication: results from the American migraine prevalence and prevention (AMPP) study. Headache 56:1635–1648

10. Mathew NT, Kurman R, Perez F (1990) Drug induced refractory headache–clinical features and management. Headache 30:634–638

11. Zeeberg P, Olesen J, Jensen R (2006) Probable medication-overuse headache: the effect of a 2-month drug-free period. Neurology 66:1894–1898

12. Bekkelund SI, Salvesen R (2002) Drug-associated headache is unrecognized in patients treated at a neurological Centre. Acta Neurol Scand 105:120–123

13. Dowson AJ (2003) Analysis of the patients attending a specialist UK headache clinic over a 3-year period. Headache 43:14–18

14. Bigal ME, Lipton RB (2008) Excessive acute migraine medication use and migraine progression. Neurology 71:1821–1828

15. Jonsson P, Hedenrud T, Linde M (2011) Epidemiology of medication overuse headache in the general Swedish population. Cephalalgia 31:1015–1022

16. Straube A, Pfaffenrath V, Ladwig KH, Meisinger C, Hoffmann W, Fendrich K et al (2010) Prevalence of chronic migraine and medication overuse headache in Germany–the German DMKG headache study. Cephalalgia 30:207–213

17. Cupini LM, De Murtas M, Costa C, Mancini M, Eusebi P, Sarchielli P et al (2009) Obsessive-compulsive disorder and migraine with medication-overuse headache. Headache 49:1005–1013

18. Atasoy HT, Unal AE, Atasoy N, Emre U, Sumer M (2005) Low income and education levels may cause medication overuse and chronicity in migraine patients. Headache 45:25–31

19. Hagen K, Vatten L, Stovner LJ, Zwart JA, Krokstad S, Bovim G (2002) Low socio-economic status is associated with increased risk of frequent headache: a prospective study of 22718 adults in Norway. Cephalalgia 22:672–679

20. Lipton RB (2015) Risk factors for and Management of Medication-Overuse Headache. Continuum (Minneap Minn) 21:1118–1131

21. Grande RB, Aaseth K, Saltyte Benth J, Gulbrandsen P, Russell MB, Lundqvist C (2009) The severity of dependence scale detects people with medication overuse: the Akershus study of chronic headache. J Neurol Neurosurg Psychiatry 80:784–789

22. Lundqvist C, Benth JS, Grande RB, Aaseth K, Russell MB (2011) An adapted severity of dependence scale is valid for the detection of medication overuse: the Akershus study of chronic headache. Eur J Neurol 18:512–518

23. Lundqvist C, Aaseth K, Grande RB, Benth JS, Russell MB (2010) The severity of dependence score correlates with medication overuse in persons with secondary chronic headaches. The Akershus study of chronic headache. Pain 148:487–491

24. Radat F, Creac'h C, Guegan-Massardier E, Mick G, Guy N, Fabre N et al (2008) Behavioral dependence in patients with medication overuse headache: a cross-sectional study in consulting patients using the DSM-IV criteria. Headache 48:1026–1036

25. Meskunas CA, Tepper SJ, Rapoport AM, Sheftell FD, Bigal ME (2006) Medications associated with probable medication overuse headache reported in a tertiary care headache center over a 15-year period. Headache 46:766–772

26. Scher AI, Lipton RB, Stewart WF, Bigal M (2010) Patterns of medication use by chronic and episodic headache sufferers in the general population: results from the frequent headache epidemiology study. Cephalalgia 30:321–328

27. Lipton RB, Munjal S, Alam A, Buse DC, Fanning KM, Reed ML, et al. 2017 Migraine in America symptoms and treatment (MAST) study: baseline study methods, gender differences, and treatment patterns Headache 2018 (in press)

28. Lipton RB, Diamond S, Reed M, Diamond ML, Stewart WF (2001) Migraine diagnosis and treatment: results from the American migraine study II. Headache 41:638–645

29. The International Classification of Headache Disorders (2013) 3rd edition (beta version). Cephalalgia 33:629–808

30. Lowe B, Wahl I, Rose M, Spitzer C, Glaesmer H, Wingenfeld K et al (2010) A 4-item measure of depression and anxiety: validation and standardization of the patient health Questionnaire-4 (PHQ-4) in the general population. J Affect Disord 122:86–95

31. Lipton RB, Bigal ME, Ashina S, Burstein R, Silberstein S, Reed ML et al (2008) Cutaneous allodynia in the migraine population. Ann Neurol 63:148–158

32. Seng EK, Robbins MS, Nicholson RA (2017) Acute migraine medication adherence, migraine disability and patient satisfaction: a naturalistic daily diary study. Cephalalgia 37:955–964

33. Wells RE, Markowitz SY, Baron EP, Hentz JG, Kalidas K, Mathew PG et al (2014) Identifying the factors underlying discontinuation of triptans. Headache 54:278–289

34. Hagen K, Linde M, Steiner TJ, Stovner LJ, Zwart JA (2012) Risk factors for medication-overuse headache: an 11-year follow-up study. The Nord-Trondelag health studies. Pain 153:56–61

35. Scher AI, Buse DC, Fanning KM, Kelly AM, Franznick DA, Adams AM et al (2017) Comorbid pain and migraine chronicity: the chronic migraine epidemiology and outcomes study. Neurology 89:461–468

36. Burstein R, Yarnitsky D, Goor-Aryeh I, Ransil BJ, Bajwa ZH (2000) An association between migraine and cutaneous allodynia. Ann Neurol 47:614–624

37. Mathew NT, Kailasam J, Seifert T (2004) Clinical recognition of allodynia in migraine. Neurology 63:848–852

38. Louter MA, Bosker JE, van Oosterhout WP, van Zwet EW, Zitman FG, Ferrari MD et al (2013) Cutaneous allodynia as a predictor of migraine chronification. Brain 136:3489–3496

39. Selby G, Lance JW (1960) Observations on 500 cases of migraine and allied vascular headache. J Neurol Neurosurg Psychiatry 23:23–32

40. Guven H, Cilliler AE, Comoglu SS (2013) Cutaneous allodynia in patients with episodic migraine. Neurol Sci 34:1397–1402

41. Kalita J, Yadav RK, Misra UK (2009) A comparison of migraine patients with and without allodynic symptoms. Clin J Pain 25:696–698

15

Neurophysiological correlates of clinical improvement after greater occipital nerve (GON) block in chronic migraine: relevance for chronic migraine pathophysiology

Alessandro Viganò[1,2], Maria Claudia Torrieri[3], Massimiliano Toscano[1,4], Francesca Puledda[5], Barbara Petolicchio[1], Tullia Sasso D'Elia[2], Angela Verzina[6], Sonia Ruggiero[1], Marta Altieri[1], Edoardo Vicenzini[1], Jean Schoenen[7] and Vittorio Di Piero[1,8*]

Abstract

Background: Therapeutic management of Chronic Migraine (CM), often associated with Medication Overuse Headache (MOH), is chiefly empirical, as no biomarker predicting or correlating with clinical efficacy is available to address therapeutic choices. The present study searched for neurophysiological correlates of Greater Occipital Nerve Block (GON-B) effects in CM.

Methods: We recruited 17 CM women, of whom 12 with MOH, and 19 healthy volunteers (HV). Patients had no preventive treatment since at least 3 months. After a 30-day baseline, they received a bilateral betamethasone-lidocaine GON-B of which the therapeutic effect was assessed 1 month later. Habituation of visual evoked potentials (VEP) and intensity dependence of auditory evoked potentials (IDAP) were recorded before and 1 week after the GON-B.

Results: At baseline, CM patients had a VEP habituation not different from HV, but a steeper IDAP value than HV ($p = 0.01$), suggestive of a lower serotonergic tone. GON-B significantly reduced the number of total headache days per month ($- 34.9\%$; $p = 0.003$). Eight out 17CM patients reversed to episodic migraine and medication overuse resolved in 11 out of 12 patients. One week after the GON-B VEP habituation became lacking respect to baseline ($p = 0.01$) and to that of HV ($p = 0.02$) like in episodic migraine, while the IDAP slope significantly flattened ($p < 0.0001$). GON-B-induced reduction in headache days positively correlated with IDAP slope decrease (rho $= 0.51$, $p = 0.03$).

Conclusions: GON-B may be effective in the treatment of CM, with or without MOH. The pre-treatment IDAP increase is compatible with a weak central serotonergic tone, which is strengthened after GON-B, suggesting that serotonergic mechanisms may play a role in CM and its reversion to episodic migraine. Since the degree of post-treatment IDAP decrease is correlated with clinical improvement, IDAP might be potentially useful as an early predictor of GON-B efficacy.

Keywords: Habituation, Serotonin, Chronic migraine, Predictors, Plasticity

* Correspondence: vittorio.dipiero@uniroma1.it
[1]Headache Centre & Neurocritical Care Unit. Department of Human Neurosciences, Sapienza – University of Rome, Viale dell'Università 30, 00185 Rome, Italy
[8]University Consortium for Adaptive Disorders and Head pain – UCADH, Pavia, Italy
Full list of author information is available at the end of the article

Background

CM is a complication of episodic migraine affecting 2% of the general population [1] and most commonly encountered in tertiary headache clinics [2]. It is frequently associated with Medication Overuse Headache (MOH), a secondary headache, which could be interpreted as a comorbidity as well as a marker of poor control of the migraine itself [3, 4]. In the migraine pathology spectrum, chronic migraine (CM) represents the most severe form and its disabling effects are not only related to the physical health of patients but also reverberate on social and economic aspects. The available pharmacological treatments of CM are quite limited. Only a few drug treatments like topiramate [5] and onabotulinumtoxin A [6, 7], have an efficacy proven by randomized controlled trials. Most drugs commonly used in the treatment of CM have been investigated only by small open studies (for a review, see [8]). Management of CM patients is further complicated by poor therapeutic adherence due to the insufficient efficacy of drug therapies and their side effects [9].

Since no predictors of treatment response are available to date, preventive medications are selected by trial and error, taking into account the patients' clinical profile, drug side effects and the patients' comorbidities more so than by their efficacy differences. Each drug is commonly recommended for 4–6 months before assessing (in)efficacy and CM patients try on average 4 therapeutic lines with severe patient discomfort and frustration of the doctor. Half of patients interrupt treatment due to lack of efficacy or side effects and only about 9% achieve clinical improvement [10].

Greater occipital nerve blocks with a local anesthetic alone [11, 12] or with a steroid-local anaesthetic combination [13, 14] were found useful for CM with varying effect sizes and durations, but their mechanism of action remains elusive.

Repetition of attacks and failure of preventive therapies produce a longer exposure to headaches that might promote central sensitization and maintain migraine chronicity and possibly refractoriness [8, 15].

Understanding neurophysiological mechanisms of chronification might allow identifying biomarkers able to predict transition and remission from chronic to episodic migraine (EM).

Possible candidates could be markers of brain excitability and responsivity, such as habituation and amplitude-stimulus function of cortical evoked responses (measured by IDAP) [16, 17].

Detailed description of the lack of habituation in migraineurs has been widely reported elsewhere [17, 18]. In EM between attacks, during repeated and unmodified sensory stimulation, cortical evoked responses are characterised by a reduced initial amplitude (lower preactivation level)

and a progressive amplitude increase (i.e. hyperresponsivity) instead of a physiological habituation, regardless of the sensory modality, visual, auditory, somatosensory, laser, including cognitive potentials like contingent negative variation or P3 [19]. All evoked potentials, besides laser evoked potentials, normalize during migraine attacks [20]. Interestingly, in CM the electrophysiological pattern is similar to that of ictal EM recordings, suggesting genuine hyperexcitability and supporting the idea that CM is a sort of "never-ending attack" [21, 22]. MOH patients have an intermediate pattern between CM and EM with an increased initial response but a lack of habituation, a pattern that is found in the pre-ictal EM phase [23].

When CM patients improve and revert to EM, they acquire again the interictal electrophysiological profile consisting of a low initial response and a deficient habituation [24].

Intensity Dependence of Auditory evoked Potentials (IDAP) is chiefly modulated by activity in central brainstem-cortical serotonergic projections [25]. In interictal EM IDAP is increased reflecting low serotonergic tone, and correlates with deficient habituation [26]. So far, no IDAP data are available in CM. It is thus not known if IDAP is correlated or not with habituation as in EM nor if it changes when patients revert from CM to EM.

In this study, we aimed to evaluate changes in IDAP before and 1 week after a greater occipital nerve block (GON-B) with a steroid-local anaesthetic combination, as well as clinical changes 4 weeks after the block in CM/MOH patients without preventive therapy. Besides confirming a possible therapeutic effect, our aim was to search for a correlation between such an effect and baseline IDAP or its GON-B induced early change in order to identify a biomarker able to predict the treatment effect.

Methods

Subjects

We consecutively recruited 17 female Chronic Migraine (CM) patients with or without Medication Overuse Headache (MOH) (ICHD-III 1.3 and 8.2) in the Headache Clinic of the University Hospital of Rome, Policlinico Umberto I, according to ICHD-III criteria. We included only > 18 years old patients, who had: i) a diagnosis of Chronic Migraine (ICHD-III 1.3); ii) migraine without aura (ICHD-III 1.1) at origin; iii) no spontaneous improvement of migraine burden in the previous 6 months. Twelve of them also qualified for a diagnosis of MOH (ICHD-III 8.2).

Exclusion criteria were other neurological and psychiatric conditions (e.g. epilepsy, cerebrovascular diseases, etc.), a Beck Depression Inventory higher than 11 points, or medical contraindications to receive GON infiltration (e.g. allergies, infections, open skull defect, anticoagulant use), other chronic painful conditions. Prophylactic migraine treatment and anti-depressants were not allowed for at least three months before trial inclusion, nor were acute migraine drugs during minimum 12 h before the neurophysiological recordings.

Healthy volunteers (HV, $n = 19$) of comparable age and gender distribution, without personal or family history of migraine, neurological or psychiatric disease, use of medications acting on brain excitability or serotonin were recruited for comparative electrophysiological recordings.

The local Ethics Committee approved the study and all patients gave their written informed consent to take part in the experiment. The study was conducted in accordance with the Helsinki Declaration.

Intensity dependence of auditory evoked potentials (IDAP)

Auditory Evoked Potentials (AEPs) were recorded as recommended [27] and implemented elsewhere [28, 29]. AEPs were evoked at four different intensities (60, 70, 80 and 90 dB) in a pseudo-randomized order. For each intensity level, 90 trials were collected with a sampling frequency of 4000 Hz and sweep duration of 400 ms (50 ms before and 350 ms after the auditory stimulus). Traces were filtered offline with a 1-20 Hz bandpass filter. We identified N1 components (the maximal negative deflections between 60 and 150 ms post-stimulus) and P2 (the positive deflections between 120 and 200 ms), and measured N1P2 peak-to-peak amplitudes at each stimulus intensity. IDAP value was calculated as the linear amplitude/stimulus intensity function (ASF) slope (IDAP slope) for block averages (μV/ 10 dB).

Pattern reversal-visual evoked potentials (PR-VEPs).

PR-VEPs were performed as recommended [27], similarly to the protocol used in our previous study [30].

During uninterrupted stimulation, 250 cortical responses were recorded by a BrainVision preamplifier at a sample a rate of 4000 Hz, and divided in epochs of 300 ms after the stimulus. We identify N1 as the first negative wave occurring around 75 ms from the stimulus, P1 as a positive wave occurring after N1 at around 100 ms, N2 as a negative wave around 145 ms. Cerebral responses were divided in 5 consecutive block and the habituation was calculated as the slope interpolating the average of amplitudes in each block (habituation slope). Negative values reflect habituation (i.e. a decrement of responses over time) whereas positive values indicate lack of habituation (i.e. an increase of responses).

Anaesthetic block of GON (GON-B)

Bilateral GON blocks were performed with a 21-gauge needle, injecting suboccipitally midway between inion and mastoid, a 3 ml solution of betamethasone sodium phosphate 4 mg (2 ml) and xylocaine 2% (1 ml).

Study design

The study design is shown in Fig. 1. During the 1st visit (T-1), CM patients were enrolled and asked to fill in a 30-day headache diary (pre GON-B), recording number

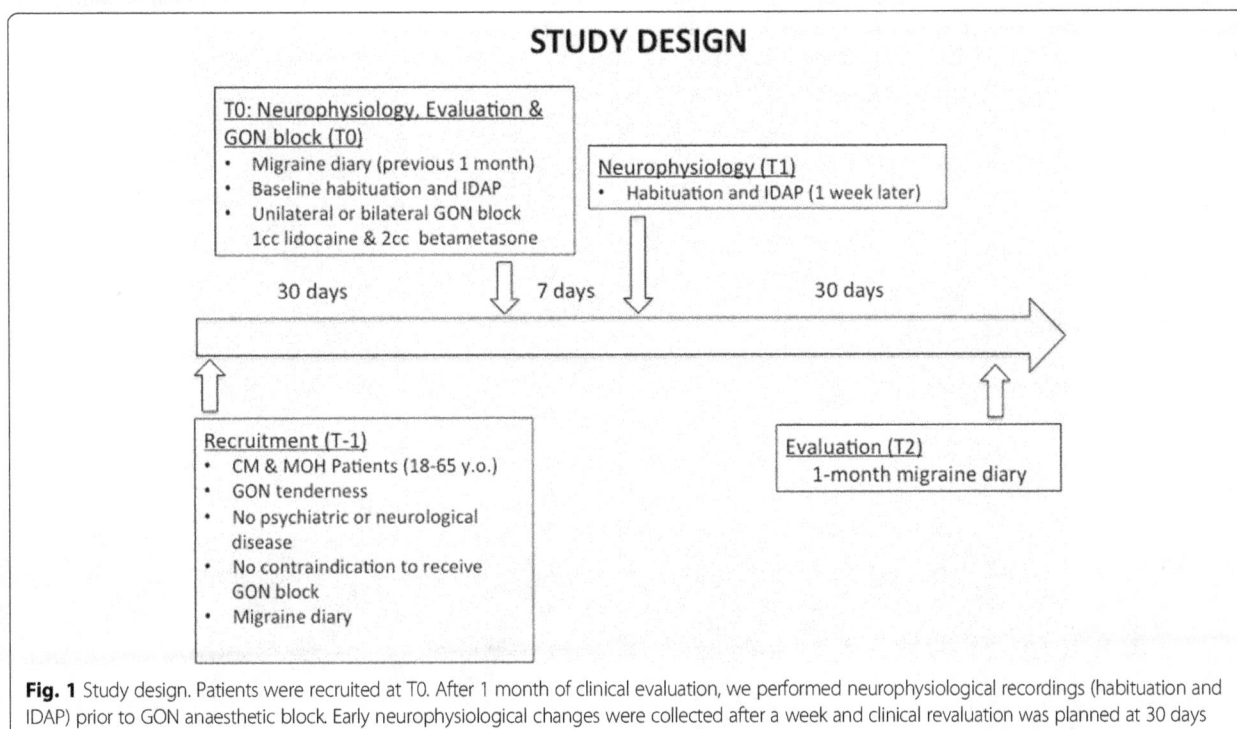

STUDY DESIGN

Fig. 1 Study design. Patients were recruited at T0. After 1 month of clinical evaluation, we performed neurophysiological recordings (habituation and IDAP) prior to GON anaesthetic block. Early neurophysiological changes were collected after a week and clinical reevaluation was planned at 30 days

and duration of attacks, as well as headache intensity of and associated symptoms using a 3-point scale from 1 (mild symptoms) to 3 (severe symptoms). Patients also recorded the number of acute medication intake.

At the 2nd visit (T0), clinical data were collected from the diary and PR-VEPs habituation and IDAP were measured. Thereafter, patients received a bilateral GON-B. Patients with acute medication overuse were not detoxified but advised to reduce their consumption of acute drugs.

PR-VEPs and IDAP were repeated after one week ±1 day (T1), and possible adverse effects of GON-B were assessed.

In women, all neurophysiological recordings were performed between day 2–10 of the luteal phase of the menstrual cycle.

Patients were clinically re-evaluated 1 month after GON-B (T2) and the post-treatment diary data were compared to the pre-treatment data.

Blinded investigators analysed the clinical and electrophysiological data (MT) and performed the statistics (AVi).

Outcome measures and statistics

We tested normal distribution of variables with Shapiro-Wilk's test. The primary clinical outcome measure was the reduction in number of total headache days (between the pre GON-B and post GON-B month). We also calculated the recovery rate from overuse of acute medication. We used Wilcoxon's rank test or Fisher's 2×2 contingency tables for clinical variables (non-normally distributed). Neurophysiological variables had a

normal distribution, and then baseline values and the changes induced by GON-B of neurophysiological tests were compared between groups with repeated measured ANOVA and Fisher's LSD test for post-hoc comparison. Since one objective of the study was to identify mechanisms related to migraine chronification and its reversal, CM patients who reversed to EM were labelled as "responders" for further sub-analyses.

We also used repeated-measures ANOVA, with Fisher's LSD test for post-hoc comparison, to compare temporal changes between pre GON-B and post GON-B in Responders (R) and Non-Responders (NR).

The correlation analysis between neurophysiological and clinical data was performed with Spearman's rho. Statistical analyses will be performed with STATISTICA 7 (StatSoft, Tulsa, Ok). Group values were represented by means ± standard deviation. Significance level was set at $p < 0.05$ after multiple comparison correction.

Results and discussion
Clinical effects of GON-B in chronic migraine

In twelve months, we recruited 20 women with CM who met the study selection criteria. Three patients dropped out since they didn't report headache diary at T2 visit. Twenty female healthy volunteers (HV) were recruited as controls, one of them dropped out as she missed a scheduled recording. Baseline characteristics of both groups are shown in Table 1. Twelve of 17 patients had also MOH, of whom seven patients overused analgesics, four triptans, one a combination of caffeine, indometacine, prochlorperazine.

Table 1 Baseline characteristics of CM patients

Parameters	Patients	Healthy volunteers	p-value
Age	32.9 ± 14.5	31.45 ± 13.94	$p = 0.63$
Gender	17 F	19 F	–
N° of headache days per month	24.88 ± 7.22	–	–
Medication Overuse Headache	12 (70%)	–	–
Type of medication overused		–	–
	Triptans: 4 (33%)		
	NSAIDs: 7 (58%)		
	Combination: 1 (8%)		
N° of acute medication per month	16.18 ± 12.31	–	–
Pain intensity (1–3 scale)	1point 0 pts		
	2 points 3 pts	–	–
	3 points 15 pts		
Habituation N1P1 at T0	0.23 ± 0.68	0.26 ± 0.63	$p = 0.53$
Habituation P1N2 at baseline	0.20 ± 0.55	0.08 ± 0.53	$p = 0.54$
IDAP at baseline	0.76 ± 0.95	0.03 ± 0.76	$p = 0.01*$

The star (*) indicates the p level after post-hoc comparison, when appropriate. Otherwise, p level indicated refers to the one obtained by the repeated measures model

In the group level analysis, the mean number of headache days decreased after the GON procedure from 24.88 ± 7.22 to 16.59 ± 10.25 ($- 34.9\%$, $p = 0.003$) (see Fig. 2). Eight out 17 CM patients reversed to episodic migraine.

The GON-B had a significant effect also in MOH patients. MOH resolved in 11 out of the 12 MOH patients. One patient, who didn't respond to GON-B, developed MOH in the month following the procedure. The clinical benefit of GON-B on stopping the medication overuse was significant (Fisher's 2×2 test, $p = 0.001$).

Neurophysiological changes at baseline and after GON-B between CM patients and HV

We tested baseline differences between HV and CM patients and changes induced by GON-B within each group by using repeated measure ANOVA model, separately for each neurophysiological variable. For N1P1 habituation, the model reported no significant difference in the model neither at baseline between groups nor in each group (HV vs. CM patients) after GON-B (repeated measure ANOVA $F(1,34) = 0.40$, $p = 0.53$). By contrast, for P1N2 we found a significant result in the model (repeated measure ANOVA $F(1,34) = 4.37$, $p = 0.04$). After post-hoc comparison, in fact, CM patients didn't differ from HV for P1N2 at baseline ($p = 0.53$), but they had a significant impairment of habituation after GON-B (0.20 ± 0.54 vs. 0.55 ± 0.72, $p = 0.01$) so that a T1 the value of habituation was significant lower in CM than in HV (CM: 0.55 ± 0.72 vs. HV: 0.08 ± 0.53, $p = 0.03$, $p = 0.02$).

As well, for IDAP, we found significant differences between HV and CM patients at baseline as well as in the CM patients before and after the GON-B (repeated measure ANOVA $F(1,34) = 12.51$, $p = 0.001$). After post-hoc comparison we found that CM patients differed from HV by a steeper IDAP slope at baseline, suggesting a lower serotonin tone (CM: 0.76 ± 0.95 vs. HV: 0.03 ± 0.76; $p = 0.01$)(see Table 1). One week after the GON-B (T1) the baseline steep IDAP slope flattened and reached negative values, indicating an inversion in serotonergic activity (pre GON-B slope: 0.76 ± 0.96 vs. post GON-B: $- 0.17 \pm 0.93$, $p < 0.0001$).

In the sub-analysis, repeated-measures ANOVA showed a difference in neurophysiological parameters between responders and non-responders after GON-B. Although habituation of N1P1 and P1N2 components did not differ neither for time or group (see Table 2), IDAP slope showed a significant decrease only in the responder group ($p = 0.004$) (see Fig. 3).

Correlations between neurophysiological and clinical changes at the group level

Furthermore, the reduction in headache days after treatment (from T0 to T2) correlated positively with the magnitude of the change in the slope of the IDAP between T0 and T1. The bigger was the flattening of IDAP slope (i.e. the higher serotonin firing), the better was the clinical response (Spearman' rho = 0.51, $p = 0.03$) (see Fig. 4). There was no correlation between the baseline IDAP slope and the reduction in headache days after GON-B (Spearman' rho = 0.31, $p = 0.25$).

Analysis of possible sources of bias

To search for possible confounding factors in our results, we searched possible differences between CM

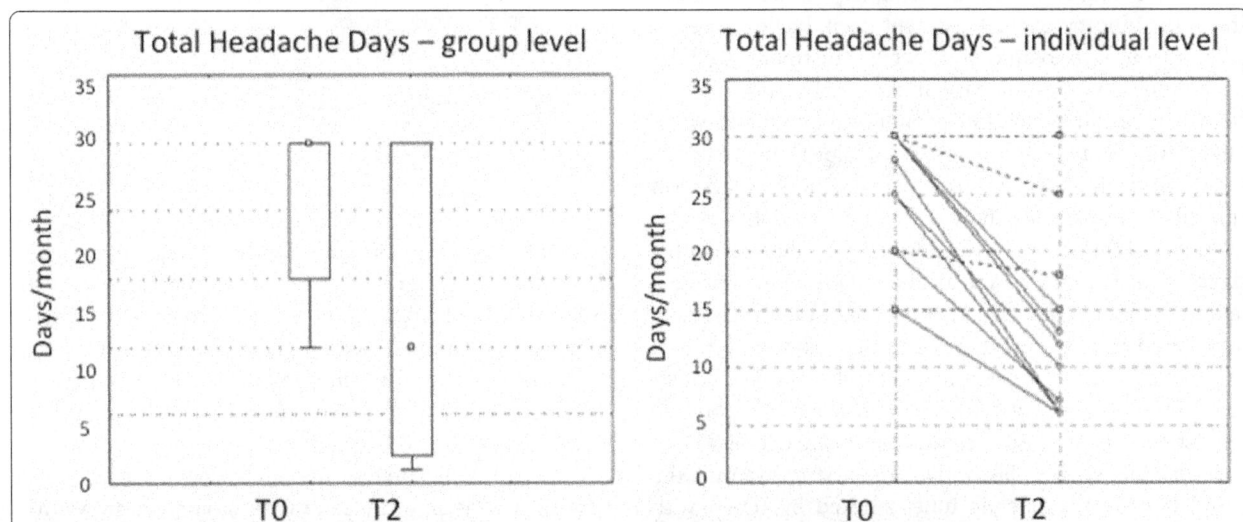

Fig. 2 Clinical effect at group and individual level. GON block was effective in reduce the average clincial burden of chronic migraine by 35%. More over we observed that after GON-B the majority of patients who responded reversed to EM. Only one case had a 15 days reduction but passed from 30 days to 15 days of headache remaining within the boundary of chronic migraine. Most of patients, who didn't respond, had no benefit (five of them are 30 days to 30 days and then superimposed in the graph). Two Responders passed from 15 days to 6 days and are superimposed in the graph. Responders are in dotted, No-responders in continuous line

Table 2 Time effect of neurophysiological parameters between Responders and Non-responders

Variables	Effect	SS	DoF	F value	p value
Habituation of N1P1	GROUP	0.03	1	0.08	0.79
	TIME	0.10	1	0.32	0.58
	TIME*GROUP	0.36	1	1.17	0.30
Habituation of P1N2	GROUP	1.01	1	2.12	0.17
	TIME	0.97	1	2.90	0.11
	TIME*GROUP	0.02	1	0.05	0.83
IDAP	GROUP	0.28	1	0.25	0.63
	TIME	6.02	1	9.66	0.008°
	TIME*GROUP	1.67	1	2.68	0.13

The symbol ° indicates the level of significance obtained by the repeated measures model

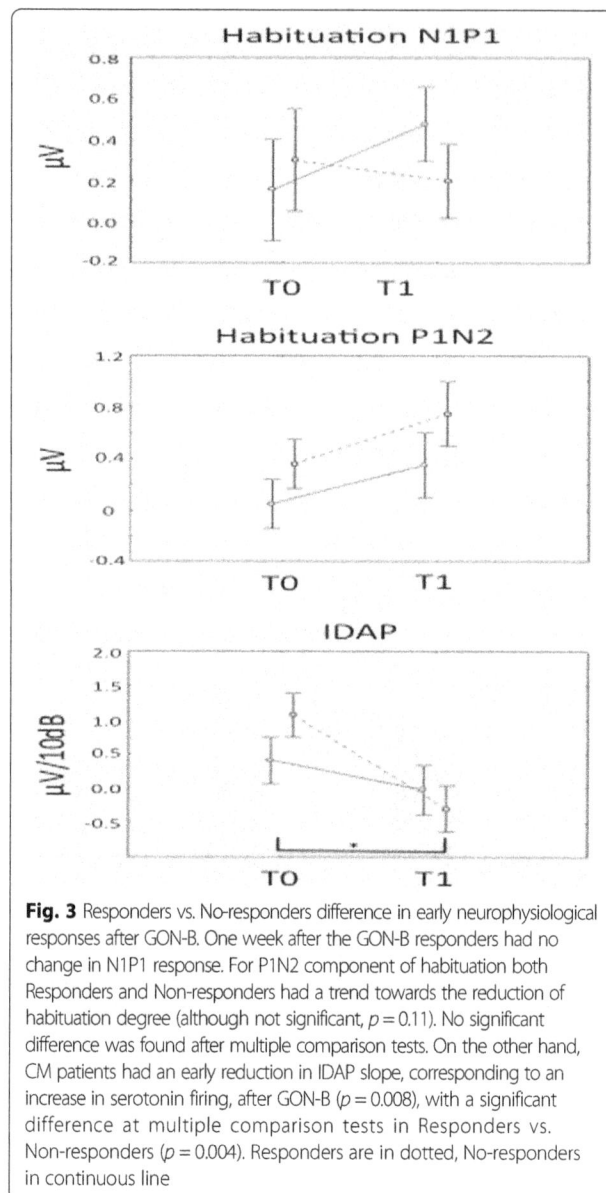

Fig. 3 Responders vs. No-responders difference in early neurophysiological responses after GON-B. One week after the GON-B responders had no change in N1P1 response. For P1N2 component of habituation both Responders and Non-responders had a trend towards the reduction of habituation degree (although not significant, $p = 0.11$). No significant difference was found after multiple comparison tests. On the other hand, CM patients had an early reduction in IDAP slope, corresponding to an increase in serotonin firing, after GON-B ($p = 0.008$), with a significant difference at multiple comparison tests in Responders vs. Non-responders ($p = 0.004$). Responders are in dotted, No-responders in continuous line

patients with and without MOH, and between responders and non-responders. VEP Habituation did not differ between CM patients with or without MOH for N1P1 (H = 0.93; $p = 0.34$) or P1N2 (H = 0.93; $p = 0.34$) components. As well, IDAP value didn't differ between CM with and without MOH (H = 0.27, $p = 0.60$). Analysing responders and non-responders using the Kruskal-Wallis test, we found no difference in age (H = 1.34; $p = 0.25$), number of anti-migraine acute medication intake (H = 0.47; $p = 0.49$), presence of MOH (Fisher 2×2 test = 0.00; df = 1; $p = 0.13$), number of headache days (H = 1.57; $p = 0.21$), VEP N1P1 habituation (H = 0.01; $p = 0.92$), P1N2 (H = 1.10; $p = 0.29$) and IDAP slopes (H = 1.93; $p = 0.16$).

Interpretation of results

Due to the low rate of response and the need to treat patients for a long time before having any clinical feedback about the efficacy of the treatment itself, having an early predictive tool to identify if a specific treatment is effective or not for a given patient is valuable information from a medical, social and economic point of view. In this study we tested if a greater occipital nerve block (GON-B) could be such a tool by assessing its long-term clinical efficacy and its short effects on brain physiology.

We found that a single GON-B produced after 1 month a clinical benefit with a 34% reduction in headache days and a return to episodic migraine in 50% of the cases. In addition, we showed that this beneficial effect was associated with a decrease of intensity dependence of auditory evoked potentials (IDAP) 1 week after the block in clinical responders, suggestive of an increase in central serotonergic tone.

To our knowledge, this study is the first to examine the correlation of serotonergic tone, indexed by IDAP, with CM and in particular its variation in association with clinical improvement. We found that patients with CM had a low baseline serotonergic tone, which increased after a clinically successful GON-B. This occurred especially in those patients who switched from a chronic form of

migraine to an episodic one. Furthermore, the degree of IDAP flattening after 1 week was directly correlated to the improvement of migraine in terms of reduction of headache days at 1 month post-GON-B. This result may thus be of some utility for clinicians who plan to perform a GON-B and like to have an early feedback of the long-term efficacy of GON-B.

The change in IDAP is not unexpected because of its strong correlation with central serotonin pathways. Migraine in general is considered since a long time to be a low serotonin disorder and in CM in particular serotonin levels are thought to be even lower on the basis of clinical (e.g. high comorbidity with depression) and biochemical data [31, 32]. Contrary to the IDAP abnormality in CM,

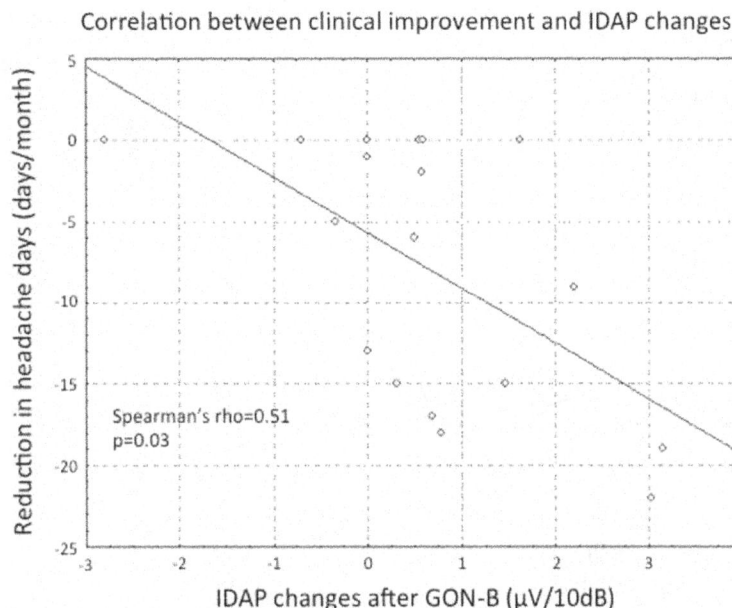

Fig. 4 Correlation analysis between clinical improvement and IDAP changes. At the group level, the reduction in IDAP value was positively correlated with the reduction of day of headache in the follow-up month. Positive IDAP values indicate that the T1 measurement was smaller than the first. The calculation for IDAP change was: IDAP change = IDAP(T0)-IDAP(T1). On the other hand for headache days calculation was: Headache reduction = days(T2)-days(T0)

we also found a normal pattern of VEP habituation in CM with or without MOH, which is consistent with previous findings and with the hypothesis that CM is a sort of a "never ending attack" [21, 33].

VEP habituation returns to the normal non-habituation pattern of episodic migraines, when patients with CM are successfully treated [24]. In line with these results, we found that habituation decreased for the PR-VEP N1P2 component with clinical improvement so that at T1 it differed from that of HV.

In previous studies of episodic migraineurs abnormal IDAP and VEP habituation were thought to be linked interictally because decreased habituation of auditory potentials may lead to a steep IDAP slope and low central serotonin activities could explain both abnormalities [26] .

A possible explanation for the dissociation between IDAP and VEP habituation changes in our study could be that in chronic migraine the apparently normal habituation pattern is due to changes in brain plasticity more than to a simple change in serotonergic tone [34, 35]. Chronic migraine is characterized by persistent hyperexcitability of sensory cortices [22], suggesting that the repetition of attacks induces plastic alterations of the excitatory-inhibitory balance that is fundamental for tuning synaptic plasticity and circuitry [36]. In this concept, inhibitory responses tend to decrease more than excitatory ones following stimulus repetition [37] and are also negatively modulated by neurotransmitters, such as acetylcholine, noradrenalin and oxytocin. The resulting disinhibition might thus promote hyperesponsivity [36].

In the presence of reduced inhibitory activity, a higher cortical preactivation level might be achieved and supported by a low serotonin activity. For this reason, the pattern of a normal habituation found in CM may actually be a "pseudo-normal habituation", related to LTD-mediated inhibitory responses more that just a "ceiling effect" as hypothesized for episodic migraine [38] and lately validated by several consistent experiments (see [17] for a review). LTD-mediated inhibition responses were found more commonly in CM and in EM with high attack frequency than in episodic migraineurs with a low frequency of attacks [39].

In patients reversing from a chronic to an episodic pattern of migraine, we observed an early flattening of the IDAP response after the GON-B, indicating that clinical improvement is likely to be associated with an increase in serotonergic firing.

Although the precise mechanism of action of GON-B is unknown, it is thought to modulate brain excitability acting on input gate at the brainstem level. Although cervical stimulation has been shown to increase directly brain serotonin [40, 41], such evidence is lacking for GON-B.

The IDAP slope flattening, and thus probably central serotonin activity, positively correlated with the reduction of total headache days after a month at group level, reinforcing a possible role of serotonin in remission from CM. Both at cortical and thalamic levels, serotonin is able to modulate the excitatory/inhibitory balance, both directly and by modifying the action of other neurotransmitters like dopamine [42–44]. Serotonin-related metaplasticity, characterized by a shift from inhibitory to excitatory activity, was already found in the hippocampus [45]. Taken together, these results corroborate the idea that serotonin may be a crucial actor in the plastic brain changes that accompany migraine chronification and reversal. In our study we provide indirect evidence for such a role, which needs to be confirmed by more direct assessments of central serotonergic neurotransmission.

Conclusions

A single greater occipital nerve block showed a good clinical response in chronic migraine patients with or without acute medication overuse. Clinical improvement, and in particular the reversal to an episodic migraine pattern was significantly associated with a decrease of intensity dependence of auditory evoked potentials (IDAP) one week after the block. As IDAP is thought to reflect central serotonergic activity and it is in addition increased at baseline in chronic migraineurs, it is likely that serotonin plays a crucial role in migraine chronification and associated plastic brain changes.

Abbreviations
ASF: amplitude/stimulus intensity function; CM: Chronic Migraine; EM: episodic migraine; GON: Greater Occipital Nerve; GON-B: Greater Occipital Nerve Block; HV: Healthy Volunteers; IDAP: intensity dependence of auditory evoked potentials; LTD: long term depression; MOH: Medication Overuse Headache; NR: Non-responders; PR-VEPs: Pattern reversal-Visual evoked potentials; R: Responders; VEP: visual evoked potentials

Acknowledgements
Authors would like to thank Mrs. Rossella Pichi for her help in organizing the different stages of the study.

Funding
This study was partially funded by Research Grant for Young Investigators (Bandi di Ateneo per l'Avvio alla Ricerca) 2017 from Sapienza – University of Rome awarded to Alessandro Viganò. The experimental protocol presented in the present paper received one of the 12 Young Against Pain Awards 2017 at SIMPAR-ISURA Congress 2017 (awarded to Alessandro Viganò).

Authors' contributions
Study design: AVi, VDP. Patients recruitment: BP, FP, EV, MA. Neurophysiological recordings: MCT, TSD, AVe, SR. GON-B injection: BP, FP. Blind evaluation of EEG traces and blind statistical analysis: MT, AVi. Results discussion and interpretation: all. Manuscript drafting: AVi. Manuscript revision: JS, VDP. All authors read and approved the final manuscript.

Competing interests
The authors declare that they have no competing interest.

Author details
[1]Headache Centre & Neurocritical Care Unit. Department of Human Neurosciences, Sapienza – University of Rome, Viale dell'Università 30, 00185 Rome, Italy. [2]Molecular and Cellular Networks Lab. Department of Anatomy, Histology, Forensic medicine and Orthopaedics, Sapienza – University of Rome, Rome, Italy. [3]Rita Levi Montalcini Department of Neuroscience, Città della Salute e della Scienza, Turin, Italy. [4]Department of Neurology, Fatebenefratelli Hospital, Rome, Italy. [5]Headache Group, Department of Basic and Clinical Neuroscience, King's College London, and NIHR-Wellcome Trust King's Clinical Research Facility, Wellcome Foundation Building, King's College Hospital, London SE5 9PJ, UK. [6]Department of Neurology, University of Perugia, Perugia, Italy. [7]Headache Research Unit. Department of Neurology, University of Liège, Citadelle Hospital, Liège, Belgium. [8]University Consortium for Adaptive Disorders and Head pain – UCADH, Pavia, Italy.

References

1. Natoli JL, Manack A, Dean B et al (2010) Global prevalence of chronic migraine: a systematic review. Cephalalgia Int J Headache 30:599–609. https://doi.org/10.1111/j.1468-2982.2009.01941.x
2. Dodick DW (2006) Clinical practice. Chronic daily headache. N Engl J Med 354:158–165. https://doi.org/10.1056/NEJMcp042897
3. Bigal ME, Serrano D, Buse D et al (2008) Acute migraine medications and evolution from episodic to chronic migraine: a longitudinal population-based study. Headache 48:1157–1168. https://doi.org/10.1111/j.1526-4610.2008.01217.x
4. Scher AI, Rizzoli PB, Loder EW (2017) Medication overuse headache: an entrenched idea in need of scrutiny. Neurology 89:1296–1304. https://doi.org/10.1212/WNL.0000000000004371
5. Silberstein SD, Lipton RB, Dodick DW et al (2007) Efficacy and safety of topiramate for the treatment of chronic migraine: a randomized, double-blind, placebo-controlled trial. Headache 47:170–180. https://doi.org/10.1111/j.1526-4610.2006.00684.x
6. Aurora SK, Dodick DW, Turkel CC et al (2010) OnabotulinumtoxinA for treatment of chronic migraine: results from the double-blind, randomized, placebo-controlled phase of the PREEMPT 1 trial. Cephalalgia Int J Headache 30:793–803. https://doi.org/10.1177/0333102410364676
7. Diener HC, Dodick DW, Aurora SK et al (2010) OnabotulinumtoxinA for treatment of chronic migraine: results from the double-blind, randomized, placebo-controlled phase of the PREEMPT 2 trial. Cephalalgia Int J Headache 30:804–814. https://doi.org/10.1177/0333102410364677
8. May A, Schulte LH (2016) Chronic migraine: risk factors, mechanisms and treatment. Nat Rev Neurol 12:455–464. https://doi.org/10.1038/nrneurol.2016.93
9. Hepp Z, Dodick DW, Varon SF et al (2017) Persistence and switching patterns of oral migraine prophylactic medications among patients with chronic migraine: a retrospective claims analysis. Cephalalgia Int J Headache 37:470–485. https://doi.org/10.1177/0333102416678382
10. Blumenfeld AM, Bloudek LM, Becker WJ et al (2013) Patterns of use and reasons for discontinuation of prophylactic medications for episodic migraine and chronic migraine: results from the second international burden of migraine study (IBMS-II). Headache 53:644–655. https://doi.org/10.1111/head.12055
11. Inan LE, Inan N, Karadaş Ö et al (2015) Greater occipital nerve blockade for the treatment of chronic migraine: a randomized, multicenter, double-blind, and placebo-controlled study. Acta Neurol Scand 132:270–277. https://doi.org/10.1111/ane.12393
12. Cuadrado ML, Aledo-Serrano Á, Navarro P et al (2017) Short-term effects of greater occipital nerve blocks in chronic migraine: a double-blind, randomised, placebo-controlled clinical trial. Cephalalgia Int J Headache 37:864–872. https://doi.org/10.1177/0333102416655159
13. Puledda F, Goadsby PJ, Prabhakar P (2018) Treatment of disabling headache with greater occipital nerve injections in a large population of childhood and adolescent patients: a service evaluation. J Headache Pain 19:5. https://doi.org/10.1186/s10194-018-0835-5

14. Afridi SK, Shields KG, Bhola R, Goadsby PJ (2006) Greater occipital nerve injection in primary headache syndromes--prolonged effects from a single injection. Pain 122:126–129. https://doi.org/10.1016/j.pain.2006.01.016

15. Martelletti P, Katsarava Z, Lampl C et al (2014) Refractory chronic migraine: a consensus statement on clinical definition from the European headache federation. J Headache Pain 15:47. https://doi.org/10.1186/1129-2377-15-47

16. Magis D, Vigano A, Sava S et al (2013) Pearls and pitfalls: electrophysiology for primary headaches. Cephalalgia Int J Headache 33:526–539. https://doi.org/10.1177/0333102413477739

17. de Tommaso M, Ambrosini A, Brighina F et al (2014) Altered processing of sensory stimuli in patients with migraine. Nat Rev Neurol 10:144–155. https://doi.org/10.1038/nrneurol.2014.14

18. Ambrosini A, de Noordhout AM, Sándor PS, Schoenen J (2003) Electrophysiological studies in migraine: a comprehensive review of their interest and limitations. Cephalalgia Int J Headache 23(Suppl 1):13–31. https://doi.org/10.1046/j.1468-2982.2003.00571.x

19. Coppola G, Di Lorenzo C, Schoenen J, Pierelli F (2013) Habituation and sensitization in primary headaches. J Headache Pain 14:65. https://doi.org/10.1186/1129-2377-14-65

20. Coppola G, Pierelli F, Schoenen J (2009) Habituation and migraine. Neurobiol Learn Mem 92:249–259. https://doi.org/10.1016/j.nlm.2008.07.006

21. Schoenen J (2011) Is chronic migraine a never-ending migraine attack? Pain 152:239–240. https://doi.org/10.1016/j.pain.2010.12.002

22. Coppola G, Schoenen J (2012) Cortical excitability in chronic migraine. Curr Pain Headache Rep 16:93–100. https://doi.org/10.1007/s11916-011-0231-1

23. Coppola G, Currà A, Di Lorenzo C et al (2010) Abnormal cortical responses to somatosensory stimulation in medication-overuse headache. BMC Neurol 10:126. https://doi.org/10.1186/1471-2377-10-126

24. Chen W-T, Wang S-J, Fuh J-L et al (2012) Visual cortex excitability and plasticity associated with remission from chronic to episodic migraine. Cephalalgia Int J Headache 32:537–543. https://doi.org/10.1177/0333102412443337

25. Wutzler A, Winter C, Kitzrow W et al (2008) Loudness dependence of auditory evoked potentials as indicator of central serotonergic neurotransmission: simultaneous electrophysiological recordings and in vivo microdialysis in the rat primary auditory cortex. Neuropsychopharmacol Off Publ Am Coll Neuropsychopharmacol 33:3176–3181. https://doi.org/10.1038/npp.2008.42

26. Ambrosini A, Rossi P, De Pasqua V et al (2003) Lack of habituation causes high intensity dependence of auditory evoked cortical potentials in migraine. Brain J Neurol 126:2009–2015. https://doi.org/10.1093/brain/awg206

27. Magis D, Ambrosini A, Bendtsen L et al (2007) Evaluation and proposal for optimalization of neurophysiological tests in migraine: part 1--electrophysiological tests. Cephalalgia Int J Headache 27:1323–1338. https://doi.org/10.1111/j.1468-2982.2007.01440.x

28. Rocco A, Afra J, Toscano M et al (2007) Acute subcortical stroke and early serotonergic modification: a IDAP study. Eur J Neurol 14:1378–1382. https://doi.org/10.1111/j.1468-1331.2007.01985.x

29. Toscano M, Viganò A, Puledda F et al (2014) Serotonergic correlation with anger and aggressive behavior in acute stroke patients: an intensity dependence of auditory evoked potentials (IDAP) study. Eur Neurol 72:186–192. https://doi.org/10.1159/000362268

30. Di Clemente L, Coppola G, Magis D et al (2009) Nitroglycerin sensitises in healthy subjects CNS structures involved in migraine pathophysiology: evidence from a study of nociceptive blink reflexes and visual evoked potentials. Pain 144:156–161. https://doi.org/10.1016/j.pain.2009.04.018

31. Panconesi A (2008) Serotonin and migraine: a reconsideration of the central theory. J Headache Pain 9:267–276. https://doi.org/10.1007/s10194-008-0058-2

32. Buse DC, Silberstein SD, Manack AN et al (2013) Psychiatric comorbidities of episodic and chronic migraine. J Neurol 260:1960–1969. https://doi.org/10.1007/s00415-012-6725-x

33. Chen W-T, Wang S-J, Fuh J-L et al (2011) Persistent ictal-like visual cortical excitability in chronic migraine. Pain 152:254–258. https://doi.org/10.1016/j.pain.2010.08.047

34. Lai T-H, Protsenko E, Cheng Y-C et al (2015) Neural plasticity in common forms of chronic headaches. Neural Plast 2015:205985. https://doi.org/10.1155/2015/205985

35. Brennan KC, Pietrobon D (2018) A systems neuroscience approach to migraine. Neuron 97:1004–1021. https://doi.org/10.1016/j.neuron.2018.01.029

36. Froemke RC (2015) Plasticity of cortical excitatory-inhibitory balance. Annu Rev Neurosci 38:195–219. https://doi.org/10.1146/annurev-neuro-071714-034002

37. Kuhlman SJ, Olivas ND, Tring E et al (2013) A disinhibitory microcircuit initiates critical-period plasticity in the visual cortex. Nature 501:543–546. https://doi.org/10.1038/nature12485

38. Coppola G, Vandenheede M, Di Clemente L et al (2005) Somatosensory evoked high-frequency oscillations reflecting thalamo-cortical activity are decreased in migraine patients between attacks. Brain J Neurol 128:98–103. https://doi.org/10.1093/brain/awh334

39. Cosentino G, Fierro B, Vigneri S et al (2014) Cyclical changes of cortical excitability and metaplasticity in migraine: evidence from a repetitive transcranial magnetic stimulation study. Pain 155:1070–1078. https://doi.org/10.1016/j.pain.2014.02.024

40. Song Z, Ultenius C, Meyerson BA, Linderoth B (2009) Pain relief by spinal cord stimulation involves serotonergic mechanisms: an experimental study in a rat model of mononeuropathy. Pain 147:241–248. https://doi.org/10.1016/j.pain.2009.09.020

41. Song Z, Meyerson BA, Linderoth B (2011) Spinal 5-HT receptors that contribute to the pain-relieving effects of spinal cord stimulation in a rat model of neuropathy. Pain 152:1666–1673. https://doi.org/10.1016/j.pain.2011.03.012

42. Meunier CNJ, Amar M, Lanfumey L et al (2013) 5-HT(1A) receptors direct the orientation of plasticity in layer 5 pyramidal neurons of the mouse prefrontal cortex. Neuropharmacology 71:37–45. https://doi.org/10.1016/j.neuropharm.2013.03.003

43. Meunier CNJ, Callebert J, Cancela J-M, Fossier P (2015) Effect of dopaminergic D1 receptors on plasticity is dependent of serotoninergic 5-HT1A receptors in L5-pyramidal neurons of the prefrontal cortex. PLoS One 10:e0120286. https://doi.org/10.1371/journal.pone.0120286

44. Yang Y-C, Hu C-C, Huang C-S, Chou P-Y (2014) Thalamic synaptic transmission of sensory information modulated by synergistic interaction of adenosine and serotonin. J Neurochem 128:852–863. https://doi.org/10.1111/jnc.12499

45. Kemp A (1991) Manahan-Vaughan D (2005) the 5-hydroxytryptamine4 receptor exhibits frequency-dependent properties in synaptic plasticity and behavioural metaplasticity in the hippocampal CA1 region in vivo. Cereb Cortex N Y N 15:1037–1043. https://doi.org/10.1093/cercor/bhh204

16

Psychological distress, neuroticism and disability associated with secondary chronic headache in the general population – the Akershus study of chronic headache

Espen Saxhaug Kristoffersen[1,2]* (iD), Kjersti Aaseth[2], Ragnhild Berling Grande[2,3], Christofer Lundqvist[2,4,5,6] and Michael Bjørn Russell[2,4]

Abstract

Background: Primary headaches are associated with psychological distress, neuroticism and disability. However, little is known about headache-related disability and psychological distress among people with secondary chronic headaches.

Methods: 30,000 persons aged 30–44 from the general population was screened for headache by a questionnaire. The responder rate was 71%. The International Classification of Headache Disorders with supplementary definitions for chronic rhinosinusitis and cervicogenic headache were used. The Hopkins Symptom Checklist-25 assessed high psychological distress, the Migraine Disability Assessment questionnaire assessed disability, and Eysenck Personality Questionnaire assessed neuroticism.

Results: Ninety-five of the 113 eligible participants (84%) completed the self-reported questionnaire. A total of 38 people had chronic post-traumatic headache, 21 had cervicogenic headache, and 39 had headache attributed to chronic rhinosinusitis, while 9 had co-occurrence of chronic post-traumatic and cervicogenic headache. Six persons had miscellaneous secondary chronic headaches. Overall, 49% of those with secondary chronic headache reported high psychological distress, which is significantly higher than in the general population. A high level of neuroticism was significantly more common in those with secondary chronic headache than in the general population. Severe headache-related disability was reported by 69%. 92 persons were followed up after 3 years. A low headache frequency was the only significant predictor of improvement of ≥ 25% in headache days. Having post-traumatic or cervicogenic headache and not headache attributed to chronic rhinosinusitis predicted an increased risk > 25% worsening of headache days or having a severe disability at 3 years follow-up.

Conclusion: Psychological distress and neuroticism were more common among people with secondary chronic headache than in the general population. Only a high headache frequency was significantly associated with increased headache disability at baseline and a poor prognosis in the long term.

* Correspondence: e.s.kristoffersen@medisin.uio.no
[1]Department of General Practice, Institute of Health and Society, University of Oslo, Box 1130 Blindern, 0318 Oslo, PO, Norway
[2]Head and Neck Research Group, Research Centre, Akershus University Hospital, Lørenskog, Norway
Full list of author information is available at the end of the article

Background

Headache, anxiety and depression are all prevalent conditions in the general population [1]. It has been suggested that anxiety, depression and neuroticism scores are associated with primary headaches [2–6]. Whether or not these factors are associated as a cause or a consequence of the headaches is still debated and personality traits and psychological problems may influence cognitive and affective functioning [3, 7, 8]. Neuroticism is often described as a personality trait that reflects the extent to which a person experiences the world as stressful, anxious, threatening, and problematic [9, 10]. Furthermore, neuroticism has been associated with depression [11].

Secondary headache after head traumas, whiplash, neck conditions or rhinosinusitis resolves in the majority of cases. The reasons why some people develop more persistent symptoms are disputed [12–16]. In addition, the pathophysiology of most of these secondary headache disorders is poorly understood [15, 16]. Both the existence of psychological distress and neuroticism are associated with chronic pain conditions and have been suggested to play important roles in the transition from acute to chronic pain in cognitive and behavioural models [9, 10, 17, 18]. Furthermore, anxiety, depression, psychological distress and neuroticism are considered to be vulnerability factors that lower the threshold at which pain is perceived as threatening, thus contributing to pain-catastrophizing and anxiety, which are associated with the progression of chronic pain [9, 10, 17, 18]. In addition, affective temperaments, personality traits, perceptions and psychological distress may significantly and negatively modify disability, treatment outcomes and long-term prognosis of patients with headache and chronic pain conditions [19–23].

However, neither anxiety, depression, neuroticism nor headache-related disability have been studied in secondary chronic headache.

The main aim of the present study was to investigate psychological distress, neuroticism and disability in people with secondary chronic headache from the general population. A secondary aim was to evaluate whether psychological distress, neuroticism or disability predicted the long-term prognosis of secondary chronic headache.

Methods

Study design, population and variables

This was a cross-sectional epidemiological survey of 30,000 representative persons aged 30–44 drawn from the general population of eastern Akershus County, Norway [24]. A postal questionnaire screened for possible chronic headache (≥15 days/last month and/or ≥ 180 days/last year). Screening-positive subjects were invited to a clinical interview at Akershus University Hospital.

The sample size was reduced to 28,871 because of error in the address list ($n = 1065$), emigration ($n = 32$), multi-handicap ($n = 28$), insufficient Norwegian language skills (n = 2) and death (n = 2). In total 71% (20,598/ 28,871) of the study population responded to the screening questionnaire. Among responders, the first questionnaire, and second and third reminders were replied to by 64%, 23% and 13%, respectively. There was no significant difference between self-reported chronic headache and response to the three reminder waves when analysed separately by sex.

Of 935 people with self-reported chronic headache, 53 persons did not consent to further contact, and 30 persons did not speak Norwegian. Among the 852 eligible, 139 declined participation and 80 could not be reached by telephone. In total, 633 participated in clinical interviews (490 as an ambulatory visit, 143 by telephone).

Figure 1 shows a flow chart of the study.The method has been described in detail elsewhere [24, 25].

After the interview, the participants filled in a self-administered questionnaire including the Hopkins Symptom Checklist-25 (HSCL-25), The Migraine Disability Assessment (MIDAS) questionnaire and the Eysenck Personality Questionnaire (EPQ) N- and L-scale. The participants also provided information on socio-demographics, height, weight, smoking status, medication-overuse and headache frequency.

Semi-structured follow-up interviews were conducted after an average of 3 years, mainly by telephone (by RBG and KAA) [26]. Among the 113 persons who fulfilled the inclusion criteria, 9 persons were not eligible because of unavailable telephone numbers, and 12 did not answer the telephone despite at least six attempts. Thus, 92 people were followed-up after 3 years.

Inclusion criteria
Secondary chronic headache.

Exclusion criteria
Secondary chronic headache exclusively due to medication overuse.

Headache classification
The International Classification of Headache Disorders (ICHD-II) was applied based on the interviews, and the diagnoses were later reclassified according to ICHD-III [27].

Chronic headache was defined as headache ≥15 days/ months for at least 3 months or ≥ 180 days/year. Chronic post-traumatic headache (CPTH) included head ($n = 24$) and whiplash ($n = 14$) traumas. Among those with CPTH caused by head injury, 20 had a mild head injury and four had a moderate to severe head injury. Cervicogenic headache (CEH) was additionally classified according to the criteria of the Cervicogenic Headache International

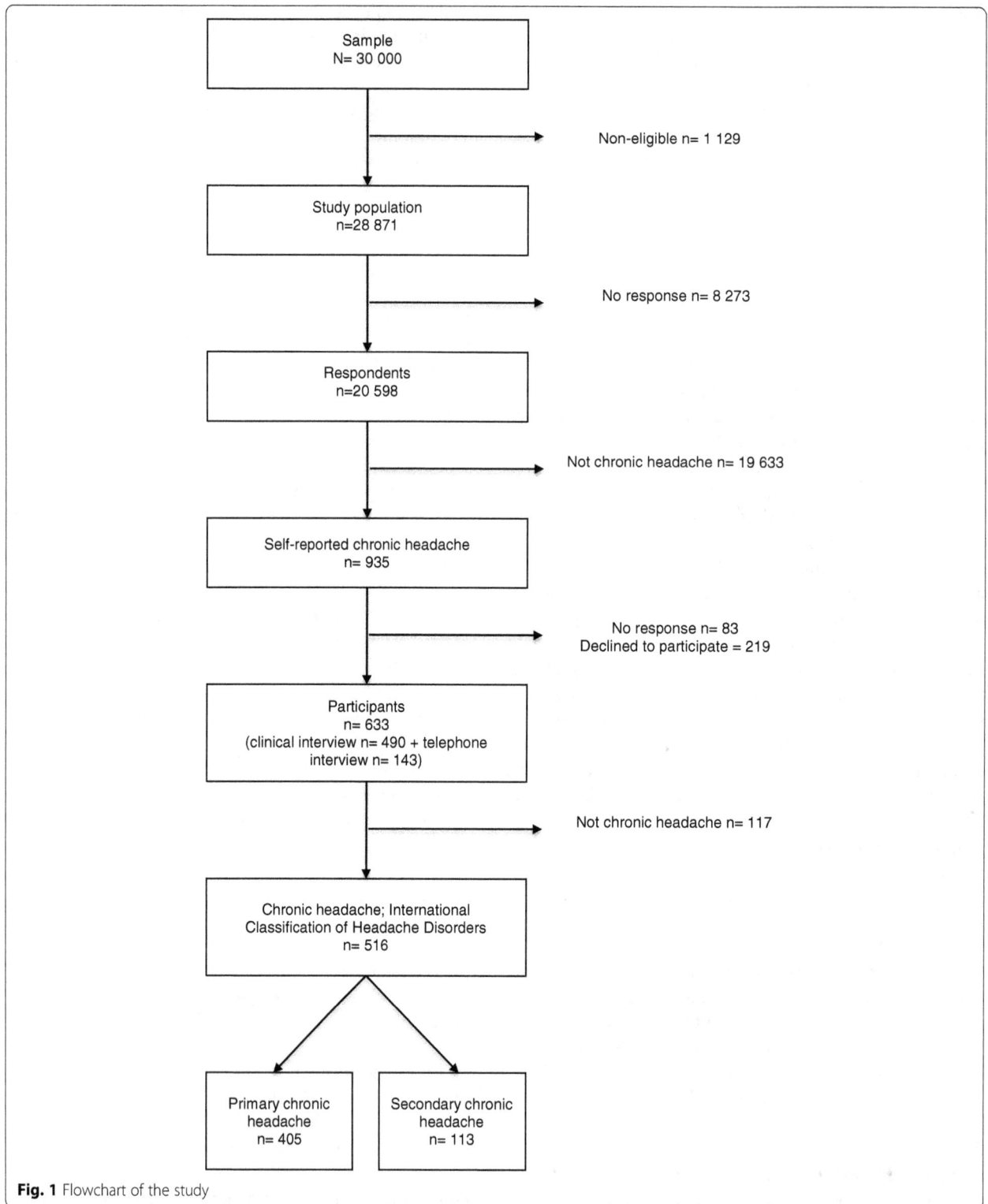

Fig. 1 Flowchart of the study

Study Group, requiring at least three criteria to be fulfilled, not including blockade of the neck due to the non-interventional nature of our study (Textbox 1a) [28]. Headache attributed to chronic rhinosinusitis (HACRS) was also, in addition, defined according to the criteria established by the American Academy of Otolaryngology – Head and Neck Surgery (Textbox 2b) adding that the symptoms had persisted for 12 weeks or more [29].

Anxiety, depression and psychological distress

The Hopkins Symptom Checklist-25 (HSCL-25) explores the symptoms of depression and anxiety and is a validated tool for measuring the level of psychological distress [30]. The HSCL-25 corresponds well to DSM-IV defined depression and anxiety disorders, depression, phobia and somatoform illness using "the Composite International Diagnostic Interview" (CIDI) as gold standard diagnostic instrument [30–32]. The 25 items are scored on a scale from 1 (not bothered) to four (extremely bothered). If 20 or more of the 25 items were answered, a mean score was calculated. High psychological distress was defined as a mean HSCL-25 score ≥ 1.67 for men and ≥ 1.75 for women [31]. Although the HSCL-25 measures anxiety and depression dimensions, "forced" two-factor analyses are in favour of a one-factor solution [31]. Thus, in the present study both the anxiety, depression and the mean total HSCL-25 scores are given, but we only used the mean total HSCL-25 score to define psychological distress which, thus, includes both anxiety disorder and depression.

Neuroticism

The Eysenck Personality Questionnaire (EPQ) is an instrument designed to measure personality dimensions or traits [33]. We used two of the four EPQ scales: the 23-item neuroticism scale (N-scale) and the 21-item lie scale (L-scale) to assess neuroticism.

The EPQ N-scale is designed to measure neurotic personality traits and symptoms of moodiness, nervousness, being easily irritated, lack of endurance, and feelings of guilt and worry [33]. The L- scale assesses dissimulation or a tendency toward social conformity [33]. Both scales are dichotomous, yes or no. 'Yes' was scored as 1 and 'no' was scored as 0.

A low N-scale score indicates a low level of neuroticism and a high L-scale score indicates a high level of social conformity. EPQ has previously been validated in Norway [34].

Headache-related disability

The Migraine Disability Assessment (MIDAS) questionnaire is a valid and widely used instrument to measure headache disability [35].

MIDAS consists of five questions concerning headache and the number of days, in the past 3 months, of activity limitations (impairment in role functioning) in three domains: schoolwork or work for pay; housework; and family, social, or leisure activities. Disability grade was scored according to MIDAS as minimal (0–5), mild (6–10), moderate (11–20) or severe (≥ 21) [35].

HSCL-25 and EPQ population controls

The age- and sex-matched HSCL-25 scores reported from the general population in this study were derived from the cross-sectional Oslo-Lofoten 2001 study [6, 36]. This study was designed to examine general health and mental health within two geographically diverse areas, one urban (Oslo) and one rural (Lofoten). The participants were interviewed with a fully structured interview that assessed a broad range of topics related to mental and physical health [6, 36].

The EPQ scores were derived from a cross-sectional Danish study of headache disorders in the general population [5]. This sample was representative of the Danish general population.

Statistical analysis

For descriptive data, proportions, means and standard deviations (SD) or 95% confidence intervals (CI) are given. Groups were compared using the t-test (continuous data) or the χ^2 test (categorical data).

Logistic regression models were used to evaluate presence of i) high psychological distress and ii) severe disability at baseline in secondary chronic headaches. Linear regression was used to investigate the association between neuroticism and secondary chronic headache. High psychological distress and neuroticism were clearly correlated with a high degree of collinearity and therefore not used in the same regression analysis. Furthermore, logistic regression was also used to evaluate i) reversion to episodic headache and ii) headache improvement ($\geq 25\%$ reduction in headache days), iii) headache worsening ($\geq 25\%$ increase in headache days), and iv) severe headache disability (MIDAS≥ 21) after 3 years follow-up. The results are presented with odds ratios (ORs) with 95% CIs.

As this was a hypothesis generating descriptive study Bonferroni corrections were not done and significance levels were set at $p < 0.05$, using two-sided test. All statistical analyses were performed using SPSS version 25.0.

Ethical issues

The Regional Committee for Medical Research Ethics and the Norwegian Social Science Data Services approved the study. All participants gave informed consent.

Results

In total 95 of the 113 eligible participants (84%) completed the self-reported questionnaire at baseline. Responders and non-responders did not differ in age, gender, or in the distribution of headache diagnoses (data not shown).

A total of 38 people had CPTH, 21 had CEH and 39 had HACRS, while 9 had co-occurrence of CPTH and CEH. Six persons had miscellaneous secondary chronic

Table 1 Descriptive statistics for all respondents with secondary chronic headache. *P*-value given for the comparison of chronic post-traumatic headache/cervicogenic headache vs. headache attributed to chronic rhinosinusitis

	All secondary chronic headaches N = 95	Post-traumatic/cervicogenic headache N = 50	Rhinosinusitis headache N = 39	(p-value for CPTH/CEH vs. HACRS)
Age, mean (SD)	38.7 (4.2)	38.9 (4.2)	38.9 (3.8)	0.82
Gender, n (%)				0.06
Female	77 (81)	37 (74)	35 (90)	
Male	18 (19)	13 (26)	4 (10)	
Education, highest attained, n (%)				0.92
≤ 15 years	75 (76)	38 (76)	30 (77)	
> 15 years	24 (25)	12 (24)	9 (23)	
Married or cohabitant, n (%)	60 (63)	32 (64)	25 (64)	0.99
Body mass index (kg/m^2), mean (SD)	26.6 (5.0)	27.4 (5.3)	25.5 (4.5)	0.11
Daily smoker, n (%)				0.93
No	57 (63)	30 (63)	24 (62)	
Yes	35 (37)	18 (37)	15 (38)	
Concomitant migraine, n (%)				0.15
No	55 (58)	32 (64)	19 (49)	
Yes	40 (42)	18 (36)	20 (51)	
Number of headache days past 3 months, mean (SD)	62.0 (27.1)	70.5 (25.4)	52.4 (24.5)	0.002
Number of medication days past month, mean (SD)	12.8 (10.8)	13.4 (11.5)	13.2 (10.3)	0.94
Medication-overuse, n (%)				0.76
No	50 (53)	26 (52)	19 (49)	
Yes	45 (47)	24 (48)	20 (51)	
HSCL-25 scores, mean (SD)				
Anxiety score, mean (SD)				
Female	1.80 (0.46)	1.88 (0.43)	1.79 (0.48)	0.37
Male	1.84 (0.49)	1.85 (0.50)	1.88 (0.56)	0.94
Depression score, mean (SD)				
Female	1.83 (0.55)	1.88 (0.59)	1.87 (0.50)	0.96
Male	1.79 (0.56)	1.76 (0.56)	1.67 (0.49)	0.77
Total score, mean (SD)				
Female	1.82 (0.48)	1.88 (0.49)	1.84 (0.44)	0.70
Male	1.81 (0.49)	1.80 (0.52)	1.75 (0.51)	0.88
HSCL-25, psychological distress, n (%)				0.40
No (< 1.67 for men and < 1.75 for women)	48 (51)	22 (45)	21 (54)	
Yes (> 1.67 for men and > 1.75 for women)	46 (49)	27 (55)	18 (46)	
EPQ N-score, mean (SD)	11.4 (5.4)	10.6 (5.5)	12.9 (4.9)	0.06
EPQ L-score, mean (SD)	10.6 (3.2)	10.4 (3.6)	10.9 (2.6)	0.5
MIDAS score, mean (SD)	66 (60)	80 (60)	44 (46)	0.005
MIDAS score (grade), n (%)				0.23
0–5 Minimal	16 (20)	6 (14)	9 (27)	
6–10 Mild	4 (5)	2 (5)	2 (6)	
11–20 Moderate	5 (6)	1 (2)	3 (9)	
> 20 Severe	55 (69)	33 (79)	19 (58)	

headaches. Those with CPTH and CEH were descriptive similar (gender, co-occurrence of migraine, medication overuse) and were also due to small groups merged for the purpose of statistical analyses. Descriptive characteristics of the sample are given in Table 1.

Psychological distress and neuroticism

The anxiety and depression HSCL-25 scores were high in secondary chronic headaches (Table 1). Mean total HSCL-25 scores for women and men were 1.82 (95% CI 1.71–1.93) and 1.81 (1.56–2.05) and thus statistically significantly higher than in the general population (women; 1.39 (1.34–1.43), men; 1.25 (1.22–1.29). In total, 46% (35–57) women and 61% (39–80) men of the sample had high psychological distress, which is statistically significantly higher than 14% (10–18) of women and 9% (6–13) of men in the general population.

Neither age, gender, headache frequency, co-occurrence of migraine, medication overuse or secondary headache diagnosis (CPTH/CEH versus HACRS) were significantly associated with high psychological distress in the multivariate regression analyses (Table 2).

Neuroticism as assessed by EPQ N-scale was significant higher in secondary chronic headache than in the general population (11.4 vs. 6.2, $p < 0.0001$). Neither age, gender, migraine, medication overuse, type of secondary chronic headache, headache frequency nor disability were significantly associated with a high level of neuroticism in bivariate and the multivariate linear regression analyses (Table 3). The EPQ L-scale was not significantly different between those with secondary chronic headache and the general population. High psychological distress and neuroticism were not associated with co-occurrence of other chronic pain conditions.

Headache disability

The mean MIDAS score was 66 (52–79) for secondary chronic headaches with a significantly higher mean score in CPTH/CEH than in HACRS (80 vs. 44, $p = 0.005$, Table 1). Almost 70% of those with secondary chronic headache were classified in the most severe disability class, i.e. approximately 80% of those with CPTH/CEH, and 60% of those with HACRS. This was statistically significant ($p = 0.05$). Only a high baseline headache frequency was associated with severe disability with an OR 4.3 (1.2–15.5, $p = 0.021$) in the multivariate regression analyses (Table 4).

Psychological distress, neuroticism and disability as predictors of headache prognosis

In total, 78 of the 92 eligible participants (85%) at 3 years follow-up had completed the self-reported questionnaire

Table 2 Odds for having high psychological distress defined as mean HSCL-25 score ≥ 1.67 for men and ≥ 1.75 for women. Logistic regression

Covariate	High psychological distress							
	Bivariate ($n = 80$–94)				Multivariable ($n = 83$)			
	n	Odds ratio	95% CI	p-value	n	Odds ratio	95% CI	p-value
Age	94	1.0	0.9–1.1	0.5	83	1.0	0.9–1.2	0.6
Gender								
Male	18	1			17	1		
Female	76	0.5	0.2–1.6	0.3	66	0.7	0.2–2.2	0.5
Headache days last 3 months								
< 80 days	50	1			47	1		
≥ 80 days	38	1.3	0.6–3.0	0.5	36	1.1	0.4–3.1	0.9
Co-occurrence of migraine								
No	54	1			48	1		
Yes	40	0.6	0.3–1.5	0.3	35	0.6	0.2–1.4	0.2
Type of headache								
HACRS	39	1			36	1		
CPTH/CEH	49	1.4	0.6–3.3	0.4	47	1.1	0.4–3.0	0.8
Medication overuse								
No	49	1			43	1		
Yes	45	2.0	0.9–4.5	0.1	40	1.9	0.8–4.8	0.2

Table 3 Linear regression analysis with variables associated with neuroticism in secondary chronic headache

| | Neuroticism Eysenck N-scale | | | | | | | |
| | Bivariate (n = 79) | | | | Multivariable (n = 72) | | | |
	N	Unstandarized coefficient	95% CI	p-value	N	Unstandarized coefficient	95% CI	p-value
Age	79	0.14	−0.15; 0.43	0.3	72	0.10	−0.23; 0.42	0.6
Gender								
Male*	16	0			15	0		
Female	63	1.34	−1.62; 4.30	0.4	57	0.88	−2.53; 4.30	0.6
Headache days last 3 months								
< 80 days*	41	0			40	0		
≥ 80 days	33	−0.77	−3.29; 1.76	0.5	32	−0.34	−3.43; 2.76	0.8
Co-occurrence of migraine								
No*	49	0			43	0		
Yes	30	0.09	−2.39; 2.55	0.9	29	−0.34	−3.10; 2.43	0.8
Type of headache								
HACRS*	32	0			30	0		
CPTH/CEH	44	−2.23	−4.65; 0.19	0.07	42	−2.10	−5.27; 1.07	0.2
Medication overuse								
No*	42	0			37	0		
Yes	37	1.73	−0.64; 4.09	0.2	35	1.72	−0.96; 4.39	0.2

*denotes reference group

Table 4 Odds for having severe disability defined as MIDAS score > 20. Logistic regression

| Covariate | Severe disability | | | | | | | |
| | Bivariate (n = 74–94) | | | | Multivariable (n = 74) | | | |
	n	Odds ratio	95% CI	p-value	n	Odds ratio	95% CI	p-value
Age	80	1.0	0.9–1.1	0.7	74	1.0	0.9–1.2	1.0
Gender								
Male	18	1			17	1		
Female	62	1.1	0.4–3.5	0.8	57	1.5	0.4–5.9	0.5
Headache days last 3 months								
< 80 days	45	1			42	1		
≥ 80 days	34	4.2	1.4–13.0	0.01	32	4.0	1.1–14.5	0.04
Co-occurrence of migraine								
No	50	1			46	1		
Yes	30	1.1	0.4–2.9	0.9	28	1.1	0.3–3.3	0.9
Type of headache								
HACRS	33	1			32	1		
CPTH/CEH	42	2.7	1.0–7.4	0.05	42	1.9	0.6–6.4	0.3
Medication overuse								
No	44	1			39	1		
Yes	36	1.3	0.5–3.5	0.5	35	1.3	0.4–4.0	0.7
HSCL-25 defined psychological distress								
No	43	1			38	1		
Yes	37	1.5	0.6–3.8	0.5	36	1.1	0.4–3.4	0.9

at baseline and were available for the predictor analyses over time.

Low headache frequency (below 75th percentile, i.e. below 80 headache days over 3 months) and non-severe disability at baseline significantly predicted reversal from chronic to episodic headache in the multivariate regression analyses (Table 5). A low headache frequency at baseline was the only predictor associated with an improvement of ≥ 25% in headache days over the follow-up time period in the multivariate regression analyses (Table 5). Having CPTH/CEH and not HACRS predicted an increased risk of ≥ 25% worsening of headache days or having a severe disability at 3 years follow-up (Table 5).

Discussion

In this large population-based study almost half of the subjects with secondary chronic headache reported high psychological distress. The main finding was that the prevalence of high psychological distress and neuroticism was higher than in the general population and that there were no differences between those with CPTH/CEH and HACRS regarding psychological distress and neuroticism. In terms of long term prognosis, we found that low headache disability, low headache frequency and having HACRS at baseline, but not psychological distress and neuroticism, predicted headache improvement.

Methodological discussion

The population-based sample in the present study was large, and the high response rate ensures representativity compare to the general population aged 30–44. The age range in our study was chosen in order to ascertain little co-morbidity of non-headache disorders and use of non-headache medications.

We used population-based reference populations for comparison to minimize selection bias. The reference populations were representative for the Danish and the Norwegian general populations regarding age, gender and marital status. The Danish reference population had a wider age range than our sample, and the data was besides collected 15 years earlier. However, the latter is probably not a source for bias, as personality traits are regarded as stable over time.

Even though the sample size of secondary chronic headache is relatively small and conferred some challenges due to reduced power in the statistical analyses, it is the largest population based sample reported so far. The sample size limited the number of variables that could be included in the multivariate analyses, and forced us to dichotomize some variables. Recall bias regarding headache days and medication days cannot be excluded, but the meticulous interview and pre-completed medication list are likely to reduce such bias.

Our study is strengthened by face-to-face interviews by headache experts as this provides more valid headache diagnoses than questionnaire-based diagnoses [37].

The majority of the participants completed a full diagnostic interview conducted by a headache expert albeit with a smaller portion by telephone. The main reason for not completing a full clinical interview was not being available for travelling to a clinical interview during an ordinary work week. However, the headache diagnoses were not significantly different in these two groups of participants. Furthermore, no significant differences between data collected at the clinic and by telephone by a trained headache expert was reported in a previous study [38].

The diagnostic criteria of CEH and HACRS have been discussed for many years. At the 1st data collection the ICHD-II criteria were available, but the criteria for CEH were vague, and HACRS was not recognized as a cause of chronic headache. Thus, to improve the diagnostic accuracy we used supplementary definitions [28, 29]. All subjects diagnosed with CEH or HACRS in the present study fulfil the new ICHD-III criteria for these chronic headaches [27]. Since two physicians conducted the investigations, inter-observer variation is a possibility. However, the headache diagnoses were equally frequent by both physicians, suggesting that inter-observer variation was low.

Psychological distress, neuroticism and disability in secondary chronic headaches

No previous study has investigated psychological distress or neuroticism for secondary chronic headache in the general population. We have previously shown that for chronic tension-type headache (CTTH) in the general population, the overall prevalence of psychological distress was 59% (53–65) for women and 43% (32–55) for men [6]. Furthermore, the mean HSCL score was 1.71 (1.60–1.82) for men with CTTH and 1.93 (1.86–2.00) for women with CTTH. Those with CTTH and co-occurrence of migraine and/or medication overuse did not have a higher level of HSCL score or psychological distress compared with those without co-occurrence of migraine and/or medication overuse [6]. These findings indicate that there are no significant differences in psychological distress between primary and secondary chronic headaches.

The prevalence of psychological distress in the Norwegian general population using the same cut-offs and age group as in the present study were 14% (10–18) for women and 9% (6–13) for men [6]. Thus, the prevalence of psychological distress is more than four times higher in people with secondary chronic headache than in the general population. A difference in psychological distress between episodic and chronic headache has been reported suggesting that the relationship between

Table 5 Multivariate logistic regression. Baseline predictors for different outcomes of secondary chronic headaches after 3 years follow-up

Covariate	No chronic headache Multivariate (n = 63)				>25% reduction in headache days Multivariate (n = 61)				>25% increase in headache days Multivariate (n = 61)				Severe disability Multivariate (n = 46)			
	N	Odds Ratio	95% CI	p-value	N	Odds Ratio	95% CI	p-value	N	Odds Ratio	95% CI	p-value	N	Odds Ratio	95% CI	p-value
Age	63	1.0	0.8–1.2	0.8	61	1.0	0.8–1.2	0.9	61	1.0	0.8–1.2	0.8	46	1.3	1.0–1.8	0.1
Gender																
Male	13	1.7	0.3–11.4	0.6	12	1.3	0.2–8.9	0.8	12	0.3	0.0–2.6	0.3	10	0.2	0.0–10.8	0.5
Female	59	1			49	1			49	1			36	1		
Headache days last 3 months																
<80 days	35	11.0	1.2–99.7	0.03	34	14.3	1.6–127.7	0.017	34	0.0	0.0–0.0	1.0	31	0.4	0.1–4.2	0.5
≥80 days	28	1			27	1			27	1			15	1		
Type of headache																
HACRS	28	2.6	0.5–13.3	0.3	27	2.5	0.5–11.9	0.3	27	0.1	0.0–0.8	0.03	26	0.1	0.0–0.8	0.035
CPTH/CEH	35	1			34	1			34	1			20	1		
Medication overuse																
No	32	1.6	0.3–7.3	0.6	30	1.6	0.4–7.0	0.5	30	0.2	0.0–1.6	0.2	24	0.1	0.0–1.6	0.1
Yes	31	1			31	1			31	1			22	1		
HSCL-25 defined psychological distress																
No	34	1.8	0.4–8.5	0.4	33	1.5	0.3–6.2	0.6	33	0.6	0.1–2.9	0.5	25	0.7	0.1–6.5	0.8
Yes	29	1			28	1			28	1			21	1		
Disability grade																
No to moderate	21	3.6	0.9–14.3	0.04	20	1.3	0.3–5.1	0.7	20	1.4	0.3–6.8	0.6	18	0.0	0.0–0.0	1.0
Severe	42	1			41	1			41	1			28	1		

psychological problems and headache depends more on headache frequency than the type of headache [3, 39, 40]. Neither in the present study nor in a study of CTTH did more headache days above 15 days increase the odds for more psychological distress [6]. Therefore, it may be the complex burden of chronic headache or an underlying vulnerability, more than the specific headache condition or additional headache days > 15 that are associated with psychological problems.

Recent reviews have estimated the global prevalence of depression and anxiety in the range 4.4–5.0% and 4.8–10.9% which is in accordance with findings from the Norwegian general population using HSCL-25 and CIDI [1, 32]. Our results thus suggest population-derived secondary chronic headache patients to lie much higher than the general population.

Whether anxiety and depression have a shared mechanism with headache, whether they represent risk factors for headache chronification or are just comorbid symptoms related to a disabling headache situation is still a matter of debate [7, 8, 27]. It may be that an improvement in headache frequency improves depression and anxiety levels or vice versa. However, independently of the causal directions of these associations, it is important always to take psychological factors into account when treating headache, as the condition is clearly associated with such factors [3, 7, 27, 39]. Thus, a best possible treatment approach for many headache sufferers includes acute and prophylactic medications and multidisciplinary treatment addressing the psychological factors such as anxiety and depression.

In the present study we report that CPTH/CEH and HACRS had similar prevalence of psychological distress despite different pathophysiological mechanisms. Furthermore, the prevalence of psychological distress was comparable to that of two other chronic headaches; chronic tension-type headache and medication-overuse headache [6, 41]. Depression and anxiety are known to be associated also with other chronic pain conditions [42–44]. However, such co-morbidity of other chronic pain did not increase the psychological distress in the present study.

The neuroticism score in secondary chronic headache reported here was comparable to that of chronic tension-type headache and chronic headache, but higher than the score reported in episodic headache [2, 5, 6]. A higher neuroticism score in primary headaches than in the general population has previously been reported with some studies suggesting a stronger association with tension-type headache than with migraine [2, 4–6]. The EPQ L-score was not significantly different from the general population and was similar to that previously reported in episodic and chronic headache [2, 5].

Disability is an important outcome as it reflects the burden and impact of diseases on daily activities [35].

Almost 70% of our participants had severe disability, suggesting that people with secondary chronic headache are among the most disabled headache patients. Surprisingly, high psychological distress, which may add to the burden of headache and pain, was not associated with increased disability.

Prognosis of secondary chronic headaches

We have previously shown that secondary chronic headaches have varying courses, depending on the subtype, with HACRS having a better long-term prognosis than CEH [26]. However, why some people develop persistent symptoms in the first place and what predicts poor prognosis in whiplash-associated traumas, mild to moderate head injuries and neck disorders is disputed partly due to inconsistent findings [12, 13, 16, 42, 45]. The lack of correspondence between severity of the traumas (whiplash and post-traumatic headache) and neck conditions (CEH) and the chronicity of symptoms has led to the assumption that psychological factors may play a crucial role in the cause and maintenance of these disorders. However, psychological factors account for only a portion of the variance in most of these studies, thereby highlighting the possible and complex bio-behavioural pathophysiology which may partly explain these conditions [42]. It has been hypothesised that a certain set of personality traits or distress makes these patients more vulnerable, with poorer adjustment to their medical condition than other people without these personality traits [10]. Our results indicate that only a high headache frequency, severe headache disability and type of secondary headache seem to influence the outcome after 3 years. However, based on the study design, it is not possible to say if personality traits or psychological distress are linked to the development of the secondary chronic headache.

Although medication overuse was not a prognostic factor or associated with neuroticism or high psychological distress, it is worthwhile to notion that about half of all patients overused acute headache medication. Whether detoxification may help these patients with other secondary headaches is still a matter of debate.

Neuroticism may influence pain sensitivity and pain perception, and hypothetically thus be involved in a possible central sensitisation in, and prognosis of, chronic pain conditions such as chronic headaches [5, 9, 46]. The results from our follow-up study do not suggest that neuroticism predicts prognosis of secondary chronic headaches. Furthermore, in this population, reported psychological distress also does not predict whether secondary chronic headaches improve or not. These findings may shed some light on the "hen and egg" issue; the headache rather than the personality characteristics seems to determine the prognosis of these secondary headaches.

Conclusion

People with secondary chronic headache have a higher psychological distress and neuroticism score than people from the general population. In terms of prognostic findings, only headache frequency and disability predicted improvement of the secondary headache, while psychological factors did not. Thus, the prime focus should be headache management, i.e. proper medication and multidisciplinary treatment addressing the psychological factors such as anxiety, depression, distress and neuroticism.

Textbox 1a. *Definition of cervicogenic headache* [28]. *It is obligatory that one or more of the phenomena Ia–Ic are present.*

Major criteria	I. Symptoms and signs of neck involvement Ia. Precipitation of head pain, similar to the usually occurring one: Ia1) by neck movement and/or sustained, awkward head positioning, and/or: Ia2) by external pressure over the upper cervical or occipital region on the symptomatic side. Ib. Restriction of the range of motion (ROM) in the neck. Ic. Ipsilateral neck, shoulder or arm pain of a rather vague, non-radicular nature, or – occasionally – arm pain of a radicular nature. II. Confirmatory evidence by diagnostic anaesthetic blockades. III. Unilaterality of the head pain, without sideshift.
Head pain characteristics	IV. Moderate-severe, non-throbbing pain, usually starting in the neck. Episodes of varying duration, or: fluctuating, continuous pain.
Other characteristics of some importance	V. Only marginal effect or lack of effect of indomethacin. Only marginal effect or lack of effect of ergotamine and sumatriptan. Female sex. Not infrequent occurrence of head or indirect neck trauma by history, usually of more than only medium severity.
Other features of lesser importance	VI. Various attack-related phenomena, only occasionally present, and/or moderately expressed when present: a) nausea, b) phono- and photophobia, c) dizziness, d) ipsilateral "blurred vision", e) difficulties swallowing, f) ipsilateral oedema, mostly in the periocular area.

Textbox 1b. *Definition of rhinosinusitis by the American Academy of Otolaryngology – Head and Neck Surgery* [29]. *Two major factors or one major and two minor factors are required for the diagnosis. Of note, facial pain requires another major factor associated with it for diagnosis, as facial pain plus two minor factors is not deemed sufficient for diagnoses of rhinosinusitis.*

Major factors

Facial pain/pressure

Nasal obstruction/blockage

Nasal discharge/purulence/discolored postnasal drainage

(Continued)

Hyposmia/anosmia

Purulence in nasal cavity on examination

Fever (acute rhinosinusitis)

Minor factors

Headache

Fever (all nonacute)

Halitosis

Fatigue

Dental pain

Cough

Ear pain/pressure/fullness

Abbreviations

CEH: Cervicogenic headache; CI: Confidence intervals; CIDI: The Composite International Diagnostic Interview; CPTH: Chronic post-traumatic headache; CTTH: Chronic tension-type headache; EPQ: Eysenck Personality Questionnaire; HACRS: Headache attributed to chronic rhinosinusitis; HSCL-25: Hopkins Symptom Checklist-25; ICHD: The International Classification of Headache Disorders; MIDAS: The Migraine Disability Assessment; ORs: Odds ratios

Acknowledgments

Akershus University Hospital kindly provided research facilities.

Funding

This study was supported by grants from the South East Norway Regional Health Authority and Institute of Clinical Medicine, Campus Akershus University Hospital, University of Oslo.

Authors' contributions

MBR had the original idea for the study and together with CL planned the overall design. RBG and KAA conducted all clinical interviews. All authors were involved in the planning and interpretation of the data analysis. ESK conducted the data analysis and prepared the initial draft. All authors have commented on, revised and approved the final manuscript.

Competing interest

The authors declare that they have no competing interests.

Author details

[1]Department of General Practice, Institute of Health and Society, University of Oslo, Box 1130 Blindern, 0318 Oslo, PO, Norway. [2]Head and Neck Research Group, Research Centre, Akershus University Hospital, Lørenskog, Norway. [3]The National Center for Epilepsy, Oslo University Hospital, Oslo, Norway. [4]Institute of Clinical Medicine, Campus Akershus University Hospital, University of Oslo, Nordbyhagen, Norway. [5]HØKH, Research Centre, Akershus University Hospital, Lørenskog, Norway. [6]Department of Neurology, Akershus University Hospital, Lørenskog, Norway.

References

1. Kessler RC, Aguilar-Gaxiola S, Alonso J, Chatterji S, Lee S, Ormel J, Ustun TB, Wang PS (2009) The global burden of mental disorders: an update from the WHO world mental health (WMH) surveys. Epidemiol Psichiatr Soc 18:23–33
2. Rasmussen BK (1992) Migraine and tension-type headache in a general population: psychosocial factors. Int J Epidemiol 21:1138–1143
3. Zwart JA, Dyb G, Hagen K, Ødegård KJ, Dahl AA, Bovim G, Stovner LJ, Odegard KJ (2003) Depression and anxiety disorders associated with headache frequency. The Nord-Trondelag health study. Eur J Neurol 10:147–152
4. Breslau N, Andreski P (1995) Migraine, personality, and psychiatric comorbidity. Headache 35:382–386
5. Ashina S, Bendtsen L, Buse DC, Lyngberg AC, Lipton RB, Jensen R (2017) Neuroticism, depression and pain perception in migraine and tension-type headache. Acta Neurol Scand 136:470–476
6. Aaseth K, Grande RB, Leiknes KA, Benth JS, Lundqvist C, Russell MB (2011) Personality traits and psychological distress in persons with chronic tension-type headache. The Akershus study of chronic headache. Acta Neurol Scand 124:375–382
7. Breslau N, Lipton RB, Stewart WF, Schultz LR, Welch KM (2003) Comorbidity of migraine and depression: investigating potential etiology and prognosis. Neurology 60:1308–1312
8. Yang Y, Ligthart L, Terwindt GM, Boomsma DI, Rodriguez-Acevedo AJ, Nyholt DR (2016) Genetic epidemiology of migraine and depression. Cephalalgia 36:679–691
9. Goubert L, Crombez G, Van Damme S (2004) The role of neuroticism, pain catastrophizing and pain-related fear in vigilance to pain: a structural equations approach. Pain 107:234–241
10. Kadimpati S, Zale EL, Hooten MW, Ditre JW, Warner DO (2015) Associations between neuroticism and depression in relation to catastrophizing and pain-related anxiety in chronic pain patients. PLoS One 10:e0126351
11. Klein DN, Kotov R, Bufferd SJ (2011) Personality and depression: explanatory models and review of the evidence. Annu Rev Clin Psychol 7:269–295
12. Atherton K, Wiles NJ, Lecky FE, Hawes SJ, Silman AJ, Macfarlane GJ, Jones GT (2006) Predictors of persistent neck pain after whiplash injury. Emerg Med J 23:195–201
13. Scholten-Peeters GG, Verhagen AP, Bekkering GE, van der Windt DA, Barnsley L, Oostendorp RA, Hendriks EJ (2003) Prognostic factors of whiplash-associated disorders: a systematic review of prospective cohort studies. Pain 104:303–322
14. Kjeldgaard D, Forchhammer H, Teasdale T, Jensen RH (2014) Chronic post-traumatic headache after mild head injury: a descriptive study. Cephalalgia 34:191–200
15. Obermann M, Naegel S, Bosche B, Holle D (2015) An update on the management of post-traumatic headache. Ther Adv Neurol Disord 8:311–315
16. Bogduk N, Govind J (2009) Cervicogenic headache: an assessment of the evidence on clinical diagnosis, invasive tests, and treatment. Lancet Neurol 8:959–968
17. Wilner JG, Vranceanu AM, Blashill AJ (2014) Neuroticism prospectively predicts pain among adolescents: results from a nationally representative sample. J Psychosom Res 77:474–476
18. Turner JA, Jensen MP, Warms CA, Cardenas DD (2002) Catastrophizing is associated with pain intensity, psychological distress, and pain-related disability among individuals with chronic pain after spinal cord injury. Pain 98:127–134
19. De Filippis S, Erbuto D, Gentili F, Innamorati M, Lester D, Tatarelli R, Martelletti P, Pompili M (2008) Mental turmoil, suicide risk, illness perception, and temperament, and their impact on quality of life in chronic daily headache. J Headache Pain 9:349–357
20. Dempster M, Howell D, McCorry NK (2015) Illness perceptions and coping in physical health conditions: a meta-analysis. J Psychosom Res 79:506–513
21. Page LA, Howard LM, Husain K, Tong J, Dowson AJ, Weinman J, Wessely SC (2004) Psychiatric morbidity and cognitive representations of illness in chronic daily headache. J Psychosom Res 57:549–555
22. Lanteri-Minet M, Radat F, Chautard MH, Lucas C (2005) Anxiety and depression associated with migraine: influence on migraine subjects' disability and quality of life, and acute migraine management. Pain 118:319–326
23. Pompili M, Serafini G, Di Cosimo D, Dominici G, Innamorati M, Lester D, Forte A, Girardi N, De Filippis S, Tatarelli R, Martelletti P (2010) Psychiatric comorbidity and suicide risk in patients with chronic migraine. Neuropsychiatr Dis Treat 6:81–91
24. Aaseth K, Grande RB, Kvaerner KJ, Gulbrandsen P, Lundqvist C, Russell MB (2008) Prevalence of secondary chronic headaches in a population-based sample of 30-44-year-old persons. The Akershus study of chronic headache Cephalalgia 28:705–713
25. Kristoffersen ES, Lundqvist C, Aaseth K, Grande RB, Russell MB (2013) Management of secondary chronic headache in the general population: the Akershus study of chronic headache. J Headache Pain 14:5
26. Aaseth K, Grande RB, Benth JS, Lundqvist C, Russell MB (2011) 3-year follow-up of secondary chronic headaches: the Akershus study of chronic headache. Eur J Pain 15:186–192
27. Headache Classification Committee of the International Headache Society (2018) The international classification of headache disorders, 3rd edition. Cephalalgia 38:1–211
28. Sjaastad O, Fredriksen TA, Pfaffenrath V (1998) Cervicogenic headache: diagnostic criteria. The Cervicogenic Headache International Study Group. Headache 38:442–445
29. Benninger MS, Ferguson BJ, Hadley JA, Hamilos DL, Jacobs M, Kennedy DW, Lanza DC, Marple BF, Osguthorpe JD, Stankiewicz JA, Anon J, Denneny J, Emanuel I, Levine H (2003) Adult chronic rhinosinusitis: definitions, diagnosis, epidemiology, and pathophysiology. Otolaryngol Head Neck Surg 129:S1–32
30. Derogatis LR, Lipman RS, Rickels K, Uhlenhuth EH, Covi L (1974) The Hopkins symptom checklist (HSCL): a self-report symptom inventory. Behav Sci 19:1–15
31. Sandanger I, Moum T, Ingebrigtsen G, Dalgard OS, Sørensen T, Bruusgaard D, Sorensen T (1998) Concordance between symptom screening and diagnostic procedure: the Hopkins symptom Checklist-25 and the composite international diagnostic interview I. Soc Psychiatry Psychiatr Epidemiol 33:345–354
32. Sandanger I, Nygård JF, Ingebrigtsen G, Sørensen T, Dalgard OS (1999) Prevalence, incidence and age at onset of psychiatric disorders in Norway. Soc Psychiatry Psychiatr Epidemiol 34:570–579
33. Eysenck HJ, SBG E (1975) Manual of the Eysenck personality questionnaire. Hodder and Stoughton, London
34. Eysenck S, Tambs K (1990) Cross-cultural comparison of personality: Norway and England. Scand J Psychol 31:191–197
35. Stewart WF, Lipton RB, Whyte J, Dowson A, Kolodner K, Liberman JN, Sawyer J (1999) An international study to assess reliability of the migraine disability assessment (MIDAS) score. Neurology 53:988–994
36. Leiknes KA, Finset A, Moum T, Sandanger I (2007) Current somatoform disorders in Norway: prevalence, risk factors and comorbidity with anxiety, depression and musculoskeletal disorders. Soc Psychiatry Psychiatr Epidemiol 42:698–710
37. Rasmussen BK, Jensen R, Olesen J (1991) Questionnaire versus clinical interview in the diagnosis of headache. Headache 31:290–295
38. Russell MB, Rasmussen BK, Thorvaldsen P, Olesen J (1995) Prevalence and sex-ratio of the subtypes of migraine. Int J Epidemiol 24:612–618
39. Lampl C, Thomas H, Tassorelli C, Katsarava Z, Lainez JM, Lanteri-Minet M, Rastenyte D, Ruiz de la Torre E, Stovner LJ, Andree C, Steiner TJ (2016) Headache, depression and anxiety: associations in the Eurolight project. J Headache Pain 17:59
40. Zebenholzer K, Lechner A, Broessner G, Lampl C, Luthringshausen G, Wuschitz A, Obmann SM, Berek K, Wober C (2016) Impact of depression and anxiety on burden and management of episodic and chronic headaches - a cross-sectional multicentre study in eight Austrian headache centres. J Headache Pain 17:15
41. Kristoffersen ES, Straand J, Russell MB, Lundqvist C (2017) Lasting improvement of medication-overuse headache after brief intervention - a long-term follow-up in primary care. Eur J Neurol 24:883–891
42. Linton SJ (2000) A review of psychological risk factors in back and neck pain. Spine (Phila Pa 1976) 25:1148–1156
43. Ohayon MM, Schatzberg AF (2003) Using chronic pain to predict depressive morbidity in the general population. Arch Gen Psychiatry 60:39–47
44. Currie SR, Wang J (2004) Chronic back pain and major depression in the general Canadian population. Pain 107:54–60
45. Yilmaz T, Roks G, de Koning M, Scheenen M, van der Horn H, Plas G, Hageman G, Schoonman G, Spikman J, van der Naalt J (2017) Risk factors and outcomes associated with post-traumatic headache after mild traumatic brain injury. Emerg Med J 34:800–805
46. Wilhelmsen I (2005) Biological sensitisation and psychological amplification: gateways to subjective health complaints and somatoform disorders. Psychoneuroendocrinology 30:990–995

17

Impact of cluster headache on employment status and job burden: a prospective cross-sectional multicenter study

Yun-Ju Choi[1], Byung-Kun Kim[2], Pil-Wook Chung[3], Mi Ji Lee[4], Jung-Wook Park[5], Min Kyung Chu[6], Jin-Young Ahn[7], Byung-Su Kim[8], Tae-Jin Song[9], Jong-Hee Sohn[10], Kyungmi Oh[11], Kwang-Soo Lee[12], Soo-Kyoung Kim[13], Kwang-Yeol Park[14], Jae Myun Chung[15], Heui-Soo Moon[3], Chin-Sang Chung[4] and Soo-Jin Cho[16*]

Abstract

Background: Cluster headaches (CH) are recurrent severe headaches, which impose a major burden on the life of patients. We investigated the impact of CH on employment status and job burden.

Methods: The study was a sub-study of the Korean Cluster Headache Registry. Patients with CH were enrolled from September 2016 to February 2018 from 15 headache clinics in Korea. We also enrolled a headache control group with age-sex matched patients with migraine or tension-type headache. Moreover, a control group including individuals without headache complaints was recruited. All participants responded to a questionnaire that included questions on employment status, type of occupation, working time, sick leave, reductions in productivity, and satisfaction with current occupation. The questionnaire was administered to participants who were currently employed or had previous occupational experience.

Results: We recruited 143 patients with CH, 38 patients with other types of headache (migraine or tension-type headache), and 52 headache-free controls. The proportion of employees was lower in the CH group compared with the headache and headache-free control groups (CH: 67.6% vs. headache controls: 84.2% vs. headache-free controls: 96.2%; $p = 0.001$). The CH group more frequently experienced difficulties at work and required sick leave than the other groups (CH: 84.8% vs. headache controls: 63.9% vs. headache-free controls: 36.5%; $p < 0.001$; CH: 39.4% vs. headache controls: 13.9% vs. headache-free controls: 3.4%; $p < 0.001$). Among the patients with CH, sick leave was associated with younger age at CH onset (25.8 years vs. 30.6 years, $p = 0.014$), severity of pain rated on a visual analogue scale (9.3 vs. 8.8, $p = 0.008$), and diurnal periodicity during the daytime ($p = 0.003$). There were no significant differences with respect to the sick leave based on sex, age, CH subtypes, and CH recurrence.

Conclusions: CH might be associated with employment status. Most patients with CH experienced substantial burdens at work.

Keywords: Cluster headache, Disability, Employment, Occupation, Sick leave, Work

* Correspondence: dowonc@naver.com
[16]Department of Neurology, Dongtan Sacred Heart Hospital, Hallym University College of Medicine, Keun Jae Bong-gil 7, Hwaseong, Gyeonggi-do 18450, South Korea
Full list of author information is available at the end of the article

Background

Cluster headache (CH) refers to trigeminal autonomic cephalalgia characterized by recurrent, severe unilateral pain and ipsilateral autonomic symptoms and has a negative impact on patient life [1]. Previous studies have shown that patients with CH report restrictions in daily living, difficulties in social-activity participation, family life, and housework; and overall life changes [2, 3]. The incidence of CH is high among young men; therefore, CH may have a significant impact on employment. A previous study showed that 30% of patients experienced absenteeism due to CH [3]. Rozen et al. reported that approximately 20% of patients with CH experienced job loss and that 8% were unemployed or were receiving disability payments [4]. However, information regarding associations among occupational status, reductions in job productivity, and sick leave with the characteristics of CH is currently limited.

In a large population-based study with patients who had headaches, 31% of participants reported that their work level was reduced by > 50% due to headaches during working hours. In addition, the mean number of absent days due to headaches was 4.2 in the past year. More than half of the patients who experienced these difficulties in the workplace reported that they were due to migraines [5]. In a Spanish study, individuals with migraines showed the lowest productivity and highest loss of workday equivalents [6]. Migraine headaches can cause serious problems; however, CH is also severe and can be expected to cause many work-related difficulties.

In this study, we analyzed the effect of CH on employment status, type of occupation, working time, difficulties including sick leave and decreases in productivity, and satisfaction with current employment. We compared patients with CH to patients with migraine or tension-type headaches (TTH) and a headache-free control group. In addition, we investigated anxiety, depression, and stress levels and analyzed all these factors as predictors of difficulties at work and sick leave.

Methods

Study design and patients

The Korean Cluster Headache Registry Study is a prospective, cross-sectional, multicenter registry study that enrolled consecutive patients with CH from 15 hospitals (13 university hospitals: eight tertiary and five secondary referral hospitals and two secondary referral general hospitals) in Korea. This study used data from patients enrolled between September 2016 and February 2018. Inclusion criteria were: CH diagnosis, episodic, chronic, or probable CH; adult age (≥ 19 years), and full understanding and agreement of the study protocol. A diagnosis of CH was performed by each investigator based on the criteria of the International Classification of Headache Disorder, 3rd Edition, beta version (ICHD-3β) [7]. Exclusion criteria were: inability to communicate in the Korean language, current enrollment in other clinical studies, and investigator's judgment of cognitive or psychological difficulty to complete the questionnaire. In this study, homemakers, students, and patients without occupational experience were also excluded (Fig. 1). The study protocol was reviewed and approved by the local ethics committee or internal review board of each participating hospital, and all procedures were in line with the Declaration of Helsinki and Good Clinical Practice guidelines (2016–396-I). All patients were enrolled after informed written consent.

Two age and sex matched control groups were enrolled. All controls were aged between 19 and 65 years, with no history of diabetes, thyroid illness, severe obesity, severe

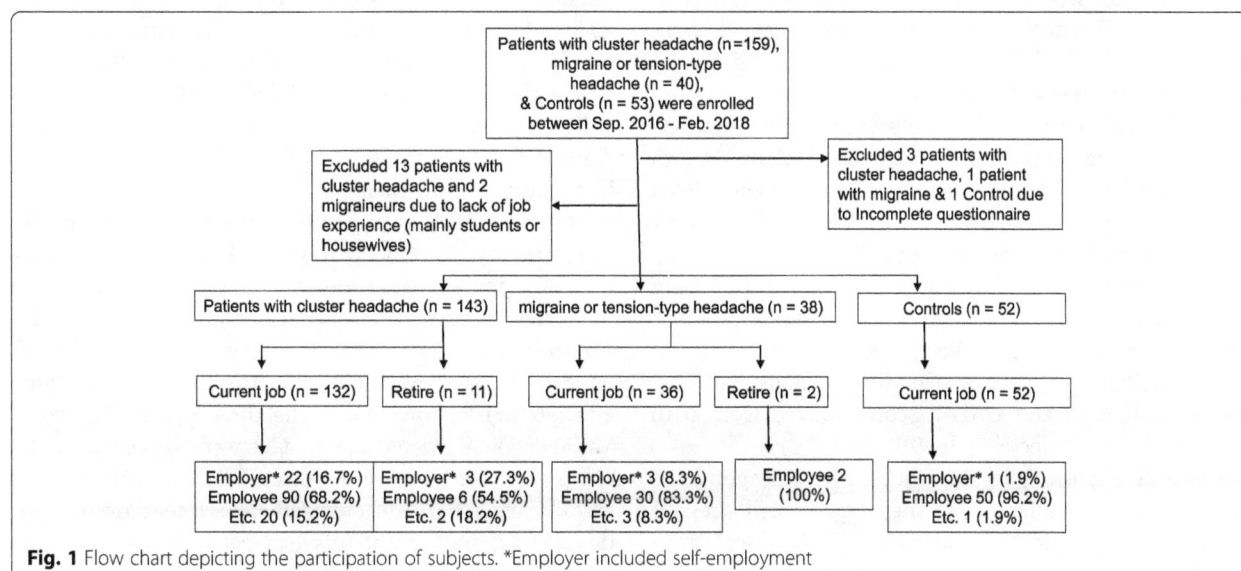

Fig. 1 Flow chart depicting the participation of subjects. *Employer included self-employment

hepatic or renal illness, malignancy, and they had the cognitive capability to complete the questionnaire. Patients with migraine or TTH were enrolled as headache controls. Healthy controls were recruited via notice board. Many were friends or relatives of patients with headaches or employees of the hospital. Additionally, healthy controls were required to be headache free (< 1 headache day per month) with no previous history of primary or secondary headache disorder based on the ICHD-3β [7]. All participants were enrolled after informed written consent.

Clinical information and cluster headache questionnaire
Demographic features included age, sex, and lifestyle factors. Lifestyle factors, such as smoking and alcohol use, were assessed in all participants.

Investigators assessed and recorded clinical information regarding the current incidence and previous history of CH in the patients. Clinical information on current headaches included the location, severity, duration, and frequency of pain; associated symptoms, and duration of headache bouts. Previous history of CH was included, such as the duration from first CH bout, frequency of cluster periods, and pattern of recurrence.

Occupation questionnaire and other parameters
All participants completed a questionnaire regarding their current employment status, shift-working time, weekly working hours, type of occupation, difficulties in working life, and satisfaction with occupation. To assess the impact of CH on occupation, any difficulties at work due to CH were assessed, such as failure to obtain or retain jobs, job changes (department or occupation), promotional disadvantage, voluntary resignation, reduction in productivity, low participation in out-of-work activities, and sick leave. We compared difficulties at work due to headaches between patients with CH and migraine or TTH, and difficulties at work were generally assessed in the headache-free controls.

Each patient completed a self-administered questionnaire assessing depression with the Patient Health Questionnaire-9 (PHQ-9), anxiety with the Generalized Anxiety Disorder-7 (GAD-7), and stress with the Short Form Perceived Stress Scale-4 (PSS 4) [8–11].

Each item on the PHQ-9 and GAD-7 was rated using a four-point scale (0 = never, 1 = several days, 2 = more than half the time, and 3 = nearly every day). Items were rated based on occurrence over the previous 2 weeks. The total PHQ-9 and GAD-7 scores ranged from 0 to 27 and 0 to 21, respectively [8, 9].

The PSS-4 consists of four items where respondents are required to rate how often they experienced stressful situations in the previous month on a Likert scale ranging from 0 to 4 (0 = never to 4 = very often). Two of the

PSS-4 items were recorded due to the reversed scale. Higher scores denoted higher stress levels [10].

Statistics
Chi-square and Student t-tests were used to compare nominal and continuous variables, respectively. Kolmogorov–Smirnov tests were performed to determine the normality of variable distribution. When normality was not confirmed, continuous variables were analyzed using the Mann-Whitney or Kruskal Wallis tests. $p < 0.05$ was considered statistically significant. Logistic regression was performed adjusting for age, sex, and PHQ-9, GAD-7, and PSS-4 scores as predictors for any difficulty at work or sick leave. Data were processed using IBM SPSS Statistics software (version 20.0 for Windows, IBM Corp., Armonk, NY, USA).

Results
We initially enrolled 159 patients with CH, 40 patients with migraine or TTH, and 53 headache-free controls. Of the 159 patients with CH, 142 (91.0%) were surveyed during the cluster period. Participants with incomplete questionnaires or without occupational experience were excluded (Fig. 1). Following this, the questionnaires of 143 patients with CH (CH, $n = 19$, episodic CH, $n = 100$; chronic CH, $n = 5$; probable CH, $n = 19$), 38 patients with migraine or TTH (chronic migraine, $n = 5$; episodic migraine, $n = 25$; chronic TTH, $n = 4$; episodic TTH, $n = 4$), and 52 controls were analyzed.

Entire study population analysis
The mean age of patients with CH was 38.1 ± 9.6 years, and 124 patients were male (86.7%); there were no differences in age and sex distribution among patients with CH, migraine or TTH, and headache-free controls (Table 1). The proportion of individuals who had retired was higher in the CH group than in the other groups (CH: 7.7%, Migraine/TTH: 5.3%, Control: 0%; $p = 0.029$). Among the 11 patients with CH who were retired, five had resigned from their job due to CH. Among the patients with CH, 25 were employers or self-employed, 96 were employees, and 22 were freelancers. The proportion of employees was lower in the CH group than in the other groups (CH: 67.6%, Migraine/TTH: 84.2%, Control: 96.2%; $p = 0.001$). There were no significant differences in shift working time, weekly working hours, and job satisfaction among the three groups (Table 1). Variable job burdens due to CH were reported in the CH group: two patients reported failure to obtain a job (1.4%), seven patients changed department or occupation (4.9%), and 17 patients had been dismissed or had voluntarily resigned (11.9%).

Table 1 Demographic characteristics, employment patterns, and satisfaction with occupation in patients with cluster headache, patients with migraine or TTH, and controls

	Cluster headache (n = 143)	Migraine or TTH (n = 38)	Controls (n = 52)	P-value
Male, n (%)	124 (86.7)	32 (84.2)	43 (82.7)	0.761
Age (year)	38.1 ± 9.6	37.6 ± 10.2	35.3 ± 8.9	0.193
Retirement, n, (%)	11 (7.7)	2 (5.3)	0 (0)	0.029
Employment status, n (%)				0.001
Employer/self-employment	25 (17.6)	3 (7.9)	1 (1.9)	
Employee	96 (67.6)	32 (84.2)	50 (96.2)	
Freelancer/others	22 (15.4)	3 (7.9)	1 (1.9)	
Shift working time, n (%)				0.781
Daytime only	96 (67.6)	25 (65.8)	34 (65.4)	
Nighttime only	5 (3.5)	3 (7.9)	2 (3.8)	
Day & Night time	23 (16.3)	5 (13.2)	6 (11.5)	
Etc	18 (12.7)	5 (13.2)	10 (19.2)	
Working hours/ week				0.151*
40 h	27 (19.6)	6 (15.8)	8 (15.4)	
40–52 h	66 (47.8)	14 (36.8)	33 (63.5)	
52–60 h	23 (16.7)	11 (28.9)	5 (9.6)	
> 60 h	22 (15.9)	7 (18.4)	6 (11.5)	
Job satisfaction, n (%)				0.295†
Satisfaction	77 (64.2)	16 (51.6)	33 (64.7)	
Neutral	38 (31.7)	11 (35.5)	17 (33.3)	
Dissatisfaction	5 (4.2)	4 (12.9)	1 (2.0)	

TTH tension-type headache
*5 patients with cluster headache did not give any information about working hours; †31 patients give no response

Analysis of the 220 employed patients

Among the participants who were currently employed, patients with CH more frequently experienced difficulties at work (CH: 84.8%, Migraine/TTH: 63.9%, Control: 36.5%; $p < 0.001$), reductions in productivity (CH: 60.6%, Migraine/TTH: 33.3%, Control: 11.5%; $p < 0.001$), low participation (CH: 36.4%, Migraine/TTH: 13.9%, Control: 5.8%; $p < 0.001$), and required sick leave (CH: 39.4%, Migraine/TTH: 13.9%, Control: 3.8%; $p < 0.001$) than patients with migraine or TTH and headache-free controls (Table 2).

Table 2 Job burden, depression, anxiety, and stress profiles in patients with cluster headache, patients with migraine or TTH, and controls among patients with current job

	Cluster headache (n = 132)	Migraine or TTH (n = 36)	Controls[a] (n = 52)	P-value
Any difficulty at work	112 (84.8)	23 (63.9)	19 (36.5)	< 0.001
Fail to get or lose job	4 (3)	1 (2.8)	7 (13.5)	0.029
Changed job	3 (2.3)	0	4 (7.7)	0.083
Promotion disadvantage	0	1 (2.8)	2 (3.8)	0.093
Voluntary resignation	10 (7.6)	0	6 (11.5)	0.036
Reduced ability	80 (60.6)	12 (33.3)	6 (11.5)	< 0.001
Low participation	48 (36.4)	5 (13.9)	3 (5.8)	< 0.001
Sick absence	52 (39.4)	5 (13.9)	2 (3.8)	< 0.001
PHQ-9	7.4 ± 6.4	6.2 ± 5.3	2.6 ± 2.5	< 0.001
GAD-7	7.3 ± 5.3	5.7 ± 4.3	1.9 ± 2.2	< 0.001
PSS-4	6.5 ± 2.9	6.4 ± 3.5	5.3 ± 2.2	0.022

TTH tension-type headache, *GAD-7* Generalized Anxiety Dirorder-7, *PHQ-9* Patient Health Questionnaire-9, *PSS-4* Perceived Stress Scale-4
[a]Any difficulty at work was generally assessed in the controls; Data was presented as n (%) or mean ± standard deviation

Multiple logistic regression, adjusting for age, sex, and PHQ-9, GAD-7, and PSS-4 scores, was used to assess any predictors for difficulties at work and found that CH and migraine or TTH were associated with increased risk (odds ratios: CH: 8.262, Migraine/TTH: 3.05). Multivariable logistic regression, adjusting for age, sex, and PHQ-9, GAD-7, and PSS-4 scores, was used to assess any predictors of sick leave and found that CH was associated with increased risk (odds ratio 15.12, Table 3).

Clinical features of patients with CH and sick leave analysis

Among the 132 patients with CH (CH, $n = 17$; episodic CH, $n = 93$; chronic CH, $n = 5$; probable CH, $n = 17$), the patients who required sick leave were younger at CH onset than those who did not (25.8 years vs. 28.7 years, $p = 0.014$). Pain severity, as measured by the visual analogue scale (VAS) was 9.3 ± 1.3 in patients with CH that required sick leave and 8.8 ± 1.2 in those who did not. Comparing sick leave with diurnal rhythms, the patients with CH with diurnal periodicity during the daytime more frequently required sick leave than those without periodicity or with periodicity during the night time (Table 4, $p = 0.003$). There was no significant difference in sick leave associated with sex, age, CH subtypes, CH recurrence, or type of employment (Table 4).

Multivariable logistic regression showed that severe pain (VAS ≥ 9) and diurnal periodicity during the daytime were significant predictors of sick leave after adjusting for age, onset age of CH, sex, PHQ-9, GAD-7, and PSS-4 scores; and cluster year (Additional file 1: Table S1).

Discussion

The purpose of this study was to investigate the employment status and job burden of patients with CH. The main findings of this study were follows: 1) more patients were self-employed and less were employees in the CH group than in the other groups; 2) patients with CH had a 8.26× increased risk of having difficulties at work and a 15.12× increased risk of requiring sick leave

compared with headache-free controls after adjusting for age, sex, and depression, anxiety, and stress levels; 3) and, in the CH group, the patients requiring sick leave were younger at CH onset and had more severe pain than those who did not require sick leave.

We found that patients with CH are more frequently self-employed than controls. This is consistent with the previous studies about the condition of CH [12–14]. One study reported that a greater proportion of patients with CH work full-time compared to controls without headaches; however, there was a high ratio of male patients with CH in that study, which may have biased the results [15]. There was no difference in working time, weekly working hours, or job satisfaction between the CH group and age-sex matched controls. The clustering of severe and painful attacks may influence patterns of employment and require greater personal responsibility; however, the reasons behind or the consequences of this pattern could not be clarified with this cross-sectional study setting.

In this study, 84.8% of patients with CH complained of difficulties in working life and over one third reported reductions in productivity and low participation. The rate of sick leave requirement in patients with CH was reported at 29.6% in Denmark, 68% in the US, and 39.4% in this study [3, 4]. The cultural environment and socioeconomic status may influence the sick leave rate, and 39.4% of patients with CH had 10× higher sick leave rates than controls. Solomon et al. found that patients with CH had significantly lower rates of social activity compared with patients with migraines, in line with our findings [16]. Indirect costs from work disability and lower participation caused by CH impose a significant socioeconomic burden on patients and society [17, 18].

Psychiatric comorbidities, such as anxiety, depression, panic attacks, or suicidal ideation are prevalent and severe in patients with CH, especially during cluster periods or chronic CH [19, 20]. Similar to the findings of previous studies, patients with CH in our study complained of higher levels of anxiety, depression, and stress

Table 3 Multivariable logistic analyses about predictors for difficulty at work and sick absence among 220 participants with current job

	Any difficulty at work		Sick leave	
	OR (95% CI)	p-value	OR (95% CI)	p-value
Age	0.94 (0.90–0.98)	0.002	0.96 (0.92–1.00)	0.041
Sex, women	0.29 (0.11–0.74)	0.010	1.80 (0.70–4.63)	0.220
Groups				
Controls	1		1	
Migraine or TTH	3.05 (1.10–8.49)	0.032	3.85 (0.67–21.98)	0.130
Cluster Headache	8.26 (3.36–20.30)	< 0.001	15.12 (3.28–69.74)	< 0.001

Adjusted for depression by Patient Health Questionnaire-9, anxiety by Generalized Anxiety Dirorder-7, stress by Perceived Stress Scale-4
TTH tension-type headache

Table 4 Difference of cluster features according to experience of sick leave among 132 CH patients with current job

	Total (n = 132)	Sick leave		p-value
		Present (n = 52)	Absent (n = 80)	
Male	115 (87.1)	42 (80.8)	73 (91.3)	0.079
Age (year)	37.2 ± 8.7	35.9 ± 8.5	38.0 ± 8.8	0.179
Onset age of CH	28.7 ± 11.2	25.8 ± 11.3	30.6 ± 10.8	0.014
Duration of cluster headache, year	7.8 ± 11.6	10.2 ± 8.5	7.4 ± 7.5	0.057
Recurrence	103 (78)	43 (82.7)	60 (75.0)	0.297
Cluster bout	117 (88.6)	48 (92.3)	69 (86.3)	0.402
Frequency of CH/day	2.1 ± 1.8	2.0 ± 1.7	2.1 ± 1.9	0.629
Duration of CH, min	104.5 ± 73.4	115.7 ± 91.0	91.0 ± 12.6	0.271
Pain severity, VAS	9.0 ± 1.2	9.3 ± 1.3	8.8 ± 1.2	0.008
Chronic CH	5 (3.8)	3 (5.8)	2 (2.5)	0.382
Probable CH	17 (12.9)	4 (7.7)	13 (16.3)	0.189
Total bouts	8.0 ± 11.6	8.2 ± 8.3	7.6 ± 7.5	0.783
Diurnal periodicity[a]				0.003
None	64 (49.6)	17 (33.3)	47 (60.3)	
Day (6:00–17:59)	33 (25.6)	20 (39.2)	13 (16.7)	
Night (18:00–05:59)	27 (20.9)	10 (19.6)	17 (21.8)	
Both time	5 (3.9)	4 (7.8)	1 (1.3)	
Employment status				0.436
Employer/self-employment	22 (16.7)	6 (11.5)	16 (20)	
Employee	90 (68.2)	38 (73.1)	52 (65)	
Freelancer/others	20 (15.2)	8 (15.4)	12 (15)	

Data was presented as n (%) or mean ± standard deviation

CH cluster headache, *VAS* visual analogue scale

[a]3 patients not give any information

when compared with patients with migraine or TTH and controls. We found higher PHQ-9, GAD-7, and PSS-4 scores in patients with CH; however, after adjustment for these confounding variables, CH still increased the risk of having difficulties at work and sick leave. This result was similar to that of a previous study that found an association between severe and persistent migraines and increased risk of work disabilities, after adjusting for mental disorders [21].

This is the first study to analyze predictors of sick leave among patients with CH. Our subgroup analysis of CH showed that sick leave was significantly associated with a younger age at CH onset, pain severity, diurnal periodicity during the daytime. Although the significance of younger age at CH onset was decreased with multivariable logistic analysis, the association between younger age at onset and increased risk for sick leave suggested that the headaches in this subgroup started before they had the opportunity to secure meaningful employment and thus these patients were more disabled by their condition when they started working and/or less able to adapt to the working environment.

This study has several limitations. First, the degree of occupational satisfaction, sick leave, and reductions in productivity were not examined using a scale. These data were collected by questionnaire; therefore, it was difficult to estimate the amount of sick leave or disability at the time the headaches were experienced based on participant recollection. Second, the headache control group included the migraine and TTH groups, and job burden may have varied among headache controls. The sex ratio among migraineurs in this study differed from that among the actual patient population, and thus our sample of patients with migraine may not have been representative. Third, headache-free controls were recruited among the relatives of patients, volunteers, and hospital staff and their families and required stricter exclusion criteria (no history of diabetes, thyroid illness, severe obesity, severe hepatic or renal illness, malignancy, and cognitive capability to complete the questionnaire). This may have led to sampling bias, which could have influenced the number of retirees in the control group. Additionally, the job burden analysis was only conducted using data from participants with current jobs. There was a disadvantage that job burden due to headache among patients who were employed was compared to overall job burden among the healthy controls. This study was conducted based on the ICHD-3β criteria and could not include a sufficient number of patients with chronic CH to analyze the impact of chronic CH. Similar to this study, the frequency of chronic CH has been reported at 3.5% in Japan [22]. These data reflect a substantial job burden for Asian patients with CH, despite the low proportion of patients with chronic CH.

Conclusions

This study reported the effect of CH on occupational factors and compared age-sex matched patients with patients with other types of headache and headache-free controls. In addition, we revealed that CH were an important predictor of work disability and need for sick leave after adjusting for psychiatric comorbidities. Furthermore, we revealed that severity of pain, younger age at CH onset, and diurnal periodicity during the daytime were associated with sick leave of CH patients.

Abbreviations
CH: Cluster headache; GAD-7: Anxiety by the generalized anxiety dirorder-7; ICHD-3β: International classification of headache disorder, 3rd edition, beta version; PHQ-9: Patient health quetionnare-9; PSS 4: Stress by short form perceived stress scale-4; TTH: Tension-type headache

Acknowledgements
Thanks to clinical research coordinator, Jung Eun Kwon for sincere cooperation during the acquisition of the data.

Funding
This study was supported by a grant from Korean Neurological Association (KNA-16-MI-09). No other financial relationships relevant to this publication were disclosed.

Authors' contributions
YJC, MKC, and SJC conceived the idea for this article. YKC, BKK, PWC, MJL, JWP, MKC, JYA, BSK, TJS, JHS, KO, KSL, SKK, JMC, and HSM contributed the acquisition of the data. KYP, MJL, and CSC performed the data analyses and data interpretations. PWC, JWP, MKC, JYA, BSK, TJS, JHS, KO, KSL, SKK, JMC, HSM, and CSC contributed with inputs to this article. SJC and YJC drafted the work and paper. BKK, PWC, MJL, JWP, MKC, JYA, BSK, TJS, JHS, KO, KSL, SKK, KYP, JMC, HSM, and CSC revised the paper for important intellectual content. All authors reviewed and approved the final manuscript. All authors agreed to be accountable aspects of the work in ensuring that questions related to the accuracy or integrity of any part of the work are appropriately investigated and resolved.

Competing interests
YJC, BKK, PWC, MJL, JWP, JYA, BSK, TJS, JHS, KO, KSL, SKK, KYP, JMC, HSM, and CSC report no conflict of interest.
MKC was involved as a site investigator for a multicenter trial sponsored by

Eli Lilly, worked an advisory member for Teva, and received lecture honoraria from Allergan Korea and Yuyu Pharmaceutical Company.
SJC was involved as a site investigator of multicenter trial sponsored by Otsuka Korea, Eli Lilly and Company, Korea BMS, and Parexel Korea Co., Ltd., and received research support from Hallym University Research Fund 2016 and Myungin Research Fund 2016.

Author details
[1]Department of Neurology, Presbyterian Medical Center, Jeonju, South Korea. [2]Department of Neurology, Eulji Hospital, Seoul, South Korea. [3]Department of Neurology, Kangbuk Samsung Hospital, Sungkyunkwan University School of Medicine, Seoul, South Korea. [4]Department of Neurology, Samsung Medical Center, Seoul, South Korea. [5]Department of Neurology, Uijeongbu St.Mary's Hospital, Uijeongbu, South Korea. [6]Department of Neurology, Severance Hospital, Seoul, South Korea. [7]Department of Neurology, Seoul Medical Center, Seoul, South Korea. [8]Department of Neurology, Bundang Jesaeng General Hospital, Daejin Medical Center, Seongnam, South Korea. [9]Department of Neurology, Ewha Womans University of Medicine, Seoul, South Korea. [10]Department of Neurology, Chuncheon Sacred Heart Hospital, Chuncheon, South Korea. [11]Department of Neurology, Korea University College of Medicine, Seoul, South Korea. [12]Department of Neurology, Seoul St. Mary's Hospital, Catholic University of Korea College of Medicine, Seoul, South Korea. [13]Department of Neurology and Institute of Health Science, Gyeongsang National University College of Medicine, Jinju, South Korea. [14]Department of Neurology, Chung-Ang University Hospital, Seoul, South Korea. [15]Department of Neurology, Inje University College of Medicine, Seoul, South Korea. [16]Department of Neurology, Dongtan Sacred Heart Hospital, Hallym University College of Medicine, Keun Jae Bong-gil 7, Hwaseong, Gyeonggi-do 18450, South Korea.

References
1. Hoffmann J, May A (2018) Diagnosis, pathophysiology, and management of cluster headache. Lancet Neurol 17:75–83. https://doi.org/10.1016/S1474-4422(17)30405-2
2. Barloese MC (2015) Neurobiology and sleep disorders in cluster headache. J Headache Pain 16:562. https://doi.org/10.1186/s10194-015-0562-0
3. Jensen RM, Lyngberg A, Jensen RH (2007) Burden of cluster headache. Cephalalgia 27:535–541
4. Rozen TD, Fishman RS (2012) Cluster headache in the United States of America: demographics, clinical characteristics, triggers, suicidality, and personal burden. Headache 52:99–113. https://doi.org/10.1111/j.1526-4610. 2011.02028.x
5. Schwartz BS, Stewart WF, Lipton RB (1997) Lost workdays and decreased work effectiveness associated with headache in the workplace. J Occup Environ Med 39:320–327
6. Castillo J, Láinez MJ, Domínguez M et al (2008) Labor productivity in migraine patients: primary care contribution to occupational medicine. J Occup Environ Med 50:895–903. https://doi.org/10.1097/JOM. 0b013e31817e9157
7. Headache Classification Committee of the International Headache Society (IHS) (2013) The International Classification of Headache Disorders, 3rd edition (beta version). Cephalalgia 33:629–808. https://doi.org/10.1177/ 0333102413485658
8. Seo JG, Park SP (2015) Validation of the patient health Questionnaire-9 (PHQ-9) and PHQ-2 in patients with migraine. J Headache Pain 16:65. https://doi.org/10.1186/s10194-015-0552-2
9. Seo JG, Park SP (2015) Validation of the generalized anxiety Disorder-7 (GAD-7) and GAD-2 in patients with migraine. J Headache Pain 16:97. https://doi.org/10.1186/s10194-015-0583-8
10. Warttig SL, Forshaw MJ, South J et al (2013) New, normative, English-sample data for the short form perceived stress scale (PSS-4). J Health Psychol 18: 1617–1628. https://doi.org/10.1177/1359105313508346
11. Lee EH, Chung BY, Suh CH et al (2015) Korean versions of the perceived stress scale (PSS-14, 10 and 4): psychometric evaluation in patients with chronic disease. Scand J Caring Sci 29:183–192. https://doi.org/10.1111/scs.12131
12. Friedman AP, Mikropoulous HE (1958) Cluster headaches. Neurology 8:653–663
13. Kudrow L (1974) Physical and personality characteristics in cluster headache. Headache 13:197–202

14. Italian Cooperative Study Group on the Epidemiology of Cluster Headache (ICECH) (1995) Case-control study on the epidemiology of cluster headache. I: etiological factors and associated conditions. Neuroepidemiology 14:123–127

15. Sjöstrand C, Russell MB, Ekbom K et al (2010) Familial cluster headache: demographic patterns in affected and nonaffected. Headache 50:374–382. https://doi.org/10.1111/j.1526-4610.2009.01426.x

16. Solomon GD, Skobieranda FG, Gragg LA (1994) Does quality of life differ among headache diagnoses? Analysis using the medical outcomes study instrument. Headache 34:143–147

17. Gaul C, Finken J, Biermann J et al (2011) Treatment costs and indirect costs of cluster headache: a health economics analysis. Cephalalgia 31:1664–1672. https://doi.org/10.1177/0333102411425866

18. Ford JH, Nero D, Kim G et al (2018) Societal burden of cluster headache in the United States: a descriptive economic analysis. J Med Econ 21:107–111. https://doi.org/10.1080/13696998.2017.1404470

19. Torkamani M, Ernst L, Cheung LS et al (2015) The neuropsychology of cluster headache: cognition, mood, disability, and qualityof life of patients with chronic and episodic cluster headache. Headache 55:287–300. https://doi.org/10.1111/head.12486

20. Jürgens TP, Gaul C, Lindwurm A et al (2011) Impairment in episodic and chronic cluster headache. Cephalalgia 31:671–682. https://doi.org/10.1177/0333102410391489

21. Kessler RC, Shahly V, Stang PE et al (2010) The associations of migraines and other headaches with work performance: results from the National Comorbidity Survey Replication (NCS-R). Cephalalgia 30:722–734. https://doi.org/10.1177/0333102410363766

22. Imai N, Yagi N, Kuroda R et al (2011) Clinical profile of cluster headaches in Japan: low prevalence of chronic cluster headache, and uncoupling of sense and behaviour of restlessness. Cephalalgia 31:628–633. https://doi.org/10.1177/0333102410391486

18

Assessment of community pharmacy professionals' knowledge and counseling skills achievement towards headache management: a cross-sectional and simulated-client based mixed study

Adeladlew Kassie Netere[1*], Daniel Asfaw Erku[1], Ashenafi Kibret Sendekie[1], Eyob Alemayehu Gebreyohannes[1], Niguse Yigzaw Muluneh[2] and Sewunet Admasu Belachew[1]

Abstract

Background: Headache is one of the most common disabling medical condition affecting over 40% of adults globally. Many patients with headache prefer to alleviate their symptom with a range of over-the-counter analgesics that are available in community medicine retail outlets (CMROs). However, data regarding how community pharmacists respond to headache presentation and their analgesic dispensing behaviors in Ethiopia is scarce. The present study aimed to assess the self-reported and actual practice of community pharmacists toward management of a headache in Gondar town, Ethiopia.

Methods: A dual-phase mixed-methods research design, including pseudo-client visits (between April 1 and 30, 2018) followed by a questionnaire-based cross-sectional study (between May 1 and 20, 2018) was conducted among CMROs in Gondar town, Ethiopia.

Results: Among the 60 pseudo-client visits, 95% of them dispensed medications. The overall counseling approach was found to be 42.6% which improved to 58.3% when the pseudo-clients demanded it. Duration (73.3%) and signs/symptoms (45%) of headache were asked before dispensing the medications. Dosing frequency (86.7%), indication (60%) and dosage form (35%) were the most discussed items. Ibuprofen (45%) and diclofenac (41.5%) were primarily added to paracetamol for better headache treatment. Effectiveness (61.7%) and cost (21.7%) were the main criteria to choose drugs. In the cross-sectional survey, 60 participants were requested and 51 of them agreed to participate (response rate of 85%). Of these participants, 64.7% agreed that managing headache symptomatically is challenging. Patient lack of confidence in dispensers (41.2%) and lack of updated medical information (31.4%) were reported as the primary barriers to counsel clients.

Conclusion: This study demonstrated the practical gaps in counseling practices and poor headache management of community pharmacies in Gondar city. National stakeholders in collaboration with academic organizations should be involved in continuous clinical training and education regarding proper counseling practices.

Keywords: Community medicine retail outlets, Counseling, Headache, Pseudo client, Ethiopia

* Correspondence: Kassieadeladlew21@gmail.com
[1]Department of Clinical Pharmacy, School of Pharmacy, College of Medicine and Health Sciences, University of Gondar, P.O. Box: 196, Chechela Street, Lideta Sub City Kebele 16, Gondar, Ethiopia
Full list of author information is available at the end of the article

Background

Headache or cephalalgia affects infrequently almost everyone [1]. The Global Burden of Disease Study 2015 (GBD2015) ranked migraine as the third highest cause for disability worldwide in persons younger than 50 years in both sexes [2]. and nearly 40% of people suffered from a headache at some time in their lives [1]. Around 15% of UK adult patients experience a migraine with a three-to-one ratio of women-to-men [1]. According to a population-based national survey of headache burdens in Ethiopia, the prevalence had been reported as migraine (17.7%), tension-type headache (TTH) (20.6%), probable medication-overuse headache (pMOH), and headache yesterday 6.4% [3]. Patients most regularly seek professional counseling from general and neurologic clinics [1, 4]. Headache challenges healthcare professionals in many ways and represents enormous social and economic burden to the health care system.; for example, 20 billion USD is lost every year in the United States for migraine [1, 2, 5].

Community pharmacists are the most accessible healthcare professionals to the public owing to their convenient location at the heart of the community and wide geographic distribution [6]. Patients with a headache successfully self-medicate by means of over-the-counter (OTC) medications that are available via CMROs [7]. This provides a unique opportunity for pharmacy staffs to play a crucial role in ensuring the quality use of medications by providing patients with counseling on the safe, correct and effective use of medicines, and solving potential drug-related problems [8, 9]. Even though CMROs can sufficiently treat minor ailments and contribute in self-care management such as headaches, still they need to be careful while recommending OTC drugs since even these drugs can cause health threats if used inappropriately [10]. Findings from developing countries showed that dispensers working in the pharmacies hardly keep sufficient knowledge and skills for effective syndrome management [11]. On the other hand, pharmacists in developed nations, such as the United Kingdom and Australia, successfully incorporated minor ailment management with other public-health programs [12–15]. In Ethiopia as in most developing countries pharmacy staff are largely confined to the traditional medication dispensing and counseling practices and once in a while delivering such public health services [16, 17] which is worsened by the absence of standard and consistence treatment (counseling) guidelines for headache and other common minor ailments [18]. Regarding self-medications and related issues, a variety of investigations were conducted in many parts of Ethiopia, though many of them used client perceptions [19, 20]. Owing to the burden of headache in Ethiopia [3], patients usually look for immediate therapy in the nearby public pharmacies. A recent study conducted by Ayele et al. identified lack of access to clinical training and poor community awareness as the most commonly cited barriers for providing public health services in CMROs such as headache management [21]. Yet, the extent to which pharmacy professionals interacts with patients for headache management is not studied in detail, and there is no published data that explores pharmacy staff knowledge and counselling skills when it comes to handling patients' request of analgesic medications. Thus, the current study aimed at assessing the knowledge and extent of community pharmacy professionals' involvement in counseling practices and overall management of a headache as well as to explore the challenges and hidden reasons that hindered professionals from delivering the standard care to the clients.

Methods

Study design and setting

A dual-phase mixed-methods research design, including a simulated client method (April, 2018) and a cross-sectional study survey (May, 2018) were employed. The study was conducted in Gondar town, Northwest Ethiopia. The town has a population of approximately 206,987 [22] and 66 community medicine retail outlets (CMROs) (40 community pharmacies and 26 drug stores). This study was reviewed and ethically approved by the Institutional Review committee of the University of Gondar, School of Pharmacy with the approval number of (UOG-SOP204/2018). The data collected were kept anonymous and no personal identifier were used.

The simulated patient (SP) study

According to Food, Medicine and Healthcare Administration and Control Authority of Ethiopia (FMHACA), community medicine retail outlets (CMROs) are mainly classified into a pharmacy, drug store (shop) and drug vendor. Gondar town's CMROs were classified by geographical locations such as Arada, Piassa, Lideta (Chechela), Maraki and Azezo sub-cities (Kifle Ketemas) and all of the community medicine retail outlets were taken as study samples. Each of the CMROs was visited once by a pseudo-patient within study period giving a total of 60 (1 in each CMROs) pseudo-patient visits. Details of the scenario (an intermittent headache) employed in the simulated study are presented in Table 1. The pharmacist was expected to rule out other medical conditions, medication history and advise the pseudo-client to take paracetamol combined with other analgesics such as nonsteroidal anti-inflammatory drugs (NSAIDS) or weak opioids like tramadol, and if inadequate and the symptom still persists advice to visit the nearby hospital or clinic.

Table 1 The scenario employed in the simulated study, Gondar, 2018

Intermittent headache	
The SP is a 20-year-old male with a complaint of an intermittent (moderate–to-severe) headache for 04 days duration. The SP is currently taking paracetamol to alleviate his symptom. Yet, he sensed that he needs a more effective treatment and, hence, visited a community pharmacy.	
The pharmacist was given the following information when asked:	The SP had no other previous or current medical condition. The SP did not drink coffee and alcohol and was non-smoker.
	The headache started 04 days back and the SP had the symptom for most of the days.
	The pain was described as mild, dull, low intensity, and affecting both sides of the head.
	Paracetamol was the only medication the SP was taking during that time.
	There were no special factors that trigger/worsen the headache.
	The patient did not visit a hospital for this cause.

The pseudo-client method

Pseudo (simulated)-patient method is a technique of assessing the service providers' (dispensers') counseling practices in CMROs by visiting the pharmacy staff after training specific patient scenario. The aim of the pseudo-client-based study was to assess the participation of CMROs dispenser staffs in the management of a self-diagnosed headache and to explore the challenges and hidden reasons that impede the delivery of standard counseling services to the clients. This method has been employed extensively and comprehensively in pharmacy practice-based researches [23, 24].

Two clinical pharmacists acted as simulated patients. A half-day long discussion and training were given to the SPs so that they will be familiar and be able to perform the given clinical scenario. They were instructed not to give and/or ask further information unless asked by the pharmacy staff so as to make sure that the information provided by each SPs is uniform across all visits. In order to avoid dependence on the human cognitive processes, which has been mentioned as a potential limitation of the simulated patient method [25], all the visits were audio recorded. Immediately after each visit, the SPs filled the data gathered into a form containing a checklist of items (such as enquiries including: client history, information provided by dispensers, self-diagnosis, medication selection process, direction for use and medical profile, aggravating and alleviating factors, and duration of headache) that were intended to assess the practice of pharmacy personnel toward the dispensing of antibiotics for the specified minor ailments. The principal investigator (AKN) compared and validated the data from the checklist against audio recordings for the purpose of quality assurance.

The cross-sectional study

A self-administered English version questionnaire was prepared and distributed to 63 community pharmacists (one in each CMRO) after securing verbal and written consent and clarification of the aim of the study. One of the working staffs of dispenser was selected randomly when there were two or more dispenser staffs during data collection. The questionnaire contains respondents' demographic factors, working hours, average client waiting time, dispensing experiences, headache management practices, and potential barriers to proper service delivery. Each questionnaire took an average of 15 min. Finally, the completed questionnaire was collected on-site by the investigators.

Data quality control, entry, analysis and interpretation

The overall data was checked for its completeness and accuracy and important variables were addressed. Data from both the simulated and the cross-sectional studies were entered into and analyzed using Statistical Package for Social Studies (SPSS) version 20.0 [26]. The results were presented as frequencies and percentages.

Operational definitions

Community medicine retail outlets in our study as described in [27]:

Pharmacy

It denotes a drug shop having the mandate to hold any medicine and medical equipment. In addition, the professional who is supposed to dispense inside the pharmacy is 'A pharmacist'. No one else is allowed to dispense according to the FMHACA of Ethiopia.

Drug store

Unlike a pharmacy, a drug store is a drug shop but the medicine to be dispensed here is restricted. That means, it is not legal to hold every medication in this medicine retail outlet. For instance: It is not allowed to hold medications like psychotropic/narcotic drugs. In addition, the professional who is supposed to dispense inside the drug store is 'A druggist'.

Pharmacists

In Ethiopia, pharmacists are professionals having a bachelor degree from private or government university. In addition, they took all the courses that one medication expert has to know at the end. The duration of the study to be a pharmacist used to be four years which has been changed to five years since 2008.

Druggists

We can use this name interchangeably with' Pharmacy technician'. In Ethiopia, those professionals having 'diploma degree' from colleges are considered druggists (i.e. it is not a university-level education). They took courses for 3 years only and it is not that much comprehensive like pharmacists..

Result

Pseudo client approach

Out of the 66 CMROs, 60 of them were visited by the pseudo-patient approach whereas the rest were non-functional (closed) during the data collection. Among the evaluated respondents, the majority ($n = 32$, 53.3%) were females. Thirty-four (56.7%) of the premises were leveled as pharmacies. Almost all the participants dispensed medications for the pseudo-patient (95%), while 3 (5%) dispensers suggested the client to consult physicians to identify the cause of a headache. More than half of the participants provided information when the pseudo-client demanded it (58.3%) and dispensed generic drugs (73.3%); ibuprofen (45%) and diclofenac (41.5%) were the most recommended ones for a headache in addition to paracetamol. Effectiveness (61.7%) and cost (21.7%) were the major reasons to choose drugs for pseudo-clients as illustrated in Table 2.

Overall professional counseling approach of the dispensers was assessed by a five-point Likert scale (poor = 1, fair = 2, good = 3, very good = 4, and excellent = 5). The mean (±SD) counseling approach of dispensers was 2.14 (0.9) which means only 42.6% of dispensers gave proper counseling. During the pseudo-client approach, most dispensers asked primarily duration ($n = 44$, 73.3%) and types of signs/symptoms ($n = 27$, 45%) of a headache before dispensed the medications. Also, 48.3% of them allowed SP to be involved in the medication-selection process. Just below half (45%) of the providers inquired signs or symptoms and around 22% asked the SPs about the type of medication previously taken. Only 5 (8.3%) dispensers asked whether they have previous or current medical condition whereas nearly 12% of them asked about their current medication profile other than paracetamol. Furthermore nobody asked about whether the pseudo-client needed additional information, the presence of allergic history, adverse drug reaction, and alleviating factors (Table 3).

Among the most commonly signposted information that every dispensary personnel should counsel every patient when dispensing pharmaceutical formulations, drug administration times (frequency) ($n = 52$, 86.7%), medication indication ($n = 36$, 60%) and dosage form ($n = 21$, 35%) were the most discussed items during interaction with the simulated patients. To the contrary, none of the dispensers discussed important items such as contraindications, drug

Table 2 Drug selections and dispensing practices of CMROs in Gondar city during pseudo-client

Variables	N (%)
Gender	
Male	28 (46.7)
Female	32 (53.3)
Community medicine retail outlets level	
Pharmacy	34 (56.7)
Drug store	26 (43.3)
Dispensers who dispensed the drug for pseudo patient	57 (95)
Dispensers send SP to consult the doctor; not dispensed drugs	3 (5)
Dispensed drugs product based on name	
Generic	44 (73.3)
Brand	13 (21.7)
Drugs were selected based on	
Effectiveness	37 (61.7)
Cost	13 (21.7)
Both effectiveness and cost	7 (11.7)
ADR	0
Availability	0
Type of drug added to PCM for headache management	
Diclofenac	25 (41.7)
Ibuprofen	27 (45)
Tramadol	3 (5)
ASA	0
Acetaminophen with tramadol combined formulation	2 (3.3)
Provision of information for the pseudo client approach	
Spontaneously	22 (36.7)
Enquired about sign and symptoms	35 (58.3)

Approach, 2018 ($N = 60$)

interactions, adverse drug reactions, adherence to treatment, and safe storage of the dispensed medications with the pseudo-clients (Fig. 1).

Cross-sectional survey

Among the 60 dispensers that were approached, 51 of them completed and returned (response rate of 85%) the questionnaire. Almost two-thirds of the respondents were male (62.7%) and ages between 22 and 30 years old (72.5%). Of the CMROs, about 60% were leveled as pharmacies. A comparable number of pharmacists and druggists participated in the study. Average work experience as a dispenser in CMROLs was 5 years (±SD = 2.9). The majority (62.7%) of the dispensers reported to work for 8–10 h per day in the pharmacies with an average of 9.1 (±1.6) hours per day. Around 70% of participants reported that the average waiting time of clients in the dispensary was 5.2 (±2.34) minutes. Only one respondent

Table 3 Questions and patient history's required by the provider during encounter

Items	Responses	
	Yes (%)	No (%)
SPs age was asked during dispensing	6 (10)	54 (90)
The provider let SP to be involved in the medication-selection process	29 (48.3)	28 (46.7)
The provider asked whether SP needed additional information	0	57 (95)
The provider personnel asked about the presence of specific conditions that could affect diagnosis or recommended treatment	3 (5)	54 (90)
Starting time of headache	13 (21.7)	44 (73.3)
Location of pain	1 (1.7)	56 (93.3)
Magnitude (intensity) of pain	4 (6.7)	53 (88.3)
Duration of headache asked	44 (73.3)	13 (21.7)
Types of typical signs/symptoms of headache asked	27 (45)	30 (50)
Current medication other than PCM asked	7 (11.7)	50 (83.3)
Previous or current medical condition asked	5 (8.3)	52 (86.7)
Type of medication history (Hx) previously taken asked	13 (21.7)	44 (73.3)
Presence of allergy history asked	0	57 (95)
Major adverse reaction (ADRs) asked	0	57 (95)
Exacerbating factors	2 (3.3)	55 (91.7)
Relieving factors	0	57 (95)

had a guideline for headache management and 11.8% of the dispensers took clinical training in their work life. Detail socio-demographic characteristics are illustrated in Table 4.

According to the survey, most of the participants (64.7%) agreed or strongly agreed that managing headache symptomatically is challenging. However, many of them agreed or strongly agreed to the importance of

syndrome-approach clinical training (52.9%) and continuous education and training (94.1%) to solve such challenges. In addition, a higher number of respondents (54.9%) agreed or strongly agreed that clients should involve in medication selection process (Table 5).

As to the respondents' reports, only one-third (33.3%) of the clients had very good or excellent awareness with the dispenser's role inregard to seeking additional information beyond what they have already obtained, and one-fourth (25.5%) were aware of generic and brand products (Table 6). The majority (66.7%) of dispensers reported that clients preferred brand products while other clients considered effectiveness ($n = 17$, 33.3%) and both price and effectiveness ($n = 15$, 29.4%) for choosing the medications. High proportions (78.4%) of community pharmacists and druggists recommended paracetamol for a non-examined headache, whereas, 60.8% of dispensers referred clients (who are taking paracetamol and in need of better treatment) to hospital or clinic. Less number of respondents recommended diclofenac (17.6%) and tramadol (13.7%). Lack of client interest towards professional counseling (41.2%) and lack of updated medical information provided by dispensers (31.4%) were the main potential barriers to counsel clients (Table 7).

Discussion

The present study evaluated the counseling manners and headache management practices of CMROs dispensers without a prescription in Gondar city. Essential variations concerning information provision and headache management practices of dispensers were discovered by comparing results found from the pseudo-client visits and the cross-sectional survey. Based on the SPs findings, the overall counseling approach was found to be 42.6%; however, it was improved to 58.3% when the pseudo-client demanded it. In the same way, findings in

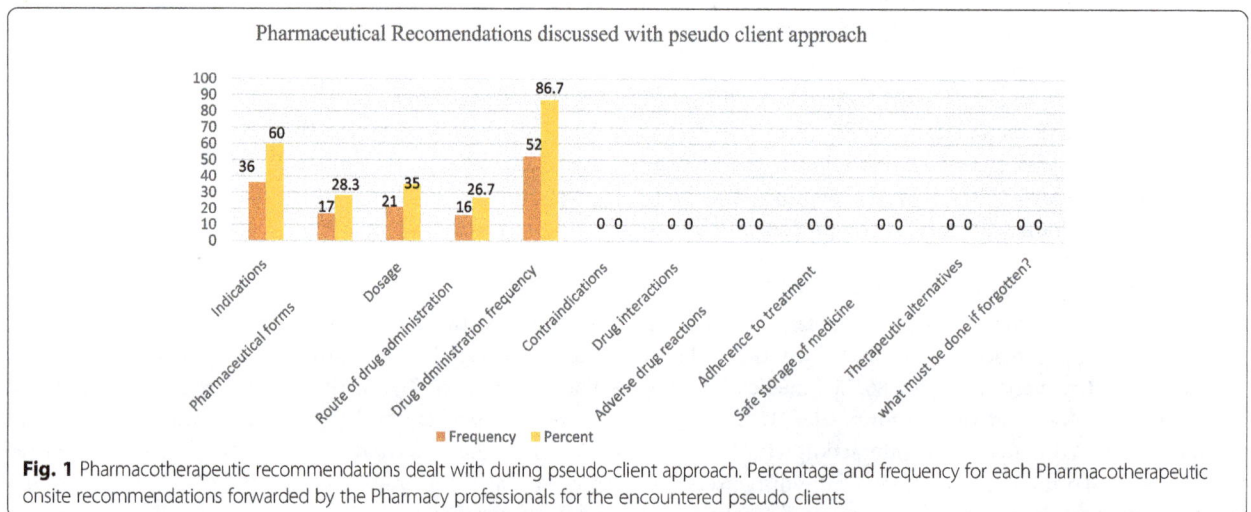

Fig. 1 Pharmacotherapeutic recommendations dealt with during pseudo-client approach. Percentage and frequency for each Pharmacotherapeutic onsite recommendations forwarded by the Pharmacy professionals for the encountered pseudo clients

Table 4 Socio-demographic characteristics of participants, (N = 51)

Characteristics	N (%)	Mean (±SD)
Sex		
Male	32 (62.7)	
Female	19 (37.3)	
Age in years		
22–30	37 (72.5)	29.7 (±4.1)
31–40	13 (25.5)	
>40	1 (2)	
Work experience in (years)		
<1 years	2 (3.9)	5 (±2.9)
1–5 years	32 (62.7)	
>5 years	17 (33.3)	
Length of working time (in hours)		
1–8 h	19 (37.3)	9.1 (±1.6)
8–10 h	32 (62.7)	
Average client waiting time (in minutes)		
1–5 min	35 (68.6)	5.2 (±2.34)
6–10 min	16 (31.4)	
Educational qualification		
Pharmacist	26 (51)	
Druggist	25 (49)	
Level of drug retail outlet		
Pharmacy	27 (52.9)	
Drug store	24 (47.1)	
Dispensers who had guideline for headache management		
Yes	1 (2)	
No	50 (98)	
Dispensers took clinical training in their work life		
Yes	6 (11.8)	
No	45 (88.2)	

Riyadh, Saudi Arabia showed that the counseling level was found to be 43% even though it was enhanced when SPs demanded more information [28]. Depending on the type of investigation methodologies, the stated advising levels fluctuated from 8 to 100% in the worldwide literature [29]. Based on this, the reasons for such poor counseling practices might be multifactorial. The main challenges include lack of interest, poor experiences, knowledge and communication skills, and lack of standard counseling guideline.

In the real dispensing practices, 95% of dispensers provided medications for the pseudo-customers who were taking paracetamol while three dispensers advised the client to consult the physicians for identifying the cause of a headache without any further professional trail to help. This study is quite comparable with the study done

in Saudi Arabia [28]. Contrarily, in the cross-sectional survey, 60.8% of participants referred the client to the hospital. This indicates that community pharmacists were not dispensing drugs based on knowledge and guidelines rather they sold for only cheesing money. Since most of CMROs are established for profit, no matter what the cause is, they sell every product without any hesitations. Moreover, unless they are profitable, their survival will be jeopardized and mainly unserved customers might disclose them to others clients that they do not serve well.

Concerning headache management using OTC medications, analgesics such as non-steroidal anti-inflammatory drugs (NSAIDs), acetaminophen, and weak opioids like tramadol are suggested as first-line drugs. Nevertheless, 64.7% of participants in the cross-sectional survey agreed that managing headache symptomatically is challenging, 78.4% of dispensers recommended acetaminophen for a non-examined headache, and about 40% of them added diclofenac, tramadol, and ibuprofen to paracetamol for better treatment. On the other hand, in the SPs approach, 95% of the participants primarily added Ibuprofen (45%), diclofenac (41.5%) and tramadol (5%) to acetaminophen for a headache management, though dispensers reported that customers chose brand products in the survey. Higher proportions of the dispensers selected the medications based on their effectiveness (61.7%) and cost (21.7%) which had similarities with survey results. In contrast, a pilot study in Brazil reported sodium dipyrone was the most recommended medication [30]. Even though customers do want brand products, suppliers rarely made them available for the community so that acetaminophen, ibuprofen, and diclofenac would be the first choice, since these drugs are safe, effective, readily available and affordable for most of the local customers.

During the pseudo-client approach, headache duration and signs or symptoms, medication profile and previous or current medical conditions were inquired by the dispensers. It is very important that dispensers pursue relevant evidence about clients' history and compliant characteristic which enables them to choose appropriate pharmacotherapeutic alternatives for customers. However, forwarding many questions towards clients requires strong communication skills and knowledge, and increases client confidence and counseling satisfaction on dispensers. Such types of questions are highly supported by many comparative findings [31, 32].

Though higher proportions of participants (54.9%) in the cross-sectional survey agreed with the clients' involvement of medication selection, smaller number of dispensers practically allowed the pseudo-client to be involved with their medication selection process. Surprisingly, nobody asked about whether the pseudo-client needed additional information, the presence of allergic

Table 5 Belief of dispensers on headache management challenges and solutions

Items	Number	Strongly disagree/Disagree (%)	Neutral (%)	Agree/strongly agree (%)
Managing headache symptomatically is challenging	51	9 (17.7)	9 (17.6)	33 (64.7)
Syndrome approach clinical training is important for treating headache	51	11 (21.5)	13 (25.5)	27 (52.9)
Continuous education and training improves challenges to treat headache	51	0	2 (3.9)	49 (94.1)
Patients should be involved in drug selection process	51	14 (27.4)	9 (17.6)	28 (54.9)

history, adverse drug reaction history, and alleviating factors of a headache. Since self-medications are retailed without any prescription dispensers thought that many questions might discourage the patients form taking the medications [33]. Furthermore, in order to provide additional information and understand typical allergic history and adverse drug reactions providers should be trained for such types of evidence and clients' interest. The survey revealed that clients' absence of interest on dispensers and lack of updated medication information were found to be the major challenges for better counseling. However, 95% of respondents reported that the community was award of the role of community pharmacists in headache management.

When dispensing pharmaceutical formulations, there are important points that every dispenser should acknowledge and counsel the clients during providing drugs. However, the findings of this study revealed that only a few of the dispensers informed the clients about drug administration times (frequency), medication indication, dosage (strength), pharmaceutical forms, and route of drug administration during interaction with the simulated patients. To the contrary, none of the dispensers discussed important items such as contraindications, drug interactions, adverse drug reactions, adherence to treatment, and safe storage of the dispensed medications with the pseudo client. The findings of this study were similar to previous studies with regard to the rare provision of essential information by community pharmacists on precautions, adverse effects, drug interactions, contraindications, and safe storage [23, 24, 34]. But a Saudi study reported somewhat different results where 97% of the SPs visits provided information about dose, whereas a very small number of SPs were counseled on precaution. To the contrary, about half of the respondents never counseled on the side effects and drug interactions [28]. As explained earlier most of

the provided counseling was superficial, easy and common that any health professionals might provide for every client. Mainly dispensers merely focus particularly on sales rather than counseling, because detailed discussions need further professional skills and extensive knowledge to deliver. Moreover, most of the patients do not seek more detailed information. Rather they need only what they want to know.

Strength and limitations of the study

Every pseudo-client visit was audio-recorded to reduce the challenges associated with the human cognitive processes in conducting SP studies. After all, this study showed the real gap between the practical services and the theoretical expectations of community pharmacies. However, we used a convenience sampling method in only Gondar city. Therefore, generalizations of the study findings to other regions and populations should be with caution as it might lead to under or over representations. In addition, because only a specific case scenario was employed that leads to specific replies, it may not comprehensively assess the professionals' competency towards a headache management. Moreover, because of the pseudo-client visit and the cross-sectional survey was conducted at different times, the respondents might not be the same and the responses to the self-administered questionnaire depended on the respondents' trustworthiness which is subjected to socially desirable responses.

Conclusions

Community pharmacists, being one of the most easily accessible health professionals in the community, are uniquely positioned to treat and manage minor ailments such as headache in their practice areas. According to findings from this study, community pharmacies demonstrated a very poor and inadequate skill headache management.

Table 6 Community awareness's and approaches towards CMROs

Items	Number	Poor/ fair (%)	Good (%)	Very good/ excellent (%)
Community awareness towards the role of community medicine retail outlets in headache management	51	5 (9.8)	29 (56.9)	17 (33.3)
Patients' interest to get additional information beyond you provide	51	20 (39.2)	14 (27.5)	17 (33.3)
Communities awareness of generic and brand name of drugs	51	25 (50)	13 (25.5)	13 (25.5)

Table 7 Dispensers and clients drug selection and counseling barriers

Items	N (%)
Type of product preferred by clients	
Generic	17 (33.3)
Brand	34 (66.7)
What do client matters to choose their medication	
Price	5 (9.8)
Effectiveness	17 (33.3)
Price and effectiveness	15 (29.4)
Effectiveness and safety	10 (19.6)
Price, effectiveness and safety	4 (7.8)
Drugs recommended for non-examined headache	
Paracetamol	40 (78.4)
Diclofenac	5 (9.8)
Ibuprofen	3 (5.9)
Tramadol	3 (5.9)
Aspirin (ASA)	0
What would you do for a headache patient taking paracetamol who wanted better treatment	
Diclofenac	9 (17.6)
Ibuprofen	4 (7.8)
Tramadol	7 (13.7)
Refer to nearby hospital	31 (60.8)
Aspirin (ASA)	0
Potential barriers to counsel the clients	
High patient load	6 (11.8)
Shortage of time	3 (5.9)
Lack of un updated information	16 (31.4)
Patients lack of awareness to be counseled	5 (9.8)
Patient lack of interest	21 (41.2)

Providing continuous clinical training and educational interventions are needed in order to mitigate the knowledge and skill gap. One suggestion is providing a hands-on evidence-based summary of headache management in their practice areas by academic institution and other stakeholders. Large scale studies that can explore community pharmacists' involvement in managing headache in community pharmacies and that further could assess clients' (purchasers') level of satisfaction towards the community pharmacy service particularly regarding headache management is recommended to identify practice barriers and to better inform regulatory bodies.

Abbreviations
ADR: Adverse Drug reaction; CMROs: Community medicine retail outlets; FMHACA: Food, Medicine, Healthcare Administration and Control Authority; GBD: Global Burden of Disease; Hx: History; MOH: Ministry of health; NSAIDs: Nonsteroidal anti-inflammatory drugs; OTC: Over the counter; PCM: Paracetamol; PCs: Pseudo clients; SD: Standard Deviation; SPs: Simulated patients; SPSS: Statistical Package of Social Sciences; TTH: Tension type headache; UK: United Kingdom; USD: United States Dollar

Acknowledgements
We would like to thank the study participants for their valuable information and time.

Authors' contributions
AKN and SAB contributed in conceptualization, project administration, formal analysis, investigation, methodology, supervision, data curation, resources, writing and original draft of the manuscript and writing, review and editing of the final manuscript. DAE, AKS, EAG, NYM and AKN contributed in formal analysis, methodology, data curation, writing and original draft of the manuscript. All authors of this manuscript read and approved the final version of this manuscript.

Ethics approval and consent to participate
This study was reviewed and ethically approved by the Institutional Review committee of University of Gondar, School of Pharmacy with the approval number of SOP204/2018. The data collected was kept anonymous and recorded in such a way that the identity of the involved pharmacy professionals could not be known. The exit interviews were conducted where a third-party could not overhear questions and answers so as to ensure privacy and confidentiality of clients. The information obtained from the study was not disclosed to the third body. Only coded numbers were used to identify study participants.

Competing interests
The authors declare that there is no competing interest.

Author details
[1]Department of Clinical Pharmacy, School of Pharmacy, College of Medicine and Health Sciences, University of Gondar, P.O. Box: 196, Chechela Street, Lideta Sub City Kebele 16, Gondar, Ethiopia. [2]Department of Psychiatry, University of Gondar, Chechela Street, Lideta Sub City Kebele 16, Gondar, Ethiopia.

References
1. Steiner TJ, Macgregor EA, Davies PTG (2007) Guidelines for all healthcare professionals in the diagnosis and management of migraine, tension-type, cluster and medication-overuse headache, 3rd edn (1st revision). British Association for the Study of Headache
2. International Headache Society (IHS) (2018) The International Classification of Headache Disorders (ICHD-III). 3rd edition. Cephalalgia 38(1):1–211
3. Zebenigus M, Tekle-Haimanot R, Dawit K, Worku DK et al (2017) The burden of headache disorders in Ethiopia: national estimates from a population-based door-to-door survey. J Headache Pain 18:58. https://doi.org/10.1186/s10194-017-0765-7
4. Steiner TJ, Scher AI, Stewart WF, Kolodner K, Liberman J, Lipton RB (2003) The prevalence and disability burden of adult migraine in England and their relationships to age, gender and ethnicity. Cephalalgia 23:519–527
5. Gahir KK, Larner AJ (2004) What role do community pharmacists currently play in the management of headache? A hospital based perspective. Int J Clin Pract 58(3):257–259

6.   Chua SS et al (2006) Response of community pharmacists to the presentation of back pain: a simulated patient study. Int J Pharm Pract 14:171–178

7.   Steiner TJ, Lange R, Voelker M (2003) Aspirin in episodic tension-type headache: placebo controlled dose-ranging comparison with paracetamol. Cephalalgia 23:59–66

8.   Berger K et al (2005) Counselling quality in community pharmacies: implementation of the pseudo customer methodology in Germany. J Clin Pharm Ther 30:45–57

9.   Schneider CR et al (2009) Measuring the assessment and counseling provided with the supply of nonprescription asthma reliever medication: a simulated patient study. Ann Pharmacother 43:1512–1518

10. Alonzo HGA, Cristiana L, Corrêa CL, FAD Z (2001) Analgesics, antipyretics and non-steroidal anti-inflammatory drugs: epidemiological data on six intoxication control centers in Brazil. Rev Bras Toxicol 14:49–54

11. Hussain A, Ibrahim M (2012) Management of diarrhoea cases by community pharmacies in 3 cities of Pakistan. East Mediterr Health J 18(6):635–640

12. Sewak NP, Cairns J (2011) A modeling analysis of the cost of a national minor ailments scheme in community pharmacies in England. IJPP 19(s1):50

13. United-Kingdom Department of Health (2005) Choosing health through pharmacy–a programme for pharmaceutical public health 2005–2015

14. Pharmaceutical Service Negotiating committee (2005) NHS community pharmacy contractual framework enhanced service: minor ailment service, pp 9–11

15. Benrimoj S, Frommer M (2004) Community Pharmacy in Australia. Aust Health Rev 28(2):238–246

16. Surur AS, Getachew E, Teressa E, Hailemeskel B, Getaw NS, Erku DA (2017) Self-reported and actual involvement of community pharmacists in patient counseling: a cross-sectional and simulated patient study in Gondar, Ethiopia. Pharm Pract 15(1):890. https://doi.org/10.18549/PharmPract.2017. 01.890 PMID: 28503225

17. Erku DA, Mekuria AB, Surur AS, Gebresillassie BM (2016) Extent of dispensing prescription-only medications without a prescription in community drug retail outlets in Addis Ababa, Ethiopia: a simulated-patient study. Drug Healthc Patient Saf 8:65–70

18. Sumia S, Mohamed A, Mahmoud AA (2014) The role of Sudanese community pharmacists in patients' self-care. Int J Clin Pharm 36:412–419. https://doi.org/10.1007/s11096-013-9911-8 PMID: 24442644

19. Ayalew MB (2017) Self-medication practice in Ethiopia: a systematic review. Patient Prefer Adherence 11:401–413. https://doi.org/10.2147/PPA.S131496 PMID: 28280312

20. Hailemichael W, Sisay M, Mengistu G (2016) Assessment of the knowledge, attitude, and practice of self-medication among Harar health sciences college students, Harar, eastern Ethiopia. J Drug Deliv Ther 6:31–36

21. Ayele AA, Mekuria AB, Tegegn HG, Gebresillassie BM, Mekonnen AB, Erku DA (2018) Management of minor ailments in a community pharmacy setting: findings from simulated visits and qualitative study in Gondar town, Ethiopia. PLoS One 13(1):e0190583. https://doi.org/10.1371/journal.pone.0190583

22. Complete report on 2007 Ethiopian census. Central statistical agency. http:// www.csa.gov.et/census-report/complete-report/census-2007. Accessed 28 Jul 2018

23. Gokcekus L, Toklu HZ, Demirdamar R, Gumusel B (2012) Dispensing practice in the community pharmacies in the Turkish republic of northern Cyprus. Int J Clin Pharm 34(2):312–324

24. Bin Abdulhak A, Al Tannir M, Almansor M et al (2011) Non prescribed sale of antibiotics in Riyadh, Saudi Arabia: a cross sectional study. BMC Public Health 11(1):538

25. Werner JB, Benrimoj SI (2008) Audio taping simulated patient encounters in community pharmacy to enhance the reliability of assessments. Am J Pharm Educ 72:136 PMID: 19325956

26. IBM Corp (2012) IBM SPSS statistics for windows, version 21.0. IBM Corp. Released, Armonk

27. Belachew SA, Tilahun F, Ketsela T, Achaw Ayele A, Kassie Netere A, Getnet Mersha A et al (2017) Competence in metered dose inhaler technique among community pharmacy professionals in Gondar town, Northwest Ethiopia: knowledge and skill gap analysis. PLoS One 12(11):e0188360. https://doi.org/10.1371/journalpone.0188360

28. Alaqeel S, Abanmy NO (2015) Counselling practices in community pharmacies in Riyadh, Saudi Arabia: a cross-sectional study. BMC Health Serv Res 15:557. https://doi.org/10.1186/s12913-015-1220-6

29. Puspitasari HP, Aslani P, Krass I (2009) A review of counseling practice on prescription medicines in community pharmacies. Res Soc Adm Pharm 5: 197–210

30. Santos AP, Mesquita AR, Oliveira KS, Lyra DP Jr (2013) Assessment of community pharmacists' counselling skills on headache management by using the simulated patient approach: a pilot study. Pharm Pract 11(1):3–7

31. Smiley T. The role of the pharmacist in identification, referral, and management of migraine headache. CE Compliance Centre National Continuing Education Program December 2005

32. Berger K, Eickhoff C, Schulz M (2005) Counselling quality in community pharmacies: implementation of the pseudo customer methodology in Germany. J Clin Pharm Ther 30(1):45–57

33. Nair K, Dolovich L, Cassels A, McCormack J, Levine M, Gray J et al (2002) Whatpatients want to know about their medications: focus group study of patient and clinician perspectives. Can Fam Physician 48:104–110

34. Al-Mohamadi A, Badr A, Bin Mahfouz L, Samargandi D (2013) Dispensing medications without prescription at Saudi community pharmacy: extent and perception. Saudi Pharm J 21(1):13–18

19

Patients' perspective on the burden of migraine in Europe: a cross-sectional analysis of survey data in France, Germany, Italy, Spain, and the United Kingdom

Pamela Vo[1], Juanzhi Fang[2], Aikaterini Bilitou[3], Annik K. Laflamme[1] and Shaloo Gupta[4*]

Abstract

Background: Migraine is a distinct neurological disease that imposes a significant burden on patients, society, and the healthcare system. This study aimed to characterize the incremental burden of migraine in individuals who suffer from ≥4 monthly headache days (MHDs) by examining health-related quality of life (HRQoL), impairments to work productivity and daily activities, and healthcare resource utilization (HRU) in the EU5 (France, Germany, Italy, Spain, United Kingdom).

Methods: This retrospective cross-sectional study used data from the 2016 National Health and Wellness Survey (NHWS; $N = 80,600$). Short-Form 36-Item Health Survey, version 2 (SF-36v2) physical and mental component summary scores (PCS and MCS), Short-form-6D (SF-6D), and EuroQoL (EQ-5D), impairments to work productivity and daily activities (Work Productivity and Activity Impairment Questionnaire (WPAI), and HRU were compared between migraine respondents suffering from ≥4 MHDs ($n = 218$) and non-migraine controls ($n = 218$) by propensity score matching using sociodemographic characteristics. Chi-square, T-tests, and Mann-Whitney tests were performed to determine significant differences between the groups after propensity score matching.

Results: HRQoL was lower in migraine individuals suffering from ≥4 MHDs compared with non-migraine controls, with reduced SF-36v2 PCS (46.00 vs 50.51) and MCS (37.69 vs 44.82), SF-6D health state utility score (0.62 vs 0.71), and EQ-5D score (0.68 vs 0.81) (for all, $p < 0.001$). Respondents with migraine suffering from ≥4 MHDs also reported higher levels of absenteeism from work (14.43% vs 9.46%; $p = 0.001$), presenteeism (35.52% vs 20.97%), overall work impairment (38.70% vs 23.27%), and activity impairment (44.17% vs 27.75%) than non-migraine controls (for all, $p < 0.001$). Additionally, HRU was significantly higher for individuals with ≥4 MHDs compared to their matched controls. Consistently, migraine subgroups (4–7 MHDs, 8–14 MHDs and CM) had lower HRQoL, greater overall work and activity impairment, and higher HRU compared to non-migraine controls.

Conclusions: Migraine of ≥4 MHDs was associated with poorer HRQoL, greater work productivity loss, and higher HRU compared with non-migraine controls. The findings of the study suggest that an unmet need exists among individuals suffering from ≥4 MHDs in the EU5 suggesting the need for effective prophylactic treatments to lessen the humanistic and economic burden of migraine.

Keywords: Activity impairment, Burden, Healthcare resource use, Health-related quality of life, Migraine, Work impairment

* Correspondence: shaloo.gupta@kantarhealth.com
[4]Kantar Health, New York, NY 10010, USA
Full list of author information is available at the end of the article

Background

Migraine is a distinct neurological disease, associated with recurrent and often debilitating headaches of moderate to severe intensity and accompanied by neurological symptoms (sensory and dysautonomic symptoms including nausea, vomiting, photophobia, or phonophobia) that exact a personal, economic, and societal burden on a global scale [1]. Migraine has been categorized into 2 major types: migraine with aura and migraine without aura. The former accounts for around 30% of the patients and involves transient visual, sensory, and aphasic or motor disturbances that occur before or during migraine attacks [2]. A single migraine attack typically disrupts patient's life and can consist of premonitory (≤48 h), aura (5–60 min), headache (4–72 h), and resolution/postdrome (≤48 h) phases [3]. Migraine generally starts during puberty and is most prevalent between 30 and 49 years of age [4]. Migraine affects approximately > 10% of the adult population globally [5], is 2–3 times more common in women than men, and tends to run in families and has a genetic trend [6].

Migraine can be immensely disabling [7] and impacts a patient's functional ability and health-related quality of life (HRQoL) during, immediately after, and between migraine episodes [8].

Migraine was the sixth leading cause of disability-adjusted life years (DALYs) worldwide for the age group 25 to 39 years in the 2015 Global Burden of Disease (GBD) study [9]. The GBD 2016 study reported migraine as the first leading cause of years lived with disability (YLDs) worldwide in both males and females for the age group 15 to 49 years, demonstrating that the burden is higher in the groups of prime productivity [10]. In fact, migraine-attributed YLDs were much higher in comparison to other neurological diseases such as epilepsy (ranked 29th) and Alzheimer disease (ranked 26th) [11].

The burden associated with migraine is underestimated even in developed countries despite its high prevalence and severity [12]. Although the prevalence of migraine in individuals suffering from ≥4 monthly headache days (MHDs) is lower when compared to <3MHDs [13], the burden is higher [14]. Studies based on sociodemographic [15] and general health characteristics of migraine [16, 17], HRQoL [18, 19], work productivity loss and activity impairment (WPAI) [17], and healthcare resource utilization (HRU) [17] have been conducted before. Furthermore, a number of studies across multiple countries have studied the impact of chronic and episodic migraine on HRQoL, WPAI, and HRU [7, 18, 20–23]. However, there is paucity of data on HRQoL, WPAI, and HRU for the entire spectrum of migraine in the EU5 (France, Germany, Italy, Spain, and the United Kingdom) especially in the population with migraine who suffer from ≥4MHDs and may be eligible for prophylactic treatment [13, 24–29].

Therefore, the primary objective of this study was to characterize the incremental burden of migraine in those experiencing ≥4 MHDs from patients' perspective in terms of HRQoL, work and activity impairment, and HRU compared with non-migraine controls among the EU5. The secondary objective was to characterize the burden of migraine from the perspective of migraine patients experiencing ≥4 MHDs from the EU5 by frequency of migraine (eg, 4–7, 8–14, and ≥15 MHDs) compared with non-migraine controls.

Methods

Sample

The sample for this retrospective, cross-sectional study was taken from the 2016 National Health and Wellness Survey (NHWS; $N = 80,600$) from adults in the EU5. All respondents were aged 18 years or older, consented to participate in the survey, and could read and write the primary language of the country at the time of the survey.

Respondents to this NHWS are members of MySurvey.com or its partners, which are opt-in survey panels, who were recruited through opt-in e-mail, co-registration with MySurvey.com partners, eNewsletter campaigns, banner placements, and both internal and external affiliate networks. All potential panelists must register with the panel through a unique e-mail address and password and complete an in-depth demographic registration profile. In countries where Internet penetration among the elderly was not considered sufficient to provide an adequate sample of the elderly population (Spain and Italy), telephone recruitment using quota sampling (age and gender) was used to supplement online recruitment, and those without access to the internet were invited to complete the survey using a computer in a private center. The protocol and questionnaire for the NHWS were reviewed for exemption by Pearl Institutional Review Board (IRB) and determined to be exempt from IRB review for the periods the data used in the current study; all respondents provided informed consent.

Of the 16,340 survey respondents who reported experiencing migraine in the past 12 months, a randomly selected subsample of 1680 respondents (10%) completed the migraine module with additional questions on migraine characteristics and of these, 771 respondents reported a physician-diagnosed migraine. Such random subsampling enabled inclusion of respondents with different conditions to provide detailed information while limiting the average interview length and respondent's burden. As the objective was to evaluate the burden of migraine in respondents with ≥4 MHDs, respondents who did not experience migraines in the past month or did not provide a frequency of MHDs or reported rare migraine (≤3 MHDs) were excluded from the study ($n =$

553) and 218 respondents were included for the study (Fig. 1).

The study sample (respondents who self-reported a physician-diagnosis of migraine) who completed the migraine module and indicated that they experienced migraines of at least 4 MHDs were matched by propensity scores to those without migraines (controls) using sociodemographic characteristics (see below). Furthermore, respondents were categorized according to the frequency of migraines (MHDs): non-migraine controls, people with migraine of 4 to 7 MHDs (4–7 EM), 8 to 14 MHDs (8–14 EM), and 15 or more MHDs (CM) [3].

Measures

Sociodemographic characteristics

The demographic characteristics collected included country of residence (i.e., France, Germany, Italy, Spain, and the United Kingdom), age in years, gender (male or female), employment status (yes vs no), annual household income (below median vs above median vs decline to answer), marital status (married or living with partner vs not), and level of education (completed university education vs not).

General health characteristics

Body mass index (BMI) was calculated from reported height and weight and reported as underweight (< 18.5 kg/ m^2), normal weight (18.5 to < 25.0 kg/m^2), overweight (25 to < 30.0 kg/m^2), obese (30.0 kg/m^2 and above), or decline to answer. Other general characteristics collected were cigarette smoking (current vs former vs never); alcohol use (yes vs no); vigorously exercised in past 30 days (yes vs no); and the Charlson Comorbidity Index (CCI) [30]. CCI weights the presence of various conditions [eg, diabetes, liver disease, connective tissue disease, chronic pulmonary disease, metastatic tumor, moderate/severe renal disease, peripheral vascular disease, myocardial infarction, congestive heart failure, diabetes with end organ damage, leukemia, dementia, and human immunodeficiency virus infection/acquired immune deficiency syndrome (HIV/ AIDS)] and sums the result. The greater the total index score, the greater is the comorbid burden on the patient.

Health-related quality of life

SF-36v2 The 2016 NHWS included the 4-week recall period of the revised Medical Outcomes Study 36-Item Short-Form Survey Instrument (SF-36v2), which is a multipurpose, generic health status instrument that consists of 36 questions [31]. Two SF-36 summary scores were calculated, physical component summary (PCS) and mental component summary (MCS) scores, with higher scores indicating better HRQoL. In addition

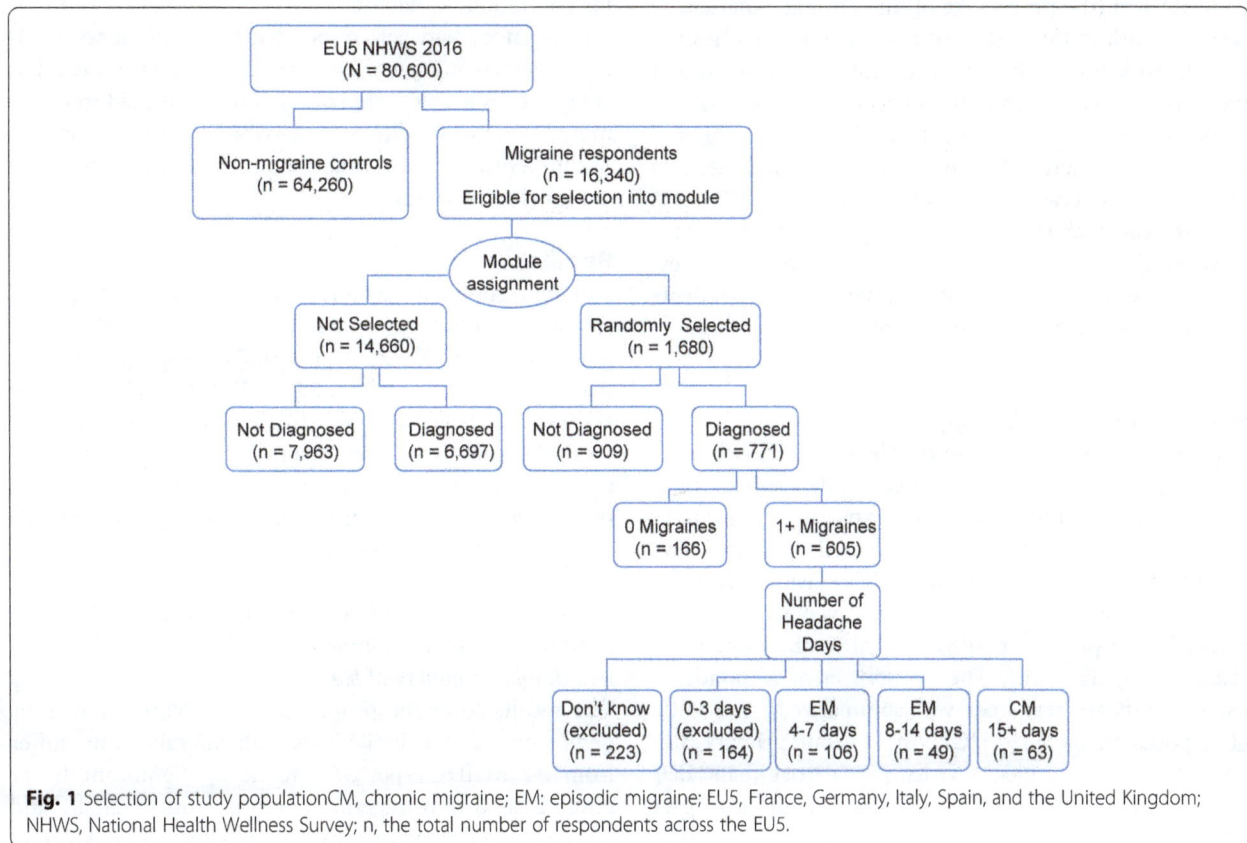

Fig. 1 Selection of study population. CM, chronic migraine; EM: episodic migraine; EU5, France, Germany, Italy, Spain, and the United Kingdom; NHWS, National Health Wellness Survey; n, the total number of respondents across the EU5.

to generating profile and summary PCS and MCS scores, the SF-36v2 can also be used to generate health state utilities, similar to those derived from the EuroQoL EQ-5D (EQ-5D). This is achieved through the application of the Short-Form Six-Dimension (SF-6D), which takes 6 items from the survey.

The SF-6D is a preference-based single index measure for health using UK general population values [32]. The SF-6D index has interval scoring properties and yields summary scores on a theoretical scale of 0 to 1. Higher scores indicate better health status. The EQ-5D Index score is a preference-based measure of health on a theoretical scale of 0 to 1, in which 1 represents full health and 0 being death. It is derived from responses to the 5-level EQ-5D version (EQ-5D-5 L), a widely used survey instrument that measures health in 5 dimensions, which was included in the questionnaire for this study [33].

Work productivity and activity impairment
Loss of productivity and activity impairment were assessed using the General Health version of the Work Productivity and Activity Impairment (WPAI-GH) questionnaire [34], a 6-item validated instrument that consists of 4 metrics: absenteeism (the percentage of work time missed because of one's health in the past 7 days), presenteeism (the percentage of impairment experienced while at work in the past 7 days because of one's health), overall work productivity loss (overall work impairment measured by combining absenteeism and presenteeism to determine the total percentage of missed time), and activity impairment (the percentage of impairment in daily activities because of one's health in the past 7 days). Only respondents who reported being full-time, part-time, or self-employed provided the data for absenteeism, presenteeism, and overall work impairment. All respondents completed the activity impairment questionnaire.

Healthcare resource utilization
HRU was defined by visits to different medical providers or healthcare system (i.e., Emergency department [ED] or hospital) 6 months before survey participation due to any medical conditions, not only migraine specific. Several types of healthcare provider (HCP) visits were summarized and analyzed as the presence versus absence of a visit in the prior 6 months as well as the number of visits during that time. The proportion of respondents using healthcare resources was summarized. The HRU of respondents included HCP visits overall, primary care provider visits, neurologist visits, psychiatrist visits, ED/urgent care visits, and hospitalization in the past 6 months.

Matching
As the objective of the study was to estimate the incremental burden associated with migraine, the propensity score of respondents with migraine was compared with that of those without migraine (controls) using demographic and comorbidities data. This procedure was conducted separately within each country and for those with 4–7 EM, 8–14 EM, and CM to limit the risk that respondents differ from controls on matching characteristics within the smaller migraine subgroups.

Logistic regressions including sociodemographic and health variables (age, sex, marital status, income, education, smoking status, alcohol use, exercise behavior, BMI category, and CCI [estimate of comorbidity burden]) were conducted. Using a greedy matching algorithm, respondents' regression-estimated probabilities were used to match each case to a single control with no reuse of controls. Matching was constrained so that each respondent with migraine was matched to a non-migraine control from the same country.

Data analysis plan
All data management and analyses were performed in SPSS 23.0, and SAS 9.4. The sample was characterized by the variables listed in the variables section using descriptive statistics, including frequencies and percentages for categorical variables, and means, standard deviations for continuous variables.

Differences between respondents diagnosed with migraine versus non-migraine controls were examined. For categorical variables, chi-square tests were used to determine significant differences, whereas t-tests or the Mann-Whitney tests, where appropriate, were used for continuous variables.

Results
Among respondents who reported a physician-diagnosed migraine, suffer from ≥4 MHDs, and completed the migraine module ($N = 218$), 67 (30.7%) respondents were from the United Kingdom, 59 (27.1%) from Germany, 39 (17.9%) from France, 31 (14.2%) from Italy, and 22 (10.1%) respondents from Spain. The demographic characteristics for respondents diagnosed with migraine and pre-matched and post-matched non-migraine controls are represented in Table 1.

Comparison of respondents with migraine and its subgroups with non-migraine controls
Health-related quality of life
The results from the propensity score matched analysis demonstrated that individuals with migraine who suffer from ≥4 MHDs reported statistically significant lower HRQoL than non-migraine controls, both mentally and physically, as measured by the SF-36v2. The MCS in

Table 1 Demographic characteristics for respondents diagnosed with migraine and pre-matched and post-matched non-migraine controls

		Diagnosed with migraine, $N = 218$	Pre-matched non-migraine controls, $N = 64,260$	Post-matched non-migraine controls, $N = 218$
Gender, n (%)	Male	45 (20.64)	31,275 (48.7)***	44 (20.18)
	Female	173 (79.36)	32,985 (51.3)	174 (79.82)
Country, n (%)	France	39 (17.89)	15,524 (24.2)	39 (17.89)
	Germany	59 (27.06)	16,635 (25.9)	59 (27.06)
	United Kingdom	67 (30.73)	15,616 (24.3)	67 (30.73)
	Italy	31 (14.22)	8868 (13.8)	31 (14.22)
	Spain	22 (10.09)	7617 (11.9)	22 (10.09)
Marital status, n (%)	Married or living with partner	131 (60.09)	39,943 (62.2)	131 (60.09)
Household income, n (%)	Low	63 (28.90)	16,219 (25.2)	57 (26.15)
	Medium	100 (45.87)	28,743 (44.7)	108 (49.54)
	High	36 (16.51)	12,462 (19.4)	38 (17.43)
	Decline to answer	19 (8.72)	6836 (10.6)	15 (6.88)
Level of education, n (%)	Completed university education	87 (39.91)	22,958 (35.7)	90 (41.28)
Employment status, n (%)	Yes	136 (62.39)	34,640 (53.9)*	131 (60.09)
	No	82 (37.61)	29,620 (46.1)	87 (39.91)
BMI, n (%)	Underweight (< 18.5 kg/m^2)	4 (1.83)	1947 (3.0)	4 (1.83)
	Normal weight (18.5 to < 25.0 kg/m^2)	87 (39.91)	26,935 (41.9)	83 (38.07)
	Overweight (25 to < 30.0 kg/m^2)	66 (30.28)	21,002 (32.7)	75 (34.40)
	Obese (30.0 kg/m^2 and above)	48 (22.02)	11,135 (17.3)	48 (22.02)
	Decline to answer	13 (5.96)	3241 (5.0)	8 (3.67)
Smoking status, n (%)	Current	66 (30.28)	14,886 (23.2)*	67 (30.73)
	Former	66 (30.28)	20,420 (31.8)	70 (32.11)
	Never	86 (39.45)	28,954 (45.1)	81 (37.16)
Use of alcohol, n (%)	Yes	153 (70.18)	49,749 (77.4) *	148 (67.89)
	No	65 (29.82)	14,511 (22.6)	70 (32.11)
Vigorous exercise in past 30 days, n (%)	Yes	126 (57.80)	40,342 (62.8)	121 (55.50)
	No	92 (42.20)	23,918 (37.2)	97 (44.50)
Age [mean ± SD]	Years	43.25 ± 13.48	16.57 ± 49.79***	44.73 ± 16.09
CCI [mean ± SD]		0.53 ± 1.04	0.82 ± 0.33***	0.44 ± 1.01

Note: Chi-square tests were used for categorical variables, whereas t-tests were used for continuous variables
p-values for pre-matched non-migraine controls vs migraine group: *$p < 0.05$, *** $p \leq 0.001$
BMI, Body mass index; *CCI*: Charlson Comorbidity Index; *SD*, standard deviation

those with migraine was significantly lower than that in non-migraine controls (37.7 vs 44.8, respectively; $p < 0.001$; Fig. 2). Furthermore, the PCS score of migraine respondents was significantly lower than that of non-migraine controls (46.0 vs 50.5, respectively; $p < 0.001$; Fig. 2), this represents an incremental difference of 7.1 in MCS and 4.5 in PCS which is greater than the previously reported MCS and PCS mean for a minimally important difference of 3 [35]. Respondents with migraine also reported significantly lower SF-6D (0.62 vs 0.71, $p < 0.001$) and EQ-5D (0.68 vs 0.81, $p < 0.001$) health utility scores than the non-migraine controls (Fig. 3); this represents an incremental difference of 0.09 which is greater than the previously reported mean for a minimally important difference of 0.041 [36]. The significant decrement in PCS and MCS scores was noted

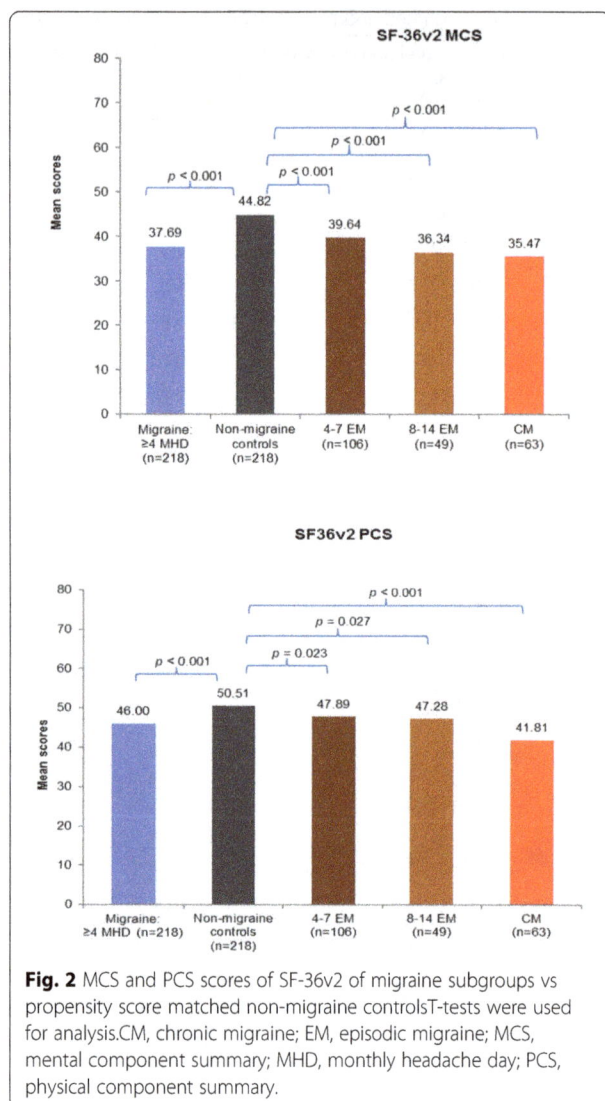

Fig. 2 MCS and PCS scores of SF-36v2 of migraine subgroups vs propensity score matched non-migraine controlsT-tests were used for analysis.CM, chronic migraine; EM, episodic migraine; MCS, mental component summary; MHD, monthly headache day; PCS, physical component summary.

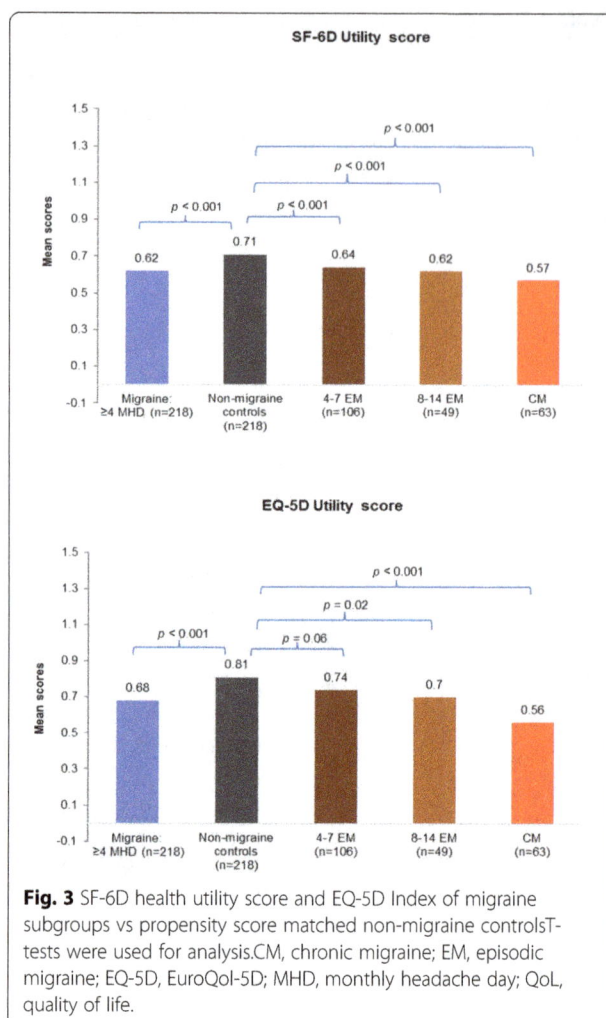

Fig. 3 SF-6D health utility score and EQ-5D Index of migraine subgroups vs propensity score matched non-migraine controlsT-tests were used for analysis.CM, chronic migraine; EM, episodic migraine; EQ-5D, EuroQol-5D; MHD, monthly headache day; QoL, quality of life.

across migraine frequency subgroups compared to non-migraine controls suggesting that migraine impacts HRQoL irrespective of frequency (Fig. 2). Furthermore, an increase in the number of MHDs was associated with worse SF-6D utility and EQ-5D health status scores compared to non-migraine controls (Fig. 3).

Work productivity impairment and activity impairment

Respondents with migraine when compared with non-migraine controls reported significantly higher absenteeism (14.4% vs 9.5%, respectively; $p = 0.001$; Fig. 4) and presenteeism (35.5% vs 21.0%, respectively; $p < 0.001$; Fig. 4). Higher incremental presenteeism vs non-migraine controls were noted across the migraine sample irrespective of migraine frequency (Fig. 4). Among employed respondents, the total work productivity impairment including both absenteeism, presenteeism, and among all respondents activity impairment was significantly higher in those

with migraine than non-migraine controls (38.7% vs 23.3% and 44.2% vs 27.8%, respectively; Fig. 5).

Healthcare resource utilization

HRU was significantly higher in the migraine sample compared with non-migraine controls (Table 2). In the past 6 months before completion of questionnaire, the mean number of total HCP visits (8.5 vs 5.1; $p < 0.001$) and ED visits (0.46 vs 0.21; $p = 0.011$) reported by the migraine sample were significantly higher than non-migraine controls. In particular, the mean general/family practitioner visits (3.1 vs 1.7; $p < 0.001$), neurologist visits (0.19 vs 0.05, $p < 0.001$), and psychiatrist visits (0.85 vs 0.15; $p < 0.001$) were significantly higher for the migraine sample when compared with the non-migraine controls. A significantly higher proportion of migraine respondents compared with non-migraine controls had at least one visit to a general/family practitioner (77.1% vs 67.4%; $p = 0.025$), neurologist (13.8% vs 3.7%; $p < 0.001$), and psychiatrist (13.3% vs. 3.2%; $p < 0.001$) in the prior 6 months.

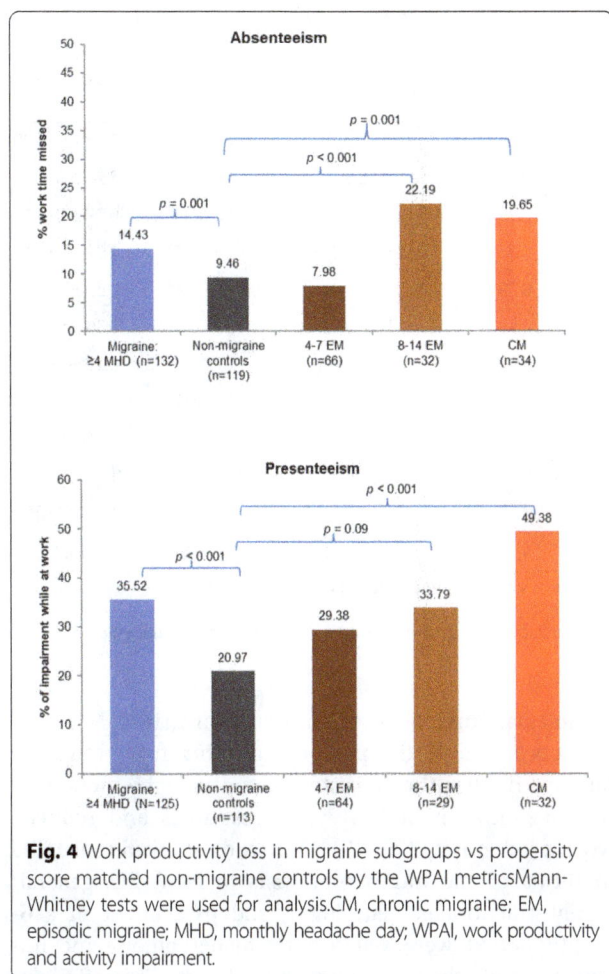

Fig. 4 Work productivity loss in migraine subgroups vs propensity score matched non-migraine controls by the WPAI metricsMann-Whitney tests were used for analysis.CM, chronic migraine; EM, episodic migraine; MHD, monthly headache day; WPAI, work productivity and activity impairment.

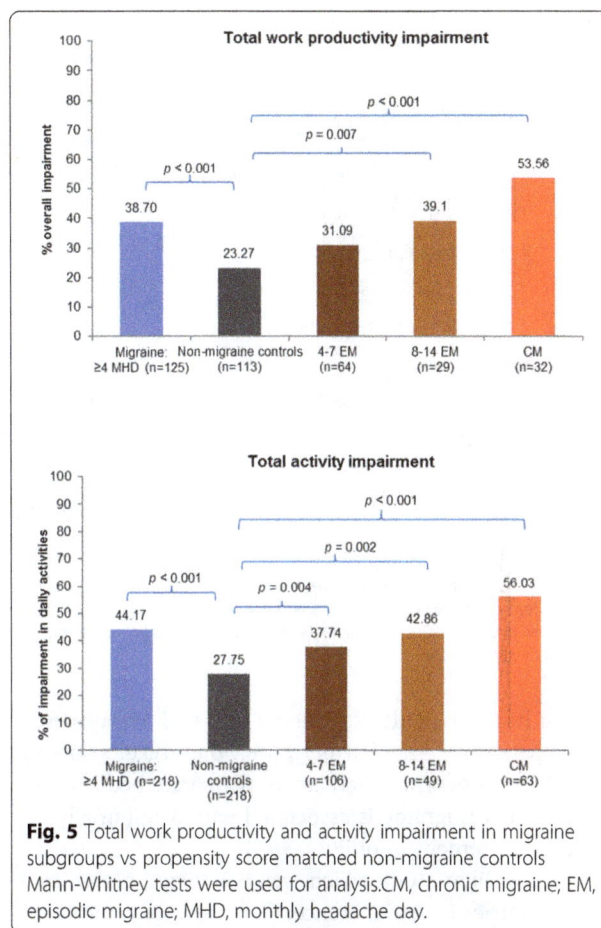

Fig. 5 Total work productivity and activity impairment in migraine subgroups vs propensity score matched non-migraine controls Mann-Whitney tests were used for analysis.CM, chronic migraine; EM, episodic migraine; MHD, monthly headache day.

The mean number of hospitalizations in a 6-month period prior to survey was also higher among those with migraine, although marginally significant, compared with non-migraine controls (0.18 vs 0.11; $p = 0.056$). The proportion of respondents who reported at least one ED visit was significantly higher in the migraine group than non-migraine control (20.6% vs. 12.4%; $p = 0.02$) whereas the proportion hospitalized (12.8% vs. 7.3% $p = 0.056$) was higher but marginally significant.

Discussion

The study used responses from patients of a randomly selected subsample who completed the migraine module (10%), and also reported a physician-diagnosed migraine with ≥4 MHDs (Fig. 1); a patient population that is often deemed eligible for prophylactic treatment in clinical trials and practice. The analysis showed that after propensity score matching of the subgroups based on demographic and health characteristics, those suffering from migraine of at least 4 MHDs had significantly lower HRQoL, increased work and activity impairment, and higher HRU than their

non-migraine matched controls. The incremental burden due to migraine was demonstrated in all domains of life across migraine frequency subgroups in the migraine spectrum with ≥4 MHDs (4–7 EM, 8–14 EM, and CM), suggesting that every migraine attack is associated with burden impacting the well-being, productivity, and HRQoL of individuals affected. This study used the self-reported data from the 2016 NHWS to provide evidence on multiple dimensions of HRQoL, WPAI, and HRU. The NHWS is a validated recurrent survey conducted across multiple countries and multiple therapy areas using standardized questionnaires to study disease-associated burden [37–40]. The methodology used ensures representativeness of the general population and is, hence, useful to understand the overall disease burden within a country.

The poorer HRQoL observed in our study in terms of lower physical, mental, and overall health status (utility scores) in those with migraine compared with non-migraine controls is consistent with previous published studies [41, 42]. Similar studies using SF-36 showed migraine to be associated with lower HRQoL in terms of physical functioning, bodily pain, general health perception, vitality, social functioning, emotional role, and

Table 2 Healthcare resource utilization in the past 6 months among people with migraine and its subgroups vs propensity score matched non-migraine controls across EU5

HRU	Migraine (n = 218)	Non-migraine controls(n = 218)	4–7 EM (n = 106)	8–14 EM (N = 49)	CM(N = 63)
Number of any HCP visits [mean ± SD]	8.48 ± 10.89***	5.13 ± 6.86	7.25 ± 7.29	7.06 ± 7.64	11.65 ± 16.30
Number of general/ family practitioner visits [mean ± SD]	3.08 ± 3.39***	1.67 ± 1.93	3.05 ± 3.38*	2.94 ± 3.42	3.24 ± 3.43*
Number of neurologist visits [mean ± SD]	0.19 ± 0.54***	0.05 ± 0.29	0.20 ± 0.59***	0.16 ± 0.51*	0.19 ± 0.47***
Number of psychiatrist visits [mean ± SD]	0.85 ± 4.48***	0.15 ± 0.86	0.36 ± 1.22**	0.41 ± 1.58*	2.02 ± 7.98***
Number of ED visits [mean ± SD]	0.46 ± 1.20*	0.21 ± 0.79	0.27 ± 1.06	0.61 ± 1.24**	0.67 ± 1.33**
Number of hospitalizations [mean ± SD]	0.18 ± 0.54	0.11 ± 0.53	0.12 ± 0.38	0.16 ± 0.43	0.30 ± 0.78*
Visited any HCP [n, %]	204 (93.58%)	193 (88.53%)	100 (94.3%)	44 (89.8%)	60 (95.2%)
Visited general /family practitioner [n, %]	168 (77.06%)*	147 (67.43%)	83 (78.3%)*	34 (69.4%)	51 (81.0%)*
Visited neurologist [n, %]	30 (13.76%)***	8 (3.67%)	14 (13.2%)***	6 (12.2%)*	10 (15.9%)***
Visited psychiatrist [n, %]	29 (13.30%)***	7 (3.21%)	11 (10.4%)**	5 (10.2%)*	13 (20.6%)***
ED visits [n, %]	45 (20.64%)*	27 (12.39%)	12 (11.3%)	15 (30.6%)**	18 (28.6%)**
Hospitalization [n, %]	28 (12.84%)	16 (7.34%)	11 (10.4%)	7 (14.3%)	10 (15.9%)*

Note: Chi-square tests were used to analyze categorical variables, whereas Mann-Whitney tests were used to analyze continuous variables

p -values for non-migraine controls vs any other group: *$p < 0.05$, **$p < 0.01$, *** $p \leq 0.001$

CM, chronic migraine; ED, emergency department; EM, episodic migraine; HCP, healthcare provider i.e. any physician; HRU, healthcare resource utilization; SD, standard deviation

mental health in Turkish patients [43] and Malaysian female patients [44]. Furthermore, our results of the SF-6D in those with migraine vs their matched controls showed that migraine is associated with a minimally important decrement in utility.

The Eurolight study which was conducted across multiple countries (Austria, France, Germany, Italy, Lithuania, Luxembourg, Netherlands, Spain, and UK) showed that migraine is associated with personal impact that affects personal, work, housework and social activities in both men and women who suffer from migraine [8] and therefore significant economic burden to the society [45]. .The American Migraine Prevalence and Prevention (AMPP) and other international studies have also shown that migraine impacts all aspects of life and that the burden increases with frequency [7, 46].

The present study showed higher levels of absenteeism (1.5-fold), presenteeism (1.7-fold), work productivity impairment (1.7-fold), and activity impairment (1.6-fold) in those suffering from at least 4 MHDs compared with non-migraine matched controls. This is consistent to previously published studies reporting that migraine can result in substantial loss in useful time and productivity, especially in the form of presenteeism (impaired productivity while at work) [8, 45].

The high burden of migraine is depicted as DALYs and YLDs in the Global Burden Disease study, 2015 especially in those younger than 50 years among whom migraine is in the leading causes of disability [9, 11]. The WHO considers a day lived with severe migraine as disabling as a day lived with dementia, quadriplegia or acute psychosis and more disabling than blindness,

paraplegia, angina or rheumatoid arthritis. Migraine impacts not only the persons suffering from migraine but also the healthcare system and society by incremental consumption of healthcare resources and reduced work productivity [25, 45]. Our study showed that HRU in terms of the number of visits to HCP, ED, general/family practitioner, neurologist, and psychiatrist in a 6-month period were significantly higher among the migraine sample than non-migraine controls. These findings are consistent with previous studies in Europe and the US conducted in the overall migraine population where ED visits, hospitalizations, and medicines are among the major cost drivers, while the presence of certain symptoms and/or comorbidities leads to further increase in direct costs [7, 17, 25]; as the frequency and severity of migraine increased, the HRU and economic impact to the healthcare system also increased. It should be noted that the low neurologist visit frequency in our study (13.8%) were similar to previous European studies [13, 27], indicating the lack of specialist healthcare availability in Europe.

Previous European studies have estimated the total cost of migraine at between €18 and €27 billion [45, 47]; these studies refer to the total migraine population and are based on prevalence-based calculations and extrapolation of rough estimates on HRU and costing across multiple countries [45, 47]. Country-specific cost of illness studies are needed to provide a more granular approach into the cost of migraine, especially in those who suffer from at least 4 migraine days per month and are often eligible for prophylaxis. It has been estimated that 77% to 93% of all costs associated with migraine are indirect and attributed to impaired or lost work productivity

[47, 48]. Previous studies have often looked at the overall population with migraine, the majority of whom suffer from less than 4 MHDs, and, therefore, the total costs associated with migraine may be underestimated.

The findings of the current study revealed that migraine is associated with high burden for those suffering from ≥4 MHDs affecting not only the sufferers (health status and HRQoL) but indirectly the society, employers, and healthcare system [7, 20, 21, 25]. Furthermore, the study also reported the overall prescription medication use for 4–7 EM, 8–14 EM, and CM subgroups were 49.1%, 46.9%, and 68.3%, respectively. That means that, 50.9% of 4–7 EM, 53.1% of 8–14 EM, and 31.7% of CM subgroups are not being treated even when suffering with ≥4 MHDs. Patients need to be treated with medications which result in reduction of migraine frequency and thus have a substantial impact on improving HRQoL, increasing work productivity, and reducing both activity impairment and associated HRU. Given that the prevalence of migraine peaks in those aged 30 to 49 years—an age of prime productivity on a personal, social and professional level—it is important to address the high unmet need for those affected.

Limitations

There are several limitations that should be noted and which are inherent to these type of studies [49, 50]. .All data are patient-reported via an online panel-based sample and therefore certain biases may exist, therefore caution needs to be taken when interpreting the data.

Despite using the method of administration and randomization to achieve representativeness of the study sample to that of the general population, some bias may still be introduced; this may be due to the inherent differences across different countries as well as access restriction for specific segments of population such as elderly, institutionalized, and those with severe comorbidities and disabilities. Certain efforts were employed to minimize this such as by telephone recruitment where internet access may be limited. The survey responses were self-reported, and data could not be independently verified. The survey questions were relatively benign, and the survey was confidential, diminishing the incentive to misrepresent one's reporting. All analyses were run in aggregate and no individual-level analysis was conducted.

The self-reported nature of the NHWS is associated with potential corresponding biases such as inaccurate recall and false reporting (whether intentional or unintentional). For example, diagnoses of migraine or other comorbidities (eg, those used in the comorbidity index) were self-reported and are not verified by a physician or medical record. However, questions on year of diagnosis and type of diagnosing physician were also asked which minimizes the probability of false reporting. There is an inherent recall bias to some

of the questions that require retrospectively to report outcomes such as HRU. However, major events like an emergency room visit or hospitalization are less likely to be subjected to inaccurate recall compared to a visit to the general practitioner. However, the panel does take adequate measures to minimize intentionally false HRU reporting. For instance, limiting ranges for the number of visits so extreme values aren't possible, checking for respondents speeding through the survey, or using adaptive questioning to reduce the complexity of the questions.

While measured variables were accounted for in matching and regression, there is the possibility of groups differing on unmeasured variables that may have an impact on outcomes. Although we have tried to match the 2 sample groups by using propensity score matching across different variables (age, gender, BMI, and other factors used), variables that were not considered and could have impacted the analysis may still exist.

Conclusions

The findings of the current study reveal that there is an incremental burden due to migraine on HRQoL (mental, physical, and health status), work productivity (both presenteeism and absenteeism), and the utilization of healthcare resources among those who suffer from migraine ≥4 MHDs in comparison to the matched non-migraine controls in the EU5. Moreover, migraine is undertreated as the patients did not have access to appropriate healthcare, suggesting that effective management and preventive treatments are needed to lessen the frequency and burden of migraine.

Abbreviations

BMI: Body mass index; CCI: Charlson comorbidity index; DALYs: Disability-adjusted life years; ED: Emergency department; EQ-5D: Euroqol-5D; EU5: France, Germany, Italy, Spain and the UK; GBD: Global Burden of Disease; HCP: Healthcare provider; HRQoL: Health-related quality of life; HRU: Healthcare resource use; IRB: Institutional Review Board; MCS: Mental component summary; MHDs: Monthly headaches days; NHWS: National Health and Wellness Survey; PCS: Physical component summary; SF 36 v2: Short-Form 36-Item Health Survey version 2; WPAI: Work productivity loss and activity impairment; WPAI-GH: Work productivity and activity impairment; YLDs: Years lived with disability

Acknowledgements

Medical writing support was provided by Uma Dasam and Ramu Periyasamy, Ph.D., Indegene Pvt. Ltd.

Funding

This study was sponsored by Novartis Pharma AG, Switzerland.

Authors' contributions

PV, JF, AB, AKL, and SG conceived and designed the study. SG analyzed the data. PV, JF, AB, AKL and SG interpreted the results and helped write the paper. All authors read and approved the final manuscript.

Competing interests

SG is an employee of Kantar Health, which conducted the NHWS and received funding to analyze and develop the manuscript from Novartis. PV, JF and AKL are employees of Novartis, which funded the current study. AB was a Novartis employee at the time of the study completion and manuscript preparation.

Author details

[1]Novartis Pharma AG, Fabrikstr. 12, CH-4002 Basel, Switzerland. [2]Novartis Pharmaceuticals Corporation, One Health Plaza, East Hanover, NJ 07936-1080, USA. [3]Novartis Global Services Centre, Patient Access Services, Dublin, Ireland. [4]Kantar Health, New York, NY 10010, USA.

References

1. (2013) The International Classification of Headache Disorders, 3rd edition Copyright. ßInternational Headache Soc. doi: https://doi.org/10.1177/0333102417738202
2. Donnet A, Daniel C, Milandre L et al (2012) Migraine with aura in patients over 50 years of age: the Marseille's registry. J Neurol 259:1868–1873. https://doi.org/10.1007/s00415-012-6423-8
3. Headache Classification Subcommittee of the International Headache Society (2004) The International Classification of Headache Disorders: 2nd edition. Cephalalgia 24 Suppl 1:9–160.
4. Lipton RB, Bigal ME, Diamond M et al (2007) Migraine prevalence, disease burden, and the need for preventive therapy. Neurology 68:343–349. https://doi.org/10.1212/01.wnl.0000252808.97649.21
5. Woldeamanuel YW, Cowan RP (2017) Migraine affects 1 in 10 people worldwide featuring recent rise: a systematic review and meta-analysis of community-based studies involving 6 million participants. J Neurol Sci 372:307–315. https://doi.org/10.1016/j.jns.2016.11.071
6. Burstein R, Noseda R, Borsook D (2015) Migraine: multiple processes. complex pathophysiology J Neurosci 35:6619–6629. https://doi.org/10.1523/JNEUROSCI.0373-15.2015
7. Blumenfeld AM, Varon SF, Wilcox TK et al (2011) Disability, HRQoL and resource use among chronic and episodic migraineurs: results from the international burden of migraine study (IBMS). Cephalalgia 31:301–315. https://doi.org/10.1177/0333102410381145
8. Steiner TJ, Stovner LJ, Katsarava Z et al (2014) The impact of headache in Europe: principal results of the Eurolight project. J Headache Pain 15(31). https://doi.org/10.1186/1129-2377-15-31
9. GBD 2015 DALYs and HALE Collaborators NJ, Arora M, Barber RM et al (2016) Global, regional, and national disability-adjusted life-years (DALYs) for 315 diseases and injuries and healthy life expectancy (HALE), 1990–2015: a systematic analysis for the Global Burden of Disease Study 2015. Lancet 388:1603–1658. https://doi.org/10.1016/S0140-6736(16)31460-X
10. Steiner TJ, Stovner LJ, Vos T et al (2018) Migraine is first cause of disability in under 50s: will health politicians now take notice? J Headache Pain 19:17. https://doi.org/10.1186/s10194-018-0846-2
11. Vos T, Allen C, Arora M et al (2016) Global, regional, and national incidence, prevalence, and years lived with disability for 310 diseases and injuries, 1990–2015: a systematic analysis for the global burden of disease study 2015. Lancet 388:1545–1602. https://doi.org/10.1016/S0140-6736(16)31678-6
12. Cevoli S, D'Amico D, Martelletti P et al (2009) Underdiagnosis and undertreatment of migraine in Italy: a survey of patients attending for the first time 10 headache centres. Cephalalgia 29:1285–1293. https://doi.org/10.1111/j.1468-2982.2009.01874.x
13. Radtke A, Neuhauser H (2009) Prevalence and burden of headache and migraine in Germany. Headache 49:79–89. https://doi.org/10.1111/j.1526-4610.2008.01263.x
14. Ford JH, Jackson J, Milligan G et al (2017) A real-world analysis of migraine: a cross-sectional study of disease burden and treatment patterns. Headache J Head Face Pain 57:1532–1544. https://doi.org/10.1111/head.13202
15. Buse DC, Manack AN, Fanning KM et al (2012) Chronic migraine prevalence, disability, and sociodemographic factors: results from the American migraine prevalence and prevention study. Headache 52:1456–1470. https://doi.org/10.1111/j.1526-4610.2012.02223.x
16. Stokes M, Becker WJ, Lipton RB et al (2011) Cost of health care among patients with chronic and episodic migraine in Canada and the USA: results from the international burden of migraine study (IBMS). Headache 51:1058–1077. https://doi.org/10.1111/j.1526-4610.2011.01945.x
17. Edmeads J, Mackell JA (2002) The economic impact of migraine: an analysis of direct and indirect costs. Headache 42:501–509
18. Sharma K, Remanan R, Singh S (2013) Quality of life and psychiatric co-morbidity in Indian migraine patients: a headache clinic sample. Neurol India 61:355–359. https://doi.org/10.4103/0028-3886.117584
19. Ayzenberg I, Katsarava Z, Sborowski A et al (2014) Headache-attributed burden and its impact on productivity and quality of life in Russia: structured healthcare for headache is urgently needed. Eur J Neurol 21:758–765. https://doi.org/10.1111/ene.12380
20. Wang S-J, Wang P-J, Fuh J-L et al (2013) Comparisons of disability, quality of life, and resource use between chronic and episodic migraineurs: a clinic-based study in Taiwan. Cephalalgia 33:171–181. https://doi.org/10.1177/0333102412468668
21. Berra E, Sances G, De Icco R et al (2015) Cost of chronic and episodic migraine. A pilot study from a tertiary headache Centre in northern Italy. J Headache Pain 16:532. https://doi.org/10.1186/s10194-015-0532-6
22. Raggi A, Giovannetti AM, Schiavolin S et al (2014) Validating the migraine-specific quality of life questionnaire v2.1 (MSQ) in Italian inpatients with chronic migraine with a history of medication overuse. Qual Life Res 23:1273–1277. https://doi.org/10.1007/s11136-013-0556-9
23. Stuginski-Barbosa J, Dach F, Bigal M, Speciali JG (2012) Chronic pain and depression in the quality of life of women with migraine - a controlled study. Headache J Head Face Pain 52:400–408. https://doi.org/10.1111/j.1526-4610.2012.02095.x
24. Andrée C, Stovner LJ, Steiner TJ et al (2011) The Eurolight project: the impact of primary headache disorders in Europe. Description of methods. J Headache Pain 12:541–549. https://doi.org/10.1007/s10194-011-0356-y
25. Bloudek LM, Stokes M, Buse DC et al (2012) Cost of healthcare for patients with migraine in five European countries: results from the international burden of migraine study (IBMS). J Headache Pain 13:361–378. https://doi.org/10.1007/s10194-012-0460-7
26. Fernández-de-Las-Peñas C, Hernández-Barrera V, Carrasco-Garrido P et al (2010) Population-based study of migraine in Spanish adults: relation to socio-demographic factors, lifestyle and co-morbidity with other conditions. J Headache Pain 11:97–104. https://doi.org/10.1007/s10194-009-0176-5
27. Allena M, Steiner TJ, Sances G et al (2015) Impact of headache disorders in Italy and the public-health and policy implications: a population-based study within the Eurolight project. J Headache Pain 16:100. https://doi.org/10.1186/s10194-015-0584-7
28. D'Amico D, Bussone G (2003) Disability and migraine: recent outcomes using an Italian version of MIDAS. J Headache Pain 4:s42–s46. https://doi.org/10.1007/s101940300008
29. Mesas AE, González AD, Mesas CE et al (2014) The association of chronic neck pain, low back pain, and migraine with absenteeism due to health problems in Spanish workers. Spine (Phila Pa 1976) 39:1243–1253. https://doi.org/10.1097/BRS.0000000000000387
30. Charlson ME, Pompei P, Ales KL, MacKenzie CR (1987) A new method of classifying prognostic comorbidity in longitudinal studies: development and validation. J Chronic Dis 40:373–383
31. Maruish ME (Ed.) (2011) User's manual for the SF-36v2 Health Survey (3rd ed.). Lincoln, RI: QualityMetric Incorporated.
32. Brazier J, Roberts J, Deverill M (2002) The estimation of a preference-based measure of health from the SF-36. J Health Econ 21:271–292

33. Herdman M, Gudex C, Lloyd A et al (2011) Development and preliminary testing of the new five-level version of EQ-5D (EQ-5D-5L). Qual Life Res 20: 1727–1736. https://doi.org/10.1007/s11136-011-9903-x

34. Reilly MC, Zbrozek AS, Dukes EM (1993) The validity and reproducibility of a work productivity and activity impairment instrument. Pharmacoeconomics 4:353–365

35. Swigris JJ, Brown KK, Behr J et al (2010) The SF-36 and SGRQ: validity and first look at minimum important differences in IPF. Respir Med 104:296–304. https://doi.org/10.1016/j.rmed.2009.09.006

36. Walters SJ, Brazier JE (2005) Comparison of the minimally important difference for two health state utility measures: EQ-5D and SF-6D. Qual Life Res 14:1523–1532

37. Meneghini LF, Lee L, Gupta S, Preblick R (2018) The association of hypoglycaemia severity and clinical, patient-reported and economic outcomes in US patients with type 2 diabetes using basal insulin. Diabetes Obes Metab. https://doi.org/10.1111/dom.13208

38. Arima K, Gupta S, Gadkari A et al (2018) Burden of atopic dermatitis in Japanese adults: analysis of data from the 2013 National Health and wellness survey. J Dermatol. https://doi.org/10.1111/1346-8138.14218

39. Ding B, DiBonaventura M, Karlsson N, Ling X (2017) A cross-sectional assessment of the prevalence and burden of mild asthma in urban China using the 2010, 2012, and 2013 China National Health and wellness surveys. J Asthma 54:632–643. https://doi.org/10.1080/02770903.2016.1255750

40. Balp M-M, Vietri J, Tian H, Isherwood G (2015) The impact of chronic Urticaria from the Patient's perspective: a survey in five European countries. Patient 8:551–558. https://doi.org/10.1007/s40271-015-0145-9

41. Lipton RB, Hamelsky SW, Kolodner KB et al (2000) Migraine, quality of life, and depression: a population-based case-control study. Neurology 55:629–635

42. Lipton R, Liberman J, Kolodner K et al (2003) Migraine headache disability and health-related quality-of-life: a population-based case-control study from England. Cephalalgia 23:441–450. https://doi.org/10.1046/j.1468-2982.2003.00546.x

43. Arslantas D, Tozun M, Unsal A, Ozbek Z (2013) Headache and its effects on health-related quality of life among adults. Turk Neurosurg 23:498–504. https://doi.org/10.5137/1019-5149.JTN.7304-12.0

44. Shaik MM, Hassan NB, Tan HL, Gan SH (2015) Quality of life and migraine disability among female migraine patients in a tertiary Hospital in Malaysia. Biomed Res Int 2015:1–9. https://doi.org/10.1155/2015/523717

45. Stovner LJ, Andrée C, Committee ES (2008) Impact of headache in Europe: a review for the Eurolight project. J Headache Pain 9:139–146. https://doi.org/10.1007/s10194-008-0038-6

46. Munakata J, Hazard E, Serrano D et al (2009) Economic burden of transformed migraine: results from the American migraine prevalence and prevention (AMPP) study. Headache 49:498–508. https://doi.org/10.1111/j.1526-4610.2009.01369.x

47. Olesen J, Gustavsson A, Svensson M et al (2012) The economic cost of brain disorders in Europe. Eur J Neurol 19:155–162. https://doi.org/10.1111/j.1468-1331.2011.03590.x

48. Linde M, Gustavsson A, Stovner LJ et al (2012) The cost of headache disorders in Europe: the Eurolight project. Eur J Neurol 19:703–711. https://doi.org/10.1111/j.1468-1331.2011.03612.x

49. Goren A, Liu X, Gupta S et al (2013) Quality of life, activity impairment, and healthcare resource utilization associated with atrial fibrillation in the US National Health and wellness survey. Am. https://doi.org/10.1371/journal.pone.0071264

50. Kalsekar I, Wagner J-S, Dibonaventura M, et al (2012) Comparison of health-related quality of life among patients using atypical antipsychotics for treatment of depression: results from the National Health and Wellness Survey. ??? 10:1 . doi: https://doi.org/10.1186/1477-7525-10-81

A PRISMA-compliant systematic review of the endpoints employed to evaluate symptomatic treatments for primary headaches

D. García-Azorin[1*], N. Yamani[2,3], L. M. Messina[4,5], I. Peeters[6], M. Ferrili[7], D. Ovchinnikov[8,9], M. L. Speranza[10], V. Marini[10], A. Negro[11], S. Benemei[12], M. Barloese[13,14] and on behalf of the European Headache Federation School of Advanced Studies (EHF-SAS)

Abstract

Background: Primary headache are prevalent and debilitating disorders. Acute pain cessation is one of the key points in their treatment. Many drugs have been studied but the design of the trials is not usually homogeneous. Efficacy of the trial is determined depending on the selected primary endpoint and usually other different outcomes are measured. We aim to critically appraise which were the employed outcomes through a systematic review.

Methods: We conducted a systematic review of literature focusing on studies on primary headache evaluating acute relief of pain, following the PRISMA guideline. The study population included patients participating in a controlled study about symptomatic treatment. The comparator could be placebo or the standard of care. The collected information was the primary outcome of the study and all secondary outcomes. We evaluated the studied drug, the year of publication and the type of journal. We performed a search and we screened all the potential papers and reviewed them considering inclusion/exclusion criteria.

Results: The search showed 4288 clinical trials that were screened and 794 full articles were assessed for eligibility for a final inclusion of 495 papers. The studies were published in headache specific journals (58%), general journals (21.6%) and neuroscience journals (20.4%).
Migraine was the most studied headache, in 87.8% studies, followed by tension type headache in 4.7%. Regarding the most evaluated drug, triptans represented 68.6% of all studies, followed by non-steroidal anti-inflammatories (25.1%). Only 4.6% of the papers evaluated ergots and 1.6% analyzed opioids.
The most frequent primary endpoint was the relief of the headache at a determinate moment, in 54.1%. Primary endpoint was evaluated at 2-h in 69.9% of the studies. Concerning other endpoints, tolerance was the most frequently addressed (83%), followed by headache relief (71.1%), improvement of other symptoms (62.5%) and presence of relapse (54%). The number of secondary endpoints increased from 4.2 (SD = 2.0) before 1991 to 6.39 after 2013 (*p = 0.001*).

(Continued on next page)

* Correspondence: davilink@hotmail.com
[1]Headache Unit Neurology Department, Hospital Clínico Universitario Valladolid, Avda. Ramón y Cajal 3, 47005 Valladolid, Spain
Full list of author information is available at the end of the article

(Continued from previous page)

Conclusion: Headache relief has been the most employed primary endpoint but headache disappearance starts to be firmly considered. The number of secondary endpoints increases over time and other outcomes such as disability, quality of life and patients' preference are receiving attention.

Keywords: Primary headaches, Clinical trials, Acute, Triptans, Non-steroidal anti-inflammatory, Prisma-guidelines, Endpoints

Background

Primary headaches are the most prevalent neurological disorders and the main neurological cause of years lived with disability, particularly in the middle age group under 50 years old adults, in which migraine is the first cause of disability [1]. They represent also one of the main neurological disorders regarding economical costs [2], and symptomatic treatment accounts for the biggest part of them [3].

Also for trials, success is a matter of perspective and depends mainly on expectations. An intervention is considered efficacious if it reaches a predefined endpoint, thus the careful definition of every endpoint is critical. Not only concerning patients' satisfaction and relief, but also in order to reach the approval from the regulatory authorities, such as the European Medicines Agency (EMA) and the Food and Drug Administration (FDA).

In the field of headache, traditional endpoints in chronic headaches have been related to the decrease in number of days with headache, changes related to pain intensity, analgesics uptake and emergency department visits. Nowadays novel factors such as quality of life or work absenteeism begin to be taken into account.

Regarding symptomatic therapies, many outcomes have been proposed. The International Headache Society (IHS) created guidelines in order to harmonize studies evaluating acute treatment. The first version was published in 1991 [4], a second edition arrived in 2000 [5] and the last dates from 2012 [6]. Every edition added new proposed outcomes and instructions about how every endpoint should be measured. Table 1 presents the list of outcomes mentioned in the three versions of IHS Guidelines.

As shown in Table 1, the recommended main endpoint has changed over time from headache relief to complete pain freedom. This was motivated by the fact that placebo response in headache relief could be substantial, over 30%, whereas pain freedom placebo response is just around 9% [7]. Despite their utility, adherence to these guidelines seemed to be low, just 31% of the studies addressing acute treatment ascribed to them in the 2002–2008 period [8].

Table 1 Recommended endpoints from IHS guidelines for migraine drug trials according to the edition

1st edition (published in 1991)	2nd edition (published in 2000)	3rd edition (published in 2012)
Number of attacks resolved within 2h	**Pain-free after 2h**	**Percentage of patients free of pain at 2h**
		Incidence of relapse
Duration of headache	Sustained pain-free 24h	Sustained pain freedom
		Total migraine freedom
Severity of headache	Headache intensity	Intensity of headache
Global rating of attack severity	Disability	Headache relief
		Time to meaningful relief
		Time to pain freedom
Escape medication	Rescue medication	Rescue medication
Global evaluation of medication	Global evaluation of medication	Global evaluation of medication
		Global impact (disability and quality of life)
Presence of nausea and vomiting		Migraine-associated symptoms
	Adverse events	Adverse events
	Patients preference	Preference to treatment
		Treatment of relapse
	Consistency of effect.	

In bold, the recommended primary endpoint

Patient preference has received little and intermittent attention. The triptan-era brought many studies trying to assess what patients value most, and complete relief of pain, a fast onset of action and lack of recurrence were the preferred endpoints. Non-clinical endpoints such as productivity, disability, direct costs, and quality of life have also been considered recently [9], considering headache as a multidimensional disease.

As we mentioned above, the criteria for success have been defined by expert consensus, and patients' opinions are not usually considered. The concept of Patient Related Outcome Measure (PROM) defines self-reported measures about symptoms, functional status and perceptions from a patient perspective [10]. This novel approach is receiving growing attention and identifying patients' preferences might help to create realistic outcomes, considering patients expectations [11, 12].

We aimed to critically appraise the employed outcomes by conducting a systematic review. The study population included patients with acute primary headache; we considered all the possible interventions pursuing the resolution of the headache episode. Studies employed placebo or the standard of care as comparator. We analyzed every employed outcome.

Methods

We conducted a systematic review of literature focusing on studies on primary headache addressing the acute relief of pain, following the PRISMA guidelines [13].

Search criteria

The target population was primary headache sufferers, the study population included patients participating in a controlled study about the symptomatic treatment for the relief of the headache episode. The intervention was compared with placebo or the standard of care. The collected information was the employed outcome of the study, differentiating between primary and secondary endpoints.

We did not restrict the search in time, considering all available articles until the search. We reviewed studies in all the European languages. Age of participants or the country in which the study took place was not limited.

We included studies addressing the acute treatment for primary headaches providing information about primary and secondary endpoints. The inclusion criteria were: 1) clinical trials comparing with placebo or standard of care, 2) studies conducted in humans, 3) with full text availability.

We excluded studies if they were: 1) not original researches, 2) not focusing on treatment and addressing other issues, 3) studying therapies that are not suitable for self administration by patients, such as intravenous therapies, 4) performed on emergency department setting, 5) not providing information about the relief of pain, 6) focused on secondary headaches.

Search strategy

The employed source was MEDLINE database. The search was performed on April 22nd 2018 and included all the studies. The electronic strategy of search was designed in order to include the primary headaches and all the possible acute therapies.

The strategy of search combined terms such as primary headache, migraine, tension-type, trigeminal, hemicrania, cluster, Short-lasting Unilateral neuralgiform headache with conjunctival injection and tearing (SUNCT) and Short-lasting unilateral neuralgiform headache attacks with cranial autonomic symptoms (SUNA) by the use of boolean operators, combining with the available therapies. We employed truncations and wildcards to optimize the search. The employed command is available in Appendix section. We included common analgesics such as acetaminophen/paracetamol or metamizol, non-steroidal anti-inflammatory drugs (NSAIDs), triptans, anti-emetics (if employed for pain relief), opioids, ergot derivatives, caffeine, magnesium, oxygen, devices that could be easily employed by patients at home and novel drugs such as lasmiditan or gepants, screening all the possible results.

Database creation and included variables

We created a database with all the potential studies. Two investigators peer reviewed independently all the abstracts and selected them according to inclusion and exclusion criteria. Results were compared and in cases with lack of agreement the rest of the team decided by consensus if the study should be included or not. After that, a different investigator reviewed the full document, addressing the final eligibility if information about the endpoint was provided and excluding the paper in the opposite case.

As we were not specifically reviewing the results of the interventions, we listed the different interventions considering the different primary and secondary outcomes employed in each study, the year of publication and the evaluated drug. We generated an electronic database employing Microsoft Excel.

We considered the risk of publication bias so we included only the information contained in the material and methods section or in the study protocol, in order to avoid lack of information. We tried to minimize the bias of missing articles using a wide search strategy, employing MeSH terms in the search and fully evaluating many of the papers in order to obtain firm evidence.

Statistical description and analysis

We present the data as frequency for categorical variables and means and their standard deviation or medians and Inter Quartile Range (IQR) for quantitative data. For analytical purposes, we classified the journals into three groups: Headache specific journals, neuroscience journals and general medicine journals. All the journals included in each group can be consulted in the Appendix. We also divided the time into 4 periods considering the date when the IHS official guidelines for symptomatic studies were published, being the intervals: before 1991, 1992–2000, 2001–2012 and after 2013. We employed SPSS v20.0 IBM for the statistical analysis employing the pertinent test for each type and distribution of variable.

Results

We present the number of identified articles, those screened and those that fulfilled inclusion and exclusion criteria in the PRISMA flow chart (Fig. 1).

We included 495 papers in the final analysis. 58% of the studies were published in headache specific journals, 20.4% in neuroscience journals and 21.6% in general journals. The specific journals that showed most articles were *Headache* with 156 papers, *Cephalalgia* with 112, *Neurology* 36, *European Neurology* 19 and *Journal of Headache and Pain* with 15.

Regarding the year of publication, the mode was 2005 and the median was 2003, with decreasing the number of papers after 2010 (Fig. 2). The pattern of publication differed comparing Headache Journals, which showed a median year of publication of 2004 (IQR 1998–2009) and general neurology journals, which had a median year of 2003 (IQR 1997–2006) and general medicine journals, whose distribution had a median of 2001 (IQR 1995–2007), $p = 0.05$. (Fig. 2).

Addressed headaches

The evaluated headache according IHS classification were migraine in 87.8%, with 22 studies addressing specifically menstrual migraine, 4.7% of the studies were focused on tension type headache, 3.6% analyzed trigeminoautonomal cephalalgias, 2 studies included patients with both migraine and tension type and 19 studies mentioned primary headaches without additional specifications. We did not find any trial on patients with other primary headaches.

Studied drugs

The most frequently evaluated group of drugs was triptans, representing 68.6% of the studies. Sumatriptan was the most studied, counting 115 papers and representing 45,1% of the triptan articles, followed by rizatriptan (37 studies, 14.5%), zolmitriptan (33, 12.9%), almotriptan (27, 10.8%), eletriptan (20, 7.8%), frovatriptan (10, 3.9%),

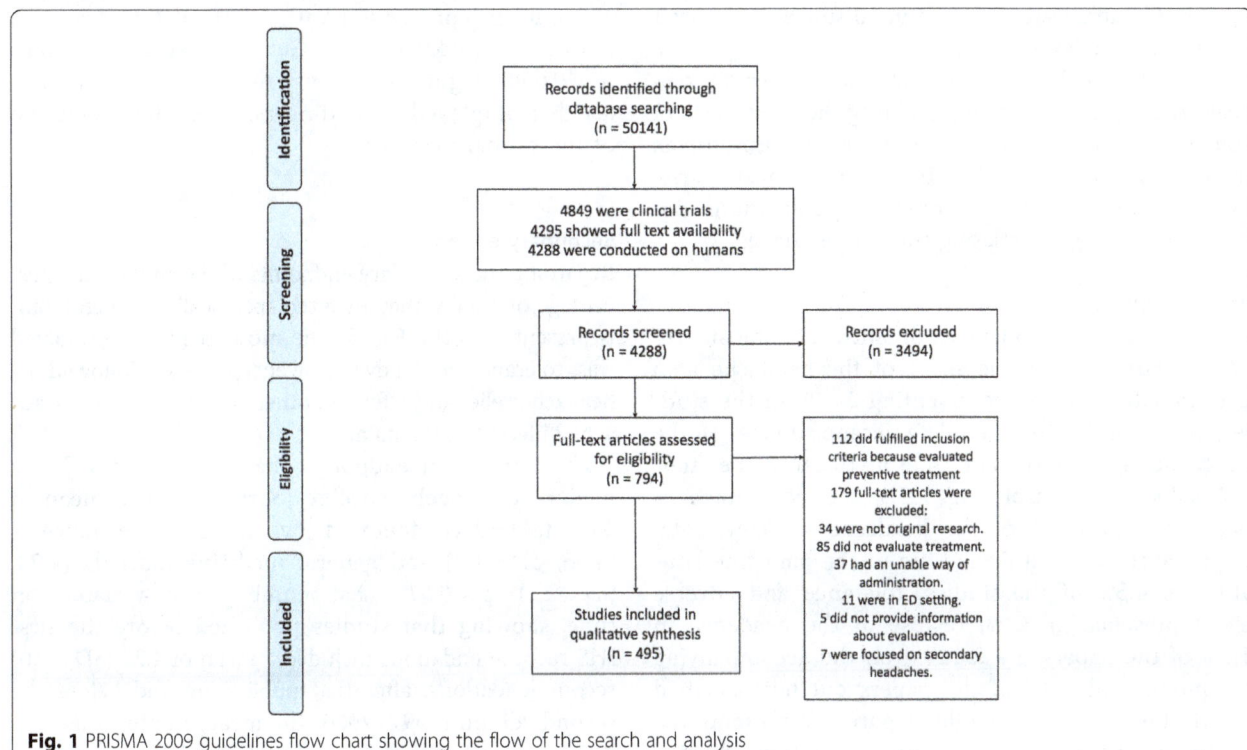

Fig. 1 PRISMA 2009 guidelines flow chart showing the flow of the search and analysis

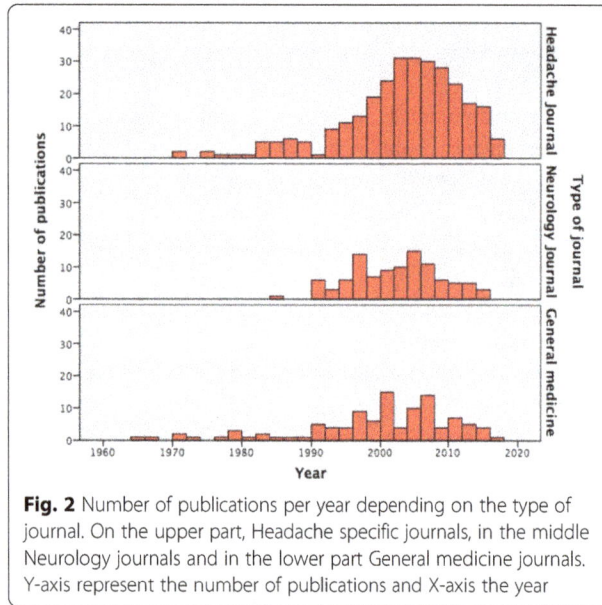

Fig. 2 Number of publications per year depending on the type of journal. On the upper part, Headache specific journals, in the middle Neurology journals and in the lower part General medicine journals. Y-axis represent the number of publications and X-axis the year

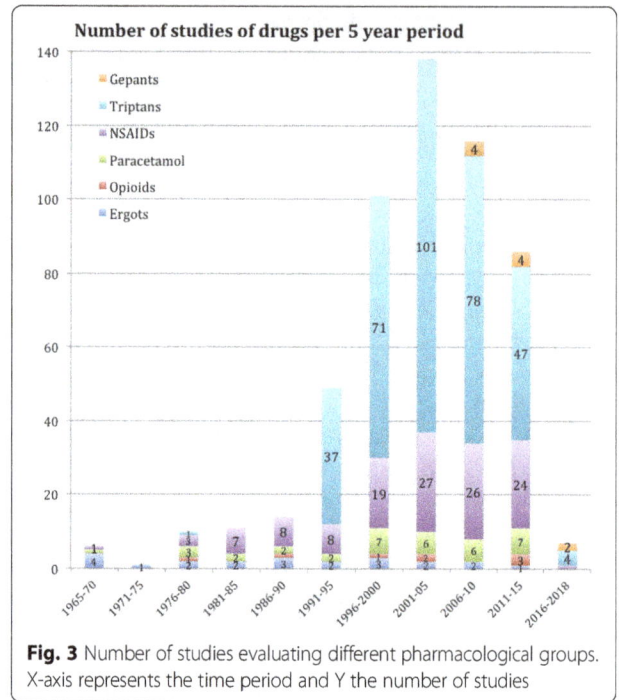

Fig. 3 Number of studies evaluating different pharmacological groups. X-axis represents the time period and Y the number of studies

naratriptan (6, 2.4%), avitriptan (3, 1.2%) and 4 studies did not specify the triptan clearly.

Non-steroidal anti-inflammatories were analyzed in 25,1% of the studies. Naproxen was the most frequently evaluated, in 31 studies (26,9% of NSAID studies), followed by acetylsalicylic acid in 27 (23.5%), ibuprofen in 17 (14.8%), diclofenac in 10 (8,7%) and dexketoprofen and COX-2 inhibitors with 9 studies each (7.8%). Paracetamol or acetaminophen were evaluated in 7.4% of the studies. Only 4.6% of the papers analyzed ergots and 1.6% studied opioids. Gepants were evaluated in 10 studies and only 1 Lasmiditan matched our criteria.

Up to 30.9% of the studies evaluated at least two different analgesics, naproxen-sumatriptan being the most frequent combination in 18 studies and dexketoprofen-frovatriptan in 4. 70.6% of the studies included a placebo arm. Figure 3 presents the number of publications per 5-year period differentiating the studied drug.

Primary endpoints

Concerning the primary endpoints, the most frequent endpoint was the relief of the headache at a determinate moment, representing 54.1% of the studies, followed by the complete disappearance of the headache at a determinate time in 16.2% of the studies, subjective variables in 7.2%, the percentage of patients with relief of the headache in 5,9%, total migraine freedom in 5.3%, time to the pain free situation in 4.5% of the studies, tolerance and adverse event presence in 3.1%, relapse of the headache in 1.2% of the papers, 1% focused on the accompanying symptoms and 2.8% of the papers did not specified clearly the primary endpoint. Figure 4 represents the evolution of the primary endpoint over time, divided

in 5-year intervals and showing the percentage of each primary endpoint in each time frame.

The time when the primary endpoint was evaluated was 120 min in 69.9% of the studies. In studies evaluating tension type headache and migraine, the percentage ascended to 74.6%. 65.3% of the Neuroscience journals analyzed the primary endpoint at 120 min, in comparison with 58.9% of the Headache journals and 44.9% of the General Medicine journals ($p = 0.008$). Figure 5 presents the percentage of studies that employed each time point in the evaluation of the primary endpoint.

Secondary endpoints

Regarding the secondary endpoints of the studies, the percentage of studies that analyzed specifically each endpoint is presented in the Fig. 6. The most frequently evaluated was tolerance and adverse event presence followed by headache relief and effect on other symptoms of the headache different to the pain.

The number of endpoints that were addressed was higher in headache specific journals, with a mean of 4.89 (SD = 2.1), followed by neuroscience journals (4.56, SD = 1.8) and general medicine journals (4.23, SD = 2.1), $p = 0.01$. That number also variated on time, showing that studies published before the first IHS recommendations included a mean of 4.20 (SD = 2.0) recommendations; after that publication and before the second edition (1991–2000) the mean number was 4.76 (SD = 1.9) and after the second IHS guidelines the mean

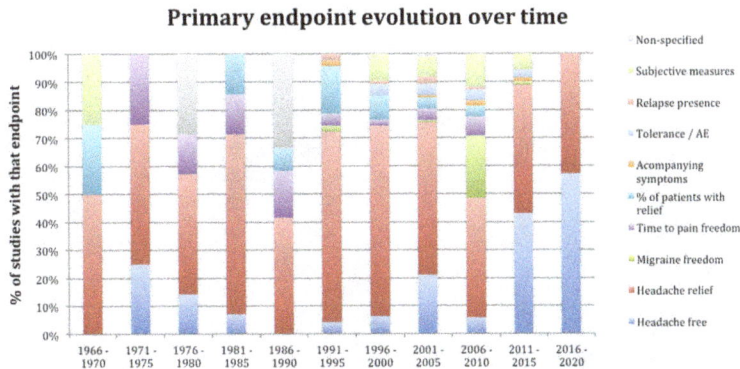

Fig. 4 Percentage of studies with a determinate primary endpoint per 5-year periods. Y-axis shows the percentages per each endpoint of the total studies of each period, X-axis shows the different periods. AE = Adverse Events

number was 4.5 (SD = 2.0) (2000–2012 period) and after the publication of the third IHS guidelines (from 2013 to present) the mean number of fulfilled endpoints was 6.39 (SD = 2.1), ($p = 0.001$).

The percentage of studies that fulfilled all the IHS recommendations was of 10.8% for the first version, 8.2% for the second version and 4.5% for the third one. Figure 7 represents the percentage of studies that analyzed each efficacy endpoint over time. Endpoints evaluating functionality were addressed in 33% of the studies. Patients' preference was considered only in 4.98% of the studies and the global evaluation of the drug in 5.1% of the papers.

Discussion

In this study, we systematically reviewed all the randomized controlled studies evaluating acute therapies for the treatment of primary headaches. We addressed not only

which headaches and drugs under analysis, but also the way they were evaluated, considering if IHS recommendations were fulfilled.

The vast majority of the studies took place in migraine patients. The low prevalence of other primary headaches difficult its study in controlled trials, nevertheless other prevalent conditions such as Tension Type Headache or Cluster Headache seem to be underrepresented. In line with the previous finding, migraine-specific therapies were the most frequently studied. Triptans and NSAIDs aggregated the majority of the studies, even when many other analgesics are used in other painful conditions, most of them have not been properly analyzed specifically in headache.

The most frequently used main endpoint determining the success has been headache relief in the majority of studies. We observed that recently, other endpoints proposed by the IHS guidelines start to be systematically addressed, specifically complete freedom of pain or disappearance of all migranous symptoms. Dealing with an exquisitely subjective condition as pain could be hard. The wide inter-individual variability and the high risk of placebo effect, with the subsequent possibility of false positive or false negative results, are well-known. As IHS guidelines recommend, it is desirable to employ total headache disappearance instead of relief, as the improvement implicates considerable subjectivity.

Two hours is the period defined as critical in the resolution of the headache such as migraine or tension type headache and most of the studies adhere to it. Only a minority of studies employs the time to the disappearance of the headache, probably because of the complexity in its evaluation and a more complicated statistical analysis. Many other endpoints were usually addressed, mainly tolerance, effect on other symptoms associated with the headache and relapse presence.

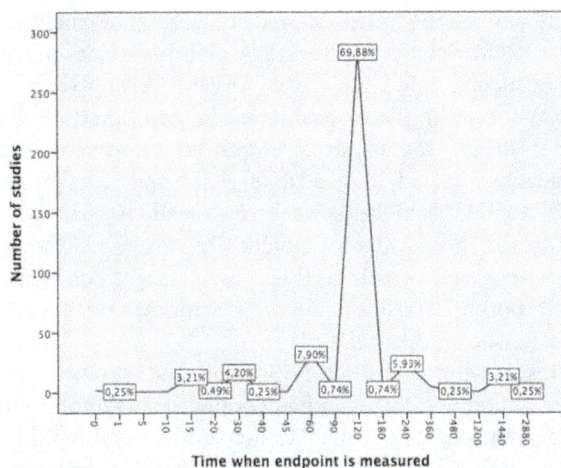

Fig. 5 Percentage of studies evaluated at each determined time. X-axis shows the predefined time points. Y-axis represents the number of papers. Percentage of the total appears squared

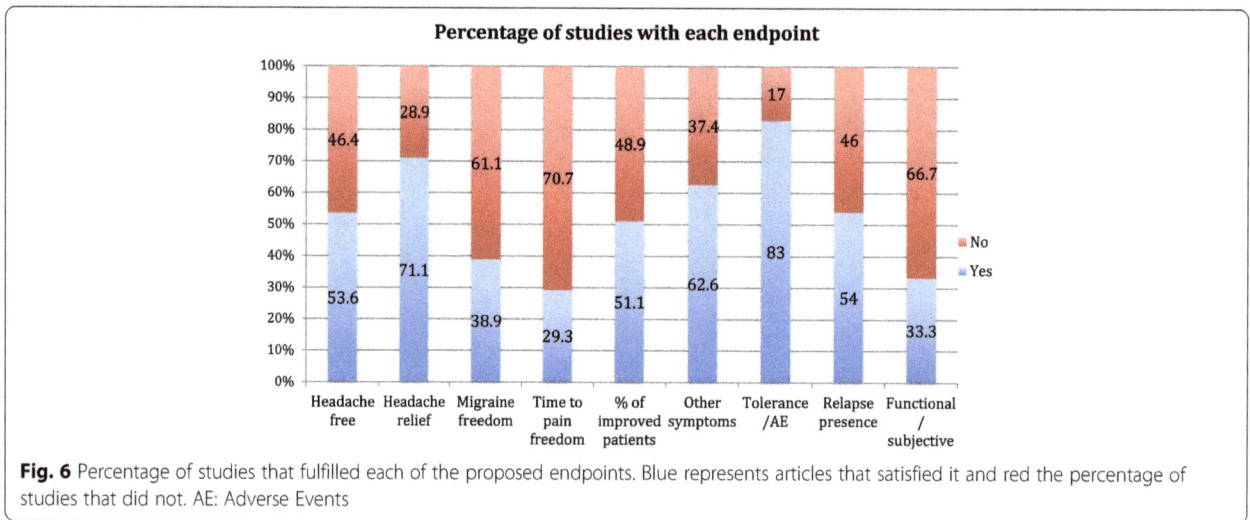

Fig. 6 Percentage of studies that fulfilled each of the proposed endpoints. Blue represents articles that satisfied it and red the percentage of studies that did not. AE: Adverse Events

The number of studies clearly increases with the arrival of the triptans, multiplying the number of publications in a 10-fold in comparison with the pre-triptan era. Sumatriptan is the most studied drug so far, present in 23.2% of all the trials indexed in PubMed. In the post-triptan era we have found a progressive decrease of publication rate of studies, which could be increased in the near future with the arrival of new agents such as lasmiditan [14] and the gepants [15]. We have found also an increasing tendency over time to publish in headache specific journals in comparison with the past, when general medicine journals represented the preferred target for publication.

Concerning the cost, difficulty and bureaucracy that conducting a randomized control trial (RCT) implicates, many drugs that we use in our daily practice have not been properly studied. Nowadays, companies support most of the studies and "orphan"

drugs do not attract great interest. Something similar can be noticed in headaches with a low prevalence, in which the number of existing RCT's is low or even non-existent. In our study, almost 88% of the studies were of migraine. Funding agencies and researchers should be encouraged to evaluate drugs in orphan indications as well.

One of the most surprising findings was the low number of studies evaluating opioids, considering how frequently patients employ them in the real world studies. We only found 8 studies, representing 1,6% of all the studies. This could be partly explained because 5 additional studies were excluded because they took place in the Emergency Department Setting or they implicated administration routes such as intravenous or intramuscular. It is well known that opioid consumption has been associated with chronification of some headaches and that they are considered one of the main causes of overuse of analgesics [16, 17] nevertheless studies evaluating their efficacy in headache relief and safety are surprisingly scarce. Many of them were evaluated in combination with other drugs, the majority employed improvement of headache instead of headache relief and their adherence to IHS guidelines was even lower. As far as this study did not evaluate specifically results of the trials, we cannot defend their use, which concerning their potential risks, should be cautious until better and newer studies take place.

Despite the fact that IHS published 3 editions of the guidelines for studies evaluating symptomatic treatment, most of the studies do not follow them completely. Adherence to the guideline is important not only because it assures the quality of the study but also ensures comparability of data. For example, the time when the main endpoint was evaluated was

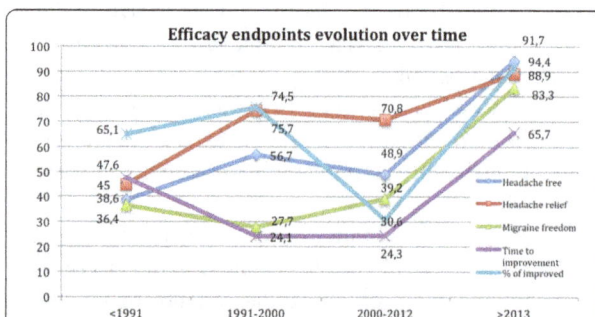

Fig. 7 Percentage of studies addressing the recommended efficacy endpoints per period, dividing X-axis in the periods pre-IHS recommendations and after each version. Y-axis represents the percentage of studies. Considered endpoints are: complete headache resolution, headache relief, complete migraine resolution, time to the improvement, and percentage of improved patients

not 120 min in up to 30% of the studies. We found a hopeful trend, as newer studies are conducted with a closer adherence to guidelines, including a higher number of endpoints and showing an increasing percentage of efficacy endpoints being measured, especially in headache specific journals, which showed statistically significant differences subscribing more IHS guidelines. It may be truth that the burden of headache is a frequent topic in headache journals; nevertheless excellence in trial designs and reports should be mandatory no matter the journal of publication.

Considering the functional limitation and quality of life impairment that most of the headaches implicate, exploring the ability to work or act normally has also been specifically evaluated. As primary headaches do not implicate mortality, the morbidity and indirect cost due to functional impairment is gaining attention, so addressing it specifically may give additional data of the positive effect of a treatment. Only a third of the studies considered this type of endpoints, so their presence still should be increased.

Personal and social burden of headache disorders is significant. Disability and health-related quality of life have been increasingly used to help patient and clinicians make better decisions regarding headache treatment and their presence in research tends to grow. Novel tools are PROMs [18] that focus on patient perspective, therapeutic preference, and satisfaction with treatments. PROMs may be an indirect indicator of efficacy, as patients will not probable feel satisfied with inefficacious or poorly tolerated treatments [19]. Nevertheless, just 10% of the published studies considered these outcomes. IHS guidelines encourage authors to employ them since the year 2000 [5] and they represent one of the strategic objectives for research in the European Community.

In line with our findings, studies fulfilling IHS guidelines reflect better the real efficacy of drugs. They employ more precise endpoints such as disappearance of the headache; they focus on other headache symptoms that can be as debilitating as the headache itself, and they start taking into account other aspects related with patient perspective. In our opinion, IHS guidelines should be the reference in future studies addressing headache specific treatments.

Concerning methodology, even though our study does not analyze specifically data there is an inherent risk of bias. Selection bias is possible if some studies did not have a title or were under Mesh classification. Further, in some cases it was difficult to identify the main variable or the time when it was evaluated. In those cases, we decided to leave that variable empty, which happened in 2.6% of the

studies for the primary endpoint and 18.2% of the studies concerning the temporal evaluation. However, we believe the impact of this to be minimal on the final results.

Conclusion

Headache relief has been the most employed primary endpoint; nevertheless, as IHS guidelines recommend, better efficacy endpoints like headache disappearance start to be preferred. We found a promising increase in the number of secondary endpoints, considering also disability, quality of life and patients' preference, so future studies should subscribe them in order to warrant quality and homogeneity.

Triptans completely changed the panorama in symptomatic drug studies and their arrival improved the way RCTs are conducted in headache, nevertheless studies should subscribe guidelines in order to allow comparability as well.

To date, most of the studies took place in migraine patients but analyzing a small proportion of all the available drugs. In the future, orphan drugs and drugs with insufficient information, such as opioids, should be also evaluated and other prevalent and rare conditions should be studied in a randomized controlled setting.

Appendix I

Command employed in the search.

((((((((((((primary headache*) OR primary headache disorder[MeSH Terms]) OR migraine) OR tension-type) OR trigeminal) OR hemicrania) OR cluster) OR sunct) OR suna) OR ""Short Lasting Unilateral Neuralgiform Headache Attacks"")) AND (((((((((telcagepant) OR ubrogepant) OR Olcegepant) OR gepant*)) OR (((((""Anti-Inflammatory Agents, Non-Steroidal""[Mesh]) OR (((((((((((((((((naproxen*) OR aspirin*) OR salicylic*) OR salicylic) OR ((paracetamol*) OR paracetamol)) OR acetaminophen*) OR ((indomethacin*) OR Indomethacin)) OR ((dexketoprofen) OR dexketoprophen)) OR celecoxib*) OR rofecoxib*) OR diclophenac) OR ketoprofen*) OR ketorolac*) OR ibuprofen*) OR Excedrin) OR Perdolan) OR Dafalgan) OR Lonarid) OR Panadol))) OR (((((((((((domperidone) OR metoclopramide*) OR ((metamizol*) OR metamizol)) OR ((codein*) OR codeine)) OR tramadol*) OR morphin*) OR oxycodon*) OR ergot*) OR ergot) OR triptan*) OR triptan)) OR ((((lasmiditan) OR caffein*) OR magnesium*) OR ((oxygen*) OR oxygen))))) OR ((((((((((Pulsante) OR gammacore) OR Transcranial direct-current stimul*) OR springTMS) OR cefaly) OR transcranial magnetic stimul*) OR vagal nerve stimul*) OR Sphenopalatine Ganglion Stimul*) OR caloric vestibular stimul*) OR Occipital nerve stimul*) OR Transcutaneous Supraorbital Neuro Stimul*)

Appendix II

Table 2 Name of the journal according to each group

	Kind of Journal			Total
	Headache J	Neuro J	General J	
Acta Neurol Scand	0	3	0	3
Adv Ther	0	0	1	1
Am J Emerg Med	0	0	3	3
Am J Med	0	0	1	1
Ann Emerg Med	0	0	3	3
Ann Neurol	0	1	0	1
Arch Intern Med	0	0	2	2
Arch Neurol	0	7	0	7
Arq Neuropsiquiatr	0	1	0	1
BMC Neurol	0	1	0	1
Br J Clin Pharmacol	0	0	1	1
Br J Prev Soc Med	0	0	1	1
Br Med J	0	0	1	1
Br Med J (Clin Res Ed)	0	0	1	1
Brain Res Bull	0	1	0	1
Cephalalgia	112	0	0	112
Clin Drug Investig	0	0	1	1
Clin Neuropharmacol	0	1	0	1
Clin Pharmacol Ther	0	0	2	2
Clin Ther	0	0	16	16
CNS Drugs	0	5	0	5
Curr Med Res Opin	0	0	12	12
Drug Dev Ind Pharm	0	0	1	1
Drug Ther Bull	0	0	1	1
Drugs	0	0	1	1
Eur J Neurol	0	8	0	8
Eur J Pain	0	1	0	1
Eur Neurol	0	19	0	19
Expert Rev. Clin Pharmacol	0	0	1	1
Expert Rev. Neurother	0	1	0	1
Gynecol Endocrinol	0	0	1	1
Headache	156	0	0	156
Heart Dis	0	0	1	1
Int J Clin Pract	0	0	3	3
Int J Neurosci	0	1	0	1
Intern Med	0	0	1	1
J Chin Med Assoc	0	0	1	1
J Clin Pharmacol	0	0	1	1
J Clin Pharmacol J New Drugs	0	0	1	1
J Coll Gen Pract	0	0	1	1
J Emerg Med	0	0	1	1
J Headache Pain	15	0	0	15

A PRISMA-compliant systematic review of the endpoints employed to evaluate symptomatic treatments...

217

Table 2 Name of the journal according to each group *(Continued)*

	Kind of Journal			Total
	Headache J	Neuro J	General J	
J Int Med Res	0	0	6	6
J Intern Med	0	0	2	2
J Neurol	0	1	0	1
J Neurol Neurosurg Psychiatry	0	1	0	1
J Pain	1	0	0	1
J Pharm Pharmacol	0	0	1	1
JAMA	0	0	4	4
Lancet	0	0	6	6
Lancet Neurol	0	3	0	3
Mayo Clin Proc	0	0	3	3
MedGenMed	0	0	3	3
N Engl J Med	0	0	2	2
Neurol Sci	0	9	0	9
Neurology	0	36	0	36
Obstet Gynecol	0	0	4	4
Pain Med	1	0	0	1
Pain Physician	1	0	0	1
Pain Pract	1	0	0	1
Pediatr Neurol	0	1	0	1
Pediatrics	0	0	3	3
Pharmacoeconomics	0	0	5	5
Phytother Res	0	0	1	1
Postgrad Med	0	0	1	1
Postgrad Med J	0	0	1	1
QJM	0	0	1	1
Sci Transl Med	0	0	1	1
Singapore Med J	0	0	1	1
Value Health	0	0	2	2
Total	287	101	107	495

Acknowledgements
This manuscript is a product of the program School of Advanced Science promoted by the European Headache Federation (EHF-SAS).

Funding
The School of Advanced Studies (SAS) of the European Headache Federation supported the publication of this study.

Authors' contributions
All authors participated in the design of the study. LM and IP reviewed the abstracts. DGA, MF, DO, ME, MV reviewed the full papers. DGA and NY created the draft. AN, SB and MB reviewed and corrected the full draft. DGA, NY, LM, IP, MF, DO, ME, MV are Junior Fellows of EHF-SAS. AN, SB and MB are Senior Fellows of EHF-SAS. All authors read and approved the final manuscript.

Competing interests
The authors declare that they have no competing interests.

Author details
[1]Headache Unit Neurology Department, Hospital Clínico Universitario Valladolid, Avda. Ramón y Cajal 3, 47005 Valladolid, Spain. [2]Danish Headache Centre and Department of Neurology, University of Copenhagen, Rigshospitalet Glostrup, Copenhagen, Denmark. [3]Headache Department, Iranian Center of Neurological Research Neuroscience Institute, Tehran University of Medical Sciences, Tehran, Iran. [4]Child Neuropsychiatry School, University of Palermo, Palermo, Italy. [5]U.O. Neuropsychiatry - ARNAS Civico, PO Di Cristina, Palermo, Italy. [6]Neurology Department, University Hospital of Brussels, Brussels, Belgium. [7]Headache Center, Bambino Gesù Children Hospital IRCCS, Rome, Italy. [8]Pavlov First Saint Petersburg State Medical University, Saint Petesburg, Russia. [9]Almazov National Medical Research Centre, Saint Petesburg, Russia. [10]Internal Medicine Department, Sant'Andrea Hospital, Rome, Italy. [11]Regional Referral Headache Centre, Sant'Andrea

Hospital, Department of Clinical and Molecular Medicine, Sapienza University, Rome, Italy. [12]Headache Centre, Careggi University Hospital, University of Florence, Florence, Italy. [13]Danish Headache Center, Department of Neurology, Rigshospitalet-Glostrup, University of Copenhagen, Copenhagen, Denmark. [14]Department of Clinical Physiology and Nuclear Medicine, Center for Functional and Diagnostic Imaging, Hvidovre Hospital, Copenhagen, Denmark.

References

1. Steiner TJ, Stovner LJ, Vos T et al (2018) Migraine is first cause of disability in under 50s: will health politicians now take notice? J Headache Pain 19(1):17
2. Osumili B, McCrone P, Cousins S et al (2018) The economic cost of patients with migraine headache referred to specialist clinics. Headache 58:287–294
3. GBD 2015 Disease and Injury Incidence and Prevalence Collaborators. Global, regional, and national incidence, prevalence, and years lived with disability for 310 diseases and injuries, 1990–2015: a systematic analysis for the Global Burden of Disease Study 2015. Lancet. 2015;388:1545–602
4. Bloudek LM, Stokes M, Buse DC et al (2012) Cost of health care for patients with migraine in five European countries: results from the international burden of migraine study (IBMS). J Headache Pain 13(5):361–378
5. Committee on Clinical Trials in Migraine. Guidelines for Controlled Trials of Drugs in Migraine. First ed Cephalalgia 1991;11(1):1-12
6. Bendtsen L, Bigal M, Cerbo R, Diener H, Holroyd K, Lampl C et al (2009) Guidelines for controlled trials of drugs in tension-type headache: second edition. Cephalalgia 30(1):1–16
7. Tfelt-Hansen P, Pascual J, Ramadan N, Dahlöf C, Damico D, Diener H-C et al (2012) Guidelines for controlled trials of drugs in migraine: third edition. A guide for investigators. Cephalalgia 32(1):6–38
8. Macedo A, Farré M, Baños J-E (2006) A meta-analysis of the placebo response in acute migraine and how this response may be influenced by some of the characteristics of clinical trials. Eur J Clin Pharmacol 62(3):161–172
9. Hougaard A, Tfelt-Hansen P (2010) Are the current IHS guidelines for migraine drug trials being followed? J Headache Pain 11(6):457–468
10. Lipton RB, Hamelsky SW, Dayno JM (2002) What do patients with migraine want from acute migraine treatment? Headache 42(s1):3–9
11. Bigal M, Rapoport A, Aurora S, Sheftell F, Tepper S, Dahlof C (2007) Satisfaction with current migraine therapy: experience from 3 centers in US and Sweden. Headache 47(4):475–479
12. Patrick DL, Martin ML, Bushmell DM, Pesa J (2003) Measuring satisfaction with migraine treatment: expectations, importance, outcomes, and global ratings. Clin Ther 25(11):2920–2935
13. Díez FI, Straube A, Zanchin G (2007) Patient preference in migraine therapy. J Neurol 254(2):242–249
14. Liberati A, Altman DG, Tetzlaff J, Mulrow C, Gotzsche PC, Ioannidis JPA et al (2009) The PRISMA statement for reporting systematic reviews and meta-analyses of studies that evaluate healthcare interventions: explanation and elaboration. BMJ 339:b2700. https://doi.org/10.1136/bmj.b2700
15. Ferrari MD et al (2010) Acute treatment of migraine with the selective 5-HT1F receptor agonist lasmiditan – a randomised proof-of-concept trial. Cephalalgia 30(10):1170–1178
16. Connor KM, Shapiro RE, Diener HC et al (2009) Randomized, controlled trial of telcagepant for the acute treatment of migraine. Neurology 73:970–977
17. Diener HC, Limmroth V (2004) Medication-overuse headache: a worldwide problem. Lancet Neurol 3:475–483
18. Bigal ME, Lipton RB (2009) Excessive opioid use and the development of chronic migraine. Pain 142:179–182
19. Marshall S, Haywood K, Fitzpatrick R (2006) Impact of patient-reported outcome measures on routine practice: a structured review. J Eval Clin Pract 12(5):559–568

21

Validation of a self-reported instrument to assess work-related difficulties in patients with migraine: the HEADWORK questionnaire

Alberto Raggi[1]*[iD], Venusia Covelli[2], Erika Guastafierro[1], Matilde Leonardi[1], Chiara Scaratti[1], Licia Grazzi[3], Marco Bartolini[4], Giovanna Viticchi[4], Sabina Cevoli[5], Giulia Pierangeli[5,6], Gioacchino Tedeschi[7], Antonio Russo[7], Piero Barbanti[8,9], Cinzia Aurilia[8], Carlo Lovati[10], Luca Giani[10], Fabio Frediani[11], Paola Di Fiore[11], Francesco Bono[12], Laura Rapisarda[12] and Domenico D'Amico[3]

Abstract

Background: The degree to which work-related difficulties are recognized in headache research is poor and often carried out with inadequate information such as "reduced ability to work as usual", which do not capture at all the variety of difficulties and the factors that impact over them. The aim of this paper is to present the validation of the HEADWORK questionnaire, which addresses the amount and severity of difficulties in work-related tasks and the factors that impact over them.

Methods: We developed a set of items based on a previous literature review and patients' focus groups and tested it on a wide set of patients with episodic and chronic migraine attending eight different Italian headache centers. HEADWORK factor structure was assessed with exploratory and confirmatory factor analysis; internal consistency and construct validity were addressed as well.

Results: The validation sample ($N = 373$) was mostly composed of patients with episodic migraine without aura (64.3%) and of females (81%). Factor analysis retrieved two different scales: "Work-related difficulties", composed of eleven items which explain 67.1% of the total variance, and "Factors contributing to work difficulties", composed of six items which explain 52.1% of the total variance. Both HEADWORK subscales have good measurement properties, with higher scores being associated to higher disability, lower quality of life, lower productivity, higher headache frequency and pain intensity.

Conclusions: HEADWORK is a 17-item, two-scale questionnaire addressing the impact of migraine on work-related difficulties in terms of difficulties in general or specific skills, and the factors contributing to these difficulties, defined as negative impact on work tasks. It can be used to address disability weights for the purpose of calculating the burden of migraine, and to assess the balance between therapeutic and side effects of medication on productivity.

Keywords: Work, Employment, Disability evaluation, Episodic migraine, Chronic migraine, Medication overuse headache, Validation study

---

* Correspondence: alberto.raggi@istituto-besta.it
[1]Neurology, Public Health and Disability Unit, Fondazione IRCCS Istituto
Neurologico Carlo Besta, Milan, Italy
Full list of author information is available at the end of the article

Background

Episodic Migraine (EM) and Chronic Migraine (CM) have a considerable impact on patients' daily lives in terms of personal suffering, reduced quality of life (QoL) and disability [1–7], with female and CM sufferers reporting higher disability [8]. In particular, CM frequently presents with medication overuse headache (MOH): as shown in some literature findings, an average of 62.6% (ranging from 50.5% to 68%) of patients with CM present MOH [9–12] and whether MOH is a consequence or a cause of CM has not been clarified [13]. Migraine disorders determine a considerable burden on societies, which is usually addressed in terms of reduced work productivity and cost [14–18]. The most recent studies on the cost of headache disorders, and of EM and CM in particular, showed that most of the cost of such conditions is due to indirect cost, i.e. to reduced work productivity [14, 15, 19]. When addressing the issue of indirect cost, two elements have to be acknowledged: the lost workdays (absenteeism) and the workdays in which people with migraine worked with reduced productivity (presenteeism). Presenteeism is the main driver of migraine cost and burden: in fact, for each lost workday, patients with EM and CM work three to four days with reduced productivity [20, 21], and the cost associated to presenteeism is higher than that associated to absenteeism [14, 15, 22]. Therefore, addressing presenteeism in terms of both frequency of days and impaired productivity is of importance to measure the burden of EM and CM.

While absenteeism can be addressed with a simple and direct question, presenteeism may involve difficulties with the interpretation of content. In fact, the degree to which migraine headaches impact over work-related tasks can be highly variable and is underlined by three elements: a) headache severity, b) the kind of activity or the multiplicity of activities, that constitute one's own job profile, and c) the context in which one's own job is carried out. The last two elements may allow the identification of the different tasks and activities as well of contextual elements of the job in terms of interpersonal relationships, and of physical elements that might act as triggers of migraine headaches. A literature review was specifically devoted to understanding the degree to which work-related difficulties are recognized and considered in headache research [23]. In brief, this review was grounded on a previous work in which the International Classification of Functioning, Disability and Health (ICF) [24] was used as a term of reference to describe a set of difficulties that are relevant to migraineurs. Fourteen topics, that could be referred to difficulties with work-related activities, were transformed into MESH terms and were used to search for relevant publications in which these difficulties were experienced by patients with EM, CM, chronic

daily headache or MOH. A total of 23 publications were selected and the results showed that there was poor recognition of the topic of work-related difficulties, which was limited to a restricted set of activities such as problem solving, speaking, driving and on "remunerative employment". The latter topic was generally expressed in terms of reduced ability to "perform job activities" or of reduced ability to "work as usual", and the meaning of these definitions was less than clear in available literature. The presence of contextual elements was a completely neglected issue.

The main reason for the paucity of information on this topic is, in our opinion, the lack of patient-reported outcome measures (PROMs) specifically aimed to capture the presence, the severity and the type of work-related difficulties in patients with EM and CM. We therefore launched an initiative to develop a new questionnaire, the HEADWORK Questionnaire. Given the paucity of literature data, we ran a qualitative study with the aim of exploring which were the most relevant difficulties experienced by patients with their work activities and which were the factors that contributed most to these difficulties, getting indications directly from employed patients with EM and CM. In this qualitative study we ran three focus groups with 14 patients, that were asked to discuss the main issues that constitute difficulties with work-related activities and factors that contributed to these activities [25]. The results of this qualitative study showed that 27 were the most relevant themes reported by patients, and that they referred to: activities (e.g. reading, writing, speaking), personal factors (e.g. attention, stress), correlated symptoms (e.g. pain, being numb), and contextual elements (e.g. office, colleagues, noise, light). The joint results of the literature review, and of this qualitative analysis enabled us to define a set of relevant themes which referred to 13 activities and 12 factors impacting on these difficulties that were used to develop the preliminary version of the HEADWORK Questionnaire. The aim of this paper is to validate this new questionnaire and report its measurement properties.

Methods

Participants

Adult patients, i.e. 18 or older, were enrolled for the validation study between June 2016 and October 2017 among those attending eight different Italian headache centers. The main inclusion criterion was the clinical diagnosis of one of the different migraine form according to the International Classification of Headache Disorders, 3-beta version (ICHD-3Beta) [26], namely EM without and with aura (i.e. codes 1.1 or 1.2 of the ICHD-3Beta), and CM, with or without associated MOH (i.e. code 1.3 with or without associated code 8.2 of the ICHD-3Beta). When available, headache diaries were also used for diagnostic purposes. The other inclusion criterion was the fact of being currently employed (or on sick leave) as main occupation and being paid for the activity at the time of enrolment, i.e. no students, retired people or people working on a voluntary basis were included. Both outpatients and inpatients were enrolled. Exclusion criteria, evaluated by the treating neurologist (LG and DD at Fondazione Istituto Neurologico C. Besta IRCCS; MB and GV at Università Politecnica delle Marche; SC and GP at IRCCS Istituto delle Scienze Neurologiche di Bologna; GT and AR at University of Campania "Luigi Vanvitelli"; PB and CA at IRCCS San Raffaele Pisana; CL and LG at Ospedale L. Sacco, University of Milan; FF and PDF at San Carlo Borromeo Hospital; FB and LR at Magna Graecia University of Catanzaro) on the basis of patient evaluation and accurate history taking, were the following: a) presence of cognitive impairments hampering protocol completion (e.g. severe attention deficits); b) anamnesis of cerebrovascular diseases or brain tumors; c) psychiatric disorders of psychotic area; d) other clinical comorbidities in which pain might be of similar or higher impact on daily activities as compared to migraine (e.g. rheumatic diseases, low back pain and other musculoskeletal chronic conditions).

Participation to the study was on a voluntary basis and all patients were asked to provide written consent before inclusion. The study was approved by the Ethical Committees of the coordinating center, Neurological Institute C. Besta (protocol approval number 07/2016, January 13, 2016) and subsequently ratified by all participating centers (Università Politecnica delle Marche, Ancona; IRCCS Istituto delle Scienze Neurologiche di Bologna, Bologna; University of Campania "Luigi Vanvitelli", Naples; IRCCS San Raffaele Pisana, Rome; Luigi Sacco Hospital-University of Milan, Milan; San Carlo Borromeo Hospital, Milan; Magna Graecia University of Catanzaro, Catanzaro).

Protocol

The protocol included the collection of socio-demographic data, and the administration of self-reported tools: the preliminary 25-item version of the HEADWORK questionnaire, the Migraine Disability Assessment schedule (MIDAS) [27, 28], the World Health Organization 12-items Disability Assessment Schedule (WHODAS-12) [29], and the Migraine Specific Quality of Life Questionnaire (MSQ) [30]. The MIDAS was chosen as it is the most commonly used outcome measure in headache research and it provides useful information on days with headache and average pain severity; the WHODAS-12 was chosen in reason of the approach to conceptualization of difficulties due to health reason (see also below) as limitations due to a health condition. Finally, since we were interested in ascertaining that HEADWORK's content was closer to a disability than to a QoL measure, we decided to rely on the MSQ as it migraine-specific and it is valid for use both EM and CM [21–23].

In the socio-demographic section, besides common information on gender, age, marital status and education, a set of employment-related items were included. Specifically, patients were asked on the overall duration of their career and duration of their career in the current company (in case of self-employed, we asked how long they have been were self-employed), on the amount of weekly worked hours, on the dimension of the company (1–9, 10–49, 50–249 or 250+ employed people), and on their current job classification according to the following definitions: apprentice/consultant, office/manual worker, executive/manager, private practice, other. Finally, patients were asked to provide – with reference to the last 30 days – the number of days they did not work due to migraine, the number of days they worked with reduced ability due to headache, and they were invited to give an estimate of their overall work performance, expressed as percentage on a 1–99% scale (of course referred to the days with reduced ability).

The items tested in this version of the HEADWORK questionnaire, defined on the basis of the results of the previous literature review and patients' input [23, 25] were revised by a small panel of 12 patients (with both EM and CM) and 8 clinicians that were asked to judge the items and report any problematic issues, namely difficulties in understanding the content of each item. Specifically, patients were asked to judge if in their opinion it was possible to misunderstand what was written, and not if they experienced the phenomenon described in the different items. None of the items was judged as unclear and minor changes were made, in particular: "Solving organizational problems at work" was rephrased from the original "Solving work problems" to focus not on generic outcomes in term of productivity or result of the job done, but on "procedural" issues, i.e. the way in which daily problems with the organization of what has to be done are handled; "Starting a new work task" was rephrased from the original "Starting to work", as the first version was felt as too much generic and could be taken in a too much broad sense (e.g. starting a work career).

Once items were finalized, they were grouped into two section. The first section included 13 items addressing different work tasks and work-related activities. Patients were asked to report how much of a difficulty they had with each activity using a five-point response scale, ranging between 1 (no difficulty) and 5 (I cannot do it). Examples of these items include talking and interacting with other people, reading and writing abilities. The second section included 12 items addressing the factors that possibly limit patients' ability with work-related activities and prevented them to perform these activities. Patients were invited to answer on a five-point scale (ranging between 1-no limitations, and 5-complete limitation): examples of these items include negative attitudes of colleagues and environmental triggers, such as noise or smell. For both the section, items had to be answered thinking back to the last 30 days and. The option "not applicable" was left in case an activity or a factor was not of relevance for respondents' jobs or was not part of the workplace features. There are different reasons for choosing a 5-point scale. First, odd number of items' response enable to use the central value for those cases in which patients feel a non-mild impact but do not wish to move closer to the maximum value: as we did not use an "agree vs. not agree" scale, we did not carry the risk of leaving a central option meaning "not taking position". Second, we preferred the 5-item options as it is easier to fill in compared to the 7-item one. In fact, in the 7-item option there are two steps between the lowest (or highest) value and the central one, which are difficult to label. Third, we intended to ground our measure on the definition of disability endorsed by the ICF [24] and operationalized with the WHODAS i.e. limitation in carrying out daily activities due to the presence of a health condition. The content of HEADWORK is close to such a definition, as the activities that are limited by migraine headaches are work-related ones.

The MIDAS [27, 28] is composed of seven questions referred to the preceding three months. The first two questions investigate the impact of headache on work, in terms of missed workdays and of work with at least half reduction, the third and fourth apply the same scheme to household work, and the fifth addresses missed leisure/family/social activities due to headache. Responses are given in terms of days with missed or reduced activities. The sixth question is on the number of days with headache and the seventh is on average pain intensity. MIDAS is scored based on the first five question by simply summing up the days: four severity grades are available, i.e. minimal (0–5), mild (6–10), moderate (11–20), and severe (≥21) disability.

The WHODAS-12 is the short version of the original 36-items WHODAS 2.0. It investigates the same domains as the original version (i.e. understanding and communicating, getting around, self-care, getting along with people, life activities, and participation in society), and accounts for 81% of the variation of the original full questionnaire. Patients are asked to respond to 12 questions referred to daily activities, and they report how much of a difficulty they experienced during the previous 30 days, due to their health condition. Answers have to be rated on a 5-point scale (no problems – complete problems/cannot do the activity), and WHODAS-12 score ranges between 0 and 100, with higher scores reflecting greater disability [29].

The MSQ is a migraine-specific measure of health-related QoL [30]. The questionnaire is composed of 14 items that form three scales, namely role-restriction (RR),

role-prevention (RP) and emotional function (EF): each scale has a 0–100 score, with lower scores indicating lower health-related QoL. Items refer to different daily activities or social situations, and patients have to rate how frequently migraine determined an impact on these activities, thinking back to the previous four weeks, using a 6-point scale from never to always. The MSQ has mostly been used with patients with EM, but it has also been validated in those with CM [31, 32].

Data analyses
Continuous variables were reported as means and standard deviations (SD), categorical variables as frequencies and percentages. Data were analyzed with SPSS 19.0.

Factor structure and item reduction
The approach to the definition of the HEADWORK questionnaire's factor structure involved an exploratory factor analysis (EFA) on 70% of the sample, followed by a confirmatory factor analysis (CFA) on the remaining 30% and, later on, on the whole sample.

Prior to carrying out the EFA, we transformed the "not applicable" items into missing and evaluated symmetry indexes: items that were clearly asymmetric (i.e. with symmetry index ≥2.58) were eliminated from the dataset. We also looked at the inter-correlation between items, separately within the two sections of HEADWORK, and removed those items with an overall inter-item correlation index below .300. We also removed those items that showed correlation indexes >.800 with at least two other items in each of the two sections of HEADWORK (i.e. more than 10% of the total number of items), to avoid, or at least limit, the risk of multicollinearity or singularity problems [33]. Suitability of data for factor analysis was assessed with Bartlett's test of sphericity (BTS), adequate if $P < .05$ [33], and with Kaiser-Meyer-Olkin Measure of Sampling Adequacy (KMO), adequate if > 0.70 [33, 34]. EFA was carried out using principal component extraction and direct Oblimin rotation to extract data, as we reasonably expected that, should EFA define more than one factor, they might have been significantly correlated each other.

Three steps to item reduction were followed. First, we deleted items that did not load into any factor (i.e. with factor loadings <.400) as they gave no contribution to questionnaire's structure. Second, items loading into more than one factor (i.e. with factor loadings >.40) were deleted as they would determine high instability to the factor structure of the questionnaire. Third, we looked at scale reliability information, namely inter-item correlation, item-total correlation and Cronbach's Alpha: we deleted items that were either too much correlated (i.e. coefficient > .800) with at least two other items, or that

Validation of a self-reported instrument to assess work-related difficulties in patients...

223

showed a low item-total correlation (i.e. coefficient < .300), or that would make Alpha increase if deleted.

The ratio between Chi^2 and degrees of freedom (Chi^2/d.f.) and the Root Mean Square Error of Approximation (RMSEA) were used as model fit indices for CFA: Chi^2/d.f. < 3 and RMSEA < 0.08 were considered acceptable [34].

Internal consistency

Internal consistency was assessed using Cronbach's Alpha coefficient, item-total correlation after correcting for overlap (i.e. removing the item from the total score), and the average inter-item correlation. Scales were considered to have a good reliability if Cronbach's alpha was >.70 [35], if item-total correlation indexes were > 0.40, and if average inter-item correlations were comprised between 0.30 and 0.70 [36].

Construct validity

Construct validity was tested in different ways. First, by correlating the two HEADWORK scales with WHODAS-12, MSQ, and MIDAS sores, headache frequency, and average pain severity in the previous three months, the amount of lost workdays and of workdays in which productivity was impaired, and with the estimated average productivity in days worked with reduced productivity. We used Pearson's correlation, and expected that HEADWORK scales: a) were directly correlated with all the other variables (with the exclusion of MSQ scores, and with the estimated average productivity, where an inverse correlation is expected), and with correlation coefficients < .700; b) had a stronger correlation with the WHODAS-12 than with the MSQ scores, as the construct underlining HEADWORK is the amount and severity of difficulties with work-related activities; c) had a stronger correlation with the average pain severity and the average work ability than with the variables related to frequency of headache, workdays lost and days worked with reduced productivity. Significance was set with alpha = 0.0023 after Bonferroni correction and two-tailed testing.

The second approach to the evaluation of construct validity, was made by testing the differences in HEADWORK scales between males and females, between patients with EM and CM, between patients working more than 40 h/week and those working less, and between patients employed in medium/large companies and those employed in small ones. We used Student's t-test and expected that females, patients with CM, those working more than 40 h/week and those employed in larger companies might experience higher difficulties. Significance was set with alpha = 0.0125 after Bonferroni correction and two-tailed testing. We also tested HEADWORK scales across patients with different degrees of education, and across patients with different types of contract using One-Way ANOVA and Bonferroni post-hoc test. We expected that those with lower education and those with

higher-level positions (i.e. employers, private practitioners or people with executive roles vs. those with temporary jobs and office/manual workers) might experience higher difficulties.

For cross-sectional comparisons, Hedges' g was used as a measure of effect size (ES): ES around or higher than 0.5 indicate a medium effect; ES around of higher than 0.8 indicate a large effect. Data were expressed as means and 95% Confidence Intervals (95% C.I.).

Results

Sample description

A total of 377 patients were enrolled in the study. However, four records showed important incompleteness of HEADWORK questionnaire, and further eleven did not have complete MIDAS, WHODAS-12 or MSQ. Therefore, 373 questionnaires were used to address the factor structure of HEADWORK, and 362 to address measurement properties. Table 1 reports the main socio-demographic information of the validation sample ($N = 373$). Most of enrolled patients (280) had EM, and most of them (240) had EM without aura. The remaining 93 patients had CM, and most of them (71) had comorbidity to MOH. None of the EM patients had MOH. On average, it was a highly educated sample, as 41.8% completed university studies and mostly composed of females (81%). On average, in the previous month patients with EM lost one day of work and worked 5–7 days with migraine (approximately with 55–60% of their ability), while those with CM lost 3–4 days and worked 14–17 days with migraine (approximately with 50% of their ability). MIDAS scores, days with headache and WHODAS-12 scores were higher among those with CM than in those with EM, indicating higher a disability level, while MSQ scores were lower, indicating a lower quality of life.

Factor analysis

Additional file 1: Tables S1-S4 report the results of items' distribution with regard to the amount of not applicable ones and, after transformation into missing, of inter-item correlation and asymmetry, as well as the full inter-item correlation matrix. Among those of the first section of the preliminary version of HEADWORK, two items were excluded from the EFA: Managing work stress, due to high asymmetry; Reaching the workplace due to high correlation (>.800) with two other items (Moving from one place to another; Driving a car). From the second section, five items were deleted as they showed high asymmetry: Having to work on shifts rotation; Side effect of symptomatic drugs; Side effect of prophylactic drugs; Feeling dazed/numb; Work stress.

The EFA carried out on 70% of the sample showed that, for both the first and the second section of the HEADWORK Questionnaire, a single factor was found: with regard to the first section, it explained 68.1% of the

Table 1 Sociodemographic characteristics of the HEADWORK validation sample

	EM (N = 280)	CM (N = 93)	All patients (N = 373)
Female gender	224 (80%)	78 (83.9%)	302 (81%)
Age	42.1 ± 10.0	44.0 ± 9.2	42.6 ± 9.8
Education level			
Up to secondary	39 (13.9%)	18 (19.4%)	57 (15.3%)
High	109 (52.4%)	51 (54.8%)	160 (42.9%)
University degree or higher	132 (47.1%)	24 (25.8%)	156 (41.8%)
Company size			
Small (1–49 employed)	108 (38.7%)	35 (37.6%)	143 (38.3%)
Medium-Large (50+ employed)	171 (61.1%)	58 (62.4%)	229 (61.7%)
Type of contract			
Stage/Other temporary	16 (5.7%)	3 (3.2%)	19 (5.7%)
Office/Manual worker	186 (66.4%)	63 (67.7%)	249 (74.3)
Executive/Manager	9 (3.2%)	5 (5.4%)	14 (4.2%)
Private Practice/Employer	37 (13.2%)	16 (17.2%)	53 (15.8%)
Duration of career	19.1 ± 10.5	21.3 ± 10.9	19.7 ± 10.6
Career in the present company	13.2 ± 9.8	14.1 ± 9.8	13.5 ± 9.8
Weekly worked hours	39.3 ± 10.8	36.9 ± 9.9	38.9 ± 10.6
Workdays lost in the previous month	1.0 ± 2.0	3.8 ± 6.0	1.7 ± 3.6
Days worked with headache in the previous month	6.5 ± 5.7	16.8 ± 7.8	8.8 ± 7.6
Average productivity (%)	56.4 ± 23.0	51.6 ± 21.0	55.1 ± 22.7
MIDAS score	27.5 ± 23.8	101.3 ± 60.3	41.8 ± 45.3
Days with headache/3 months	18.9 ± 11.3	61.7 ± 15.6	27.7 ± 21.2
Average pain intensity	7.2 ± 1.7	7.8 ± 1.6	7.3 ± 1.7
WHODAS-12	24.6 ± 17.0	41.2 ± 19.6	28.0 ± 18.7
MSQ-RR	51.6 ± 20.3	30.2 ± 18.9	47.2 ± 21.8
MSQ-RP	65.3 ± 22.0	43.2 ± 22.3	60.8 ± 23.7
MSQ-EF	62.9 ± 27.8	34.4 ± 27.7	57.1 ± 30.0

Notes. EM episodic migraine, *CM* chronic migraine, *MOH* medication overuse headache, *MIDAS* migraine disability assessment, *WHODAS-12* 12-items WHO disability assessment, *MSQ* migraine specific quality of life questionnaire, *RR* role restriction, *RP* role prevention, *EF* emotional function

variance of the questionnaire, while for the second section it explained 49.9%. The CFA, carried out on the remaining 30% of the sample confirmed the factor structure for the first section of HEADWORK, with a similar amount of explained variance (64.7%) and adequate fit indices. With regard to the second section, the scale had an average inter-item correlation that was not satisfactory (.379) and one of the item that was previously included (Need to take an excessive amount of symptomatic drugs) was critical. It showed inadequate factor loading (.353) and its elimination made Cronbach's Alpha to increase. It was therefore deleted, and

the new CFA showed better fit indices, including a higher average inter-item correlation (.423) and explained a higher proportion of variance (53% instead of 47.8%). Additional file 1: Tables S5-S9 show the full factor structure and the reliability analysis for both sections, separately for EFA and CFA.

Table 2 reports the results of the factor analysis carried out over the whole sample. Both sections were composed of one factor, which accounted for 67.1%, and 52.1% of variance, respectively, with good internal consistency and fit indices. Thus, the first HEADWORK scale, which we named "Work-related difficulties", is composed of eleven items with a theoretical range 11–55: actually, it ranged between 11 and 53 and its mean was 31.4 (SD 9.0). The second HEADWORK scale, which we named "Factors contributing to work difficulties", is composed of six items with a theoretical range 6–30: actually, it ranged between 6 and 29 and its mean was 15.8 (SD 5.0).

Construct validity

Table 3 reports the results of correlations between HEADWORK scales and WHODAS-12, MSQ, MIDAS scores, headache frequency and average pain severity in the previous three months, the amount of lost workdays in the previous month, the amount of workdays in which productivity was impaired and the estimated average productivity in those days. All correlations were significant, with the exception of the first HEADWORK scale (Work-related difficulties), and the number of days with reduced productivity, and all correlations were in the expected direction. As expected, HEADWORK scales were more strongly correlated with the WHODAS-12 than with MIDAS and MSQ scores and also with the average pain severity and the average work ability rather than with frequency of headache, workdays lost and days worked with reduced productivity.

Table 4 reports the results of Student's *t*-test in assessing the differences in HEADWORK scales between males and females, between patients with EM and CM, between patients working more than 40 h/week and those working less, and between patients employed in medium/large companies and those employed in small ones. Consistently with our expectations, females and patients with CM showed higher scores at both HEADWORK scales, than males and EM patients, with medium to large ES. Contrary to our expectations, people working less than 40 h per week showed higher scores than those working less only at HEADWORK "Factors contributing to work difficulties" scale, with a small ES, while no differences were found for the subscale "Work-related difficulties". With regard to company size, the results were in line with our expectation, but no significant differences were detected. Finally, the

Validation of a self-reported instrument to assess work-related difficulties in patients...

225

Table 2 Factor analysis and reliability data of HEADWORK questionnaire (N = 373)

	Loadings	Item Mean ± SD	Item-Total Correlation	Alpha if item excluded
Section A: Work-related difficulties KMO= .938; BTS, P<.001; Eigenvalue: 7.377 (67.1% of variance) Alpha= .950; Inter-item R= .636; Average Item-total R= .775 Chi^2= 131.2; d.f.= 44; Chi2/d.f.= 2.98; RMSEA=0.047				
Paying attention to work tasks	.883	2.94 ± 0.97	.851	.942
Solving organizational problems at work	.876	2.96 ± 1.04	.832	.943
Starting a new work task	.865	2.87 ± 1.03	.818	.943
Dealing with work problems	.851	2.95 ± 0.96	.830	.943
Reading and writing	.822	2.90 ± 1.05	.784	.945
Using the PC	.795	3.13 ± 0.98	.753	.946
Answering the phone	.765	2.67 ± 1.01	.754	.946
Driving a car	.762	2.81 ± 1.13	.745	.946
Moving from one place to another	.760	2.75 ± 1.07	.741	.946
Talking and interacting with other people	.756	2.86 ± 0.88	.743	.946
Understanding what is said	.684	2.46 ± 0.99	.677	.949
Section B: Factors contributing to work difficulties KMO = .830; BTS, P < .001; Eigenvalue: 3.127 (52.1% of variance) Alpha = .808; Inter-item R = .412; Average Item-total R = .570 Chi^2 = 20.1; d.f. = 9; Chi^2/d.f. = 2.23; RMSEA = 0.050				
Noise in the workplace	.840	2.94 ± 1.06	.715	.744
Smell in the workplace	.767	2.58 ± 1.20	.627	.762
Brightness of workplace	.765	2.75 ± 1.07	.676	.752
Extended working hours	.652	2.72 ± 1.10	.579	.774
Negative attitudes of colleagues	.428	2.17 ± 1.04	.424	.806
Air conditioning	.419	2.19 ± 1.15	.400	.809

Notes. KMO Kaiser-Meyer-Olkin Measure of Sampling Adequacy, *BTS* Bartlett's Test of Sphericity, *d.f.* degrees of freedom, *RMSEA* Root Mean Square Error of Approximation, *SD* standard deviation

Table 3 Correlation analysis between HEADWORK scales, patient-reported outcomes, headache frequency, pain intensity and productivity indexes (N = 362)

	Work-related difficulties	Factors contributing to work difficulties
WHODAS-12	.607*	.565*
MSQ-RR	−.593*	−.537*
MSQ-RP	−.586*	−.522*
MSQ-EF	−.496*	−.465*
MIDAS	.443*	.394*
Headache Frequency/ 3 months	.247*	.296*
Average pain severity	.367*	.301*
N. of lost workdays	.256*	.206*
N. of days worked with hampered productivity	.123	.220*
Average productivity	−.522*	−.342*

*Notes. *P < .0023. WHODAS-12* 12-items WHO disability assessment, *MSQ* migraine specific quality of life questionnaire, *RR* role restriction, *RP* role prevention, *EF* emotional function, *MIDAS* migraine disability assessment

results of One-Way ANOVA testing HEADWORK scales across patients with different degrees of education, and across patients with different types of contract showed no significant differences, also in this case contrary to our expectation.

Discussion

With this paper we present the validation of the HEADWORK questionnaire, a 17-item PROM specifically designed to assess the impact of EM and CM on work-related tasks and the factors that may contribute to such difficulties. Our results showed that the different dimensions regarding the negative influence of migraine on work activities, i.e. the amount and severity of difficulties in work-related tasks and the factors that impact over them, can be measured by two distinct scales. The first scale, named "Work-related difficulties", is composed of eleven item dealing with the degree to which migraine headaches determine a difficulty in general skills, such as solving organizational problems or starting a new work task, or in specific tasks, e.g. using the computer or talking and interacting with other people. The

Table 4 Independent sample t-test assessing differences in HEADWORK scales based on gender, migraine type, amount of weekly worked hours and company size

Variable			Mean (95% CI)	t-test (*P*-value)	ES
Gender	Work-related difficulties	Males (*N* = 71)	27.1 (25.2–29.1)	4.41 (<.001)	0.59
		Females (*N* = 302)	32.3 (31.3–33.4)		
	Factors contributing to work difficulties	Males (*N* = 71)	12.8 (11.7–13.9)	5.66 (<.001)	0.77
		Females (*N* = 302)	16.5 (15.9–17.0)		
Migraine type	Work-related difficulties	EM (*N* = 280)	30.5 (29.5–31.6)	3.43 (.001)	0.45
		CM (*N* = 93)	34.5 (32.5–36.5)		
	Factors contributing to work difficulties	EM (*N* = 280)	15.2 (14.6–15.8)	4.57 (<.001)	0.59
		CM (*N* = 93)	18.1 (17.1–19.0)		
Amount of weekly worked hours	Work-related difficulties	Up to 40 h/week (*N* = 247)	31.7 (30.6–32.9)	1.20 (.23)	0.13
		> 40 h/week (*N* = 115)	30.5 (28.8–32.2)		
	Factors contributing to work difficulties	Up to 40 h/week (*N* = 247)	16.2 (15.6–16.9)	2.61 (.009)	0.28
		> 40 h/week (*N* = 115)	14.8 (13.9–15.7)		
Company size	Work-related difficulties	Up to 49 employees (*N* = 143)	30.1 (28.6–31.6)	2.01 (.045)	0.22
		50+ employees (*N* = 229)	32.1 (30.9–33.3)		
	Factors contributing to work difficulties	Up to 49 employees (*N* = 143)	15.1 (14.3–16.0)	1.78 (.075)	0.20
		50+ employees (*N* = 229)	16.1 (15.4–16.8)		

Notes. 95% CI 95% Confidence Interval, *EM* episodic migraine, *CM* chronic migraine. Significance set with alpha = 0.0023 after Bonferroni correction

second scale, named "Factors contributing to work difficulties" is composed by six item, and addresses the degree to which some factors, such as noise of brightness of workplace, or the attitudes of colleagues, negatively impact on difficulties with work-related tasks. Thus, with the validation process, we reduced the amount of items from the initial number of 25 to the final number of 17, and both HEADWORK subscales showed good measurement properties, with higher scores being associated to higher impact levels.

The assessment of migraine-related impact on work-place activities is a relevant research and healthcare topic because migraine is recognized as one of the most burdensome diseases [37–42]. Of notice, the studies published on the Global Burden of Disease (GBD) confirmed that migraine is more prevalent among females and in both sexes in the most productive age, and acknowledged migraine as the seventh position in the rank of top causes of Years Lived with a Disability (YLDs) in 2010, and then to the sixth in 2013, and eventually to the second in 2016 [37–39]. Such an increased in GBD ranking is likely due to the fact that MOH was kept distinct from migraine in the first GBD reports, while in the newly published GBD study, the burden of MOH was partly assigned to migraine and partly to tension-type headache, with the result that migraine ascended to the second rank in the causes of YLD, being responsible for 5.6% of all YLDs [41]. The reasons for such a change are shareable, as MOH is a complication of a pre-existing headache disorder and it does not occur

otherwise [42, 43]. Thus we think that it is correct to assume that there is continuity in terms of disease burden between EM and CM with MOH, the impact over work-related tasks being the main domain for negative impact [44, 45]. Our results are in line with such a hypothesis: HEADWORK scores were higher in CM patients for both scales, as compared to their episodic counterpart (with medium to large ES): these findings can be explained by different aspects characterizing CM patients, i.e. higher headache frequency, more severe pain intensity, but mainly the presence of MOH, which in fact was present in most patients of this group. MOH is present in more than 60% of CM patients, as shown by previous literature findings [9–12] and is presumed to be a concause of CM development [13], but is a distinct feature as not all CM patients present with MOH. Mixing primary and secondary headaches may be problematic but, in our opinion, the problem is mostly taxonomic, as HEADWORK is intended to capture work-related difficulties due to the presence of EM and CM, irrespectively from the presence of MOH. It has also to be noted that the single item of the preliminary version of our questionnaire addressing MOH (i.e. Need to take an excessive amount of symptomatic drugs) was not retained in the final version: so, we believe that HEADWORK can be used by both the two subgroups of CM patients, with and without MOH.

HEADWORK is intended to fill in the existing gap on the measurement and better understanding of reduced productivity, a task that presents relevant challenges. As far as we know, three are the main available instrument for this task: the Migraine Work and Productivity Loss Questionnaire (MWPLQ) [46, 47], the MIDAS, and the Work Productivity and Activity Impairment (WPAI) [48]. The MWPLQ is the only migraine-specific tool to assess difficulties in the workplace [46, 47]. It is aimed at measuring the impact of migraine headache on work, in terms of hours of work lost or of hours worked with migraine symptoms, which also includes a set of questions assessing the different activities and influencing factors. These items included difficulty in getting to work, working in proximity to environmental triggers of migraine symptoms, difficulty in handling physical aspects of jobs, visual tasks, mental aspects, and interpersonal issues at work. A grading of limitations in each investigated activity is required, on a 6-point scale, from "no difficulty" to "so much difficulty couldn't do at all". This questionnaire was developed to assess the positive impact of acute medications: all questions are focused on in the most recent headache attack, and some of them specifically ask the number of hours missed before and after the medication was taken. The MIDAS includes two questions on the number of days with total or partial impairment in work activities experienced in the previous three months. The question on days with 50% or more impairment in work activities does not allow to capture the whole range of possible productivity reduction which may be lower than 50% [14, 15, 49]. Addressing the full range of limitation is more relevant than missed workdays in migraine patients, as it is the main driver of migraine cost and burden [14, 15, 20–22, 45]. Furthermore, the value of MIDAS seems problematic in those patients with high frequency migraine and CM, because patients are likely to approximate responses to MIDAS questions by multipliers of 5 or 10 [21]. Finally, the WPAI is a generic instrument addressing the negative impact of different diseases on work productivity [48]. Questions of the WPAI investigate the number of lost working hours and of hours worked with partial productivity limitations (as assessed on a 10 point scale) in the past seven days, and includes two questions inquiring how much did the underlining health condition affected productivity while working – as well as it affected other regular daily activities – on a 10-point scale (from "no effect" to "completely prevented from working"). A migraine-specific version of this tool can be found on the developer's website [50] and its use has been suggested by recent guidelines for randomized trials in CM [51].

In synthesis, the different available PROMS that can be used in migraine patients are not comparable to HEADWORK, as none of them systematically enable to address a set of activities that are relevant to carrying out work-related tasks. The MWPLQ includes some "qualitative" information on the different types of activities and

on influencing factors in the work-place, and both the MWPLQ and the WPAI include questions on the degree of impairment while continuing to perform work activities with migraine. However, the MWPLQ has the specific aim to assess difficulties in relation to the use of an acute medication: therefore, the main focus is the amount of time with difficulties in productivity before and after the intake of medication during a single migraine attack. Despite the WPAI was recently used to address the role of nausea and vomiting in determining the economic burden of migraines [52] and in a RCT on the anti-CGRP antibody fremanezumab in CM (data reported at the 2017 International Headache Congress [53]), it has never been formally validated for migraine patients to date. Finally, the time-frame of reference of these questionnaires may be too long (such as the three-month period for MIDAS which may determine reporting bias, particularly in CM patients [21]) or too short (such as the most recent headache episode for MWPLQ, and the previous seven days for WPAI) in order to assess clinically meaningful data for epidemiological and outcome research. On the contrary, the HEADWORK questionnaire is likely to give an appropriate insight on the different dimensions of work-place difficulties in subjects with migraine in a clinical relevant period of time (one month). It addresses not only the degree of work-related limitations, but also the impact on specific work tasks, and the evaluation of whole range of possible degree of impairment (by a scale from "no difficulty" to "I cannot do it"), thus offering an evaluation of the reduced work productivity while experiencing a migraine episode, which is the most relevant driver of the total costs of migraine [14, 15, 19]. In reason of these features, we recommend it is used as a measure of migraine impact over work activities, to produce work-related disability weights in studies evaluating the burden of EM and CM, and as a secondary outcome measure in clinical research.

Some of the results we found were expectable and represent a confirmation of the content of HEADWORK items. Among these, our study confirmed that women and CM patients showed a higher difficulties in work activities and reported more factors contributing to these difficulties than men and episodic migraine patients. In addition to this, the fact that HEADWORK questionnaire showed higher correlation indexes with the WHODAS-12 than with the MSQ and with the MIDAS, was expected in consideration of the similarity in the formulation of item and questionnaire construct.

Other results shed light on the value and novelty of HEADWORK as a measure of impact on work-related activities under different aspects. First, the fact that headaches frequency showed higher correlation with the scale "Factors contributing to work difficulties" than with the scale "Work-related difficulties". Second, the fact that headache intensity showed higher correlations than headache frequency with HEADWORK scales. This is somehow novel, as one could expect that the presence of an higher number of headaches is a factor associated to the presence of more difficulties, while pain intensity is generally considered as a secondary outcome. Third, the fact that both HEADWORK scales showed little correlation with the number of lost workdays and with the number of days worked with reduced productivity. This aspect constitutes a step forward in the understanding of migraine impact, because previously used parameters, such as absenteeism and presenteeism, may provide only an indirect information on the extent of work-related difficulties: what cannot be inferred with such indirect procedures is the extent of reported limitations with reference to the specificity of the task constituting one's own work duty. HEADWORK fills in this gap, and the little correlation with commonly used indicators, such as the number of lost workdays and the number of days worked with reduced productivity, is a proof of the fact that the content of HEADWORK is not transposable with them. The strong correlation between the HEADWORK scales and the self-reported productivity in the days worked with reduced ability is a further confirmation of the unique information produced by HEADWORK questionnaire. In our opinion, all of these aspects show the ability of HEADWORK to disentangle the problems due to migraine as a disease – which is accompanied by an ensemble of socio-cultural representation, such as the need to use drugs to function, and stigma (which is particularly affected by the ability to work [54]) – and the presence of single headaches, which may have a "more or less" severe impact depending on several factors. These factors can be connected to the subjective response to therapies, but also to the features of the context in which the person works, in terms, for example, of environmental triggers (like noise or light) or of possibility to quit working or attitudes of colleagues.

Some limitations have to be acknowledged. Sample size was wide enough, as showed by KMO and BTS, but was entirely derived from specialty headache centers: the primary effect of this was the high presence of patients with CM (around 25%) compared to what could be expectable based on the epidemiological presentation of this condition. Second we did not test the stability of the questionnaire, i.e. whether few days after the first administration patients would report similar responses. Similarly, sensitivity to change, i.e. the degree to which changes in patients' responses are consistent with changes in the disease profile, was not addressed as a longitudinal design would be needed. Such an aspect is of particular relevance, and might constitute important information for clinicians and patients in the process of

decision making on the best therapeutic options. In fact, it will be very interesting to understand what may be the main drivers of HEADWORK scales change, considering the potential role of different variables, such as frequency (which is generally considered as the major outcome measure in headache research – but showed a modest correlation with HEADWORK scores), or severity of headaches, but also presence of treatment-related side effects, particularly such those that may have an important role on work-place activities and productivity, such as somnolence, sedation dizziness or fatigue, and which are relatively common with preventive anti-migraine medications. Third, the questionnaire is not designed to distinguish the impact of migraine on work-related aspects in ictal and interictal phases as patients are required to fill in HEADWORK with reference to the previous 30 days, thus taking into account good and bad days. Fourth, headache diaries were used when available, but we do not have track of how many patients had. Diagnosis was clinical and based on ICHD-3Beta criteria for EM with and without aura and CM with and without MOH: however, we cannot exclude mixed diagnoses, i.e. presence of tension-type headaches, for some cases. Finally, among the next steps to further on implement HEADWORK, the definition of cut-off scores is surely the most relevant one. Further clinical and labor-related aspects would however be needed to perform such a task. Frequency of access to emergency departments, recurrence of relapses into MOH and presence of comorbidities, that have been showed to negatively impact on disability and QoL [55], may be relevant clinical indicators, and presence of disability benefits and – prospectively – risk of unemployment may be relevant labour-related indicators for grading of HEADWORK questionnaire.

Conclusions

We presented the validation of the HEADWORK questionnaire, a brief questionnaire which addresses the impact of migraine on work-related difficulties in terms of presence, and severity, of difficulties in general and specific skills, and it also addresses the factors contributing to these difficulties, defined as negative impact on work tasks. It has been validated in patients with episodic and chronic migraine and it can be used in all populations of employed persons, either adults or adolescents. HEADWORK is composed of 17 items that are grouped in two scales, both of them with good measurement properties, where higher scores reflect the presence of severe difficulties on one side, and of more interfering factors contributing to these difficulties on the other side.

We propose HEADWORK as a feasible way to produce reliable work-related disability weights in studies evaluating the burden of episodic and chronic migraine in epidemiological and clinical research. Further studies are needed to prove its role as an outcome tool, and its ability to assess the balance between therapeutic effects and side effects of given treatment interventions on work performance and productivity. Future studies are also needed to test the validity of HEADWORK in other headache disorders, such as tension-type headache.

Additional file

Additional file 1: Table S1. Full inter-item correlation on HEADWORK first section (Work-related difficulties). Table S2. Items' average score, percentage of not applicable and missing items, item asymmetry index inter-item correlation for HEADWORK first section (Work-related difficulties). Table S3. Full inter-item correlation on HEADWORK section B (Factors contributing to work difficulties). Table S4. Items' average score, percentage of not applicable and missing items, item asymmetry index inter-item correlation for HEADWORK section B (Factors contributing to work difficulties). Table S5. EFA on HEADWORK section A (Work-related difficulties). Table S6. EFA on HEADWORK section B (Factors contributing to work difficulties). Table S7. CFA on HEADWORK section A (Work-related difficulties). Table S8. CFA on HEADWORK section B (Factors contributing to work difficulties). Table S9. second CFA on HEADWORK section B (Factors contributing to work difficulties). (DOCX 39 kb)

Abbreviations

95% C.I.: 95% Confidence Intervals; BTS: Bartlett's Test of Sphericity; CFA: Confirmatory factor analysis; Chi2/d.f.: ratio between Chi2 and degrees of freedom; CM: Chronic Migraine; EF: Emotional function; EFA: Exploratory factor analysis; EM: Episodic Migraine; ES: Effect size; GBD: Global Burden of Disease; ICF: International Classification of Functioning, Disability and Health; ICHD-3Beta: International Classification of Headache Disorders, 3-beta version; KMO: Kaiser-Meyer-Olkin Measure of Sampling Adequacy; MIDAS: Migraine Disability Assessment schedule; MOH: Medication Overuse Headache; MSQ: Migraine Specific Quality of Life Questionnaire; MWPLQ: Migraine Work and Productivity Loss Questionnaire; PROMs: Patient-reported outcome measures; QoL: Quality of life; RMSEA: Root Mean Square Error of Approximation; RP: Role-prevention; RR: Role-restriction; SD: Standard deviation; WHODAS-12: World Health Organization 12-items Disability Assessment Schedule; WPAI: Work Productivity and Activity Impairment; YLDs: Years Lived with a Disability

Funding
The study was partially supported by Allergan.

Authors' contributions
ARaggi study conception and design, data analysis and interpretation, manuscript drafting and revision. VC: data collection, data analysis and interpretation, manuscript drafting and revision. EG: data collection, data analysis and interpretation, manuscript drafting and revision. ML: data interpretation, manuscript revision. CS: data collection, data analysis and interpretation, manuscript drafting and revision. LGrazzi: data collection, data interpretation, manuscript revision. MB: data collection, data interpretation, manuscript revision. GV: data collection, data interpretation, manuscript revision. SC: data collection, data interpretation, manuscript revision. GP: data collection, data interpretation, manuscript revision. GT: data collection, data interpretation, manuscript revision. ARusso: data collection, data interpretation, manuscript revision. PB: data collection, data interpretation, manuscript revision. CA: data collection, data interpretation, manuscript revision. CL: data collection, data interpretation, manuscript revision. LGiani: data collection, data interpretation, manuscript revision. FF: data collection, data interpretation, manuscript revision. PDF: data collection, data interpretation, manuscript revision. FB: data collection, data interpretation, manuscript revision. LR: data collection, data interpretation,

manuscript revision. DD: study conception and design, data collection, data interpretation, manuscript drafting and revision. All authors read and approved the final manuscript.

Ethics approval and consent to participate
The study was approved by the Ethical Committees of the coordinating center, Neurological Institute C. Besta (protocol approval number 07/2016, January 13, 2016) and subsequently ratified by all participating centers (Università Politecnica delle Marche, Ancona; IRCCS Istituto delle Scienze Neurologiche, Bologna; University of Campania "Luigi Vanvitelli", Naples; IRCCS San Raffaele Pisana, Rome; Luigi Sacco Hospital-University of Milan, Milan; San Carlo Borromeo Hospital, Milan; Magna Graecia University of Catanzaro, Catanzaro).
Participation to the study was on a voluntary basis: all patients provided written consent before inclusion.

Competing interests
The authors declare that they have no competing interests.

Author details
[1]Neurology, Public Health and Disability Unit, Fondazione IRCCS Istituto Neurologico Carlo Besta, Milan, Italy. [2]e-Campus University, Novedrate, Italy. [3]Headache and Neuroalgology Unit, Fondazione IRCCS Istituto Neurologico Carlo Besta, Milan, Italy. [4]Clinica di Neurologia, Università Politecnica delle Marche, Ancona, Italy. [5]IRCCS Istituto delle Scienze Neurologiche di Bologna, Bologna, Italy. [6]DIBINEM - Alma Mater Studiorum, Università di Bologna, Bologna, Italy. [7]Headache Center, Department of Medical, Surgical, Neurological, Metabolic and Aging Sciences, University of Campania "Luigi Vanvitelli", Naples, Italy. [8]Headache and Pain Unit, Department of Neurological, Motor and Sensorial Sciences. IRCCS San Raffaele Pisana, Rome, Italy. [9]San Raffaele University, Rome, Italy. [10]Neurology Unit, Headache Center, Ospedale L, Sacco University of Milan, Milan, Italy. [11]Neurological and Stroke Unit Department, Headache Center, ASST Santi Paolo e Carlo, San Carlo Borromeo Hospital, Milan, Italy. [12]Headache Center, Institute of Neurology, Magna Graecia University of Catanzaro, Catanzaro, Italy.

References
1. Abu Bakar N, Tanprawate S, Lambru G, Torkamani M, Jahanshahi M, Matharu M (2016) Quality of life in primary headache disorders: a review. Cephalalgia 36:67–91
2. D'Amico D, Grazzi L, Usai S, Leonardi M, Raggi A (2013) Disability and quality of life in headache: where we are now and where we are heading. Neurol Sci 34:S1–S5
3. Raggi A, Giovannetti AM, Quintas R, D'Amico D, Cieza A, Sabariego C, Bickenbach JE, Leonardi M (2012) A systematic review of the psychosocial difficulties relevant to patients with migraine. J Headache Pain 13:595–606
4. Lantéri-Minet M, Duru G, Mudge M, Cottrell S (2011) Quality of life impairment, disability and economic burden associated with chronic daily headache, focusing on chronic migraine with or without medication overuse: a systematic review. Cephalalgia 31:837–850
5. D'Amico D, Grazzi L, Usai S, Raggi A, Leonardi M, Bussone G (2011) Disability in chronic daily headache: state of the art and future directions. Neurol Sci 32:S71–S76
6. Buse DC, Rupnow MF, Lipton RB (2009) Assessing and managing all aspects of migraine: migraine attacks, migraine-related functional impairment, common comorbidities, and quality of life. Mayo Clin Proc 84:422–435
7. Stovner LJ, Hagen K, Jensen R, Katsarava Z, Lipton R, Scher A, Steiner T, Zwart JA (2007) The global burden of headache: a documentation of headache prevalence and disability worldwide. Cephalalgia 27:193–210
8. Buse DC, Manack AN, Fanning KM, Serrano D, Reed ML, Turkel CC, Lipton RB (2012) Chronic migraine prevalence, disability, and sociodemographic factors: results from the American migraine prevalence and prevention study. Headache 52:1456–1470

9. Ahmed F, Zafar HW, Buture A, Khalil M (2015) Does analgesic overuse matter? Response to OnabotulinumtoxinA in patients with chronic migraine with or without medication overuse. Springerplus 4:589

10. Rojo E, Pedraza MI, Muñoz I, Mulero P, Ruiz M, de la Cruz C, Barón J, Rodríguez C, Herrero S, Guerrero AL (2015) Chronic migraine with and without medication overuse: experience in a hospital series of 434 patients. Neurologia 30:153–157

11. Aurora SK, Dodick DW, Turkel CC, RE DG, Silberstein SD, Lipton RB, Diener HC, Brin MF, PREEMPT 1 Chronic Migraine Study Group (2010) OnabotulinumtoxinA for treatment of chronic migraine: results from the double-blind, randomized, placebo-controlled phase of the PREEMPT 1 trial. Cephalalgia 30:793–803

12. Rendas-Baum R, Bloudek LM, Maglinte GA, Varon SF (2013) The psychometric properties of the migraine-specific quality of life questionnaire version 2.1 (MSQ) in chronic migraine patients. Qual Life Res 22:1123–1233

13. Negro A, Martelletti P (2011) Chronic migraine plus medication overuse headache: two entities or not? J Headache Pain 12:593–601

14. D'Amico D, Grazzi L, Curone M, Leonardi M, Raggi A (2017) Cost of medication overuse headache in Italian patients at the time-point of withdrawal: a retrospective study based on real data. Neurol Sci 38:S3–S6

15. Linde M, Gustavsson A, Stovner LJ, Steiner TJ, Barré J, Katsarava Z, Lainez JM, Lampl C, Lantéri-Minet M, Rastenyte D, Ruiz de la Torre E, Tassorelli C, Andrée C (2012) The cost of headache disorders in Europe: the Eurolight project. Eur J Neurol 19:703–711

16. Burton WN, Landy SH, Downs KE, Runken MC (2009) The impact of migraine and the effect of migraine treatment on workplace productivity in the United States and suggestions for future research. Mayo Clin Proc 84:436–445

17. Stovner LJ, Hagen K (2006) Prevalence, burden, and cost of headache disorders. Curr Opin Neurol 19:281–285

18. Stang P, Cady R, Batenhorst A, Hoffman L (2001) Workplace productivity. A review of the impact of migraine and its treatment. Pharmacoeconomics 19:231–244

19. Gustavsson A, Svensson M, Jacobi F, Allgulander C, Alonso J, Beghi E, Dodel R, Ekman M, Faravelli C, Fratiglioni L, Gannon B, Jones DH, Jennum P, Jordanova A, Jönsson L, Karampampa K, Knapp M, Kobelt G, Kurth T, Lieb R, Linde M, Ljungcrantz C, Maercker A, Melin B, Moscarelli M, Musayev A, Norwood F, Preisig M, Pugliatti M, Rehm J, Salvador-Carulla L, Schlehofer B, Simon R, Steinhausen HC, Stovner LJ, Vallat JM, Van den Bergh P, van Os J, Vos P, Xu W, Wittchen HU, Jönsson B, Olesen J, CDBE2010Study Group (2011) Cost of disorders of the brain in Europe 2010. Eur Neuropsychopharmacol 21:718–779

20. Landy SH, Runken MC, Bell CF, Higbie RL, Haskins LS (2011) Assessing the impact of migraine onset on work productivity. J Occup Environ Med 53: 74–81

21. Raggi A, Grazzi L, Grignani E, Leonardi M, Sansone E, Scaratti C, D'Amico D (2018) The use of MIDAS in patients with chronic migraine and medication-overuse headache: should we trust it? Neurol Sci 39:S125–S127

22. Raggi A, Leonardi M, Scaratti C, Sansone E, Grazzi L, D'Amico D (2018) Gender and education inequalities in the cost of medication-overuse headache. Neurol Sci 39:S117–S119

23. Raggi A, Covelli V, Leonardi M, Grazzi L, Curone M, D'Amico D (2014) Difficulties in work-related activities among migraineurs are scarcely collected: results from a literature review. Neurol Sci 35:S23–S26

24. World Health Organization (2001) The international classification of functioning, disability and health. World Health Organization, Geneva

25. Scaratti C, Raggi A, Leonardi M, Grazzi L, D'Amico D (2015) Work-related difficulties in patients with episodic and chronic migraine: a study protocol to define relevant themes. Neurol Sci 36:S174

26. Headache Classification Committee of the International Headache Society (2013) The international classification of headache disorders, 3rd edition (beta version). Cephalalgia 33:629–808

27. Stewart WF, Lipton RB, Whyte J, Dowson A, Kolodner K, Liberman JN, Sawyer J (1999) An international study to assess reliability of the migraine disability assessment (MIDAS) score. Neurology 53:988–994

28. D'Amico D, Mosconi P, Genco S, Usai S, Prudenzano AM, Grazzi L, Leone M, Puca FM, Bussone G (2001) The migraine disability assessment (MIDAS) questionnaire: translation and reliability of the Italian version. Cephalalgia 21:947–952

29. Federici S, Bracalenti M, Meloni F, Luciano JV (2017) World Health Organization disability assessment schedule 2.0: an international systematic review. Disabil Rehabil 39:2347–2380

30. Martin BC, Pathak DS, Sharfman MI, Adelman JU, Taylor F, Kwong WJ, Jhingran P (2000) Validity and reliability of the migraine-specific quality of life questionnaire (MSQ version 2.1). Headache 40:204–215

31. Raggi A, Giovannetti AM, Schiavolin S, Leonardi M, Bussone G, Grazzi L, Usai S, Curone M, Di Fiore P, D'Amico D (2014) Validating the migraine-specific quality of life questionnaire v2.1 (MSQ) in Italian inpatients with chronic migraine with a history of medication overuse. Qual Life Res 23:1273–1277

32. Bagley CL, Rendas-Baum R, Maglinte GA, Yang M, Varon SF, Lee J, Kosinski M (2012) Validating migraine-specific quality of life questionnaire v2.1 in episodic and chronic migraine. Headache 52:409–421

33. Field A (2009) Discovering statistics using SPSS, third edn. Sage, London

34. Hu L, Bentler PM (1994) Cutoff criteria for fit indexes in covariance structure analysis: conventional criteria versus new alternatives. Struct Equ Modeling 6:1–55

35. Bland JM, Altman DG (1997) Cronbach's alpha. BMJ 314:572

36. Nunnally JC, Bernstein I (1994) Psychometric theory, 3rd edn. McGraw-Hill, New York

37. Leonardi M, Raggi A (2013) Burden of migraine: international perspectives. Neurol Sci 34:S117–S118

38. Vos T, Flaxman AD, Naghavi M et al (2012) Years lived with disability (YLD) for 1160 sequelae of 289 diseases and injuries 1990–2010: a systematic analysis for the global burden of disease study 2010. Lancet 380:2163–2196

39. Global Burden of Disease Study (2013) Collaborators (2015) global, regional, and national incidence, prevalence, and years lived with disability for 301 acute and chronic diseases and injuries in 188 countries, 1990–2013: a systematic analysis for the global burden of disease study 2013. Lancet 386:743–800

40. Steiner TJ, Stovner LJ, Birbeck GL (2013) Migraine: the seventh disabler. J Headache Pain 14:1

41. GBD (2016) Disease and injury incidence and prevalence collaborators (2017) global, regional, and national incidence, prevalence, and years lived with disability for 328 diseases and injuries for 195 countries, 1990–2016: a systematic analysis for the global burden of disease study 2016. Lancet 390:1211–1259

42. Steiner TJ, Stovner LJ, Vos T, Jensen R, Katsarava Z (2018) Migraine is first cause of disability in under 50s: will health politicians now take notice? J Headache Pain 19:17

43. Headache Classification Committee of the International Headache Society (2018) The international classification of headache disorders, 3rd edition. Cephalalgia 38:1–211

44. D'Amico D, Grazzi L, Curone M, Di Fiore P, Proietti Cecchini A, Leonardi M, Scaratti C, Raggi A (2015) Difficulties in work activities and the pervasive effect over disability in patients with episodic and chronic migraine. Neurol Sci 36: S9–S11

45. Munakata J, Hazard E, Serrano D, Klingman D, Rupnow MF, Tierce J, Reed M, Lipton RB (2009) Economic burden of transformed migraine: results from the American migraine prevalence and prevention (AMPP) study. Headache 49:498–508

46. Lerner DJ, Amick BC 3rd, Malspeis S, Rogers WH, Santanello NC, Gerth WC, Lipton RB (1999) The migraine work and productivity loss questionnaire: concepts and design. Qual Life Res 8:699–710

47. Davies GM, Santanello N, Gerth W, Lerner D, Block GA (1999) Validation of a migraine work and productivity loss questionnaire for use in migraine studies. Cephalalgia 19:497–502

48. Reilly MC, Zbrozek AS, Dukes EM (1993) The validity and reproducibility of a work productivity and activity impairment instrument. Pharmacoeconomics 4:353–365

49. Pradalier A, Auray JP, El Hasnaoui A, Alzahouri K, Dartigues JF, Duru G, Henry P, Lantéri-Minet M, Lucas C, Chazot G, Gaudin AF (2004) Economic impact of migraine and other episodic headaches in France: data from the GRIM2000 study. Pharmacoeconomics 22:985–999

50. Reilly MC (2016) WPAI:Migraine. Available at: http://www.reillyassociates.net/WPAI-MIGRAINE_English_US_V2.doc. Accessed 23 Aug 2018

51. Tassorelli C, Diener HC, Dodick DW, Silberstein SD, Lipton RB, Ashina M, Becker WJ, Ferrari MD, Goadsby PJ, Pozo-Rosich P, Wang SJ; International Headache Society Clinical Trials Standing Committee (2018) Guidelines of the international headache society for controlled trials of preventive treatment of chronic migraine in adults. Cephalalgia 38: 815–832

52. Gajria K, Lee LK, Flores NM, Aycardi E, Gandhi SK (2017) Humanistic and economic burden of nausea and vomiting among migraine sufferers. J Pain Res 10:689–698

53. Lipton RB, Gandhi SK, Fitzgerald YPP, Cohen JM, Yang RH, Aycardi E (2017) The positive impact of fremanezumab on work productivity and activity impairment in patients with chronic migraine. In: Cephalalgia 37:S328-S329; meeting abstract PO-01-182

54. Young WB, Park JE, Tian IX, Kempner J (2013) The stigma of migraine. PLoS One 8:e54074

55. D'Amico D, Sansone E, Grazzi L, Giovannetti AM, Leonardi M, Schiavolin S, Raggi A (2018) Multimorbidity in patients with chronic migraine and medication overuse headache. Acta Neurol Scand E-Pub on Aug 14:2018. https://doi.org/10.1111/ane.13014

22

Practical and clinical utility of non-invasive vagus nerve stimulation (nVNS) for the acute treatment of migraine: a post hoc analysis of the randomized, sham-controlled, double-blind PRESTO trial

Licia Grazzi[1,13]*, Cristina Tassorelli[2,3], Marina de Tommaso[4], Giulia Pierangeli[5], Paolo Martelletti[6], Innocenzo Rainero[7], Pierangelo Geppetti[8], Anna Ambrosini[9], Paola Sarchielli[10], Eric Liebler[11], Piero Barbanti[12] and on Behalf of the PRESTO Study Group

Abstract

Background: The PRESTO study of non-invasive vagus nerve stimulation (nVNS; gammaCore®) featured key primary and secondary end points recommended by the International Headache Society to provide Class I evidence that for patients with an episodic migraine, nVNS significantly increases the probability of having mild pain or being pain-free 2 h post stimulation. Here, we examined additional data from PRESTO to provide further insights into the practical utility of nVNS by evaluating its ability to consistently deliver clinically meaningful improvements in pain intensity while reducing the need for rescue medication.

Methods: Patients recorded pain intensity for treated migraine attacks on a 4-point scale. Data were examined to compare nVNS and sham with regard to the percentage of patients who benefited by at least 1 point in pain intensity. We also assessed the percentage of attacks that required rescue medication and pain-free rates stratified by pain intensity at treatment initiation.

Results: A significantly higher percentage of patients who used acute nVNS treatment ($n = 120$) vs sham ($n = 123$) reported a $\geq$ 1-point decrease in pain intensity at 30 min (nVNS, 32.2%; sham, 18.5%; $P = 0.020$), 60 min (nVNS, 38.8%; sham, 24.0%; $P = 0.017$), and 120 min (nVNS, 46.8%; sham, 26.2%; $P = 0.002$) after the first attack. Similar significant results were seen when assessing the benefit in all attacks. The proportion of patients who did not require rescue medication was significantly higher with nVNS than with sham for the first attack (nVNS, 59.3%; sham, 41.9%; $P = 0.013$) and all attacks (nVNS, 52.3%; sham, 37.3%; $P = 0.008$). When initial pain intensity was mild, the percentage of patients with no pain after treatment was significantly higher with nVNS than with sham at 60 min (all attacks: nVNS, 37.0%; sham, 21.2%; $P = 0.025$) and 120 min (first attack: nVNS, 50.0%; sham, 25.0%; $P = 0.018$; all attacks: nVNS, 46.7%; sham, 30.1%; $P = 0.037$).

(Continued on next page)

* Correspondence: licia.grazzi@istituto-besta.it
[1]Neuroalgology Unit, Carlo Besta Neurological Institute and Foundation, Milan, Italy
[13]Department of Fondazione IRCCS Istituto Neurologico C. Besta, U.O. Neurologia III – Cefalee e Neuroalgologia, Via Celoria 11, 20133 Milan, Italy
Full list of author information is available at the end of the article

(Continued from previous page)

Conclusions: This post hoc analysis demonstrated that acute nVNS treatment quickly and consistently reduced pain intensity while decreasing rescue medication use. These clinical benefits provide guidance in the optimal use of nVNS in everyday practice, which can potentially reduce use of acute pharmacologic medications and their associated adverse events.

Keywords: Neuromodulation, Vagus nerve stimulation, Post hoc analysis, Migraine, Rescue medication, Pain intensity

Background

Non-invasive vagus nerve stimulation (nVNS; gamma-Core®; electroCore, Inc., Basking Ridge, NJ, USA) (Fig. 1) is a safe and effective treatment for patients with migraine [1–4]. The therapy is practical, flexible, and easy to use, with the lack of drug-drug interactions allowing its use as a complement to existing treatments [5, 6]. nVNS reduces the need for pharmacologic therapies and their related side effects in the treatment of migraine [7, 8]. In the PRospectivE Study of nVNS for the acute Treatment Of migraine (PRESTO), nVNS was superior to sham for the majority of end points including pain freedom, pain relief, and ≥ 50% responder rates at various time points [4]. Adverse events were minimal and mostly mild in severity [4]. The PRESTO trial provided Class I evidence that for patients with an episodic migraine, nVNS significantly increases the probability of having mild pain or being pain-free 2 h post stimulation.

In this post hoc analysis, we provide further insight into the practical utility of acute nVNS treatment through the reporting of clinically relevant end points that extend beyond the traditional key end points recommended for pivotal clinical trials by the International Headache Society (IHS) [9]. The objectives of this analysis were to evaluate the likelihood of experiencing at least a 1-point decrease in pain intensity while reducing

the need for rescue medication and to assess whether treatment of a migraine attack when the pain is mild affects the efficacy of nVNS.

Methods

Study design

The methods for the prospective, double-blind, randomized, sham-controlled, multicenter PRESTO study were previously reported (ClinicalTrials.gov identifier: NCT02686034) [4]. The study took place at 10 Italian sites from January 11, 2016, through March 31, 2017, and consisted of three 4-week periods: 1) run-in, 2) double-blind, and 3) open-label periods. During the run-in period, patients received their standard medications. In the double-blind period, patients were randomly assigned to either nVNS or sham treatment. During the open-label period, all patients received nVNS treatment. Patients were instructed to treat up to 5 migraine attacks with nVNS or sham during the double-blind period and up to 5 additional attacks with nVNS during the open-label period. Only one attack could be treated within a 48-h period.

Study population

Patients were 18 to 75 years of age and had a previous diagnosis of migraine with or without aura according to the *International Classification of Headache Disorders, 3rd edition* criteria (*ICHD-3*) [10]. Key exclusion criteria included history of secondary headache, another significant pain disorder, uncontrolled hypertension, botulinum toxin injections in the last 6 months, and head or neck nerve blocks in the last 2 months.

Intervention

Within 20 min of migraine pain onset, patients self-administered two bilateral 120-s stimulations (ie, 1 stimulation each to the right and left cervical branch of the vagus nerve) (Fig. 2). If pain did not decrease 15 min after nVNS administration, the bilateral stimulations were repeated. At 120 min, an optional additional set of stimulations was repeated if the patient was not pain-free, and optional rescue medication could be used. Any rescue medication use before the 120-min assessment was considered treatment failure. Patients

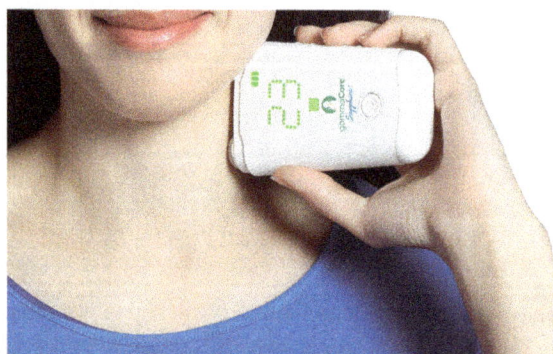

Fig. 1 The Non-invasive Vagus Nerve Stimulation Device. Note: A previous model of the nVNS device was used by patients in the PRospectivE Study of nVNS for the acute Treatment Of migraine (PRESTO) trial. Image provided courtesy of electroCore, Inc. Abbreviation: nVNS, non-invasive vagus nerve stimulation

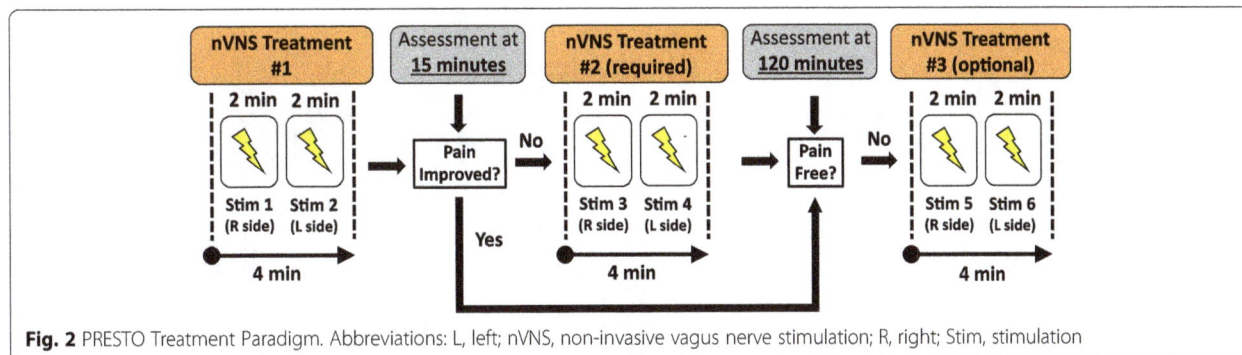

Fig. 2 PRESTO Treatment Paradigm. Abbreviations: L, left; nVNS, non-invasive vagus nerve stimulation; R, right; Stim, stimulation

maintained preventive migraine medication use at a stable dose and frequency during the 2 months before enrollment and throughout the study. No new preventive medication was permitted during the study.

End points

The percentage of patients with a ≥ 1-point reduction in pain intensity on a 4-point scale (0, *no pain*; 1, *mild pain*; 2, *moderate pain*; 3, *severe pain*) was measured at 30, 60, and 120 min after the first treated attack of the double-blind and open-label periods. Rescue medication use and pain-free rates at 30, 60, and 120 min stratified by initial pain intensity were evaluated for the first treated attack of both periods. Similar analyses were performed for all attacks for both periods.

Statistical analyses

All analyses were evaluated in the *intent-to-treat (ITT) population*, defined as patients who treated at least one migraine attack in the double-blind period. Proportions of patients with pain reductions of ≥1 point and proportions of patients who did not use rescue medication were estimated for the first attack using logistic regression models adjusted for baseline pain score, preventive medication use, and presence of aura. *P*-values for comparisons between the nVNS and sham groups were from the covariate-adjusted logistic regression models. Pain-free rates for the first attack were presented as proportion and 95% exact binomial confidence interval (CI). *P*-values for comparison of pain-free rates for the first attack between the nVNS and sham groups in the double-blind period were from the chi-square test or Fisher exact test, as appropriate. To estimate proportions of all attacks that achieved ≥1-point pain reductions and proportions of all attacks not requiring rescue medication, generalized linear mixed-effects regression models adjusted for baseline pain score, preventive medication use, and presence of aura were used. Odds ratios and 95% CIs for comparisons of rates between the nVNS and sham groups for all attacks were from the covariate-adjusted generalized linear mixed-effects

regression models; *P*-values were from resulting F tests. To estimate pain-free rates for all attacks, unadjusted generalized linear mixed-effects regression models were used; *P*-values comparing nVNS with sham were from resulting F tests. All data were analyzed using SAS® 9.4 (SAS Institute Inc., Cary, NC, USA).

Results

Patients

Full details on patient disposition, demographics, and baseline characteristics in the PRESTO study were reported previously [4]. A total of 285 patients with episodic migraine were enrolled, with 248 randomly assigned to the nVNS (*n* = 122) and sham (*n* = 126) groups. The ITT population consisted of 120 patients randomized to receive nVNS and 123 patients randomized to receive sham. Patients were < 50 years of age at migraine onset, with a frequency of 3 to 8 attacks per month. Demographic and baseline characteristics were similar between the nVNS and sham groups. More patients in the nVNS group than in the sham group initiated treatment when attack intensity was severe (first attack: nVNS, 23.5%; sham, 15.1%; all attacks: nVNS, 25.1%; sham, 17.6%). A total of 238 patients (nVNS, *n* = 117; sham, *n* = 121) completed the open-label period.

≥1-point reduction in pain intensity

Acute nVNS treatment provided clinically meaningful and significant benefits vs sham in the double-blind period. For the first treated attack (Fig. 3A), percentages of patients who recorded a ≥ 1-point reduction in pain intensity were significantly greater in the nVNS group than in the sham group at 30 min (nVNS, 32.2%; sham, 18.5%; *P* = 0.020), 60 min (nVNS, 38.8%; sham, 24.0%; *P* = 0.017), and 120 min (nVNS, 46.8%; sham, 26.2%; *P* = 0.002). For all treated attacks (Fig. 3B), significantly more ≥1-point pain improvements were seen with nVNS than with sham at 60 min (nVNS, 33.3%; sham, 22.2%; *P* = 0.010) and 120 min (nVNS, 39.4%; sham, 26.4%; *P* = 0.006).

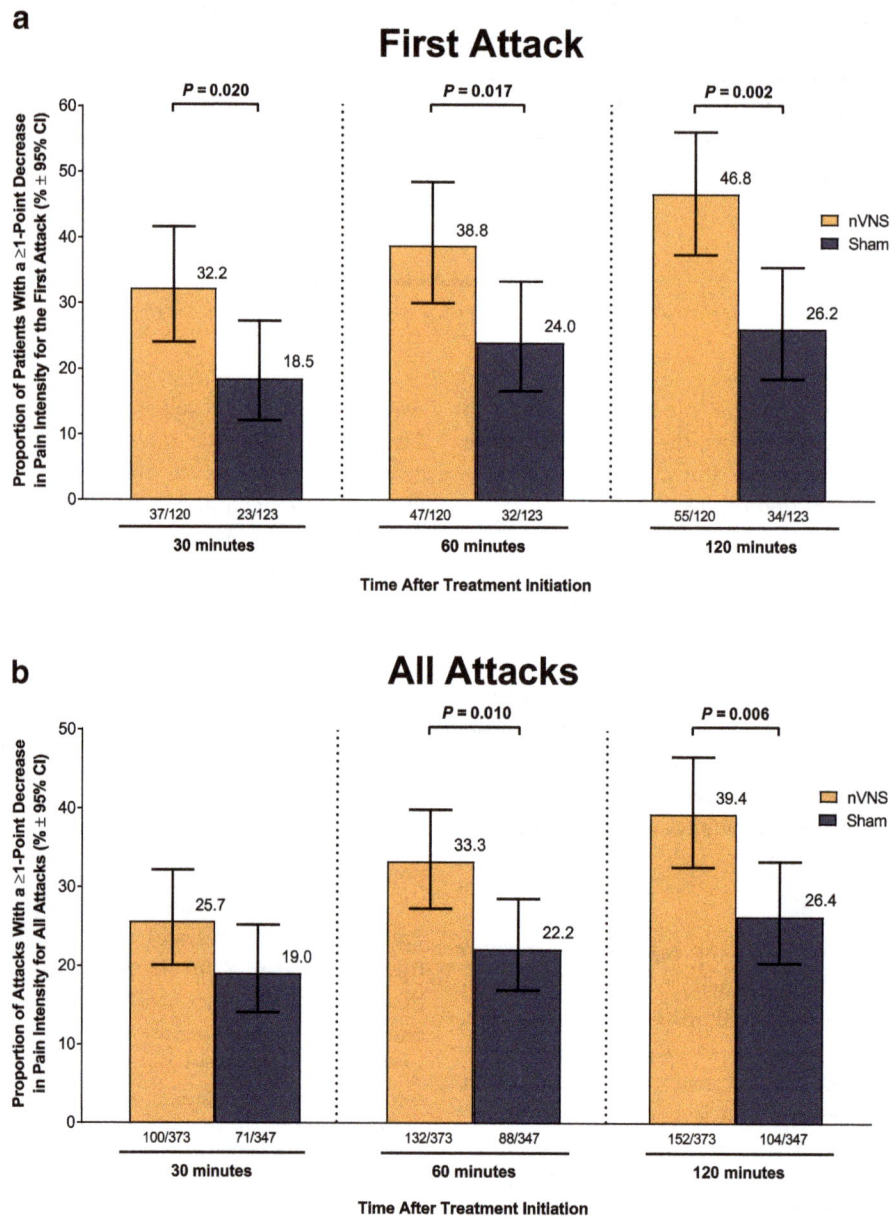

Fig. 3 ≥1-Point Reduction in Pain Intensity at 30, 60, and 120 Minutes for (**a**) First Attack and (**b**) All Attacks

Percentage of patients not requiring rescue medication

The proportion of patients who did not use rescue medication was significantly higher with nVNS than with sham for the first attack (nVNS, 59.3%; sham, 41.9%; $P = 0.013$) and for all attacks (nVNS, 52.3%; sham, 37.3%; $P = 0.008$) (Fig. 4).

Pain-free rates by initial pain intensity levels

Differences in pain-free rates between nVNS and sham were more pronounced in patients who initiated treatment when their attack was mild than for those who waited until the pain was moderate or severe to treat

their attack. The percentage of patients who successfully aborted a mild first migraine attack was significantly higher with nVNS than with sham at 120 min (nVNS, 50.0%; sham, 25.0%; $P = 0.018$) (Fig. 5A). When all mild attacks were considered, the percentages that became pain-free remained significantly higher with nVNS than with sham at 60 min (nVNS, 37.0%; sham, 21.2%; $P = 0.025$) and at 120 min (nVNS, 46.7%; sham, 30.1%; $P = 0.037$) (Fig. 5B). When the initial pain was severe, the percentage of all treated attacks that were aborted was significantly higher with nVNS than with sham at 30 min (nVNS, 4.4%; sham, 0.0%; $P < 0.0001$)

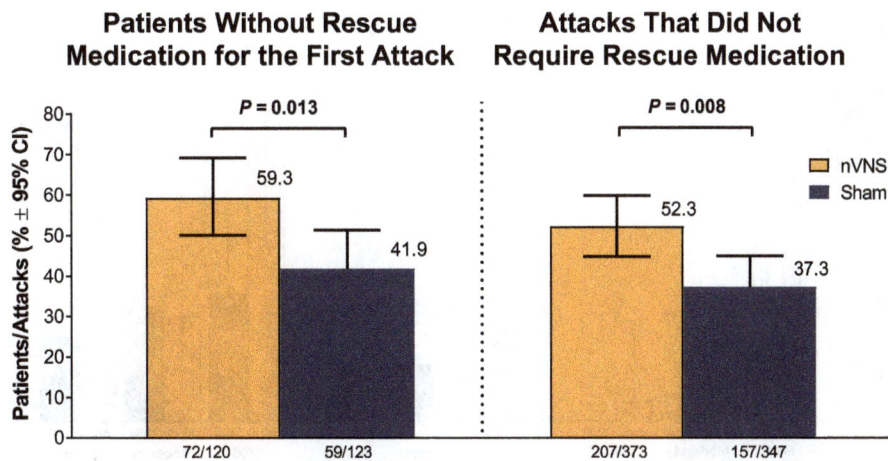

Fig. 4 Rescue Medication Use. Models are adjusted for the patients' baseline pain score, use of preventive therapies, and presence of aura; data for number of patients are unadjusted numbers. Abbreviation: nVNS, non-invasive vagus nerve stimulation

(Fig. 5B). The statistical benefit of nVNS vs sham in treating these severe attacks at 30 min may not be reliable given that the sham group had a proportion size of zero. When the initial pain intensity was moderate or severe, pain-free rates were not significantly different between the nVNS group and the sham group, though they were generally higher in the nVNS group at all time points.

Clinical utility outcomes in the open-label period

Therapeutic benefits observed in the nVNS group at 120 min during the double-blind period (ie, ≥1-point reductions in pain, decreases in rescue medication use, and improvements in pain-free rates by initial pain level) were sustained in the 4-week open-label period during which all patients received nVNS (Table 1).

Discussion

Treatment with nVNS consistently led to clinically relevant reductions in pain while reducing the need for rescue medication for the first and all attacks. The ability of nVNS to offer measurable pain relief for patients without increasing their exposure to pharmacologic adverse events or medication overuse provides a practical rationale for its early use as an acute treatment [11]. Patients who initiated their treatment when their migraine was mild were more likely to abort their attacks than those who treated when their pain was more severe, a finding consistent with clinical studies that demonstrated the efficacy of pharmacologic therapies during early stages of migraine attacks [12, 13] and when pain was still mild [14–18]. The combination of efficacy and tolerability with nVNS might provide patients with the confidence to initiate treatment earlier in their attacks compared with pharmacologic options that, in clinical experience, are often initiated when

the pain is more severe because of concerns with drug availability, overuse, and adverse events [14, 19–21].

Findings from mechanistic studies further support the initiation of nVNS treatment as early as possible to facilitate greater reductions in pain [22, 23]. Early nVNS treatment may reduce central excitability by blunting subsequent neurotransmitter release associated with severe migraine pain [23]. Two additional animal models demonstrated that nVNS inhibited expression of proteins associated with central sensitization of trigeminal neurons and reduced susceptibility to cortical spreading depression [24, 25]. These findings provide the mechanistic rationale for optimizing treatment response with early nVNS administration, before these neurophysiological activities are established.

Migraine may share common mechanistic pathways and latent causes with comorbid pain disorders such as fibromyalgia, chronic pelvic pain, and myofascial pain syndromes [26, 27]. Consistent with IHS recommendations, the PRESTO study excluded patients with such disorders although they are frequently seen in clinical practice [4, 9, 26]. Improvements in fibromyalgia symptoms have been observed in patients receiving pharmacologic migraine medication [26], suggesting that other effective migraine therapies such as nVNS could also have expanded benefits for these difficult-to-treat patients. In mechanistic studies, nVNS was shown to suppress pain markers that are not necessarily specific to migraine [22–24, 28, 29]. This potential broader effect on pain is further supported by a proof-of-concept study of adjunctive implantable VNS for fibromyalgia, which demonstrated improvement in pain, overall wellness, and physical function for 5 patients implanted with VNS [30]. These mechanistic and clinical insights suggest that evaluation of nVNS as a possible treatment for patients with migraine and comorbidities such as fibromyalgia is warranted.

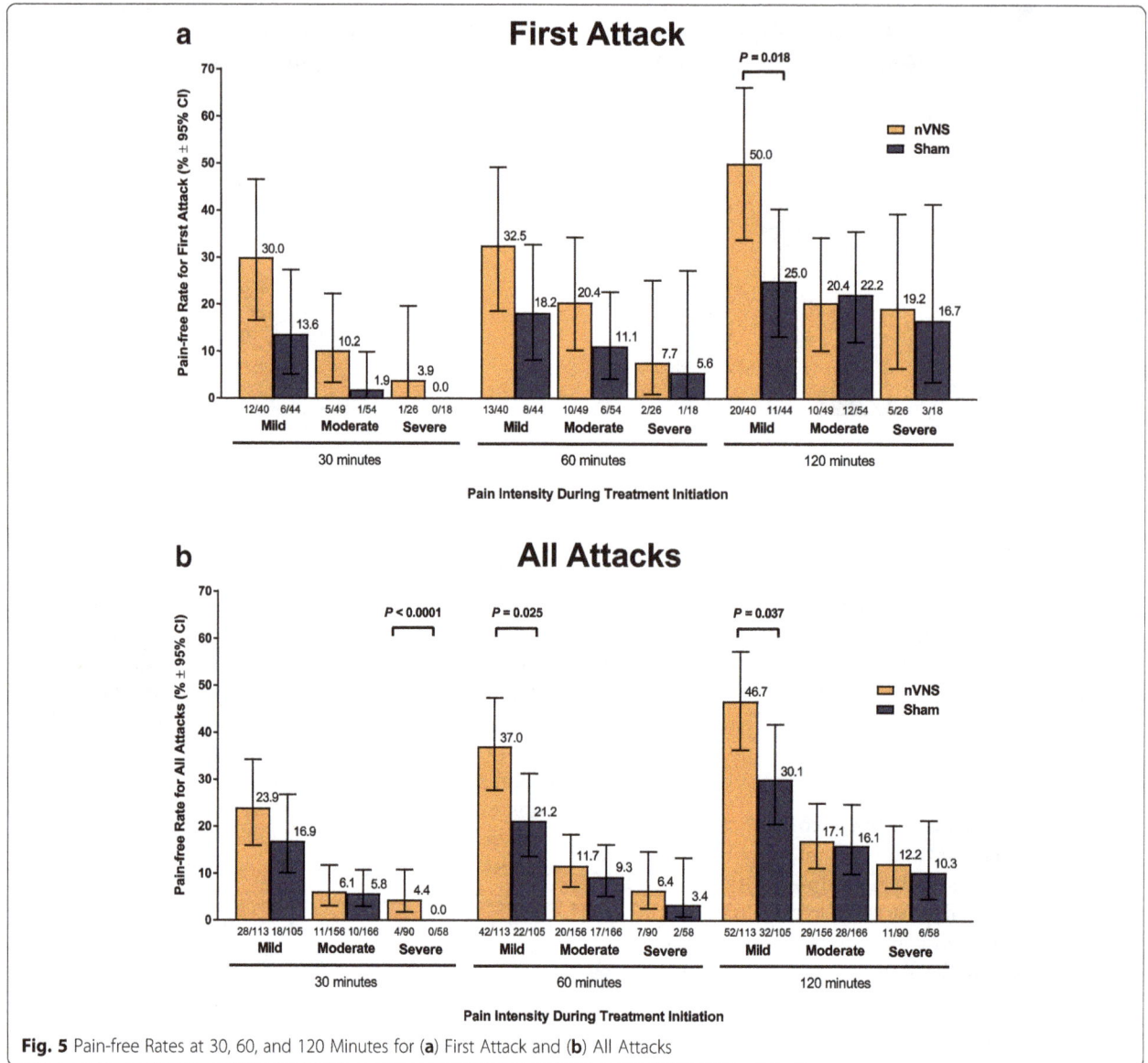

Fig. 5 Pain-free Rates at 30, 60, and 120 Minutes for (**a**) First Attack and (**b**) All Attacks

Post hoc analyses of clinical trials can be criticized for the use of less-rigorous methods or nonrepresentative subsets of a larger population [31–33]. We performed these post hoc analyses on the entire study population, which allowed the identification of a subpopulation of subjects who were more likely to respond to nVNS (ie, those who treat the attack when pain is mild). The findings are further strengthened by the analysis of data collected during the observational open-label phase [11]. There are currently no guidelines on the study design of neuromodulation devices in migraine, and well-controlled studies must rely only on the recommendations of the IHS for controlled trials of drugs [9]. These pharmacologic guidelines may be suboptimal for studies of neuromodulation devices because of the differing mechanisms of action

and interventional targets. Our findings suggest that rigorous post hoc analyses of well-controlled clinical trials could inform future guidelines for neuromodulation devices. Although the end points in this analysis are not the previously reported primary or key secondary end points recommended by the IHS, they provide additional insight into the practical clinical utility of nVNS in relieving pain while reducing rescue medication use.

A limiting factor of the PRESTO trial was that the sham device, which delivered an appreciable electrical signal, appears to have had some level of vagal activation [34]. The design of sham devices for neuromodulation studies is inherently difficult because a compromise must be reached between maintaining blinding with a noticeable stimulation and minimizing an active effect.

Table 1 Summary of Clinical Utility Outcomes at 120 Minutes After Treatment Initiation (Double-blind and Open-label Periods)

End Point	Pain Intensity at Treatment Initiation	Double-blind Period		Open-label Period
		nVNS	Sham	nVNS
First Attack				
% ≥1-point pain improvement	–	46.8**	26.2	42.9
% without rescue medication	–	59.3*	41.9	49.1
% pain-free response	Mild	50.0*	25.0	56.9
	Moderate	20.4	22.2	14.8
	Severe	19.2	16.7	23.3
All Attacks				
% ≥1-point pain improvement	–	39.4**	26.4	41.8
% without rescue medication	–	52.3**	37.3	49.7
% pain-free response	Mild	46.7*	30.1	48.6
	Moderate	17.1	16.1	13.8
	Severe	12.2	10.3	14.6

*$P < 0.05$ vs sham in the double-blind period
**$P < 0.01$ vs sham in the double-blind period
Abbreviation: *nVNS* non-invasive vagus nerve stimulation

A sham device that produces an active signal could obscure the actual effects of the verum device, thus reducing the opportunity to demonstrate therapeutic benefits above that of the sham device. We believe that the sham signal in the PRESTO study likely provided a detectable degree of active treatment effects that potentially masked some of the differences between the nVNS and sham groups in the current analysis [34].

nVNS is a practical treatment option with considerable clinical utility in the acute treatment of migraine. The likelihood that nVNS will quickly reduce pain by at least 1 point and decrease the use of rescue medication highlights its favorable risk-benefit profile [1–3, 9]. Significant reductions in the use of acute pharmacologic therapies for the nVNS group in this analysis may encourage patient confidence and adherence to nVNS as it provides an opportunity to minimize or avoid the potential limitations associated with traditional acute migraine medications, including drug-drug interactions, pharmacologic adverse events, and medication overuse [35–37]. nVNS offers flexibility, efficacy, and established safety and tolerability that may encourage earlier use than is typically seen with conventional acute therapies. Although demonstrated to be beneficial, pharmacologic treatments are often reserved for pain that is more severe because of a range of issues, including medication-related tolerability and a potentially insufficient availability of other acute medications [4, 38]. This analysis supports nVNS as a practical and effective alternative that can be used frequently and as early in an attack as desired to decrease migraine pain while reducing the need for rescue medication and minimizing drug-related adverse events.

Conclusions

These data highlight clinically important benefits of nVNS as an acute treatment of migraine. nVNS decreased pain by at least 1 point while reducing rescue medication use in most migraine attacks. Unlike most pharmacologic options, nVNS has the flexibility to be used alone or as adjunctive therapy for multiple attacks without risk of pharmacologic interactions and adverse events. These benefits, along with its convenience and ease of use, make nVNS an appealing practical option for the acute treatment of migraine.

Abbreviations

CI: confidence interval; ICHD-3: International Classification of Headache Disorders, 3rd edition; IHS: International Headache Society; ITT: intent-to-treat; L: left; nVNS: non-invasive vagus nerve stimulation; PRESTO: Prospective study of nVNS for the acute treatment of migraine; R: right; Stim: stimulation

Acknowledgements

The authors acknowledge all co-investigators, research nurses, study sites, and electroCore study team members. Statistical analyses for the study were conducted by Candace McClure, PhD, and Lisa Thackeray, MS, of North American Science Associates Inc. (Minneapolis, MN, USA). Medical writing support was provided by Mark Skopin, PhD, of MedLogix Communications, LLC, in cooperation with the authors.
Co-investigators:
The PRESTO Study Group.
Coinvestigators are listed by study site: 1. Headache Science Centre, National Neurological Institute C. Mondino Foundation and University of Pavia: **Cristina Tassorelli, MD, PhD (Principal Investigator)**; Vito Bitetto (Subinvestigator); Roberto De Icco, MD (Subinvestigator); Daniele Martinelli, MD (Subinvestigator); Grazia Sances, MD (Subinvestigator); Monica Bianchi, MD (Research Nurse); 2. Carlo Besta Neurological Institute and Foundation: **Licia Grazzi, MD (Principal Investigator)**; Anna Maria Padovan (Subinvestigator); 3. University of Bari Aldo Moro: **Marina de Tommaso, MD, PhD (Principal Investigator)**; Katia Ricci (Subinvestigator); Eleonora Vecchio, MD, PhD (Subinvestigator); 4. IRCCS Istituto delle Scienze Neurologiche di Bologna: **Pietro Cortelli, MD, PhD (Principal Investigator)**; Sabina Cevoli, MD, PhD (Subinvestigator); Giulia Pierangeli, MD, PhD (Subinvestigator);

Rossana Terlizzi, MD (Subinvestigator); 5. Sapienza University of Rome: **Paolo Martelletti, MD, PhD (Principal Investigator)**; Andrea Negro, MD (Subinvestigator); Gabriella Addolorata Chiariello (Research Nurse); 6. University of Turin: **Innocenzo Rainero, MD, PhD (Principal Investigator)**; Paola De Martino, MD, PhD (Subinvestigator); Annalisa Gai, MD (Subinvestigator); Flora Govone, MD (Subinvestigator); Federica Masuzzo, MD (Subinvestigator); Elisa Rubino, MD, PhD (Subinvestigator); Maria Claudia Torrieri, MD (Subinvestigator); Alessandro Vacca, MD (Subinvestigator); 7. University Hospital of Careggi: **Pierangelo Geppetti, MD, PhD (Principal Investigator)**; Alberto Chiarugi, MD, PhD (Subinvestigator); Francesco De Cesaris (Subinvestigator); Simone Li Puma (Subinvestigator); Chiara Lupi (Subinvestigator); Ilaria Marone (Subinvestigator); 8. IRCCS Neuromed: **Anna Ambrosini, MD, PhD (Principal Investigator)**; Armando Perrotta, MD, PhD (Subinvestigator); 9. Santa Maria della Misericordia Hospital: **Paola Sarchielli, MD, PhD (Principal Investigator)**; Laura Bernetti, MD (Subinvestigator); Ilenia Corbelli, MD, PhD (Subinvestigator); Michele Romoli, MD (Subinvestigator); Simone Simoni, MD (Subinvestigator); Angela Verzina, MD (Subinvestigator); 10. IRCCS San Raffaele Pisana: **Piero Barbanti, MD, PhD (Principal Investigator)**; Cinzia Aurilia, MD (Subinvestigator); Gabriella Egeo, MD, PhD (Subinvestigator); Luisa Fofi, MD (Subinvestigator).

electroCore Study Team: **Eric Liebler (Senior Vice President, Neurology)**; Annelie Andersson (Senior Director, Clinical Director); Lia Spitzer (Senior Director, Clinical/Study Manager); Juana Marin, MD (Clinical Advisor, Safety Monitor); Candace McClure, PhD (North American Science Associates Inc., Statistician); Lisa Thackeray, MS (North American Science Associates Inc., Statistician), Maria Giovanna Baldi (Monitor); Daniela Di Maro (Monitor).

Funding
This study was sponsored by electroCore, Inc.

Authors' contributions
Licia Grazzi, MD, Cristina Tassorelli, MD, PhD, and Eric Liebler contributed to the PRESTO study design and provided detailed input into the development of the manuscript. All primary investigators were involved in participant recruitment and treatment for the PRESTO study. All authors participated in data collection, interpretation, and validation and had full access to all study data. Cristina Tassorelli, MD, PhD and Eric Liebler were involved in data analysis. Data analysis support from North American Science Associates was funded by electroCore, Inc. Licia Grazzi, MD and Eric Liebler drafted and revised the manuscript for content in cooperation with all authors. All authors reviewed, critiqued, and contributed to revision of the manuscript content and provided approval of the final manuscript draft to be submitted to the *Journal of Headache and Pain*. Professional medical writing and editorial support (i.e., technical editing, copyediting, preparation of tables and figures, and clerical assistance) from MedLogix Communications, LLC, was funded by electroCore, Inc. The principal author, Licia Grazzi, MD takes responsibility for the data, analyses and interpretation, and conduct of the research.

Competing interests
L. Grazzi has received consultancy and advisory fees from Allergan S.p.A. and electroCore, Inc. C. Tassorelli has consulted for Allergan S.p.A.; electroCore, Inc.; Eli Lilly and Company; and Novartis AG and has received research grants from the European Commission and the Italian Ministry of Health. She is also a principal investigator or collaborator for RCTs sponsored by Alder BioPharmaceuticals Inc.; Eli Lilly and Company; and Teva Pharmaceutical Industries Ltd. M. de Tommaso has received advisory fees from Allergan S.p.A.; Neopharmed; and Pfizer Inc. G. Pierangeli has nothing to disclose. P. Martelletti has received research grants, advisory board fees, or travel fees from ACRAF; Allergan S.p.A.; Amgen Inc.; electroCore, Inc.; Novartis AG; and Teva Pharmaceutical Industries Ltd. I. Rainero has received consultancy fees from electroCore, Inc., and Mylan N.V. and research grants from the European Commission -- Horizon 2020. He is also a principal investigator for RCTs sponsored by Axovant Sciences Ltd. and TauRx Pharmaceuticals Ltd. P. Geppetti has received consultancy fees from Allergan S.p.A.; electroCore, Inc.;

Evidera; Novartis AG; Pfizer Inc.; and Sanofi S.p.A. and research grants from Chiesi Farmaceutici S.p.A. He is also a principal investigator for RCTs sponsored by Eli Lilly and Company; Novartis AG; and Teva Pharmaceutical Industries Ltd. A. Ambrosini has received consultancy fees from Almirall, S.A., and travel grants from Allergan S.p.A.; Almirall, S.A.; and Novartis AG. P. Sarchielli has received clinical study fees from Allergan S.p.A. E. Liebler is an employee of electroCore, Inc., and receives stock ownership. P. Barbanti has received consultancy fees from Allergan S.p.A.; electroCore, Inc.; Janssen Pharmaceuticals, Inc.; Lusofarmaco; and Visufarma and advisory fees from Abbott Laboratories and Merck & Co., Inc.

Author details
[1]Neuroalgology Unit, Carlo Besta Neurological Institute and Foundation, Milan, Italy. [2]Headache Science Centre, IRCCS C. Mondino Foundation, Pavia, Italy. [3]Department of Brain and Behavioral Sciences, University of Pavia, Pavia, Italy. [4]Neurophysiology and Pain Unit, University of Bari Aldo Moro, Bari, Italy. [5]IRCCS Istituto delle Scienze Neurologiche di Bologna, Bologna, Italy. [6]Department of Clinical and Molecular Medicine, Sapienza University, Rome, Italy. [7]Department of Neuroscience, University of Turin, Turin, Italy. [8]Headache Centre, University Hospital of Careggi, Florence, Italy. [9]IRCCS Neuromed, Pozzilli (IS), Italy. [10]Neurologic Clinic, Santa Maria della Misericordia Hospital, Perugia, Italy. [11]electroCore, Inc, Basking Ridge, NJ, USA. [12]Headache and Pain Unit, IRCCS San Raffaele Pisana, Rome, Italy. [13]Department of Fondazione IRCCS Istituto Neurologico C. Besta, U.O. Neurologia III – Cefalee e Neuroalgologia, Via Celoria 11, 20133 Milan, Italy.

References
1. Barbanti P, Grazzi L, Egeo G, Padovan AM, Liebler E, Bussone G (2015) Non-invasive vagus nerve stimulation for acute treatment of high-frequency and chronic migraine: an open-label study. J Headache Pain 16:61. https://doi.org/10.1186/s10194-015-0542-4
2. Goadsby PJ, Grosberg BM, Mauskop A, Cady R, Simmons KA (2014) Effect of noninvasive vagus nerve stimulation on acute migraine: an open-label pilot study. Cephalalgia 34(12):986–993. https://doi.org/10.1177/0333102414524494
3. Kinfe TM, Pintea B, Muhammad S, Zaremba S, Roeske S, Simon BJ, Vatter H (2015) Cervical non-invasive vagus nerve stimulation (nVNS) for preventive and acute treatment of episodic and chronic migraine and migraine-associated sleep disturbance: a prospective observational cohort study. J Headache Pain 16:101. https://doi.org/10.1186/s10194-015-0582-9
4. Tassorelli C, Grazzi L, de Tommaso M, Pierangeli G, Martelletti P, Rainero I, Dorlas S, Geppetti P, Ambrosini A, Sarchielli P, Liebler E, Barbanti P, Group PS (2018) Noninvasive vagus nerve stimulation as acute therapy for migraine: the randomized PRESTO study. Neurology 91(4):e364–e373. https://doi.org/10.1212/WNL.0000000000005857
5. Buse DC, Serrano D, Reed ML, Kori SH, Cunanan CM, Adams AM, Lipton RB (2015) Adding additional acute medications to a triptan regimen for migraine and observed changes in headache-related disability: results from the American migraine prevalence and prevention (AMPP) study. Headache 55(6):825–839. https://doi.org/10.1111/head.12556
6. Lipton RB, Buse DC, Serrano D, Holland S, Reed ML (2013) Examination of unmet treatment needs among persons with episodic migraine: results of the American migraine prevalence and prevention (AMPP) study. Headache 53(8):1300–1311. https://doi.org/10.1111/head.12154
7. Puledda F, Goadsby PJ (2017) An update on non-pharmacological neuromodulation for the acute and preventive treatment of migraine. Headache 57(4):685–691. https://doi.org/10.1111/head.13069
8. Puledda F, Messina R, Goadsby PJ An update on migraine: current understanding and future directions. J Neurol 264(9):2031–2039. https://doi.org/10.1007/s00415-017-8434-y
9. Tfelt-Hansen P, Pascual J, Ramadan N, Dahlof C, D'Amico D, Diener HC, Hansen JM, Lanteri-Minet M, Loder E, McCrory D, Plancade S, Schwedt T (2012) Guidelines for controlled trials of drugs in migraine: third edition. A guide for investigators. Cephalalgia 32(1):6–38. https://doi.org/10.1177/0333102411417901

Practical and clinical utility of non-invasive vagus nerve stimulation (nVNS) for the acute treatment...

239

10. Headache Classification Committee of the International Headache Society (IHS) (2018) The International Classification of Headache Disorders, 3rd edition. Cephalalgia. 38(1):1–211.

11. Martelletti P, Barbanti P, Grazzi L, Pierangeli G, Rainero I, Geppetti P, Ambrosini A, Sarchielli P, Tassorelli C, Liebler E, de Tommaso M (2018) Consistent effects of non-invasive vagus nerve stimulation (nVNS) for the acute treatment of migraine: additional findings from the randomized, sham-controlled, double-blind PRESTO trial [abstract MTIS2018-060]. Cephalalgia 28(1S):43. https://doi.org/10.1177/0333102418789865

12. Cady R, Elkind A, Goldstein J, Keywood C (2004) Randomized, placebo-controlled comparison of early use of frovatriptan in a migraine attack versus dosing after the headache has become moderate or severe. Curr Med Res Opin 20(9):1465–1472. https://doi.org/10.1185/030079904x2745

13. Luciani R, Carter D, Mannix L, Hemphill M, Diamond M, Cady R (2000) Prevention of migraine during prodrome with naratriptan. Cephalalgia 20(2):122–126. https://doi.org/10.1046/j.1468-2982.2000.00030.x

14. Goadsby PJ, Zanchin G, Geraud G, de Klippel N, Diaz-Insa S, Gobel H, Cunha L, Ivanoff N, Falques M, Fortea J (2008) Early vs. non-early intervention in acute migraine-'Act when mild (AwM)'. A double-blind, placebo-controlled trial of almotriptan. Cephalalgia 28(4):383–391. https://doi.org/10.1111/j.1468-2982.2008.01546.x

15. Mathew NT, Finlayson G, Smith TR, Cady RK, Adelman J, Mao L, Wright P, Greenberg SJ (2007) Early intervention with almotriptan: results of the AEGIS trial (AXERT early migraine intervention study). Headache 47(2):189–198. https://doi.org/10.1111/j.1526-4610.2006.00686.x

16. Freitag FG, Finlayson G, Rapoport AM, Elkind AH, Diamond ML, Unger JR, Fisher AC, Armstrong RB, Hulihan JF, Greenberg SJ (2007) Effect of pain intensity and time to administration on responsiveness to almotriptan: results from AXERT 12.5 mg time versus intensity migraine study (AIMS). Headache 47(4):519–530. https://doi.org/10.1111/j.1526-4610.2007.00756.x

17. Foley KA, Cady R, Martin V, Adelman J, Diamond M, Bell CF, Dayno JM, Hu XH (2005) Treating early versus treating mild: timing of migraine prescription medications among patients with diagnosed migraine. Headache 45(5):538–545. https://doi.org/10.1111/j.1526-4610.2005.05107.x

18. Becker WJ, Findlay T, Moga C, Scott NA, Harstall C, Taenzer P (2015) Guideline for primary care management of headache in adults. Can Fam Physician 61(8):670–679

19. Rapoport AM (2008) Acute and prophylactic treatments for migraine: present and future. Neurol Sci 29(Suppl 1):S110–S122. https://doi.org/10.1007/s10072-008-0901-x

20. Ozturk V (2013) Acute treatment of migraine. Noro Psikiyatr Ars 50(Suppl 1):S26–s29. https://doi.org/10.4274/Npa.y7299

21. Pilgrim AJ (1991) Methodology of clinical trials of sumatriptan in migraine and cluster headache. Eur Neurol 31(5):295–299. https://doi.org/10.1159/000116757

22. Akerman S, Simon B, Romero-Reyes M (2017) Vagus nerve stimulation suppresses acute noxious activation of trigeminocervical neurons in animal models of primary headache. Neurobiol Dis 102:96–104. https://doi.org/10.1016/j.nbd.2017.03.004

23. Oshinsky ML, Murphy AL, Hekierski H, Jr., Cooper M, Simon BJ (2014) Noninvasive vagus nerve stimulation as treatment for trigeminal allodynia. Pain 155 (5):1037–1042. doi:https://doi.org/10.1016/j.pain.2014.02.009

24. Chen SP, Ay I, de Morais AL, Qin T, Zheng Y, Sadeghian H, Oka F, Simon B, Eikermann-Haerter K, Ayata C (2016) Vagus nerve stimulation inhibits cortical spreading depression. Pain 157(4):797–805. https://doi.org/10.1097/j.pain.0000000000000437

25. Hawkins JL, Cornelison LE, Blankenship BA, Durham PL (2017) Vagus nerve stimulation inhibits trigeminal nociception in a rodent model of episodic migraine. Pain Rep 2(6):e628. https://doi.org/10.1097/pr9.0000000000000628

26. Giamberardino MA, Affaitati G, Martelletti P, Tana C, Negro A, Lapenna D, Curto M, Schiavone C, Stellin L, Cipollone F, Costantini R (2015) Impact of migraine on fibromyalgia symptoms. J Headache Pain 17:28. https://doi.org/10.1186/s10194-016-0619-8

27. Yuan H, Silberstein SD (2016) Vagus nerve and vagus nerve stimulation, a comprehensive review: part I. Headache 56(1):71–78. https://doi.org/10.1111/head.12647

28. Vecchio E, Bassez I, Ricci K, Tassorelli C, Liebler E, de Tommaso M (2018) Effect of non-invasive vagus nerve stimulation on resting-state electroencephalography and laser-evoked potentials in migraine patients: mechanistic insights. Front Hum Neurosci 12:366

29. de Tommaso M (2012) Prevalence, clinical features and potential therapies for fibromyalgia in primary headaches. Expert Rev Neurother 12(3):287–295; quiz 296. https://doi.org/10.1586/ern.11.190

30. Lange G, Janal MN, Maniker A, Fitzgibbons J, Fobler M, Cook D, Natelson BH (2011) Safety and efficacy of vagus nerve stimulation in fibromyalgia: a phase I/II proof of concept trial. Pain Med 12(9):1406–1413. https://doi.org/10.1111/j.1526-4637.2011.01203.x

31. Curran-Everett D, Milgrom H (2013) Post-hoc data analysis: benefits and limitations. Curr Opin Allergy Clin Immunol 13(3):223–224. https://doi.org/10.1097/ACI.0b013e3283609831

32. Elliott HL (1996) Post hoc analysis: use and dangers in perspective. J Hypertens Suppl 14 (2):S21-24; discussion S24-25

33. Srinivas TR, Ho B, Kang J, Kaplan B (2015) Post hoc analyses: after the facts. Transplantation 99(1):17–20. https://doi.org/10.1097/tp.0000000000000581

34. Moeller M, Schroeder CF, May A (2018) Comparison of active and "sham" non-invasive vagal nerve stimulation on lacrimation in healthy volunteers. Headache 58(S2):195. https://doi.org/10.1111/head.13306

35. Martelletti P (2017) Acute treatment of migraine: quo vadis? Expert Opin Pharmacother 18(11):1035–1037. https://doi.org/10.1080/14656566.2017.1329821

36. Thorlund K, Toor K, Wu P, Chan K, Druyts E, Ramos E, Bhambri R, Donnet A, Stark R, Goadsby PJ (2017) Comparative tolerability of treatments for acute migraine: a network meta-analysis. Cephalalgia 37(10):965–978. https://doi.org/10.1177/0333102416660552

37. Sabato D, Lionetto L, Martelletti P (2015) The therapeutic potential of novel anti-migraine acute therapies. Expert Opin Investig Drugs 24(2):141–144. https://doi.org/10.1517/13543784.2015.983223

38. Goadsby PJ (2008) The 'Act when Mild' (AwM) study: a step forward in our understanding of early treatment in acute migraine. Cephalalgia 28(Suppl 2):36–41. https://doi.org/10.1111/j.1468-2982.2008.01689.x

Permissions

All chapters in this book were first published in TJHP, by BioMed Central; hereby published with permission under the Creative Commons Attribution License or equivalent. Every chapter published in this book has been scrutinized by our experts. Their significance has been extensively debated. The topics covered herein carry significant findings which will fuel the growth of the discipline. They may even be implemented as practical applications or may be referred to as a beginning point for another development.

The contributors of this book come from diverse backgrounds, making this book a truly international effort. This book will bring forth new frontiers with its revolutionizing research information and detailed analysis of the nascent developments around the world.

We would like to thank all the contributing authors for lending their expertise to make the book truly unique. They have played a crucial role in the development of this book. Without their invaluable contributions this book wouldn't have been possible. They have made vital efforts to compile up to date information on the varied aspects of this subject to make this book a valuable addition to the collection of many professionals and students.

This book was conceptualized with the vision of imparting up-to-date information and advanced data in this field. To ensure the same, a matchless editorial board was set up. Every individual on the board went through rigorous rounds of assessment to prove their worth. After which they invested a large part of their time researching and compiling the most relevant data for our readers.

The editorial board has been involved in producing this book since its inception. They have spent rigorous hours researching and exploring the diverse topics which have resulted in the successful publishing of this book. They have passed on their knowledge of decades through this book. To expedite this challenging task, the publisher supported the team at every step. A small team of assistant editors was also appointed to further simplify the editing procedure and attain best results for the readers.

Apart from the editorial board, the designing team has also invested a significant amount of their time in understanding the subject and creating the most relevant covers. They scrutinized every image to scout for the most suitable representation of the subject and create an appropriate cover for the book.

The publishing team has been an ardent support to the editorial, designing and production team. Their endless efforts to recruit the best for this project, has resulted in the accomplishment of this book. They are a veteran in the field of academics and their pool of knowledge is as vast as their experience in printing. Their expertise and guidance has proved useful at every step. Their uncompromising quality standards have made this book an exceptional effort. Their encouragement from time to time has been an inspiration for everyone.

The publisher and the editorial board hope that this book will prove to be a valuable piece of knowledge for researchers, students, practitioners and scholars across the globe.

List of Contributors

Christian Wöber
Department of Neurology, Medical University of Vienna, Vienna, Austria

Çiçek Wöber-Bingöl
Dr Gönül Bingöl-Dr Muammer Bingöl Çocuk ve Ergen Başağrısı Derneği, Istanbul, Turkey

Derya Uluduz, Tuna Stefan Aslan, Uğur Uygunoglu and Aksel Siva
Neurology Department, Cerrahpaşa School of Medicine, Istanbul University, Istanbul, Turkey

Ahmet Tüfekçi
Neurology Department, Recep Tayyip Erdoğan University School of Medicine, Rize, Turkey

Selen Ilhan Alp
Neurology Department, Namık Kemal University School of Medicine, Tekirdağ, Turkey

Taşkın Duman and Fidan Sürgün
Neurology Department, Mustafa Kemal University School of Medicine, Hatay, Turkey

Gülser Karadaban Emir
Neurology Department, Sıtkı Kocaman University School of Medicine, Mugla, Turkey

Caner Feyzi Demir and Ferhat Balgetir
Neurology Department, Fırat University School of Medicine, Elazığ, Turkey

Yeliz Bahar Özdemir
Department of Physical Medicine and Rehabilitation, Marmara University Medical School, Istanbuk, Turkey

Tanja Auer
Department of Child and Adolescent Psychiatry, Medical University of Vienna, Vienna, Austria

Timothy J. Steiner
Department of Neuromedicine and Movement Science, NTNU Norwegian University of Science and Technology, Edvard Griegs Gate, Trondheim, Norway
Division of Brain Sciences, Imperial College London, London, UK

Delphine Magis, Kevin D'Ostilio, Marco Lisicki and Jean Schoenen
Headache Research Unit, University Department of Neurology CHR, CHU de Liège, Boulevard du 12ème de Ligne 1, 4000 Liège, Belgium

Chany Lee
Department of Biomedical Engineering, Hanyang University, 222 Wangsimni-ro, Seongdong-gu, Seoul 04763, South Korea

Xue-Ying Wang, Hui-Ru Zhou, Sha Wang, Chao-Yang Liu, Guang-Cheng Qin, Qing-Qing Fu and Li-Xue Chen
Laboratory Research Center, The First Affiliated Hospital of Chongqing Medical University, Chongqing, China 1st You Yi Road, Yu Zhong District, Chongqing 400016, China

Ji-Ying Zhou
Department of Neurology, The First Affiliated Hospital of Chongqing Medical University, Chongqing, China

Stephen Landy
Baptist Medical Group Headache Clinic, University of Tennessee Medical School, 6029 Walnut Grove, Suite 210, Memphis, TN 38120, USA

Sagar Munjal and Elimor Brand-Schieber
Promius Pharma, a subsidiary of Dr Reddy's Laboratories, 107 College Road East, Princeton, NJ 08540, USA

Alan M. Rapoport
The David Geffen School of Medicine at UCLA, 4255 Jefferson Avenue, Suite 27, Woodside, CA 94062, USA

Marco Lisicki, Kevin D'Ostilio, Alain Maertens de Noordhout, Jean Schoenen and Delphine Magis
Headache Research Unit, University Department of Neurology CHR, CHU de Liège, Boulevard du 12eme de Ligne 1, 4000 Liege, Belgium

Gianluca Coppola and Vincenzo Parisi
G. B. Bietti Foundation IRCCS, Research Unit of Neurophysiology of Vision and Neuro-Ophthalmology, Rome, Italy

Felix Scholtes
Departments of Neurosurgery and Neuroanatomy, University of Liège, Liege, Belgium

Stephen Landy
Baptist Medical Group Headache Clinic, University of Tennessee Medical School, 6029 Walnut Grove, Suite 210, Memphis, TN 38120, USA

Sagar Munjal and Elimor Brand-Schieber
Promius Pharma, LLC, a subsidiary of Dr. Reddy's Laboratories, 107 College Road East, Princeton, NJ 08540, USA

Alan M. Rapoport
The David Geffen School of Medicine at UCLA, 4255 Jefferson Avenue, Suite 27, Woodside, CA 94062, USA

Giannapia Affaitati and Maria Adele Giamberardino
Headache Center, Geriatrics Clinic, Department of Medicine and Science of Aging and Ce.S.I.-Met, G. D'Annunzio University of Chieti, 66100, Chieti, Italy

Raffaele Costantini
Institute of Surgical Pathology, G. D'Annunzio University of Chieti, Chieti, Italy

Claudio Tana
Internal Medicine and Critical Subacute Care Unit, Medicine Geriatric-Rehabilitation Department, University-Hospital of Parma, Via Antonio Gramsci 14, 43126 Parma, Italy

Domenico Lapenna and Cosima Schiavone
Department of Medicine and Science of Aging, G. D'Annunzio University of Chieti, Chieti, Italy

Francesco Cipollone
Medical Clinic, G. D'Annunzio University of Chieti, Chieti, Italy

Xin Zhang, Yang Yang, Hai-Yan Nan, Ying Yu, Qian Sun, Lin-Feng Yan, Bo Hu, Jin Zhang, Guang-Bin Cui and Wen Wang
Department of Radiology and Functional and Molecular Imaging Key Lab of Shaanxi Province, Tangdu Hospital, the Military Medical University of PLA Airforce (Fourth Military Medical University), 569 Xinsi Road, Xi'an, Shaanxi Province 710038, China

Yu-Jie Dai
Department of Radiology and Functional and Molecular Imaging Key Lab of Shaanxi Province, Tangdu Hospital, the Military Medical University of PLA Airforce (Fourth Military Medical University), 569 Xinsi Road, Xi'an, Shaanxi Province 710038, China
Department of Obstetrics and Gynecology, Xijing Hospital, the Military Medical University of PLA Airforce (Fourth Military Medical University), 15 West Changle Road, Xi'an, Shaanxi Province 710032, China
Department of Clinical Nutrition, Xijing Hospital, the Military Medical University of PLA Airforce (Fourth Military Medical University), 15 West Changle Road, Xi'an, Shaanxi Province 710032, China

Bi-Liang Chen
Department of Obstetrics and Gynecology, Xijing Hospital, the Military Medical University of PLA Airforce (Fourth Military Medical University), 15 West Changle Road, Xi'an, Shaanxi Province 710032, China

Zi-Yu Qiu and Yi Gao
Student Brigade, the Military Medical University of PLA Airforce (Fourth Military Medical University), 169 West Changle Road, Xi'an, Shaanxi Province 710032, China

Kun Wang and Xiaofeng Wang
State Key Laboratory of Genetic Engineering, Collaborative Innovation Center for Genetics and Development, School of Life Sciences, Fudan University, Shanghai 200438, China
Human Phenome Institute, Fudan University, Shanghai 201203, China

Jiucun Wang and Li Jin
State Key Laboratory of Genetic Engineering, Collaborative Innovation Center for Genetics and Development, School of Life Sciences, Fudan University, Shanghai 200438, China
Human Phenome Institute, Fudan University, Shanghai 201203, China
Six Industrial Research Institute, Fudan University, Shanghai 200433, China

Weilin Pu
Ministry of Education Key Laboratory of Contemporary Anthropology, Department of Anthropology and Human Genetics, School of Life Sciences, Fudan University, Shanghai 200438, China

Menghan Zhang, Yi Wang and Xiaoyu Liu
Ministry of Education Key Laboratory of Contemporary Anthropology, Department of Anthropology and Human Genetics, School of Life Sciences, Fudan University, Shanghai 200438, China
Human Phenome Institute, Fudan University, Shanghai 201203, China

Yi Li and Yanyun Ma
Ministry of Education Key Laboratory of Contemporary Anthropology, Department of Anthropology and Human Genetics, School of Life Sciences, Fudan University, Shanghai 200438, China
Human Phenome Institute, Fudan University, Shanghai 201203, China
Six Industrial Research Institute, Fudan University, Shanghai 200433, China

Bin Qiao
Institute of Cardiovascular Disease, General Hospital of Jinan Military Region, Jinan 250022, Shandong, China

Longli Kang
Key Laboratory of High Altitude Environment and Genes Related to Diseases of Tibet Autonomous Region, School of Medicine, Xizang Minzu University, Xianyang 712082, China

Andrew M. Blumenfeld
Headache Center of Southern California, The Neurology Center, 6010 Hidden Valley Road, Carlsbad, CA 92024, USA

Richard J. Stark
Monash University and Alfred Hospital, Melbourne, VIC, Australia

Marshall C. Freeman
Headache Wellness Center, Greensboro, NC, USA

Amelia Orejudos and Aubrey Manack Adams
Allergan plc, Irvine, CA, USA

Louise S. Mose
Department of Neurology, Hospital Southwest Jutland, Esbjerg, Denmark
The Research Unit of Health Science, Hospital of Southwest Jutland, Esbjerg and Department of Regional Health Research, University of Southern Denmark, Odense, Denmark

Bibi Gram
The Research Unit of Health Science, Hospital of Southwest Jutland, Esbjerg and Department of Regional Health Research, University of Southern Denmark, Odense, Denmark

Susanne S. Pedersen
Department of Psychology, University of Southern Denmark, Odense, Denmark.
Department of Cardiology, Odense University Hospital, Odense, Denmark

Birgit Debrabant
Epidemiology, Biostatistics and Biodemography Department of Public Health, University of Southern Denmark, Odense, Denmark

Rigmor H. Jensen
Danish Headache Centre, Department of Neurology, Rigshospitalet-Glostrup, University of Copenhagen, Copenhagen, Denmark

Jair Lozano-Cuenca and Carlos M. Villalón
Departamento de Farmacobiología, Cinvestav-Coapa, Tenorios 235, Col. Granjas-Coapa, Deleg. Tlalpan, 14330 Ciudad de México, México

Abimael González-Hernández
Departamento de Farmacobiología, Cinvestav-Coapa, Tenorios 235, Col. Granjas-Coapa, Deleg. Tlalpan, 14330 Ciudad de México, México
Departamento de Neurobiología del Desarrollo y Neurofisiología, Instituto de Neurobiología, Universidad Nacional Autónoma de México, Campus UNAM, Juriquilla, México

Bruno A. Marichal-Cancino
Departamento de Farmacobiología, Cinvestav-Coapa, Tenorios 235, Col. Granjas-Coapa, Deleg. Tlalpan, 14330 Ciudad de México, México
Departamento de Fisiología y Farmacología, Centro de Ciencias Básicas, Universidad Autónoma de Aguascalientes, Ciudad Universitaria, 20131 Aguascalientes, Ags, México

Antoinette MaassenVan Den Brink
Division of Vascular Medicine and Pharmacology, Erasmus University Medical Center, P.O. Box 2040, 3000, CA, Rotterdam, The Netherlands

Eric P. Baron
Center for Neurological Restoration - Headache and Chronic Pain Medicine, Department of Neurology, Cleveland Clinic Neurological Institute, 10524 Euclid Avenue, C21, Cleveland, OH 44195, USA

Joshua Eades
Tilray, 1100 Maughan Rd, Nanaimo, BC V9X 1J2, Canada

Philippe Lucas
Tilray, 1100 Maughan Rd, Nanaimo, BC V9X 1J2, Canada
Social Dimensions of Health, University of Victoria, 3800 Finnerty Rd, Victoria, BC V8P 5C2, Canada
Canadian Institute for Substance Use Research, 2300 McKenzie Ave, Victoria, BC V8N 5M8, Canada

Olivia Hogue
Section of Biostatistics, Department of Quantitative Health Sciences, Cleveland Clinic Lerner Research Institute, 9500 Euclid Avenue, JJN3, Cleveland, OH 44195, USA

Todd J. Schwedt and David W. Dodick
Mayo Clinic, 5777 East Mayo Boulevard, Phoenix, AZ 85054, USA

Aftab Alam and Sagar Munjal
Promius Pharma, 107 College Rd East, Princeton, NJ 08540, USA

Michael L. Reed and Kristina M. Fanning
Vedanta Research, 23 Tanyard Ct, Chapel Hill, NC 27517, USA

Dawn C. Buse
Albert Einstein College of Medicine, 1250 Waters Place, 8th Floor, Bronx, NY 10461, USA

Richard B. Lipton
Montefiore Medical Center, The Saul R. Korey Department of Neurology, Albert Einstein College of Medicine, 1165 Morris Park Avenue, Rousso Building, Room 332, Bronx, NY 10461, USA

Barbara Petolicchio, Sonia Ruggiero, Marta Altieri and Edoardo Vicenzini
Headache Centre and Neurocritical Care Unit. Department of Human Neurosciences, Sapienza – University of Rome, Viale dell'Università 30, 00185 Rome, Italy

Alessandro Viganò
Headache Centre and Neurocritical Care Unit. Department of Human Neurosciences, Sapienza – University of Rome, Viale dell'Università 30, 00185 Rome, Italy
Molecular and Cellular Networks Lab. Department of Anatomy, Histology, Forensic medicine and Orthopaedics, Sapienza – University of Rome, Rome, Italy

Tullia Sasso D'Elia
Molecular and Cellular Networks Lab. Department of Anatomy, Histology, Forensic medicine and Orthopaedics, Sapienza – University of Rome, Rome, Italy

Maria Claudia Torrieri
Rita Levi Montalcini Department of Neuroscience, Città della Salute e della Scienza, Turin, Italy

Massimiliano Toscano
Headache Centre and Neurocritical Care Unit. Department of Human Neurosciences, Sapienza – University of Rome, Viale dell'Università 30, 00185 Rome, Italy
Department of Neurology, Fatebenefratelli Hospital, Rome, Italy

Vittorio Di Piero
Headache Centre and Neurocritical Care Unit. Department of Human Neurosciences, Sapienza – University of Rome, Viale dell'Università 30, 00185 Rome, Italy
University Consortium for Adaptive Disorders and Head pain – UCADH, Pavia, Italy

Francesca Puledda
Headache Group, Department of Basic and Clinical Neuroscience, King's College London, and NIHR-Wellcome Trust King's Clinical Research Facility, Wellcome Foundation Building, King's College Hospital, London SE5 9PJ, UK

Angela Verzina
Department of Neurology, University of Perugia, Perugia, Italy

Jean Schoenen
Headache Research Unit. Department of Neurology, University of Liège, Citadelle Hospital, Liège, Belgium

Espen Saxhaug Kristoffersen
Department of General Practice, Institute of Health and Society, University of Oslo, Blindern, 0318 Oslo, PO, Norway
Head and Neck Research Group, Research Centre, Akershus University Hospital, Lørenskog, Norway

Kjersti Aaseth
Head and Neck Research Group, Research Centre, Akershus University Hospital, Lørenskog, Norway

Ragnhild Berling Grande
Head and Neck Research Group, Research Centre, Akershus University Hospital, Lørenskog, Norway
The National Center for Epilepsy, Oslo University Hospital, Oslo, Norway

Michael Bjørn Russell
Head and Neck Research Group, Research Centre, Akershus University Hospital, Lørenskog, Norway
Institute of Clinical Medicine, Campus Akershus University Hospital, University of Oslo, Nordbyhagen, Norway

Christofer Lundqvist
Head and Neck Research Group, Research Centre, Akershus University Hospital, Lørenskog, Norway
Institute of Clinical Medicine, Campus Akershus University Hospital, University of Oslo, Nordbyhagen, Norway
HØKH, Research Centre, Akershus University Hospital, Lørenskog, Norway
Department of Neurology, Akershus University Hospital, Lørenskog, Norway

Yun-Ju Choi
Department of Neurology, Presbyterian Medical Center, Jeonju, South Korea

Byung-Kun Kim
Department of Neurology, Eulji Hospital, Seoul, South Korea

Pil-Wook Chung
Department of Neurology, Kangbuk Samsung Hospital, Sungkyunkwan University School of Medicine, Seoul, South Korea

Byung-Su Kim
Department of Neurology, Bundang Jesaeng General Hospital, Daejin Medical Center, Seongnam, South Korea

Tae-Jin Song
Department of Neurology, Ewha Womans University of Medicine, Seoul, South Korea

Jong-Hee Sohn
Department of Neurology, Chuncheon Sacred Heart Hospital, Chuncheon, South Korea

Kwang-Yeol Park
Department of Neurology, Chung-Ang University Hospital, Seoul, South Korea

Jae Myun Chung
Department of Neurology, Inje University College of Medicine, Seoul, South Korea

Soo-Jin Cho
Department of Neurology, Dongtan Sacred Heart Hospital, Hallym University College of Medicine, Keun Jae Bong-gil

Adeladlew Kassie Netere, Daniel Asfaw Erku, Ashenafi Kibret Sendekie, Eyob Alemayehu Gebreyohannes and Sewunet Admasu Belachew
Department of Clinical Pharmacy, School of Pharmacy, College of Medicine and Health Sciences, University of Gondar, Chechela Street, Lideta Sub City Kebele 16, Gondar, Ethiopia

Niguse Yigzaw Muluneh
Department of Psychiatry, University of Gondar, Chechela Street, Lideta Sub City Kebele 16, Gondar, Ethiopia

Pamela Vo and Annik K. Laflamme
Novartis Pharma AG, Fabrikstr. 12, CH-4002 Basel, Switzerland

Juanzhi Fang
Novartis Pharmaceuticals Corporation, One Health Plaza, East Hanover, NJ 07936-1080, USA

Aikaterini Bilitou
Novartis Global Services Centre, Patient Access Services, Dublin, Ireland

Shaloo Gupta
Kantar Health, New York, NY 10010, USA

D. García-Azorin
Headache Unit Neurology Department, Hospital Clínico Universitario Valladolid, Avda. Ramón y Cajal 3, 47005 Valladolid, Spain

N. Yamani
Danish Headache Centre and Department of Neurology, University of Copenhagen, Rigshospitalet Glostrup, Copenhagen, Denmark
Headache Department, Iranian Center of Neurological Research Neuroscience Institute, Tehran University of Medical Sciences, Tehran, Iran

L. M. Messina
Child Neuropsychiatry School, University of Palermo, Palermo, Italy
U.O. Neuropsychiatry - ARNAS Civico, PO Di Cristina, Palermo, Italy

I. Peeters
Neurology Department, University Hospital of Brussels, Brussels, Belgium

M. Ferrili
Headache Center, Bambino Gesù Children Hospital IRCCS, Rome, Italy

D. Ovchinnikov
Pavlov First Saint Petersburg State Medical University, Saint Petesburg, Russia
Almazov National Medical Research Centre, Saint Petesburg, Russia

M. L. Speranza and V. Marini
Internal Medicine Department, Sant'Andrea Hospital, Rome, Italy

A. Negro
Regional Referral Headache Centre, Sant'Andrea Hospital, Department of Clinical and Molecular Medicine, Sapienza University, Rome, Italy

S. Benemei
Headache Centre, Careggi University Hospital, University of Florence, Florence, Italy

M. Barloese
Danish Headache Center, Department of Neurology, Rigshospitalet-Glostrup, University of Copenhagen, Copenhagen, Denmark
Department of Clinical Physiology and Nuclear Medicine, Center for Functional and Diagnostic Imaging, Hvidovre Hospital, Copenhagen, Denmark

Alberto Raggi and Laura Rapisarda
Neurology, Public Health and Disability Unit, Fondazione IRCCS Istituto Neurologico Carlo Besta, Milan, Italy

Venusia Covelli
e-Campus University, Novedrate, Italy

Licia Grazzi
Headache and Neuroalgology Unit, Fondazione IRCCS Istituto Neurologico Carlo Besta, Milan, Italy

Marco Bartolini
Clinica di Neurologia, Università Politecnica delle Marche, Ancona, Italy

Sabina Cevoli
IRCCS Istituto delle Scienze Neurologiche di Bologna, Bologna, Italy

Giulia Pierangeli
IRCCS Istituto delle Scienze Neurologiche di Bologna, Bologna, Italy
DIBINEM - Alma Mater Studiorum, Università di Bologna, Bologna, Italy

Luca Giani
Neurology Unit, Headache Center, Ospedale L, Sacco University of Milan, Milan, Italy

Fabio Frediani
Neurological and Stroke Unit Department, Headache Center, ASST Santi Paolo e Carlo, San Carlo Borromeo Hospital, Milan, Italy

Francesco Bono
Headache Center, Institute of Neurology, Magna Graecia University of Catanzaro, Catanzaro, Italy

Licia Grazzi
Neuroalgology Unit, Carlo Besta Neurological Institute and Foundation, Milan, Italy
Department of Fondazione IRCCS Istituto Neurologico C. Besta, U.O. Neurologia III – Cefalee e Neuroalgologia, Via Celoria 11, 20133 Milan, Italy

Cristina Tassorelli
Headache Science Centre, IRCCS C. Mondino Foundation, Pavia, Italy
Department of Brain and Behavioral Sciences, University of Pavia, Pavia, Italy

Marina de Tommaso
Neurophysiology and Pain Unit, University of Bari Aldo Moro, Bari, Italy

Giulia Pierangeli
IRCCS Istituto delle Scienze Neurologiche di Bologna, Bologna, Italy

Paolo Martelletti
Department of Clinical and Molecular Medicine, Sapienza University, Rome, Italy

Innocenzo Rainero
Department of Neuroscience, University of Turin, Turin, Italy

Pierangelo Geppetti
Headache Centre, University Hospital of Careggi, Florence, Italy

Anna Ambrosini
IRCCS Neuromed, Pozzilli (IS), Italy

Paola Sarchielli
Neurologic Clinic, Santa Maria della Misericordia Hospital, Perugia, Italy

Eric Liebler
electroCore, Inc, Basking Ridge, NJ, USA

Piero Barbanti
Headache and Pain Unit, IRCCS San Raffaele Pisana, Rome, Italy

Index

www.ingramcontent.com/pod-product-compliance
Lightning Source LLC
Chambersburg PA
CBHW080505200326
41458CB00012B/4091